Clinical Voice Disorders

Fourth Edition

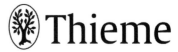

Clinical Voice Disorders
Fourth Edition

Arnold E. Aronson, PhD
Professor and Emeritus Consultant
Division of Medical Speech Pathology
Mayo Clinic
Mayo Medical College
Rochester, Minnesota

Diane M. Bless, PhD
Professor Emeritus
Department of Communicative Disorders
Department of Surgery
Division of Otolaryngology-Head and Neck Surgery
University of Wisconsin School of Medicine and Public Health
Madison, Wisconsin

Thieme
New York • Stuttgart

Thieme Medical Publishers, Inc.
333 Seventh Ave.
New York, NY 10001

Executive Editor: Timothy Y. Hiscock
Editorial Assistant: David Price
Vice President, Production and Electronic Publishing: Anne T. Vinnicombe
Production Editor: Kenneth L. Chumbley, Publication Services
Vice President, International Marketing and Sales: Cornelia Schulze
Chief Financial Officer: Peter van Woerden
President: Brian D. Scanlan
Compositor: Aptara, Inc.
Printer: Sheridan Books
Cover illustrations drawn by Markus Voll and Karl Wesker

Library of Congress Cataloging-in-Publication Data

Aronson, Arnold Elvin, 1928-
    Clinical voice disorders / Arnold E. Aronson, Diane M. Bless.—4th ed.
        p.   ;   cm.
    Includes bibliographical references and index.
    ISBN 978-1-58890-662-5 (alk. paper)
    1. Voice disorders. I. Bless, Diane M. II. Title.
    [DNLM: 1. Voice Disorders. WV 500 A769c 2009]

    RF510.A76 2009
    616.85'56—dc22
                            2008009089

Important note: Medical knowledge is ever-changing. As new research and clinical experience broaden our knowledge, changes in treatment and drug therapy may be required. The authors and editors of the material herein have consulted sources believed to be reliable in their efforts to provide information that is complete and in accord with the standards accepted at the time of publication. However, in view of the possibility of human error by the authors, editors, or publisher of the work herein or changes in medical knowledge, neither the authors, editors, nor publisher, nor any other party who has been involved in the preparation of this work, warrants that the information contained herein is in every respect accurate or complete, and they are not responsible for any errors or omissions or for the results obtained from use of such information. Readers are encouraged to confirm the information contained herein with other sources. For example, readers are advised to check the product information sheet included in the package of each drug they plan to administer to be certain that the information contained in this publication is accurate and that changes have not been made in the recommended dose or in the contraindications for administration. This recommendation is of particular importance in connection with new or infrequently used drugs. Some of the product names, patents, and registered designs referred to in this book are in fact registered trademarks or proprietary names even though specific reference to this fact is not always made in the text. Therefore, the appearance of a name without designation as proprietary is not to be construed as a representation by the publisher that it is in the public domain.

Printed in the United States of America

5 4 3 2 1

ISBN: 978-1-58890-662-5

In memory of Sylvia Zelda Aronson,
September 13, 1930–June 16, 2008,
who lives in this book.

Contents

Preface to the Fourth Edition

This fourth edition, like the first three, addresses the organic disorders of voice due to laryngeal structural changes and neurologic diseases, as well as the psychogenic voice disorders due to environmental stress and psychoneuroses and muscle tension dysphonias. This edition of *Clinical Voice Disorders* differs from previous editions by both the expansion and addition of chapters. The chapters are updated with current references and augmented with extended content. A DVD-R has been added with supplementary chapters, demonstration therapy, and interviewing. More specifically, organic evolution has been considerably expanded to include the photographs and concepts fleshed out by the late Jan Wind, PhD, in his seminal work *On the Ontogeny and the Phylogeny of the Human Larynx* (1970, Wolters-Noordhoff; out of print).

Embryology of the larynx has been amplified, along with embryology of the respiratory system, and expanded to include many more detailed drawings illustrating the embryologic stages of both systems. Anatomy and physiology of voice production was revised by Susan L Thibeault, PhD, to include information on the microstructure of the vocal fold. Chapters on spasmodic dysphonias have been combined, updated, and revised. A new chapter, by Brian E. Petty, on the singer's voice that addresses special issues related to the treatment of voice disorders in this population has been added. Psychogenic voice disorders now has extended case studies that relate personal stories behind this etiology of dysphonias and aphonias. The chapter on examination of voice disorders has been rewritten by Nathan V. Wellham, PhD. Greater descriptions of more voice therapy techniques and their underlying principles also have been included in this edition.

In this work I reassert that the study of clinical voice disorders, and their diagnosis and treatment is now more than ever a medical subspecialty that requires highly specialized education and training of the speech language pathologist in order to interface with other members of the health care team. I now believe more firmly than ever that possession of an abnormal voice is either a sign of illness or an illness in and of itself. People with voice disorders are suffering from an *illness* in every medical sense of the word, and a patient who presents himself or herself to the physician or speech language pathologist can be a major challenge to clinicians who are untrained in the differential diagnosis of abnormal voice signs and symptoms. The analysis and interpretation of abnormal voice is such an esoteric subspecialty that it requires extensive experience with hundreds of patients before the clinician is able to pick up the nuances of patient responses to questions posed about their conditions and acoustic-perceptual shadings of voice produced by specific disease states.

I believe that it is impossible to achieve such expertise from reading a book or listening to lectures. What is necessary is direct observation and practical contact with patients under the supervision of someone with extensive experience with voice disorders.

As in previous editions of this book, I prepare the student in the gross anatomy, neuroanatomy, and physiology of the respiratory, phonatory, and velopharyngeal mechanisms. My objective is to address the needs of students who will one day find themselves in clinical voice situations where they will be responsible for answering the following diagnostic and therapeutic questions.

1. What are the medical reasons responsible for this abnormal voice?

2. How can I examine this patient in a way that will lead to an answer to this all important question?

3. What kinds of information will I have to know in order to obtain a full understanding of this patient and his or her voice disorder?

4. What do I need to know in order to reduce or eliminate the abnormal voice?

In this book I will try to show how abnormal voices are important to the physician's medical diagnosis and treatment, as well as to the speech-language pathologist's assessment and treatment plan. I will try to address the speech language pathologist's role. There are highly practical reasons for the medical speech language pathologist in a medical setting to have a central role in the process, because he or she is often the person best trained to relate the abnormal voice to the structural problem or neurologic disease and thus serves as the mortar between the specialities. The etiologic diagnosis and therapy for voice disorders is a highly demanding subspecialty that requires considerable talent and skill honed by years of experience. And "you can't teach experience." An internship or residency in departments of otolaryngology and neurology would be an ideal exposure of students to the full spectrum of medical voice disorders at the elbow of a consulting physician.

In this book I will try to pass on to the student whatever pearls of wisdom I have accumulated during my nearly 50 years of experience with voice disorders in medicine.

From my practice five seminal ideas have emerged: (1) your voice is your identity; (2) when it becomes abnormal, the disorder is tantamount to an illness as devastating as any other illness; (3) dysphonia can be a sign of an organic or emotional illness, or a combination of the two; (4) the voice is complex; and (5) the study of voice is inseparable from the practice of medicine.

1. *Your voice is your identity.* Of the many meanings of voice in our lives, perhaps the most important is that it lies at the very heart of our personal identity—as indelibly implanted in our consciousness as our faces. One of our patients who had been placed on voice rest after laryngeal surgery complained poignantly that her life had become intolerable because she was unable to express her feelings or thoughts to her family. "My voice is me," she lamented. The catastrophic effects of abnormal voice on the life of the patient is a recurring theme in adult voice disorders practice. I dramatize this fact in the autobiographical expressions of a 75-year-old woman with adductor spasmodic dysphonia (see "Confessions of an Adductor Spasmodic Dysphonic" Chapter 6).

2. *When it becomes abnormal, the disorder is tantamount to an illness as devastating as any other illness.* Early textbooks on voice disorders centered upon abnormal voice as an aesthetic aberration, primarily, and not as a barrier to intelligibility, or a sign of organic disease, or psychologic disequilibrium, or as a diagnostic window that could be used to ascertain the neurologic, psychologic, general, or laryngologic health of the patient. Early textbooks had no information about the impact of voice disorders on the quality of life, on choice of occupations, or on social relationships. From its infancy, the field of voice disorders has matured into a rich cache of knowledge and lore about the supernormal, normal, and abnormal voice. The importance of its loss now can be found in its devastating effects on the average speaker's self image, as attested to by recent memoirs and scientific papers.

3. *Dysphonia as a sign.* (A) As a sign of organic illness. Voice becomes abnormal when there are pathological changes of the vocal folds or surrounding structures due to primary focal laryngeal pathology, laryngeal changes due to endocrine, and/or changes in the innervation of the laryngeal musculature secondary to neurological diseases. (B) As a sign of emotional illness. Voice becomes abnormal when there are emotional, psychological, psychiatric illnesses, or stress reflected in the voice organ. They are one of the most common causes of nonorganic voice disorders.

4. *Voice is complex.* The study of this complex phenomenon of voice is termed vocology, a term coined by Ingo Titze, PhD. Vocology has evolved from the knowledge that voice production requires a wide variety of physiological activities to produce sounds ranging from valving pulmonary air needed for a soft whisper and the hush of a baby, to loud screams for help and the intricate control needed for singing a beautiful aria. Voice production is not merely a couple of folds of tissue set into vibration by a stream of air from the lungs. Rather, this vibratory source is an exquisitely constructed biomechanical histoarchitectural structure with specific properties that are intricately connected and affected by one's internal physical and mental well-being. The study of voice now comes from a variety of disciplines including, but not limited to, communicative disorders, psychology, laryngology, bioengineering, molecular biology, theater and music, kinesiology, linguistics, physiology, neurology, and

genetics. Although difficult to ascertain when the evolution of voice study began, it is clear that when the American Speech Language Hearing Association was initially formed over 75 years ago, voice was not a major focus. Vocology was nonexistent. Stuttering, speech development, and hearing impairment dominated early curricula. Times have changed.

5. *Clinical voice disorders are no longer speech pathology's stepchild.* It has grown up into a mature adult with strong ties to the medical specialties of otolaryngology, neurology, and psychiatry. Since the last edition of this book, our medical care system has continued to offer diagnoses and treatments of many different areas of human illness, including voice disorders. The American public now is coming to expect the best, most sophisticated care available for all of its ills. The percentage of speech-language pathologists in medical clinics and hospitals continues to grow at a steady pace. Clinicians in the schools increasingly see medically fragile students, who not too many years ago would have been seen only in a hospital setting. Because of this medical connection, I continue to believe in the importance of a solid education in the basic sciences of gross and neuroanatomy and neurophysiology and in the clinical medical specialties of otolaryngology, neurology, psychiatry, and even internal medicine.

Thus, it seems clearly evident that the study of voice disorders is inseparable from the practice of medicine, and that the SLP functions as an arm of medicine, providing differential diagnostic information to the referring physician, as well as therapeutic decisions in the patient's interest. From my perspective, of all the major areas of information, organic diseases and psychological dysfunctions are the two bodies of knowledge that I must master in order to practice the specialty of clinical voice disorders competently. And that is what this book is all about—the organic and psychiatric infrastructure of normal and abnormal voice.

It is also clearly evident to me that the theory and practice of voice disorders are squarely embedded in the cardinal medical specialties of internal medicine, pediatrics, neurology, psychiatry, and otolaryngology. The skilled clinician needs to have some knowledge and working vocabulary from these disciplines, be able to work with practitioners in these medical subspecialities, and be an astute observer of behavior. The skilled clinician must also be a scholar who keeps abreast of the ever-changing concepts in the field and in the knowledge of how the wonderful human body and mind work together to produce and correct disorders of voice production.

I wish to express my gratitude to Dr. and Mrs. Muriel Kulwin for their permission to use their writings; to the late Jan Wind, MD, PhD, for his seminal work on the ontogeny and phylogeny of the human larynx, parallel in its brilliance to the research of Sir Victor Negus, MD, on the comparative anatomy and physiology of the human larynx; to our patients and medical colleagues in the departments of neurology, psychiatry, and otolaryngology; to the late Joe R. Brown, MD, Norman P. Goldstein, MD, Edward M. Litin, and Frederick L. Darley, PhD, of the Mayo Clinic; to my colleagues at the University of Wisconsin; and to Diane M. Bless, PhD, for helping edit the manuscript.

Arnold E. Aronson, PhD
Mayo Clinic, Rochester, Minnesota

Contributors

Arnold E. Aronson, PhD
Professor and Emeritus Consultant
Division of Medical Speech Pathology
Mayo Clinic
Mayo Medical College
Rochester, Minnesota

Diane M. Bless, PhD
Professor Emeritus
Department of Communicative Disorders
Department of Surgery
Division of Otolaryngology-Head and Neck Surgery
University of Wisconsin School of Medicine
    and Public Health
Madison, Wisconsin

Brian E. Petty, MA, CCC-SLP
Speech-Language Pathologist, Singing Voice Specialist
Department of Surgery
Division of Otolaryngology-Head and Neck Surgery
University of Wisconsin School of Medicine
    and Public Health
Madison, Wisconsin

Susan L. Thibeault, PhD, CCC-SLP
Assistant Professor
Department of Surgery
Division of Otolaryngology-Head and Neck Surgery
University of Wisconsin School of Medicine
    and Public Health
Madison, Wisconsin

Nathan V. Welham, PhD, CCC-SLP
Assistant Professor
Department of Surgery
Division of Otolaryngology-Head and Neck Surgery
University of Wisconsin School of Medicine
    and Public Health
Madison, Wisconsin

Chapter 1

Introduction to Clinical Voice Disorders

It is impossible to know the fundamentals of a phenomenon without having solid knowledge of its origin, development and the chain of causes, conditions and circumstances determining its actual existence.

—Kiml

♦ The Functions of the Larynx in Living Creatures

The larynx lies at the crossroads of life, a barometer of our physical and mental health, an airway through which flows life-sustaining oxygen, and a valve that protects the lungs from ingestion of foreign substances. When its powerful musculature shuts off the airway, air can be impounded in the lungs, forming a rigid thorax to support firmly the attached upper extremities during lifting and pushing. Bearing down during laryngeal closure compresses the abdominal contents for defecation, micturition, and parturition and fixation of the thoracic cage for coughing, throat clearing, and vomiting. Yet, as vital as these functions are, the larynx manages to shift deftly from protector of life to communicator, generating raw sound for articulation of intellect and as a prosodic background to language informing the outside world of its owner's personality, emotional state, and cultural heritage. It is a somewhat daunting task to attempt to write a book that provides the bases for voice assessment and treatment of this formidable organ. The mechanics of speech require integration of the respiratory, phonatory, resonatory, and articulatory musculature. Although the emphasis of this book is on voice production, we consider herein, for the most part, components of the total speech act: *respiration*, the power and driving force of sound; *phonation*, sound generated by rapid vocal fold movement driven by the exhaled air stream; and *resonation*, modification of the raw sound generated by the larynx by movement of the other articulatory structures including the velopharyngeal complex.

The larynx is a complex organ composed of cartilage, muscles, nerves, and connective tissues. The vocal folds themselves, the source of sound, are made of layers of laminated tissue, with a muscular layer in the innermost part of the folds and progressively thinner layers of softer tissues toward the epithelium. During vocalization, cells from the skin layer are destroyed and sloughed off. Vocalization causes cellular and extracellular damage to vocal fold tissues, which the body can repair with time. Factors such as genetic predisposition, internal and external vocal tissue environment, physical and mental health, and quantity and quality of vocal use are thought to contribute to the recovery rate of injured vocal fold tissue.

An important and unusual fact about the larynx is that phylogenetically it is eons older than those brain and muscle structures responsible for articulation and language. The latter are synonymous with the intellect, itself a recent vertebrate acquisition, but the larynx and voice owe a disproportionately strong allegiance to the primitive emotions, persuasive proof of which can be found in everyday experience, during emotional arousal. When we are incapable of preventing loss of cortical control over the larynx, it escapes our grasp and drags us back into its primeval depths as we laugh, cry, scream, groan, or are rendered voiceless. Have we not often witnessed such loss of intellectual speech expression as in the following experience? A professor of law, known for his razor-sharp tongue and habit of taunting and ridiculing students (who, incidentally, loved him in spite of it), rose to speak at a farewell banquet:

He stood motionless for a long time. We observed that his face was different than we had ever seen it before. It had lost its severity. It was flushed and looked pink and kind. The mouth was not a snarl. His voice, too, was different. It was soft without a trace of belligerence or sarcasm. "I cannot bid you all goodbye and leave unsaid that which is the most important thing in my life." He took a deep breath and continued, *his voice hoarse with emotion.* It grew hoarser as he struggled to eliminate the quiver, which was entering it. *He then paid tribute to his lovely wife. "I cannot in this leavetaking do other than tell you that I owe all my happiness to her, that she has . . ." He turned. Tears were running down her cheeks. Their gazes met and locked in long silence. Then without another word, he sat down"* (Nizer, 1978).

We are fascinated by the mystery of how speech and language evolved in the kingdom of the vertebrates and have struggled with a basic question: Are the structure and sound-generating properties of the human larynx mere extensions of its role in lower vertebrates, the ultimate in evolutionary refinement for the expression of ideas? That is to say, is the Darwinian belief correct, that speech is not a product of special creation but only another form of sound-making, more sophisticated because of a quantitative increase in human intelligence? Or, is speech uniquely human, de novo, different in kind, not degree, from lower animals? The answer is unknown.

Another, perhaps only slightly less difficult, question is this: Is it the monkey's and chimpanzee's intellect or anatomy that prevents speech in these primates? Some argue that the primitiveness of their laryngeal and articulatory anatomy stands in the way of speech, yet the larynges of the monkey and chimpanzee are remarkably similar in structure and method of sound production to those of humans. The fact is that human speech is not dependent upon a particularly refined larynx, for speech continues despite laryngeal tumor, paralysis, and even total laryngectomy, whereupon the esophagus or even an electronic sound generator can assume the responsibility for sound-making. Most scientists now concur that before primates could talk, a high level of abstract intelligence was required as the governing force.

A universal fact about the world of living creatures is that almost all make sounds. Insects tap surfaces, snap or rub their wings, or rub leg against wing, as in the case of the grasshopper, producing complex trains of pulses that send messages of courtship and sexual recognition. Admittedly, many lower forms produce sound accidentally, but most do so for a purpose; survival-signaling fear, aggression, mating, territoriality, and pleasure. Situation-specific use of voice in birds, for example, has been firmly categorized into mating, distress, fear, anger, terrorizing, and triumphal calls.

Negus (1929) observed that individual living creatures produce sound as both defense and offense: intimidation, cries for help and food, and decoying of prey. Sound brings and keeps the sexes together for survival of the species, attracting and repulsing the opposite sex, and protecting offspring. Sound further enables each species to keep in touch when out of sight, as in grass, in trees, at night, and in lairs or burrows. Sound also aids in the conveyance of special ideas, such as cooperation, calls to food and migration, and entertainment.

Human phonation is linked to much more than the intellectual act of speech. The human voice serves similar sublinguistic purposes of survival. The larynx is an important escape valve for the emotions—anger, grief, and affection—which are essential to the maintenance of our psychologic equilibrium.

◆ Definitions of Terms

Voice

We need to define terms used constantly in the field of voice disorders. To begin with, *voice* is an auditory perceptual term that means the audible sound produced by the larynx, which embodies such parameters as pitch, loudness, quality, and variability.

◆ *Pitch* is the perceptual correlate of frequency.

◆ *Loudness* is the perceptual correlate of intensity.

◆ *Quality* is the perceptual correlate of complexity.

◆ *Variability* is the perceptual correlate of variations of the above parameters.

Phonation

◆ *Phonation* is the physical-physiologic act of sound production: the oscillations of the vocal folds driven by the exhaled air stream. Clinical terms denoting abnormal voice are dysphonia, aphonia, and muteness.

◆ *Dysphonia* describes any voice that sounds abnormal in its psychoacoustic parameters of pitch, loudness, quality, and variability; for example, excessively high or low pitch, inadequately or excessively loud voice, aberrant quality such as hoarseness, or breathiness or voices lacking in variability and as monopitch or in some patients excessive variability.

◆ *Aphonia* refers to the absence of a laryngeal tone: sounds like whispered speech or an extreme degree of breathiness.

◆ *Muteness* is a word to describe the patient who has no voice or articulation.

Normal Voice

Frequently asked is, what is a *normal voice*? Johnson, Brown, Curtis, et al. (1965) listed several criteria:

◆ *Quality must be pleasant,* with a certain musical quality and an absence of noise, inappropriate breaks, voice perturbations, or atonality.

◆ *Pitch must be appropriate to the age and gender of the speaker.*

◆ *Loudness appropriate to the communication event,* not so weak as to be borderline intelligible or unintelligible under ordinary speaking circumstances, not so loud that it calls attention to itself, and appropriately adjusted to the context of the event be it for confidential communication, speaking in a large lecture hall, or yelling for help

♦ *Adequate flexibility*   Pitch and loudness variations are available to express emphasis, meanings, or subtleties indicating individual feelings and semantic differences.

♦ *Adequate sustainability*   Voice must meet one's social and occupational needs even when extended voice is required.

As we have become more sophisticated in our knowledge about "normal" voice production, we recognize that any normal criteria must be adjusted for different age levels.

Abnormal Voice

By definition, an *abnormal voice* is any voice that calls attention to itself, does not meet the occupational or social needs of the speaker, or is inappropriate to age, gender, or situation. Voices that attract unwanted attention are most often due to aberrant vocal qualities.

Abnormal voice qualities are often subsumed under the term *hoarseness*, most often referring to voices that are noisy, atonal, or possess odd resonance patterns. A plethora of abnormal voice quality terms has been accumulated over time, not all of which are easily identified by listeners or agreed upon (e.g., aspirate, asthenic, breathy, choppy, coarse, dull, feeble, flat, gloomy, grating, grave, growling, guttural, harsh, hoarse, hollow, husky, infantile, lifeless, loud, metallic, monotonous, muffled, nasal, neurasthenic, passive, pectoral, pinched, rough, somber, strained, strident, subdued, thick, thin, throaty, tired, toneless, tremulous, tremorous, weak, whining, and whispered).

Fairbanks (1960) tried to distill voice quality defects into three categories: harshness, breathiness, and hoarseness. The validity and reliability of these terms, however, were questioned in a study by Jensen (1965). He asked six experienced speech-language pathologists to rate the voices of cheerleaders who had different degrees and types of dysphonia and found disagreement and inconsistency among their ratings. What certain judges heard as "breathiness" others described as "hoarseness," whereas still others thought "harshness" best applied. In addition, estimations of voice quality were contaminated by severity. The study unearthed a common problem in clinical practice: individual voices were inconsistent throughout the sample, embodying more than one type of quality. The reliability of listeners' ratings of voice quality is a central issue in voice research laboratories and the clinic because of the clinical primacy of such ratings and because they are the standard against which other measures are evaluated. An extensive literature review reported by Kreiman, Gerratt, Kempster, et al. (1993) clearly documents that both intrarater and interrater reliability fluctuate greatly from study to study. They went on to demonstrate with data collected in their laboratory that even within individual clinicians, a single voice often received nearly the full range of possible ratings.

Kent (1996) attempted to define some limits to the auditory perceptual assessment of several communication prob-

lems including voice disorders. In this review article, he focuses on the variety of sources of error and bias that clinicians are susceptible to make in auditory perceptual judgments. He suggests that awareness of these threats to validity and reliability moves us toward being more clinically effective and refining use of perceptual methods. A major factor is that the assumptions on which clinical judgments are predicated are often false. Listeners do not necessarily have a common understanding of perceptual labels, use the same verbal descriptors or associated scale values to assess a given voice, have the ability to isolate judgment of one perceptual dimension from co-occurring dimensions, have uniform reliability in judging voice dimensions, or have the ability to make perceptual judgments for which the inter-judge differences are smaller than the differences needed for clinical classification or to detect changes in clinical status. This lack of defined terminology, limitless variety of voice quality, lack of reliability, and difficulties in determining specificity and sensitivity led some international voice communities, namely the Japanese Society of Logopedics and Phoniatrics, the European Research Group on the Larynx, the United Kingdom British Voice Association, and the 2002 ASHA Auditory Perceptual Judgment Consensus Conference, to independently reach similar conclusions concerning perceptual judgments of voice. They have suggested minimal standards and development of criterion-based training materials such as those routinely used in training speech-language pathologists in Australia (Oates and Russell, 1998). These issues will be discussed in some detail later in the book and the DVD accompanying the book.

Thus, what Jensen, Kreiman, and colleagues concluded experimentally is substantiated clinically that the traditional labels used to describe voice quality deviations must be viewed with skepticism; one clinician's hoarseness is another's breathiness or harshness. To keep a proper perspective, however, it should be noted that the incongruence within terminology to describe the deviant voice is not as critical as it might seem from research studies and international consensus groups on voice perception. *More important* than terminology is the clinician's ability to make similar judgments from test-to-test, to integrate perceptual, acoustic, physiologic, and psychologic dimensions of abnormal voice, to interpret the abnormal sound in light of other assessment data to determine its cause, and to develop a sensitivity to nuances of voice during therapy.

♦ *Abnormal pitch*   Pitch is the perceptual counterpart of fundamental voice frequency. Disorders of pitch refer to abnormally high or low voices.

♦ *Abnormal loudness*   Loudness is the perceptual correlate of the physical dimension of vocal intensity. The voice may be too weak or too loud.

♦ *Abnormal flexibility*   The normal voice possesses adequate pitch, loudness, and quality variability during contextual speech to convey more subtle, intellectual, and emotional meanings. In voice disorders, those fluctuations may be either inappropriately flattened, excessive, or inconsistent.

Rarely in clinical practice does abnormal voice vary along a single dimension of quality, loudness, pitch, or flexibility

(Hirano, 1981). Most of the time, even though one may predominate, they are usually present in different combinations and proportions making it often difficult for clinicians to describe the abnormality.

Abnormal Voice as a Sign of Illness

In medicine, as well as in speech-language pathology, we need to distinguish between the words *sign* and *symptom*. A sign is a physical manifestation of an illness (e.g., hoarseness, diplophonia, or unilateral vocal fold paralysis are signs). The patient's complaints of abnormal voice, pain, or discomfort are symptoms. Signs are objective findings, symptoms are the patient's subjective interpretation of what is physically occurring. Faced with someone whose voice sounds abnormal, the clinician's chief concern should be whether or not the abnormal signs and symptoms of a voice problem signify illness. Communicative or aesthetic considerations are, for the moment, secondary though in the long run no less important. From the laryngology syllabus of a medical school curriculum comes the following statement pertaining to the meaning of abnormal voice in medical practice:

> Dysphonia is not a disease but rather a sign or symptom of disease of the larynx itself or along the course of the laryngeal motor nerves. Thus, hoarseness is the cardinal sign of laryngeal involvement, often the first and only signal of dangerous disease, local or systemic, involving this area . . . . A thorough examination is necessary in all cases to ascertain the exact cause and prescribe the proper treatment . . . . The differential diagnosis may tax the ingenuity of the most exacting physician and speech pathologist since many different medical, surgical and non-organic conditions may cause disturbing dysphonia.

The cause or causes of the abnormal voices need to be established, if at all possible. A breathy voice quality that appears gradually and increases in severity may have only minor social, communicative, or aesthetic significance yet may announce the onset of a brain-stem tumor. Once the reason for the voice disorder is known and has been eliminated as a threat to the life of the individual, the communicative significance of the voice can then be considered. The modern speech clinician must be educated along medical as well as rehabilitative lines, however. Working with physicians, speech-language pathologists can contribute to the medical diagnosis of voice disorders as well as to their treatment though it must be underscored that the actual medical diagnosis is made by the physician.

Often, determining the etiology must accompany early corrective procedures frequently referred to as *facilitating approaches* or trial therapy; in many cases, necessary diagnostic information can be gained only by testing (the patient's) response to these rehabilitory measures; but in every case . . . a thoroughgoing investigation as to the cause of the defect . . . should be reopened (West, Kennedy, and Carr, 1947) before a decision is made regarding corrective devices to be employed. A search for the cause, or causes, should not be ended until the basic etiology has been uncovered; and, if at any time . . . it appears that a reappraisal of its origins would give a clearer picture of its nature, the search for the ultimate cause should be reopened (West, Kennedy, and Carr, 1947).

Abnormal Voice as a Symptom of Illness

Used properly, *symptom* refers to the patient's subjective complaint, real or imagined; whether or not the clinician thinks the voice is abnormal is independent of the patient's beliefs. Three variations on this theme occur in practice:

1. *The voice is judged defective by both clinician and patient, and both advocate a need for its investigation and therapy.* Such mutual agreement is ideal for maximum cooperation in clinical diagnosis and therapy. Both parties realize that something needs to be done about the abnormal voice and assuming patient-clinician treatment goals are matched proceed with optimal effectiveness.

2. *The clinician is convinced of a need for voice investigation and therapy, but the patient is not.* This situation arises from either (a) the clinician's unrealistic, overdetermined definition of abnormal voice and overemphasis on voice improvement or (b) the patient's indifference to or denial of a genuine problem. In either instance, covert or even overt disagreement between patient and clinician ensues, and efforts at diagnosis or therapy are met with patient disinterest, resistance, or even hostility.

3. *The patient's conviction that a voice disorder exists despite the fact that clinicians are unable to detect a major focus for concern.* Such conflicts may be a sign of patient overreaction, a sequel to recovery from laryngologic disease or laryngeal surgery, or, in the case of singers, a clinician's inability to detect the changes. Overreactions of patients are viewed as expressions of hostility, perfectionism, or depression, requiring psychologic assistance. It is also possible that the patient's voice complaint only demonstrates itself under periods of stress or fatigue or is related more to vocal effort than vocal quality making its clinical description challenging.

Abnormal Voice as a Disorder of Communication

In addition to abnormal voice as an index of health or illness, it is also valued as an instrument of communication. Within this framework, the following questions are pertinent: (1) Is the voice adequate to carry language intelligibly to the listener? (2) Are its acoustic properties aesthetically acceptable? (3) Does it satisfy its owner's occupational and social requirements? Voice, in other words, has personal, social, and economic significance. This has led recently to surgical treatment of the larynx to produce a younger, fuller voice in aged individuals. The higher one ascends the socioeconomic scale, the greater the emphasis placed on pleasant, effective voices. With few exceptions, the greater the dependence on voice for occupational and social gratification, the more devastating the effects of a voice disorder on the person. Imagine the consequences of being a singer, actor, politician, clergy member, teacher, or salesperson and not having full voice at your command. The consequences of even a relatively minor voice defect can be devastating.

◆ Voice Disorder

An abnormal-sounding voice does not always provoke individuals to seek the services of a laryngologist or speech-language pathologist. Although a voice disorder exists when quality, pitch, loudness, or flexibility differs from the voices of others of similar age, sex, and cultural group, no fixed, uniform standard of abnormal voice exists, just as no absolute criterion for normal voice can be established. Consequently, a wide range of voices accepted as normal differs based on occupational needs and cultural expectations, and many dysphonic individuals are not even aware they have a voice problem. Those individuals who do seek professional help come for a variety of reasons. Some patients request voice services because they have noticed increased effort to sing or speak even though the voice "sounds normal" for most purposes. For others, it is a change in voice and fear of laryngeal cancer that causes them to seek help. Even though the voice may not have been a good one previously, it is appropriately alarming that it has changed. Others seek help because their voice fatigues, cannot project, or does not meet their vocal needs at home or work. Although laypersons often pay little attention to the specific acoustic parameters of voice that have caught their attention, clinicians and laboratory researchers are more analytic. This can lead to differences in therapeutic goals if the clinician is not careful to identify what brought the patient to the clinic in the first place. The layperson is often more interested in easy, effortless phonation than a good quality; a singer may want to improve range without reducing vocal identity; a smoker with a rough quality may merely want to be assured he does not have laryngeal cancer.

It follows that the perceived defectiveness of any one voice will vary among listeners. It is apparent that the voice is abnormal for a particular individual when he or she judges it to be so regardless of the circumstances. Judgment implies a set of standards that are learned through experience and that are related to the judge's own aesthetic and cultural criteria. Judgment also implies that standards are not fixed, that there is opportunity for more than one conclusion. This flexibility in determining the defectiveness of voices does not alter the validity of the basic definition of voice disorders, but it does underscore the observation that vocal standards are culturally based and environmentally determined (Moore, 1971b).

The main implication of this statement is that the definition of a given voice as normal or abnormal depends upon the orientation of the person making the judgment. Child, parent, adult, employer, speech-language pathologist, and laryngologist all define normal and abnormal according to their own needs and backgrounds, an important point for the speech-language pathologist to remember, whose judgments about voice must be adjusted according to the purposes of the evaluation. The Voice Handicapped Index (VHI) recently developed by Jacobson and Benninger helps clinicians understand the patient's perspective and plan treatment accordingly.

Perkins (1971) lists five kinds of information that can be extracted from the voice. It is an indicator of the speaker's (1) physical health, (2) emotional health, (3) personality, (4) identity, and (5) aesthetic orientation. It is also (6) a carrier of connotative and denotative content. This list is important in that it tells us that voice has many meanings for both speaker and clinician and is a rich storehouse of clues to understanding the individual. It also underscores the importance of taking a careful case history to obtain the information necessary to understanding how the voice problem relates to the individual and choice of treatment.

Classifications

Etiologic

Etiology means the underlying cause or hypothesis that explains signs and symptoms. Because such a classification encourages the deepest understanding of dysphonia or aphonia, it will be the primary category used in this book. For example, a neurologic disease, such as trauma to one recurrent laryngeal nerve, is the etiology of a voice disorder. It causes a pathophysiologic condition, unilateral vocal fold paralysis, which in turn causes the abnormal voice signs of breathiness, hoarseness, reduced loudness, diplophonia, and reduced variability (Moore, 1971a).

Etiologic diagnosis of voice disorders is imperative when speech-language pathology is practiced within the framework of medicine. The teaching that voice signs, such as breathiness and hoarseness, are "disorders" in and of themselves is contrary to the purposes of educating one to understand the individual behind the abnormal voice. Attempts to change the voice alone without understanding its etiology and concomitant maintenance factors are the most common reasons for failure in diagnosis and therapy, especially within the realm of nonorganic voice signs and symptoms.

Perceptual

Voice disorders can be classified according to their acoustic perceptual attributes: quality, pitch, loudness, and flexibility. Although this system has the advantage of emphasizing the voice characteristics perceived by the listener, if used alone it has the disadvantage of failing to provide sufficient information about the underlying causes and muscular dynamics responsible for the abnormal voice.

Kinesiologic

Exemplified by the terms *vocal hyperfunction* and *vocal hypofunction*, this classification categorizes voice disorders according to whether the vocal folds overadduct or underadduct, thus closing the glottis too tightly or incompletely. Although not without merit, this classification, if used exclusively, oversimplifies the complexities of laryngeal diseases, placing excess emphasis on the degree of approximation of the glottal margins rather than on the multiple causes of such approximation defects. Furthermore, it neglects to recognize that many persons with so-called hypofunctional problems compensate by overadduction of the supraglottal structures.

Table 1.1   List of Some Etiologies of Organic Voice Disorders

Congenital Disorders	**Malignant Neoplasms**
Atresia	Squamous cell carcinoma
Cri du chat	Adenocarcinoma
Laryngomalacia	Fibrosarcoma
Subglottic stenosis	Lymphoma
Laryngeal web	Neurofibrosarcoma
Laryngeal cleft	Malignant melanoma
Papilloma	Neurolemmoma
Laryngocele	Spindle cell carcinoma
Mongolism	**Trauma**
Laryngeal saccule	Contact ulcer
Lymphangioma	Vocal nodule
Subglottic hemangioma; ectopic thyroid gland	Postintubation granuloma
Inflammation	Mucosal burns
Laryngitis	**Sulcus Vocalis**
Tuberculosis	**Presbylarynges**
Fungal laryngotracheobronchitis	**Neurologic Disorders**
Epiglottitis	Bilateral upper motor neuron (spastic) disorder
Streptococcus	Mixed lower-upper motor neuron (flaccid-spastic) disorder
Staphylococcus	Basal ganglia (hypokinetic-parkinsonism) disorder
Scarlet fever	Essential tremor
Pertussis	Cerebellar (ataxic) disorder
Typhoid fever	Basal ganglia (hyperkinetic-chorea) disorder
Histoplasmosis	Basal ganglia (hyperkinetic-dystonia) disorder
Blastomycosis	Brain-stem (palatopharyngolaryngeal myoclonus) disorder
Reflux esophagitis	Brain-stem (organic voice tremor) disorder
Metabolic Disorders	Gilles de la Tourette's disease
Hypothyroidism	Apraxia of phonation
Hyperthyroidism	Akinetic mutism
Amyloidosis	Foreign dialect syndrome
Lipoid proteinosis	Jugular foramen syndrome
Wegener's granulomatosis	Adductor spasmodic dysphonia, essential tremor type
Rheumatoid arthritis	Adductor spasmodic dysphonia, dystonia type
Benign Neoplasms	Abductor spasmodic dysphonia, essential tremor type
Papilloma	Abductor spasmodic dysphonia, dystonia type
Chondroma	
Fibroma	
Cysts	

Etiology

Organic Voice Disorders

A voice disorder is *organic* if it is caused by structural (anatomic) or physiologic disease, either a disease of the larynx itself or by remote systemic or neurologic diseases that alter laryngeal structure or function. **Table 1.1** lists various causes of organic voice disorders.

Psychogenic Voice Disorders

Common synonyms for *psychogenic* are *functional* and *nonorganic*. *Psychogenic* voice disorders include disorders of quality, pitch, loudness, and flexibility caused by psychoneuroses, personality disorders, or faulty habits of voice usage (**Table 1.2**). The voice is abnormal despite normal laryngeal anatomy and physiology.

Table 1.2   List of Etiologies of Psychogenic Voice Disorders

Emotional Stress–Musculoskeletal Tension
Voice disorders without secondary laryngeal pathology
Voice disorders with secondary laryngeal pathology
Vocal abuse
Vocal nodule
Contact ulcer
Vocal fatigue
Psychoneurosis
Conversion disorder
Mutism
Aphonia
Muscle tension dysphonia
Psychosexual conflict
Mutational falsetto (puberphonia)
Dysphonia associated with conflict of sex identification.
Iatrogenic dysphonia

Voice Disorders of Multiple Etiology

Voice disorders are complex and often do not have a single etiology. For example, spasmodic dysphonia, including adductor, abductor, and mixed adductor-abductor types, can be neurologic, psychogenic, or of unknown (idiopathic) etiology. Persons with a clear organic etiology may be so depressed by their dysphonia that the depression compounds the voice problem becoming a clear secondary etiology. Still other individuals with voice problems may present with compensatory strategies developed from an organic problem, such as laryngitis that has long since resolved, and often secondary to anatomic changes from laryngeal or other surgeries.

Incidence

The National Institute of Deafness and Communicative Disorders, a division of the National Institutes of Health, estimates 7.5 million individuals have diseases or disorders of the voice caused by overuse of the vocal folds, upper respiratory infections, vocal fold lesions, laryngeal cancer, and other laryngeal pathologies (American Speech Language Hearing Association, 2002). Differences in vocal expectations (occupational, social, and cultural) make it difficult to determine how these incidence figures relate to such factors as age, vocal use, and occupation. Interpretation of incidence figures is further complicated by differences in methodology and definitions used by investigators as to what constitutes a voice disorder. Thus, it is not surprising to see estimates of voice disorder in total population ranging from 3 to 9% (Ramig and Verdolini, 1998), in children ranging from 3 to 24% (Senturia and Wilson, 1968; Silverman and Zimmer, 1975; Yairi, Currin, Bulian, et al. 1974). Koufman and Blalock (1991) suggest at least 10% of these are functional in origin, but here, too, the estimates range widely. We will not try to rectify the reported differences but rather present some representative studies.

Statistics on the incidence of voice disorders in school-age children suggest most children with voice disorders have dysphonia related to vocal abuse, either with or without resultant vocal fold nodules or general inflammation (Cooper, 1973; Pannbacker, 1999). In contrast with the studies on adults, the studies on children have been drawn from large bases. For example, Senturia and Wilson's (1968) study of 32,500 school-aged children in St. Louis, Missouri, demonstrated 6% had voice disorders. Other studies report a somewhat higher level. Yairi, Currin, Bulian, et al. (1974), based on a study of 1500 school-age children, found an incidence of hoarseness in 13%. The highest incidence was reported by Silverman and Zimmer (1975), who found voice disorders in 23.4% of schoolchildren. Whether these differences are related to actual differences in the children tested or criteria for voice disorder could not be determined.

Many of the studies reported for adults have been done in voice centers or specific occupational settings and the numbers extrapolated to the general population. One of the few incidence studies of adults, performed by Laguaite (1972), found that of 428 patients aged 18 to 82 years, 7.2% of the males and 5% of the females had voice disorders. In his otolaryngologic practice, Brodnitz (1971), reporting on only "functional" voice disorders, found that in 1851 cases, 25.8%

had hyperfunctional (musculoskeletal tension) voice disorders, 19.7% had polyps, 15.3% had vocal nodules, 9.4% had polypoid thickening, 5.3% had contact ulcers, 4.7% had mutational voice disorders, 4.7% had spastic dysphonia, 4.4% had psychogenic aphonia, and the remaining patients had voice disorders from other causes less common.

Representative statistics on the incidence, or prevalence, of abnormal voice in otolaryngologic practice are meager. In a study of the prevalence of laryngeal pathologies in medicine according to sex, age, and occupation, Herrington-Hall, Lee, Stemple, et al. (1988) investigated 1262 patients drawn from several otolaryngologic practices. They found that the most common disorders were vocal nodules, 21.6%; edema, 14.1%; polyps, 11.4%; cancer, 9.7%; vocal fold paralysis, 8.1%; and dysphonia without laryngeal pathology, 7.9%. Laryngeal pathologies occurred mostly in the older age groups; 57% of patients were over 45 years of age, with 22.4% over age 64 years. In a study by Dobres, Lee, Stemple, et al. (1990), the most common disorders in children were subglottal tracheal stenosis, vocal nodules, laryngomalacia, nonorganic voice disorders, and vocal fold paralysis. Kaufman and colleagues have reported several studies on the prevalence of the spectrum of dysphonia (Koufman, Blalock, 1991; Koufman and Isaacson, 1991; Koufman, 1991), including one one ocupations and pathology in a otolaryngology practice. She also looked at occupation and pathology in an otolaryngology practice. She divided her adult clinical population into four primary conditions and found that the total added up to more than 100% because many patients exhibit more than one problem. She reported that the Wake Forest Voice Center population broke down into 100% infectious and inflammatory conditions, 42% vocal misuse/abuse syndromes, 39% benign and malignant growths, 17% neuromuscular disease, and 3% psychogenic disorders. Clearly, laryngeal diseases do not occur with equal frequency across age and gender. Between 60% and 80% of papillomatosis occurs in children before the age of 3 years. Spastic dysphonia usually appears between 30 and 50 years of age in females. Nodules occur frequently in children and young adult women but rarely occur in adult males. According to Dobres, Lee, Stemple, el al. (1990), vocal nodules and edema were most common in early adulthood (22 to 44 years); polyps and dysphonia, despite a normal laryngeal examination, were most common during middle adulthood (45 to 64 years); and vocal fold paralysis in late adulthood (over age 64 years). Cancer was evenly distributed between the ages of 45 to 64 and over age 64 years. In males, vocal nodules were most common between 0 and 14 years, edema between 25 and 44 years, polyps between 45 and 64 years, and vocal fold paralysis primarily after age 64 years.

No summary of the incidence and prevalence of voice disorders would be complete without some information on how the figures relate to occupation. In the total working population in the United States, ~25% have jobs that critically require voice use, and 3% of the population have occupations in which their voice is necessary for public safety (National Institute on Deafness and Other Communication Disorders, 1999). Thus, it is not surprising in clinical practice to find certain occupations where vocal abuse, emotional stress, and ambient noise are prevalent and individuals prone to develop voice disorders (e.g., classroom teachers, actors, singers, telemarketers, auctioneers, factory workers, athletic coaches, and the clergy). A landmark study by Titze, Lemke, and Montequin (1997) compared U.S. workers who rely on voice to fulfill professional tasks with their appearance in voice centers. Teachers comprise ~20% of the patient load in voice clinics though they only constitute 4% of the workforce. Sapir, Keidar, and Mathers-Schmidt (1993) and Smith, Lemke, Taylor, et al. (1998), researching voice problems in teachers, support the notion that the incidence of voice problems in teachers is high. These investigators surveyed teachers and found that one third to one half report voice problems characterized by symptoms of hoarseness, difficulty with pitch, voice fatigue, weakness, and effortful production. Elementary and secondary schoolteachers were 32 times more likely to report these symptoms than a random sample of people in other occupations. Nearly indentical results were reported in Poland (Sliwinska-Kowalska, Niebudek-Bogusz, Fisher et al, 2006). This high occurrence is unfortunate because it has also been estimated that 75% of teachers' problems could be prevented or self-rehabilitated (Voice Academy, 2003). There are several obvious factors for why teachers are at risk for developing voice problems. They use their voices for prolonged periods, often over background noise, with little recovery time. They are also exposed to upper respiratory tract infections by their close contact with children, have limited time-off for illnesses, and often work in unfavorable environments having poor acoustics, chalk dust, low humidity levels, and noisy and inefficient heating systems. Mothers of small children are also prone to develop vocal nodules. Mothers and teachers have much in common. Although mothers may not have chalk dust to contend with, they often develop voice problems secondary to vocal stress from yelling at home and during sporting events of their children.

Of 73 different occupations in the total sample, the most commonly occurring ones were retired persons, homemakers, factory workers, unemployed persons, executives or managers, teachers, students, secretaries, singers, and nurses. Factory workers were third on the list of the top five occupations with a high incidence of laryngeal pathologies. These findings are consistent with a National Institute of Neurological Disorders and Stroke (2000) report that there is evidence of an increased incidence of vocal nodules in such occupations as homemakers, teachers, singers, lawyers, salespeople, preachers, and telemarketers. It is not surprising to read that persons in "talking professions" or persons who work in factories around noise commonly have voice problems. What is surprising is that retired and unemployed persons commonly have voice problems. It may be explained in part by Smith, Gray, Dove, et al. (1997): in a study of teachers, 40% expressed concern that voice problems might adversely affect future career options, who were almost twice as likely as nonteachers to state that difficulty with voice may be a problem in pursuing their profession of choice. Retired and unemployed persons with voice problems may represent individuals who quit "talking" careers because of voice difficulties. The retired persons may also be exhibiting problems related to the anatomic and physiologic changes that co-occur with age. In Koufman's clinical population, 45% were elite vocal performers and professional voice users such as clergy and teachers and 43% were non–vocal professionals whose job performance was affected by voice.

In Dorbe's patients diagnosed as having psychogenic voice disorders, 85% were female. With respect to occupational background, 35% of psychogenic voice disorders were found in female homemakers. This gender-biased result may be skewed by the fact that, in general, females seek medical attention with greater frequency than do males.

Several factors need to be considered in interpreting incidence studies. The time, place, population, definition of voice problems, and assessment tools all affect the outcome and explain the wide variance in reported results. Ten years ago, investigators were unaware of the importance of esophageal reflux on laryngeal tissue, subtle neurologic signs often went undetected, and videostroboscopy and other means of detecting minor structural deviations and lesions were often not included in test batteries. We are left to conclude that incidence studies are sorely needed, that the incidence and types of voice problems vary across lifespan changes and occupations, and that persons working in voice-dependent occupations and those working around noisy or polluted environments are at greater risk.

◆ Summary

- The vital functions of the larynx are to protect the lungs from foreign substances, to stabilize the thoracic cage during work done with the upper extremities, and to compress the abdominal contents.

- Phonation is a secondary laryngeal function and has primitive survival, emotive, entertainment (e.g., singing), and higher linguistic purposes.

- Normal voice is one in which voice quality, pitch, loudness, and flexibility are reasonably pleasing and audible to the listener.

- Abnormal voice is defined as deviations in quality, pitch, loudness, or flexibility that may signify illness and interfere with communication or a person's occupational or social needs.

- Voice disorders are classified into organic types, which consist of dysphonias or aphonia caused by mass lesions, infections, or neurologic disease; psychogenic types, which include abnormal voice resulting from psychoneurosis, psychosis, or faulty habit patterns; or complex when the problem is multidimensional.

- The incidence of voice disorders is not well documented. It is estimated in school-age children to be 6 to 9% and possibly as high as 24%. These are mostly dysphonias caused by vocal abuse. The incidence of voice disorders in adults differs by age group, gender, occupation, and pathology, and thus contains nearly the entire spectrum of organic and psychogenic voice disorders.

References

American Speech Language Hearing Association. Incidence and prevalence of speech, voice, and language disorders in the United States. Available at http://professional.asha.org/resources/factsheets/speech voice language.cfm. Accessed October 1, 2002.

Brodnitz, F.S. (1971). Vocal rehabilitation. A manual prepared for the use of graduates of medicine. (Ed 4), Rochester, MN. Am Acad Ophthalmol Otolaryngol 75.

Cooper, M. (1973). *Modern techniques of vocal rehabilitation.* Springfield, IL: Charles C. Thomas.

Dobres, R., Lee, L., Stemple, J., Kummer, A., Kretchmer, L. (1990). Description of laryngeal pathologies in children evaluated by otolaryngologists. J Speech Hear Disord 55, 526–533.

Fairbanks, G. (1960). *Voice and articulation drillbook.* New York: Harper & Brothers.

Herrington-Hall, B.L., Lee, L., Stemple, J.C., Niemi, K.R., McHone, M.M. (1988). Description of laryngeal pathologies by age, sex, and occupation in a treatment-seeking sample. J Speech Hear Disord 53, 57–64.

Hirano, M. (1981). *Clinical examination of voice.* New York: Springer-Verlag.

Jensen, P.J. (1965). Adequacy of terminology for clinical judgment of voice quality deviation. Eye Ear Nose Throat Mon 44, 77–82.

Johnson, W., Brown, S.F., Curtis, J.F., Edney, C.W., Keaster, J. (1965). *Speech handicapped school children.* New York: Harper & Brothers.

Kent, R.D. (1996). Hearing and believing some limits to the auditory perceptual assessment of speech and voice disorders. Am J Speech Lang Pathol 5, 7–23.

Koufman, J.A. (1991). The otolaryngologic manifestations of gastroesophageal reflux disease (GERD): a clinical investigation of 225 patients using ambulatory 24-hour pH monitoring and an experimental investigation of the role of acid and pepsin in the development of laryngeal injury. Laryngoscope 101 (Suppl 53), 1–78.

Koufman, J.A., Blalock, P.D. (1982). A classification and approach to patients with functional voice disorders, Ann Otol Rhinol Laryngol 91, 372–377.

Koufman, J.A., Blalock, P.D. (1991). Functional voice disorders. Otolaryngol Clin North Am 24, 1059–1073.

Koufman, J.A., Isaacson, G. (1991). The spectrum of vocal dysfunction. Otolaryngol Clin North AM 24, 985–988.

Kreiman, J., Gerratt, B.R., Kempster, G.B., Erman, A., Berke, G.S. (1993). Perceptual evaluation of voice quality: review, tutorial, and a framework for future research. J Speech Hear Res 36, 21–40.

Laguaite, J.K. (1972). Adult voice screening. J Speech Hear Disord 37, 147–151.

Moore, G.P. (1971a). *Organic voice disorders.* Englewood Cliffs, NJ Prentice-Hall.

Moore, G.P. (1971b). Voice disorders organically based. In L.E. Travis (Ed.), *Handbook of speech pathology and audiology.* New York: Appleton-Century-Crofts.

National Institute of Neurological Disorders and Stroke. (2000). Amyotrophic lateral sclerosis fact sheet. Available at http://www.ninds.nih.gov/health and medical/pubs/als.htm. Accessed April 18, 2001.

National Institute on Deafness and Other Communication Disorders. (n.d.). Strategic plan: plain language version. Available at http://www.nidcd.nih.gov/about/director/nsrp.htm. Accessed April 23, 2001.

National Institute on Deafness and Other Communication Disorders. (1999). Disorders of vocal abuse and misuse. NIH Pub. No. 99–4375. Bethesda, MD: NIH.

Negus, V.E. (1929). *The mechanism of the larynx.* St. Louis: C. V. Mosby Co.

Nizer, L. (1978). *Reflections without mirrors.* New York: Doubleday and Co.

Oates, J., Russell, A. (1998). Learning voice analysis using an interactive multi-media package: development and preliminary evaluation. J Voice 12, 500–512.

Pannbacker, M. (1999). Treatment of vocal nodules. Am J Speech Lang Pathol 8, 201–208.

Perkins, W.H. (1971). Vocal function: a behavioral analysis. In L.E. Travis (Ed.), *Handbook of speech pathology and audiology.* New York: Appleton-Century-Crofts.

Ramig, L.O., Verdolini, K. (1998). Treatment efficacy voice disorders. Am J Speech Lang Pathol Hear Res 41, S101–S116.

Robbins, S.D. (1963). *A dictionary of speech pathology and therapy.* Cambridge, MA: Sci-Art Publishers.

Sapir, S., Keidar, A., Mathers-Schmidt, B. (1993). Vocal attrition in teachers survey findings. Eur J Disord of Commun 28, 177–185.

Senturia, B.H., Wilson, F.B. (1968). Otorhinolaryngologic findings in children with voice deviations. Preliminary report. Ann Otol Rhinol Laryngol 77, 1027–1042.

Silverman, E.M., Zimmer, C.H. (1975). Incidence of chronic hoarseness among school-age children. J Speech Hear Disord 40, 211–215.

Smith, E., Gray, S., Dove, H., Kirchner, L., Heras, H. (1997). Frequency and effects of teachers' voice problems. J Voice 11, 80–87.

Smith, E., Lemke, J., Taylor, M., Kirchner, H.L., Hoffman, H. (1998). Frequency of voice problems among teachers and other occupations. J Voice 12, 480–488.

Titze, I.R., Lemke, J., Montequin, D. (1997). Voice as an occupational tool of trade. J Voice 11, 254–259.

Voice Academy. University of Iowa, Iowa City. Iowa, and the National Center for Voice and Speech, Denver Center for Performing Arts, Denver, Co. http://www.uiowa.edu/~shcvoice.

West, R., Kennedy, L., Carr, A. (1947). *The rehabilitation of speech.* New York: Harper & Brothers.

Yairi, E., Currin, L.H., Bulian, N., Yairi, J. (1974). Incidence of hoarseness in school children over a 1 year period. J Commun Disord 7, 321–328.

Additional Reading

Hooper, C.R. (2004). Treatment of voice disorders in children. Lang Speech Hear Serv Sch 35, 320–325.

McMurray, J.S. (2003). Disorders of phonation in children. Pediatr Clin North Am 50, 363–380.

(The preceding articles provide good reviews of dysphonias in children and their treatment.)

Miller, S.Q., Madison, C.L. (1984a). Public school voice clinics, part I: a working model. Lang Speech Hear Serv Sch 15, 51–57.

Miller, S.Q., Madison, C.L. (1984b). Public school voice clinics, part II: diagnosis and recommendations—a 10-year review. Lang Speech Hear Serv Sch 15, 58–64.

(The two preceding articles are interesting for their information on incidence of voice disorders, survey methods, and procedures for setting up voice clinics in schools.)

Pannbacker, M. (1984). Classification systems of voice disorders: a review of the literature. Lang Speech Hear Serv Sch 15, 169–174. (A worthwhile article on classification of voice disorders.)

Roy, N., Merrill, R.M., Gray, S.D., Smith, E.M. (2005). Voice disorders in the general population: prevalence, risk factors, and occupational impact. Laryngoscope 115, 1988–1995.

Ilomaki, I., Maki, E., Laukkanen, A.M. (2005). Vocal symptoms among teachers with and without voice education. Logoped Phoniatr Vocol 30, 171–174.

(The preceding pair of articles provides valuable information on prevalence, risk factors, and occupational impact of voice disorders with particular focus on teachers.)

Senturia, B.H., Wilson, F.B. (1968). Otorhinolaryngologic findings in children with voice deviations. Preliminary report. Ann Otol Rhinol Laryngol 77, 1027–1042. (One of the few detailed and comprehensive laryngologic studies of school-age children with voice disorders.)

Wilson, K. (1979). Voice problems of children (2nd ed.). Baltimore: Williams & Wilkins, Co. (Pages 6 to 11 contain an excellent review of the literature on public school voice disorder surveys.)

Chapter 2

Normal Voice Development

But what am I? An infant crying in the night: An infant crying for the light: And with no language but a cry.

—Tennyson, Lord Alfred

◆ Infancy

The Postnatal Larynx

By the third month of fetal life, the larynx has the same features recognizable at birth but is a structure quite different from the adult larynx. At birth, the 2-cm-long by 2-cm-wide larynx is estimated to be one third the dimension of the adult larynx, is extremely soft and malleable, does not possess a vocal fold layer structure, and shows no sex differentiation (Bosma, 1985; Kent and Vorperian, 1995; Tucker and Tucker, 1979; Verhulst, 1987). The laryngeal evolution from this embryonic state through senescence is central to voice, swallow, and respiration. Woisard, Serrano, and Pessey (1996) divide the laryngeal developmental modifications affecting the evolution of a child's voice into topographic (laryngeal descent in the neck), morphologic (increase in volume modification of laryngeal shape), and histologic (lamina propria differentiation). The chronological voice evolution primed by the central nervous system integrates these modifications in development.

Of these three modifications, topographic evolution appears to be the most controversial. It is commonly believed that phonation is phylogenetically a recent function of the larynx, made possible by the laryngeal descent, and is the reason humans can speak. Not all evidence supports this contention. During the neonatal cry, only gross vertical movements of the larynx and mandibular movements are possible, yet Menard, Schwartz, and Boe (2004) have shown that anatomy does not prevent even the youngest speaker from producing vowels perceived as the 10 French oral vowels though they recognize that the specific configuration of the vocal tract for the newborn seems to favor the production of low and front vowels. Lieberman, Harris, Wolff, et al. (1971) have observed that these limited movements and the uniform cross-sectional configuration of the supralaryngeal tract bear a striking resemblance to those of primates. At birth, the neonate's larynx occupies a position higher in the neck, relative to the palate and mandible, than at any other time in life. In fact, it is sufficiently high that the epiglottis is in contact with the velum allowing infants to carry out the functions of breathing and feeding simultaneously (Kent and Vorperian, 1995). Almost immediately after birth, it begins its descent in the neck. Lieberman, McCarthy, Hiiemae, et al. (2001) have suggested that spatial constraints related to deglutition impose greater restrictions on the rate and degree of hyo-laryngeal descent than do adaptations for vocalization, highlighting the different functional roles of the hyoid during voicing and oral transport. From a longitudinal series of lateral radiographs taken between the ages of 1 month and 15 years, these investigators observed vocal tract shape changed markedly during ontogeny, especially in the first postnatal year and during the adolescent growth spurt. The ratio of pharynx height to oral cavity length decreased from 1.5 to 1.0 between birth and 6 to 8 years, after which it remained stable. The superoinferior spatial relations between the positions of the vocal folds, the hyoid body, the mandible, and the hard palate did not change significantly throughout the entire postnatal growth period. **Figure 2.1** shows that at birth, the lower border of the cricoid cartilage is level between cervical vertebrae 3 and 4 (C3 and C4). By age 5, the larynx has descended almost to the level of C7. Between ages 15 and 20, it remains at C7. Although this developmental phenomenon has been reported to be unique to humans, Nishimura, Mikami, Suzuki, et al. (2005) found the laryngeal descent during infancy in chimpanzee infants was similar to that in human infants. Fitch and Reby (2001) also argue that laryngeal descent is not uniquely human. Using bioacoustic analyses of red and fallow deer coupled with anatomic analyses of functional morphology, they have documented these species lower the larynx in a manner similar to that exhibited by humans. They suggest

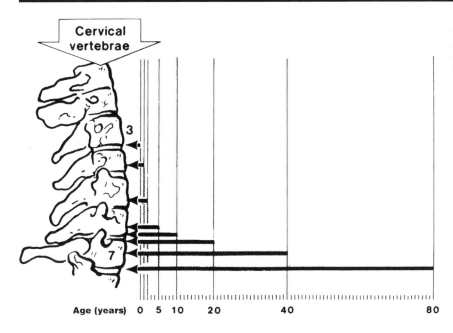

Cervical vertebrae

Age (years)   0   5   10   20   40   80

Fig. 2.1 Vertical descent of the larynx during life. The illustration demonstrates the relationship of the lower border of the cricoid cartilage to the cervical vertebrae at various ages. (Adapted from Wind, J. [1970]. On the phylogeny and the ontogeny of the human larynx. Gröningen: Wolters-Noordhoff Publishing, p. 105.)

that laryngeal descent serves to elongate the vocal tract, allowing callers to exaggerate their perceived body size by decreasing vocal-tract resonant frequencies. This exaggerated body size is consistent with work done by biologists Evans, Neave, and Wakelin (2006) who propose that a deep male voice may have once played a role in courtship and competitive behavior in humans by attracting female mates and indicating body size to male competitors. Thus, it seems clear that there is a developmental relationship between the descent of the larynx and the decrease in average voice pitch (as the pharyngeal tube elongates, it resonates lower fundamental frequencies) and that the descent is not unique to humans. Less clear is the evolutionary cause of the descent, which is currently thought to have first evolved for swallowing and secondarily for voice.

Morphologic changes begin at birth and continue throughout life. At birth, the thyroid cartilage is contiguous with the hyoid bone. The laryngeal skeleton then separates in a craniocaudal direction. The infant's epiglottis is bulky at this stage when seen superiorly. Together with the thick aryepiglottic folds, it is omega-shaped and lies over the dorsum of the tongue. During postnatal development, the epiglottis undergoes several changes, [enlarging epiglottis becomes firmer, and omega-shaped appearance is reduced,] reaching maturity at puberty (Kent and Vorperian, 1995). The configuration of the alae of the thyroid cartilage changes from a rounded shield during fetal life to an angle of ~90 to 100 degrees in the male and 120 degrees in the female at birth. During puberty, the angle in the male thyroid alae narrows to 90 degrees, whereas in the female it remains nearly the same. Increase in length of the thyroid cartilage is nearly 3 times greater in males than in females (Kahane, 1982). During the first years of life, the opening into the larynx widens, changing from its T-shape to one that is more rounded or oval.

The laryngeal airway is maintained by the circumference of the cricoid cartilage. However, the soft cartilages of the neonatal larynx and lax supporting ligaments predispose the infant's

larynx to collapse if negative air pressures become excessive within the internal vocal tract. Because the subepithelial tissues are less dense and more abundant and vascular, they have a tendency to accumulate tissue fluids, accounting for the high incidence in infants of infraglottic and supraglottic obstruction due to inflammatory edema. Ossification of the hyoid bone begins by age 2. Onset of ossification of the cartilage is controversial (Kent and Vorperian, 1995). Claassen and Kirsch (1994) suggest it begins soon after puberty when the larynx reaches its final size, which would be ~15 to 20 years of age, but Kahane (1983) and Sato, Kurita, Hirano, et al. (1990) suggest it begins around the third decade for males and fourth decade for females. It is generally agreed that the onset of ossification begins in the hyaline cartilage first with the thyroid followed by the cricoid. The hyaline and elastic arytenoid ossify later, but by the seventh or eighth decade, all the laryngeal cartilage, except the elastic epiglottis, cuneiforms, and corniculates, have ossified in males. The female larynx never completely ossifies (Claassen and Kirsch, 1994).

Vocal fold length, glottal width, and infraglottal sagittal and transverse dimensions at infancy, puberty, and adulthood are given in **Table 2.1.** The membranous and cartilaginous portions of the vocal folds are equal in length in infancy creating a proportionately larger glottis in the infant, but by adulthood, the membranous portion with greater pliability has elongated to approximately two thirds of the total glottal length. Glottal width and infraglottal dimensions also increase with age.

Histologic modifications occur coincidental with the topographic and morphologic changes contributing to the evolution of voice. Most notable are changes that occur in the delicate histoarchitecture of the vocal folds, which consist of the thyroarytenoid and mucosa. At birth, the mucosa is thicker than that in adults and, in contrast with the layered lamina propria seen in adults, the infant mucosa is uniform and does not begin forming layers until somewhere between the ages of 1 to 4 years (Hirano and Sato, 1993; Hirano, Kurita, and Nakashima, 1983; Kahane, 1988). The adult

Table 2.1 Dimensions of the Larynx*

	Infancy (mm)	Puberty (mm)	Adult Male (mm)	Adult Female (mm)
Vocal cord length	6–8	12–15	17–23	12.5–17
Membranous portion	3–4	7–8	11.5–16	8–11.5
Cartilaginous portion	3–4	5–7	5.5–7	4.5–5.5
Glottis width at rest	3	5	8	6
Maximum	6	12	19	13
Infraglottis sagittal	5–7	15	25	18
Transverse	5–7	15	24	17

Source: Ballenger, J.J. (1969). Diseases of the nose, throat and ear. Philadelphia: Lea & Febiger, p. 275.

*Measurements from other studies differ somewhat from those reported above but all concur that there is a continual increase in vocal fold length from birth to puberty with sex differences appearing between 6 and 10 years of age (Kent and Vorperian, 1995).

differentiation between lamina propria layers is evident by puberty, but the histologic modifications continue throughout life with geriatrics exhibiting thicker edematous lamina propria with decreased density of elastin and collagen fibers.

Histologic changes in the vocalis muscle are also abundant. Hirano, Kurita, and Nakashima (1983) noted that the muscle fibers were thin in newborns, fully developed by 27 years and somewhat atrophied by the fifth decade of life. The newborn infant has more type II (long prolonged contraction) than type I (short fast contraction) muscles. Type I muscles become more prominent with age contributing to increased control of vocal modifications and prolonged vocal expression (Woisard et al., 2006). Structural differences are not limited to developmental age related changes: Xue and Hao (2006), using acoustic pharyngometry to develop a database of the geometry of the vocal tract, found significant differences related to gender and race.

Infant Cries

The birth cry after the neonate has emerged from the womb signals the first conventional appearance of voice in humans. Nevertheless, human cries from the fetus in utero are known to have occurred. Thiery, Yo Le Sian, Vrijens, et al. (1973) documented such a case in a 31-year-old woman in her fifth pregnancy. When the fetal head was 3 cm above the ischial spines, the membranes ruptured, releasing 2000 mL of clear fluid. According to Thiery, "While the fetal head was being displaced to allow the drainage of as much amniotic fluid as possible, the fetus started crying. This sound was clearly heard by the mother, three physicians, and two midwives. The crying recurred six to seven times at intervals of up to 20 seconds."

Do normal infants have distinctively different cries, and, if so, are they indicative of definitive physiologic and emotional states? Is it possible to differentiate types of infant cries from acoustic spectrographic data and by listening to recordings? Are the cries of infants who are ill distinguishable from normal infant cries, based on spectrographic data and listener judgment? In perhaps the earliest comprehen-

sive study done of normal infant cries, Wasz-Höckert, Lind, Vuorenkoski, et al. (1968) obtained spectrographic and listener judgment data based on 419 cries of 351 healthy infants. Listeners were able to identify four distinctive types of cries from birth through 7 months.

1. *Birth signal*   Duration ±1 second; flat of falling melody; usually voiceless; always strained or strident; contains glottal plosives

2. *Pain signal*   Long duration; usually falling melody; high-pitched; strident

3. *Hunger signal*   Pitch rising-falling; frequent glottal plosives

4. *Pleasure signal*   Flat pitch; hypernasal; greater pitch variability than the other types of cries; rare glottal plosives; never voiceless; never strident

Because the cries are distinct LaGasse, Neal, and Lester (2005) have suggested that infant cry provides a noninvasive window into the neurologic and medical status of the infant because the acoustic characteristics of the cry from infants with neurologic damage, sudden infant death syndrome, prematurity, and various medical conditions deviate from typical cry characteristics. Robb (2003) similarly noted neuromaturational differences in cries of pre- and full-term infants. The crying episodes of full-term infants contained a greater number of bifurcations and aperiodic segments. Wermke, Mende, Manfredi, et al. (2002) interpreted their longitudinal data on complexity of cry melodies in three pairs of healthy identical twins as support that acoustic analysis of cries reflects neuromuscular maturation and is a good indication for evaluation of prespeech development. These authors recorded the twins at 8th to 9th, 15th to 17th, and 23rd to 24th weeks of postnatal development. Over the period of recording time, cry melodies were increasingly complex. An increasing coupling and tuning between melody and resonance frequencies began during the second recording period at the 15th to 17th weeks.

As early as infancy, cries illustrate a universal fact about the larynx: the true and false vocal folds respond differentially, depending upon psychophysiologic state. The pain cry is strained, tense, harsh, and forced owing to massive, tight, effortful closure of the entire laryngeal tract (i.e., it is an undifferentiated adduction of both the true and false vocal folds). The pleasure cry, more sonorous, lax, and devoid of strain of tension, is produced by the true vocal folds alone. Throughout life, the voice is smooth, clear, sonorous, devoid of strain or effort, and filled with rich inflectional patterns during pleasure and freedom from anxiety, fear, hostility, or depression. However, it is harsh, strained, and lacking in inflectional patterns during times of situational stress both in normal persons and in persons with some psychiatric illnesses. Clarici, Travan, Accardo, et al. (2002) attempted to determine if the crying of a newborn child was an alarm signal or protocommunication. Acoustic analyses comparing spontaneous cries in the cradle with pain conditions demonstrated that the newborn infants modulated the supralaryngeal tract more in cries after painful stimulus than in spontaneous cries. The authors proposed that these data supported the hypothesis that crying is protolanguage meant to communicate meaning.

In his review article on the signal functions of early infant crying, Soltis (2004) offers an interesting evolutionary perspective. He states that infant cries are in large part adaptations that maintain proximity to and elicit care from caregivers. He continues that infant cries may function as a graded signal, as evidenced by the observation that during pain-induced autonomic nervous system arousal, neural input to the larynx increases tension and cry pitch. Increases in amounts of crying during the first few months of life he claims is a human universal, and potential signal functions of this excessive crying have been hypothesized to be manipulation of parents to acquire additional resources, honest signaling of need, and honest signaling of vigor. Of these hypotheses, he suggests evidence is most consistent with excessive crying as a signal of vigor that evolved to reduce the risk of a reduction or withdrawal of parental care.

Fundamental Frequency

Life begins with a voice fundamental frequency 300 to 400 Hz above that which is ultimately achieved by adulthood. In a 1968 study of 419 cries from birth to 7 months by Wasz-Hockert et al., the measured frequencies varied according to the type of cry: 77 birth cries averaged 500 Hz, 60 pain cries between birth and 1 month averaged 530 Hz, 72 pleasure cries averaged 440 Hz. There was little difference for recordings on the same type of cry for infants between 1 and 7 months. Michelsson et al. (2002) analyzed a total of 1,836 cry signals from 172 healthy babies between 1 and 7 days old. Measuring 8–15 cry samples from each infant, the authors reported that each infant's cries varied between 450 and 520 Hz. In their sample of infants, 93% had cries with a mean Fo below 600 Hz and a range of over 200 Hz; mean value of the highest point of Fo was $583 +- 151$ Hz and the lowest point $398 +- 75$ Hz. The Fo contour was generally a rising-falling contour, and there were no significant differences in cry according to gender or age. This large-scale study is consistent with earlier cross-sectional studies completed in the 1960s: Ringel and Kuppel (1964) found that the fundamental frequency of pain cries from 10 normal infants was 413 Hz; Ostwald, Phibbs, and Fox (1968), in a study of the pain cries of five infants, obtained initial, highest, and final mean fundamental frequencies of 418 Hz, 506 Hz, and 393 Hz, respectively, for each cry.

In a longitudinal study of infant vocalizations recorded during the first 9 months of life Greene (1972) noted a progressive increase in the range of inflectional glides during cooing and babbling. The earliest appearance of the upward glide, C3-C#, was in a 2-week-old girl, whose range increased from C3 to E3 by 7 weeks of age. The voice of an infant male at 5 weeks ranged from C# to F# in one breath, and at 16 weeks his musical inflections varied, rising and falling between C2# and E. Upward glides appeared first, then rising and falling glides increased in quantity and range up to an octave at 6 to 7 months of age.

Acoustic features of comfort-state vocalization of infants 3, 5, and 9 months were studied by Kent and Murray (1982). Fundamental frequency measures were similar to those previously reported for 3-month-old infants (445 Hz), 6-month-old infants (450 Hz), and 9 month-old infants (415 Hz). Similar to cry data, the vocalizations were associated with tremor, harmonic doubling, abrupt Fo shift, vocal fry, and noise segments.

Duration

Wasz-Höckert, Lind, Vuorenkoski, et al. (1968) found that between birth and 1 month of age, pain cries (2.6 seconds) averaged approximately twice the average duration of hunger cries (1.3 seconds). The duration of cries between 1 and 7 months of age were found to be nearly identical to those recorded for newborns. Similarly, Ringel and Kuppel (1964) and Ostwald, Phibbs, and Fox (1968) both found that pain cries averaged 1.5 seconds in length. Similarly Michelsson, Eklund, Leppanen, et al. (2002) reported cry duration of 1- to 7-day-old infants was $1.4 +- 0.6$ seconds. Collectively, these figures indicate that on average, cries can be as short as 0.2 second and as long as 2.7 seconds with pain cries being longer in duration than those recorded for hunger. Duration of comfort-state vocalizations for infants 3, 6, and 9 months old is generally less than 400 milliseconds but occasionally as long as 2 seconds (Kent and Murray, 1982).

Listener Identification of Infant Cries

Apparently, listeners are able to identify birth, pain, hunger, and pleasure cries beyond chance odds, and training improves this skill. Wasz-Höckert, Lind, Vuorenkoski, et al. (1968) had 349 women identify and categorize 24 infant birth, pain, hunger, and pleasure cries. The results showed that pleasure cries were identified most accurately, followed by hunger, pain, and birth cries. However, the accuracy of judgments depended upon the rater's background. Ranked according to decreasing order of accuracy were (1) midwives; (2) children's nurses; (3) mothers; (4) registered nurses; (5) other women experienced in childcare; (6) women with no experience in child care. Overall, there was a high degree of accuracy with all raters, even though rater groups differed significantly from one another.

Hollien and Müller (1973) took issue with the conclusions of Wasz-Höckert and colleagues that certain cries are associated with specific stimulus situations and that recognizable perceptual differences exist between cries. They argued that (1) birth cries and "pleasure" vocalizations ought not to have been juxtaposed in the design of the study; (2) preselection of "typical" samples of cries for listener judgments may have biased the listeners; (3) cry duration and infant age ought to have been controlled experimentally and statistically. In their own study, Hollien and Müller recorded cries in response to pain, auditory, and hunger stimuli from four male and four female infants, aged 3 to 5 months. Two groups of mothers listened: one, the real mothers of the eight infants, and the other, mothers of infants of comparable age. Although statistical analysis proved that some of the hunger cries were correctly identified, a significant number of times, the listeners overidentified cries of all types as hunger cries, possibly revealing a bias toward judgments of this kind. From the study, the authors concluded that the acoustic characteristics of normal infant cries carry little perceptual information to the mother about the situation that evoked the cry response. However, the experimenters were less than completely confident in their conclusions, calling them "tentative" and advocating the need for "additional investigations." Moreover, as research has demonstrated significant durational differences between cries, Hollien and Müller's durational control may have eliminated an important acoustic cue in cry identification. An additional interesting finding of this study was that the mothers of the infants in the study had little difficulty recognizing which samples were produced by their own infants.

Thus, although caregiver perception of cry is far from clear, many authors suggest infant cries provide signal function that caregivers can reliably assess. This notion has been the impetus for the development of pain assessment tools for clinical assessment in the neonatal intensive care units (Bellieni, Sisto, Cordelli, et al. 2004; McNair, Ballantyne, Dionne, et al. 2004; Spence, Gillies, Harrison, et al. 2005).

Facial Expression Associated with Infant Cries

Infant cries and other vocalizations are inseparable from associated facial expressions and bodily movements. Young and Décarie (1977) coded the facial/vocal behavior and body movements of 75 male and female infants, aged 9 to 14 months, who were exposed to six different types of emotionally arousing situations. From their study, they were able to identify two main classes of vocalizations:

1. *Positive vocalizations*. Those associated with smiling facial expressions (e.g., babbling, cooing, laughing, and squealing)

2. *Negative vocalizations*. Those associated with grimacing, trembling of the lips, and frowning (e.g., harsh wailing, wailing without harsh voice quality, and soft wailing)

They then categorized these vocalizations into the following:

- *Babbling* Vocalization of low intensity, moderate pitch, and a soft-sounding sequence of consonant-vowel combinations, generally pleasurable to the listener, produced during prolonged exhalation and in quick sequence

- *Coo* Sustained, moderately high-pitched voice of moderate intensity, having a smooth onset, pleasant to the listener, and produced during prolonged exhalation

- *Laugh* Rapid repetitions of short exhalations of moderate pitch and harsh quality; pleasant to hear

- *Squeal* Extremely high-pitched, of moderate intensity, variable in duration, positive, and produced during extended exhalation

- *Harsh wail* Begins with breath-holding of sudden onset and has a rhythmic piercing sound, a definitely negative quality, and is harsh, irritating, and painful to hear

- *Soft wail* Begins with breath-holding, has a soft but negative quality

- *Wail* Hard, high-pitched, discordant

Physiologic Bases of the Infant Cry and Intonation

Little is known of the aerodynamic, respiratory, and neuromuscular bases of the infant cry. Fluctuations from periodic to aperiodic acoustic spectra in such cries have been noted by Lieberman, Harris, Wolff, et al. (1971), who attributed these variations to the infant's inability to adjust the vocal folds to rising subglottic air pressures, the soft laryngeal tissues being unable to withstand such pressures.

In normal children and adults, the fundamental frequency of the voice drops toward the end of a sustained utterance or breath group owing to the decline of infraglottal air pressure as exhalation progresses and there is less respiratory support. Lieberman (1967) traces the origins of this universal human tendency to early infancy. Citing Bosma, Lind, and Truby (1964), he notes that the shape of the fundamental frequency contour of the cry is similar to that of the typical esophageal pressure contour. The amount of expiratory muscle activity is directly related to the infant's excitability; as greater thoracic contraction produces greater subglottal air pressure, infant cries show higher fundamental frequency and intensity. The fundamental frequency falls as the breath group ends, the lungs being depleted of air at the end of the exhalation. There thus appears to be an innate physiologic basis for intonation. According to Lieberman (1967), "The infant's hypothetical innate referential breath-group furnishes the basis for the universal acoustic properties of the normal breath-group that is used to segment speech into sentences in so many languages."

Infants respond to intonation of voice before they are able to comprehend language. This was first demonstrated by Lewis (1936), who showed that a 10-month-old male and a 13-month-old female changed the fundamental frequencies of their voices depending upon whether they were playing with their mother (higher-pitched voice) or their father (lower-pitched voice). Thus, early in language development, before the actual appearance of distinctive linguistic features, intonation apparently takes on imitation and/or symbolic meaning.

Lewis identified three intonational stages in the development of language:

1. At an early stage, the child shows broad discrimination between different patterns of expression in intonation.

2. When the total pattern (phonetic form plus intonational form) emerges because of language learning, intonation, not the phonetic pattern, dominates the child's response at first.

3. Finally, the phonetic pattern becomes the dominant feature. Although the intonational pattern is subordinated, it never completely disappears.

◆ Childhood

Fundamental Frequency

Fundamental frequency reflects vibratory patterns of the vocal fold and its elasticity, length, and vocal fold shape and thickness. Fundamental frequency of children has been the focus of hundreds of research studies initiated in the 1940s and continuing into the present time, where they have been the fodder for numerous theses and dissertations (e.g. Curry,

1940, 1949; Fairbanks, Herbert and Hammond, 1949; Fuchs et al. 2007). Generally, researchers agree that Fo decreases from the 500-Hz cry of an infant to around 300 Hz for the toddler. By prepubescence, Fo drops nearly 50% to around 250 Hz (Busby and Plat, 1995; Curry, 1940; Hasek, Sadanand, and Murry, 1980; McGlone and McGlone, 1972; Smith and Gray, 2002; Stathopoulos, 2002) for both boys and girls. The most marked adolescent Fo drop occurs in boys and is thought to be related to the laryngeal growth changes resulting from hormonal secretions of adrenal androgens (Smith and Gray, 2002). Comparison of the frequency/pitch in the male at puberty and at the termination of adolescence indicates that the male voice drops approximately one octave. Curry (1940) found the median fundamental frequency in 10- and 14-year-old boys to be 269 Hz and 241 Hz, respectively, whereas in 18-year-old males the frequency descended to 137 Hz. Hollien and Malcik (1967) found the median fundamental frequency in 18-year-old males to be 126 Hz. These figures are similar to those reported by Whiteside and Hodgson (2000), Whiteside (2001), and Whiteside, Hodgson, and Tapster (2002). Thus, for males we see a nearly 50% drop from the infant cry (500 Hz) to childhood voice (250 Hz) and another 50% drop from childhood voice to adulthood (125 Hz). The change in Fo for females is less dramatic but also reaches adult maturity during puberty. McGlone and Hollien (1963) found that female voices dropped 2.4 semitones between ages 7 and 8 to 11 and 15 years. In a study of 15-, 16-, and 17-year-old females, Michel, Hollien, and Moore (1966) reported average fundamental frequencies of 207 Hz; their similarities indicating that by age 15, mutational change of voice is essentially completed in females. After pubertal changes, the voice remains fairly stable until around the sixth decade when postmenopausal voice may lower in some females and around the seventh decade when the male Fo may rise slightly.

During the transition from the child to adult voice, audible voice breaks are uncommon, and they almost always occur in males, rarely in females. Pitch breaks can span an entire octave, transcending vocal registers from high-pitched falsetto to bass. Hoarseness from chronic laryngitis is common, particularly if vocal abuse occurs during the period of voice change. If Curry's (1949) figures are indicative, there is, apparently, a high prevalence of transient dysphonia during adolescent voice change, as he found that 80% of the voices of 14-year-old boys were of hoarse-husky quality.

In brief, it seems clear that the fundamental frequency of the human voice descends with age. The most notable changes occur between birth and adolescence, paralleling the descent of the larynx in the neck and growth of the laryngeal structure. Despite hundreds of studies on fundamental frequency during childhood, data are incomplete; we do not yet have an unbroken continuity of data. Because each study varies in methodology—some employing oral reading and others contextual speech—interpretation of results must be guarded.

Frequency Range

Phonational frequency range is the difference in frequency between the lowest sustainable tone in the modal register and the highest falsetto. Studies of children's frequency (pitch is its physical correlate) ranges are incomplete, com-

plicated by mixed purposes and methodologies, some being designed for gathering musical information and others for physiologic data. Nevertheless, a picture of frequency range begins to emerge. Van Oordt and Drost (1963) studied 126 children, dividing them into two groups: birth through 5 years of age (45 children) and 6 through 16 years of age (81 children). The children aged 6 through 16 were asked to sing from an arbitrary tone up to the highest they could reach and then down to the lowest one. From this method, the researchers derived (1) highest musical tone (the highest tone having musical quality) and (2) highest physiologic tone (the highest tone attainable, regardless of musical quality or clarity). The lowest musical tone and the lowest physiologic tone were based on similar judgments. **Figure 2.2** shows the comparison between the physiologic voice (frequency) range and the musical voice (frequency) range. This figure illustrates that the physiologic voice range remains constant from ages 6 to 16 (~2½ octaves) whereas the musical voice range expands.

Developmental changes in voice are not limited to changes in frequency. Aerodynamic and acoustic results, reported by Stathopoulos and Sapienza (1997) in a cross-sectional study that included children aged 4 to 14 years and adults, show that men and 14-year-old boys function differently than women and all other groups of children. Children's respiratory values are similar to those of adults by the time they are 12 to 14 years of age.

♦ Puberty and Adolescence

Anatomy and Physiology of Adolescent Voice Change

Until puberty, the larynx is of equal size in the male and the female as discussed elsewhere in this text. As shown in **Table 2.1**, at puberty the male laryngeal growth outdistances the female particularly in the anteroposterior dimensions.

♦ By adulthood, the membranous portions of the male vocal folds range from 11.5 to 16 mm (in length, a 4- to 8-mm increase from puberty). However, on average, the female membranous vocal folds increase in length to only 8 to 11.5 mm (a 1- to 3.5-mm increase).

♦ The dimensions of the infraglottal sagittal and transverse planes grow in the male to 25 mm, respectively, and in the female to 18 mm and 17 mm, respectively.

♦ Although there is considerable gender overlap, the angle of the thyroid lamina decreases until it becomes ~90 degrees, whereas in the female larynx, the angle remains ~120 degrees.

♦ The laryngeal mucosa loses some of its transparency and becomes stronger; the epiglottis flattens, increases in size, and elevates; and the tonsils and adenoids partially atrophy.

♦ The larynx descends in the neck. The neck itself elongates. Because of the greater enlargement of the thorax in most males, there also is a more prominent increase in vital capacity than seen in females.

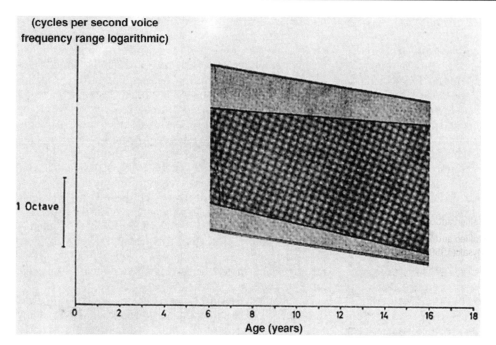

Fig. 2.2 Comparison between physiologic and musical voice frequency range. Physiologic frequency range (PVR) is represented by total area and musical frequency range (MVR) by darker area. Both are bordered by regression lines of highest and lowest registered physiologic and musical tones plotted logarithmically. (From van Oordt, H.W.A., Drost, H.A. [1963]. Development of the frequency range of the voice in children. Folia Phoniat 15, 289–298.)

Age of Onset and Duration of Adolescent Voice Change

Evidence indicates that onset of puberty occurs earlier in warmer climates and with children who are heavier in weight. In temperate climates, onset of puberty in females ranges from ages 12 to 14 and in males from ages 13 to 15. Near the Equator, onset is accelerated 1 to 2 years, and near the poles it is delayed 1 year. Onset of puberty also may be delayed in females by excessive exercise or nutritional deficiencies such as occur with anorexia and bulimia.

The average time from onset to completion of adolescent voice change is 3 to 6 months, 1 year at most. Fuchs, Froehlich, Hentschel, et al. (2007) claim that acoustic features of voice change begin appearing 5 to 7 months before onset. They divide pubertal voice change into three time periods: premutation, mutation when the voice is most unstable, and postmutation. In females, the voice change is complete by age 15 and in males by age 14 or 15. Although the onset of voice change occurs earlier in females, males and females complete the change at approximately the same age.

Adolescent Voice Frequency Change

Frequency/pitch distinction between male and female begins during puberty and continues throughout adolescence. These voice changes—the result of growth of the phonatory, resonatory, and respiratory anatomy—roughly parallel the appearance and development of the secondary sex characteristics. The pitch and quality changes that occur at puberty are more apparent in males than in females because of the greater magnitude of the pitch change, which is approximately one octave in males. The voice of males at puberty often begins with a husky quality and an unsteady

pitch, oscillating perhaps one to two tones. Although the pitch fluctuates from day to day, the general trend is downward. With time, the high tones become less steady, the low tones more stable. Fuchs, Froehlich, Hentschel, et al. (2007) reported on a 3-year longitudinal study of 21 male members of a professional boys' choir from which they concluded that acoustic analyses could be used to predict mutational change in the speaking voice because nonaudible significant changes of acoustic features appeared 5 to 7 months before mutation onset.

Stormy Voice Mutation

Stormy voice mutation refers to pervasive sudden voice breaks from high to low pitch, or the reverse, or excessively husky or hoarse voice associated with adolescent voice change. Although there may be some hoarseness or huskiness to the voice quality and increased perturbations, it should be emphasized that the majority of male adolescents have uneventful voice change.

◆ Adulthood

Fundamental Frequency

Research on the fundamental frequency of the speaking voice for the age continuum in adults is also far from complete because the instrumentation, procedures, time of day, and subject inclusion/exclusion criteria used to obtain fundamental frequency vary among studies. Despite these limitations, the fundamental frequency values obtained by independent researchers are similar within gender groups.

Table 2.2 Male Mean Fundamental Frequency (Hz) as a Function of Age Comparative Studies

Age Range (Years)	No.	Mean Fundamental Frequency (Hz)	Investigators
20–29	175	120	Hollien and Shipp (1972)
	27	119	Hanley (1951)
	157	128	Hollien and Jackson (1973)
	24	132	Philhour (1948)
	6	132	Pronovost (1942)
	103	138	Majewski, Hollien, Zalewski (1972)
30–39	175	112	Hollien and Shipp (1972)
40–49	175	107	Hollien and Shipp (1972)
	39	113	Mysak (1959)
50–59	175	118	Hollien and Shipp (1972)
60–69	175	112	Hollien and Shipp (1972)
70–79	175	132	Hollien and Shipp (1972)
	39	124	Mysak (1959)
80–89	175	146	Hollien and Shipp (1972)
	39	141	Mysak (1959)

Table 2.3 Female Mean Fundamental Frequency (Hz) as a Function of Age

Age Range (Years)	No.	Mean Fundamental Frequency (Hz)
20–29	10	227
30–39	10	214
40–49	10	214
50–59	10	214
60–69	10	209
70–79	10	206
80–90	10	197

Source: Kelley, A. (1977). Fundamental frequency measurement of female voices from twenty to ninety years of age. (Unpublished manuscript.) Greensboro, NC: University of North Carolina.

We have arbitrarily taken 69 years as a cutoff point in our discussion of adult fundamental frequency because we wish to discuss a succeeding category that might be designated "older age."

A summary of several major fundamental frequency studies, conducted in the middle of the 20th century, of the male speaking voice in adult males is found in **Table 2.2.** From this table, it can be seen that most early studies were of males within the 20- to 29-year age group. The group mean fundamental frequency for all studies within this age group is 128 Hz, and the range is 119 to 138 Hz. Similar values (Fo = 119 Hz) were reported by Naufel de Felippe, Grillo, and Grechi (2006) for males between 20 to 45 years of age without signs or symptoms of vocal problems. Studies by Hollien and Shipp (1972) and Wang, Gao, Yang, et al. (2006) show that in the seventh decade, the fundamental frequency of males begins to rise. Critics suggest studies using college student volunteers should be regarded with caution because they represented a narrow segment of the population, and this data might be different from average individuals. Hollien, Hollien, and de Jong (1997) put this argument to rest. They reported that university students were found to be slightly larger than a cohort approaching the average population, but only minor insignificant vocal differences were found.

Data on the fundamental frequency of the speaking voice in adult females indicate that as a group, their voices average 1.6 times higher than those of males. Kelley (1977) studied 70 females, aged 20 to 90 years, whose mean fundamental frequencies and ranges are given in **Table 2.3.** An important finding of this study was a strong correlation between age and Fo with fundamental frequency in females decreasing throughout the age range 20 to 70 years. These data are at variance with the results of studies by McGlone and Hollien (1963), who found no significant change in mean fundamen-

tal frequency in females from early adulthood through advanced age. In addition, Saxman and Burk (1967) found that in females, mean fundamental frequency decreases during the middle years and then increases in old age. The reason for these differences has not been adequately documented but is hypothesized to relate to changes in the anatomic structure of the vocal apparatus. Additionally, oral reading results in higher mean speaking fundamental frequencies than those for spontaneous speech (Hollien, Hollien, and de Jong, 1997) suggesting different tasks may have contributed to differences. Also, the variability between subjects is sufficiently high that it may be necessary to record larger sample sizes with enough power to take into account race, hormones, culture, age, and general health.

♦ Older Age

Having documented the decline in the fundamental frequency of the human voice from infancy through adulthood, we now ask, "What happens to the voice of the aged?" Does it attest to signs of aging organism? Can we hear differences between younger and older voices? Are there physical changes in the structure of the larynx or its innervation that might account for such voice changes? Information accumulated to date indicates an affirmative answer to all of these questions.

Physical Changes

Several studies show structural changes of both the respiratory system and the vocal folds with age. Atrophy of the intrinsic laryngeal muscles, thinning and dehydration of the laryngeal mucosa, loss of elasticity of ligaments, qualitative and quantitative changes in collagenous fibers resulting in changes in the viscoelasticity of the vocal folds, calcification of cartilages, flaccidity and bowing of the vocal folds, and edema have been documented by Ferreri (1959), Jackson and Jackson (1959), Keleman and Pressman (1955), Myerson (1976) and Sato, Hirano, and Nakashima (2002).

In a study of men and women aged 69 to 85 years, Honjo and Isshiki (1980) saw a yellowish or dark-grayish discoloration of the vocal folds in 39% of the men and 47% of the women. Edema of the vocal folds was noted in 74% of the women and 56% of men. Vocal fold atrophy was found in 67% of the men and 26% of the women, inferred from either bowing of the edges of the vocal folds, visibility of the ventricle, or prominence of the contour of the vocal processes of the arytenoid cartilages. Glottal gap was observed in 67% of the men as semicircular (22%), linear (28%), or partial (17%). However, this finding was less common in women, 58%, among whom the semicircular gap was particularly rare. Vocal sulcus was noted in ~10% of both men and women.

These authors concluded that the discoloration of the vocal folds found in approximately one half of the subjects was due to either fat degeneration or keratosis of the mucous membrane that lines the larynx. Vocal fold atrophy and glottal gap in men were attributed to senescent changes of the entire thyroarytenoid muscle and mucous membrane, and edema of the vocal folds in women was attributed to general endocrine changes after menopause. This increase in the mass of the vocal folds may be the cause for noticeable lowering of average fundamental frequency and roughness and hoarseness of voice in aged women.

Morrison and Gore-Hickman (1986) found that it is the older men with atrophy and the older women with polypoidal degeneration who usually complain about their abnormal voices. These authors found that older patients have a tendency to misuse their voices, their phonation commonly associated with hyperactivity of the ventricular folds. They speculate that this vocal misuse or abuse may have psychogenic bases or may be due to an attempt to compensate for atrophy or polypoidal changes. Thus, they raise the strong possibility that psychologic distress may make an important contribution to dysphonia in older persons, owing to tension, hypochondriasis, multiple medications and health problems, reduced finances, and depression. This neglected population, although they may not complain of depression or anger, may nevertheless be reacting to loneliness, isolation, family separation, and conflicts with spouses who are also aging.

In a study of the stroboscopic movements of the vocal folds in 20 young adult women aged 22 to 28 years and 20 older women aged 60 to 77 years, Biever and Bless (1989) found aperiodic vibration in 85% of the older women but in only 30% of the younger ones and a posterior glottal gap common to both age groups. Electroglottography (EGG) recorded on geriatrics (Higgins and Saxman (1991); Winkler and Sendlmeier, 2006) showed a decreased EGG open quotient (OQ) with increased age that was positively related to perceived age.

◆ Perceptual Studies of Voice Sound Changes

Listeners can accurately detect differences in chronological age by the sound of the voice, based on ratings of contextual speech and vowel prolongation (Ptacek and Sander, 1966; Ryan and Burk, 1974; Ryan and Capadano, 1978; Shipp and Hollien, 1969). Studies have also shown that the acoustic physical properties of voice change with advancing age (Ferrand, 2002; Kent and Burkhard, 1981; Mueller, 1997; Verdonck-de Leeuw and Mahieu, 2004; Watson, 1998). Sustained phonation in older age groups has been described as hoarse, breathy, and tremorous by Ptacek and Sander (1966), Hartman and Danhauer (1976), and Ryan and Capadano (1978), characterized by overall deterioration of the acoustic signal (Verdonck-de Leeuw and Mahieu, 2004), lowering of harmonics-to-noise ratio (Ferrand, 2002), decreases in Fo during devoicing (Watson, 1998), and increases in variability of voice onset time (VOT) (Sweeting and Baken, 1982).

The notion that voice deterioration is a given with geriatrics was challenged by Ramig and Ringel (1983), who found that whether or not the voice of an aging person was judged abnormal depended on that person's general physical health. Older subjects in poor physiologic condition had statistically significantly more jitter, shimmer, and spectral noise in their voices than did those in good physical condition. Peppard and Bless (1987) compared the voices of geriatric singers with nonsinger geriatric and young adults. They found that the voices of the geriatric singers did not deteriorate and were more like those of young adults than the voices of their aged-matched peers suggesting vocal exercises may prevent, or at least deter, age-related changes in voice production.

In a subsequent study, Ramig, Gray, Baker, et al. (2001) compared speakers' physiologic condition with listeners' ratings of age according to resting heart rate, systolic blood pressure, diastolic blood pressure, forced vital capacity, and adjusted forced vital capacity. They found no statistically significant relationship between ratings of age and actual chronologic age in patients 25 to 75 years who were in good physiologic condition but did find a statistically significant relationship between age and judgment of voices as poor in patients who were in poor condition. Listeners were more accurate in their ratings of age when judging connected speech in comparison with vowel prolongation. They were, however, more accurate in identifying aged speakers on the basis of vowel prolongation who were in poor physiologic condition in comparison with older speakers who were in good condition. Similarly, Orlikoff (1990) in his study of the relationship of age and cardiovascular health to certain acoustic characteristics of male voices noted that the phonations of atherosclerotic individuals were generally associated with greater short- and long-term variability compared with healthy elderly and that perturbation values were higher in both geriatric groups compared with their younger cohorts. These data seem to support the importance of good general health in the preservation of youthful voice in older age groups.

From these data, it can then be deduced that an older sounding voice is not inevitable as we age; how we sound may be closely tied to the general health and physiologic reserve of the person as well as vocal exercise. What also needs to be studied in greater depth, however, is the effect of psychologic changes on voice in the elderly. Physical and

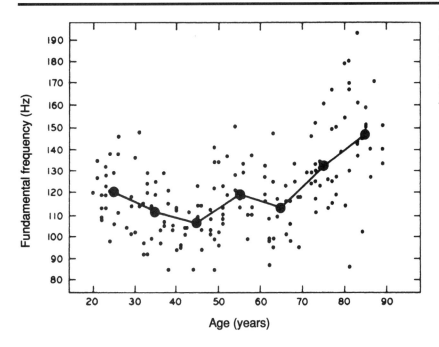

Fig. 2.3 Male fundamental frequency as a function of age. Scatterplot of the mean fundamental frequencies of the speaking voices of 175 subjects. Solid line connects mean values for each age decade. (From Hollien, H., Shipp, T. [1972]. Speaking fundamental frequency and chronologic age in males. J Speech Hear Res 15, 155–159.)

social isolation restricting the amount of daily voice use in the elderly may have deleterious effects on voice.

Fundamental Frequency

It was already noted that Hollien and Shipp (1972) demonstrated a progressive lowering of fundamental frequency in males from early adulthood to the 40- to 50-year age range, but above this range there was a reversal of this downward trend. The saucer-shaped scatterplot of 175 male subjects can be seen in **Fig. 2.3.** The same trend has been demonstrated in a study by Mysak (1959) of 12 males aged 65 to 79 years and 12 males aged 80 to 92 years. He obtained mean impromptu speaking voice fundamental frequencies of 120 Hz for the 65- to 79-year age group and 137 Hz for the 80- to 92-year age group. The males aged 80 to 92 years had statistically significantly higher fundamental frequencies than those in the 65- to 79-year age group. Similarly, in a study by Honjo and Isshiki (1980), the average fundamental frequency of 20 males aged 69 to 85 years was 162 Hz, considerably higher than that for young males (120 to 130 Hz).

Fundamental frequency of the speaking voice as a function of age in females does not follow the same trend as in males. In a group of females aged 65 to 79 years studied by McGlone and Hollien (1963), the average frequency was 196 Hz, and in another group aged 80 to 94 years, 199 Hz was the average. In the study by Kelley (1977), not only did fundamental frequency fail to rise in older-aged females, it declined. In the study by Honjo and Isshiki (1980) of 20 females aged 69 to 85 years, fundamental frequency also showed a failure to increase; it actually decreased from ~260 Hz in young females to an average of 170 Hz in the older age group. The increase in fundamental frequency in males and its failure to increase in females is hypothesized to be related to gender differences in the aging structure.

Frequency Range

A study by Hollien, Dew, and Philips (1971) of 534 subjects (332 males and 202 females) is still one of the most extensive works available on phonational frequency range in adults. The males ranged in age from 16 to 59 years and the females from 18 to 75 years. Subjects had to match voice pitches to series of pure tones downward and upward from a predetermined frequency. **Figure 2.4** shows the frequency ranges for each subject. Individual ranges extended from approximately one octave (13 semitones) to more than 4.5 octaves (55 semitones). Females produced a greater range than males, extending from nearly two frequency ranges for males and females were 38 semitones, and both groups exhibited large standard deviations. From these cross-sectional data, there appeared to be no age-related trend though others have reported it expands during puberty and reduces with old age. These ranges are slightly greater when compared with the studies of fewer subjects done by Ptacek, Sander, Maloney, and Jackson (1966), Hollien and Michel (1968), and Colton (1959). The negative consequence of vocal aging on quality of life is significant according to results of a longitudinal study completed by Verdonck-de Leeuw and Mahieu (2004) and underscores the importance of voice studies.

Developmental Changes Reflected in Other Voice Measures

Measures of fundamental frequency are not the only measures thought to reflect changes related to gender, age, race, native language, general health, and task. Because individual speakers have unique ways of achieving the same phonatory targets, neither Fo nor any other single analysis procedure is sufficient to identify age. Vocal age is effected by vocal use, biological condition, and disease. If we are to identify measures that have

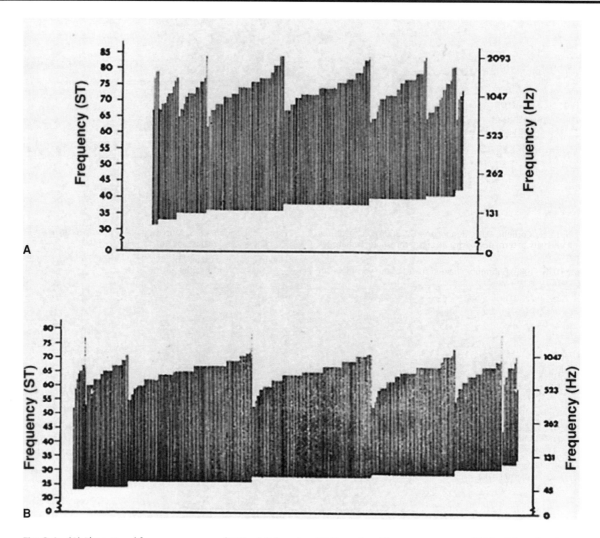

Fig. 2.4 (**A**) Phonational frequency ranges of 202 adult females. (**B**) Phonational frequency ranges of 332 adult males. (From Hollien, H., Dew, D., Philips, P. [1971]. Phonational frequency ranges of adults. J Speech Hear Res 14, 755–760.)

both specificity and sensitive to life-span changes, it is necessary to take these factors into consideration.

Knowledge of the lack of sensitivity and specificity of single vocal measures to age has led to a plethora of multidimensional analyses. As previously stated, acoustic analyses including perturbation values, phonation gaps, intensity, variability of frequency, harmonics-to-noise ratio, and dynamic range are not frequently used in the clinic. Another example, Hwa-Chen (2007, 2008) determined that speakers of tonal language had a greater frequency/intensity profile than did nontonal language speakers though their mean fundamental frequencies were similar. Gorham-Rowan and Laures-Gore (2006) reported significant age-related differences in Fo standard deviation, amplitude perturbation quotient, and noise-to-harmonic ratio. Videostroboscopic images of geriatric speakers also differed from their younger counterparts (Biever and Bless, 1989; Linville (1992, 1995); Bloch and Behrman, 2001) but when singing training was taken into account, they were similar (Peppard and Bless, 1991; Peppard, 1991; Peppard, Bless, and Milenkovic, 1988).

♦ Summary

- ♦ Birth, pain, hunger, and pleasure cries can be differentiated from one another.

- ♦ From birth, the larynx enlarges and descends in the neck, and with these growth changes the fundamental frequency (pitch) of the voice decreases.

- ♦ Male-female fundamental frequency differences are insignificant until puberty, at which time the male voice descends a full octave, whereas the female voice drops three to five semitones.

- ♦ Acoustic signs of puberty occur 3 to 4 months before its onset.

- ♦ Fundamental frequency may not be as specific or sensitive to age-related changes in the voice as other acoustic measures.

♦ In male and female adults, the fundamental frequency of the voice descends throughout life. However, in older age, the fundamental frequency of the male voice begins to ascend, whereas in the female voice it does not.

♦ The vocal folds undergo structural changes during older age, consisting of atrophy, thinning, edema, both quantitative and qualitative changes in the extracellular matrices of the vocal folds, and dehydration of the mucosa covering the vocal folds.

♦ Perceptual studies indicate listeners can identify older subjects by the sound of the voice. However, studies have also shown that the voices of older persons who are in good health are difficult to distinguish from the voices of younger speakers, as are those who participate in singing.

♦ Voice deterioration associated with aging has a significant negative impact on quality of life.

References

Bellieni, C.V., Sisto, R., Cordelli, D.M., Buonocore, G. (2004). Cry features reflect pain intensity in term newborns: an alarm threshold. Pediatr Res 55, 142–146.

Biever, D., Bless, D.M. (1989). Vibratory characteristics of the vocal folds in young adult and geriatric women. J Voice 3, 120–131.

Bloch, I., Behrman, A. (2001). Quantitative analysis of videostroboscopic images in presbylarynges. Laryngoscope 111, 2022–2027.

Bosma, J.F. (1985). Postnatal ontogeny of performance of the pharynx, larynx, and mouth. Am Rev Respir Dis 131, S10–S15.

Bosma, J.F., Lind, J., Truby, H.M. (1964). Respiratory motion patterns of the newborn infant in cry. In Kay, J.L. (Ed.), Physical diagnosis of the newly born (pp. 103–116). Report of the Forty-Sixth Ross Conference on Pediatric Research. Columbus, OH: Ross Laboratories.

Busby, P.A., Plant, G.L. (1995). Format frequency of vowels produced by preadolescent boys and girls. J Acoust Soc Am 97(4), 2603–2606.

Claassen, H., Kirsch, T. (1994). Temporal and spatial localization of type I and II collagens in human thyroid cartilage. Anat Embryol (Berl) 189, 237–242.

Clarici, A., Travan, L., Accardo, A., De Vonderweid, U., Bava, A. (2002). Crying of a newborn child: alarm signal or protocommunication? Percept Mot Skills 95, 752–754.

Colton, R.H. (1959). Some acoustic and perceptual correlates of the modal and falsetto registers. Doctoral dissertation. Gainesville: University of Florida.

Curry, E.T. (1940). The pitch characteristics of the adolescent male voice. Speech Monogr (Research Annual) 7, 48–62.

Curry, E.T. (1949). Hoarseness and voice change in male adolescents. J Speech Hear Disord 14, 23.

Evans, S., Neave, N., Wakelin, D. (2006). Relationships between vocal characteristics and body size and shape in human males: an evolutionary explanation for a deep male voice. Biol Psychol 72, 160–163.

Fairbanks, G., Herbert, E., Hammond, E. (1949). An acoustical study of vocal pitch in seven- and eight-year-old girls. Child Dev 20, 71–74.

Ferrand, C.T. (2002). Harmonics-to-noise ratio: an index of vocal aging. J Voice 16, 480–487.

Ferreri, G. (1959). Senescence of the larynx. Ital Gen Rev Otorhinolaryng 1, 640–709.

Fitch, W.T., Reby, D. (2001). The descended larynx is not uniquely human. Proc Biol Sci 268, 1669–1675.

Fuchs, M., Froehlich, M., Hentschel, B., Stuermer, I.W., Kruse, E., Knauft, D. (2007). Predicting mutational change in the speaking voice of boys. J Voice 21, 169–178.

Gorham-Rowan, M.M., Laures-Gore, J. (2006). Acoustic-perceptual correlates of voice quality in elderly men and women. J Commun Disord 39, 171–184.

Greene, M.C.L. (1972). The voice and its disorders. Philadelphia: J.B. Lippincott Co.

Hanley, J.R. (1951). An analysis of vocal frequency and duration characteristics of selected samples of speech from general American, Eastern American and Southern American dialect regions. Speech Monogr 18, 78–93.

Hartman, D., Danhauer, J. (1976). Perceptual features of speech for males in four perceived age decades. J Acoust Soc Am 59, 713–715.

Hasek, C.S., Sadanand, S., Murry, T. (1980). Acoustic attributes of preadolescent voices. J Acoust Soc Am 68, 1262–1265.

Higgins, M.B., Saxman, J.H. (1991). A comparison of selected phanatory behaviors of healthy aged and young adults. J Sp Hear Res 34, 1000–1010.

Hirano, M., Kurita, S., Nakashima, T. (1983). Growth development and aging of human vocal folds. In D.M. Bless and J.H. Abbs (Eds.), Vocal fold physiology: contemporary research and clnical issues (pp. 22–43). San Diego: College-Hill Press.

Hirano, M., Sato, K. (1993). Histological color atlas of the human larynx. San Diego: Singular Publishing Group.

Hollien, H., Dew, D., Philips, P. (1971). Phonational frequency ranges of adults. J Speech Hear Res 14, 755–760.

Hollien, H., Hollien, P.A., de Jong, G. (1997). Effects of three parameters on speaking fundamental frequency. J Acoust Soc Am 102, 2984–2992.

Hollien, H., Jackson, B. (1973). Normative data on the speaking fundamental frequency characteristics of young adult males. J Phonetics 1, 117–120.

Hollien, H., Malcik, E. (1967). Evaluation of cross-sectional studies of adolescent voice change in males. Speech Monogr 34, 80–84.

Hollien, H., Michel, J. (1968). Vocal fry as a phonational register. J Speech Hear Res 11, 600–604.

Hollien, H., Müller, E. (1973). Perceptual responses to infant crying: identification of cry types. J Child Lang 1, 89–95.

Hollien, H., Shipp, T. (1972). Speaking fundamental frequency and chronologic age in males. J Speech Hear Res 15, 155–159.

Honjo, I., Isshiki, N. (1980). Laryngoscopic and voice characteristics of aged persons. Arch Otolaryngol 106, 149–150.

Hwa-Chen, S. (2008). Voice range profiles for tonal dialect of Min. Folia Phoniatr Logo 60, 4–10.

Hwa-Chen, S. (2007). Sex differences in frequency and intensity in reading and voice range profiles for Taiwanese adult speakers. Folio Phoniatr Logo 59, 1–9.

Jackson, C., Jackson, C.L. (Eds.). (1959). Diseases of the nose, throat and ear. Philadelphia: W.B. Saunders Co.

Kahane, J.C. (1982). Growth of the human prepubertal and pubertal larynx. J Speech Hear Res 25, 446–455.

Kahane, J.C. (1983). A survey of age-related changes in the connective tissue of the human adult larynx. In D. Bless and J.H. Abbs (Eds.), Vocal fold physiology: contemporary research and clinical issues (pp. 44–49). San Diego: College-Hill Press.

Kahane, J.C. (1988). Histologic structure and properties of the human vocal folds. Ear Nose Throat J 67, 322–330.

Kelemen, G., Pressman, J.J. (1955). Physiology of the larynx. Physiol Rev 35, 506–554.

Kelley, A. (1977). Fundamental frequency measurements of female voices from twenty to ninety years of age (unpublished manuscript). Greensboro, NC: University of North Carolina.

Kent, R., Burkhard, R. (1981). Changes in the acoustic correlates of speech production. In D.S. Beasley and G.A. Davis (Eds.), Aging communication processes and disorders. New York: Grune & Stratton, pp. 47–62.

Kent, R.D., Murray, A.D. (1982). Acoustic features of infant vocalic utterances at 3, 6, and 9 months. J Acoust Soc Am 72, 353–365.

Kent, R.D., Vorperian, H.K. (1995). *Development of the craniofacial-oral-laryngeal anatomy: a review.* San Diego: Singular Publishing Group.

LaGasse, L.L., Neal, A.R., Lester, B.M. (2005). Assessment of infant cry: acoustic cry analysis and parental perception. Ment Retard Dev Disabil Res Rev 11, 83–93.

Lewis, M. (1936). *Infant speech, a study of the beginnings of language.* New York: Harcourt Brace.

Lieberman, D.E., McCarthy, R.C., Hiiemae, K.M., Palmer, J.B. (2001). Ontogeny of postnatal hyoid and larynx descent in humans. Arch Oral Biol 46, 117–128.

Lieberman, P. (1967). *Intonation, perception, and language.* Cambridge, MA: M.I.T. Press.

Lieberman, P., Harris, K.S., Wolff, P., Russell, L.H. (1971). Newborn infant cry and nonhuman primate vocalization. J Speech Hear Res 1, 718–727.

Linville, S.E. (1992). Glottal gap configurations in two age groups of women. J Sp Hear Res 35, 1209–1215.

Linville, S.E. (1995). Vocal aging. Cur Op Oto Head Neck Surg 3, 183–187.

Majewski, W., Hollien, H., Zalewski, W. (1972). Speaking fundamental frequency of Polish adult males. Phonetica 25, 119–125.

McGlone, R., Hollien, H. (1963). Vocal pitch characteristics of aged women. J Speech Hear Res 6, 164–170.

McGlone, R.E., McGlone, J. (1972). Speaking fundamental frequency of eight-year-old girls. Folia Phoniatr (Basel) 24, 313–317.

McNair, C., Ballantyne, M., Dionne, K., Stephens, D., Stevens, B. (2004). Postoperative pain assessment in the neonatal intensive care unit. Arch Dis Child Fetal Neonatal Ed 89, 537–541.

Menard, L., Schwartz, I.L., Boe, L.I. (2004). Role of vocal tract morphology in speech development: perceptual targets and sensorimotor maps for synthesized French vowels from birth to adulthood. J Speech Lang Hear Res 47, 1059–1080.

Meyerson, M.D. (1976). The effects of aging on communication. J Gerontol 31, 29–68.

Michel, J., Hollien, H., Moore, P. (1966). Speaking fundamental frequency characteristics of 15-, 16-, and 17-year-old girls. Lang Speech 9, 40.

Michelsson, K., Eklund, K., Leppanen, P., Lyytinen, H. (2002). Cry characteristics of 172 healthy 1- to 7-day-old infants. Folia Phoniatr Logop 54, 190–200.

Morrison, M.D., Gore-Hickman, T. (1986). Voice disorders in the elderly. J Otolaryngol 15, 231–234.

Mueller, P.B. (1997). The aging voice. Semin Speech Lang 18, 159–168.

Mysak, E.D. (1959). Pitch and duration characteristics of older males. J Speech Hear Res 2, 46–54.

Naufel de Felippe, A.C., Grillo, M.H., Grechi, T.H. (2006). Standardization of acoustic measures of normal voice patterns. Rev Bras Otorrinolaringol (Engl Ed) 72, 659–664.

Nishimura, T., Mikami, A., Suzuki, J., Matsuzawa, T. (2005). Descent of the larynx in chimpanzee infants. Proc Natl Acad Sci U S A 102, 6930–6933.

Orlikoff, R.F. (1990). The relationship of age and cardiovascular health to certain acoustic characteristics of male voices. J Speech Hear Res 33, 450–457.

Ostwald, P.F., Phibbs, R., Fox, S. (1968). Diagnostic use of infant cry. Biol Neonat 13, 68–82.

Peppard, R.C., Bless, D.M. (1991). Effects of aging on acoustic characteristics of singers and nonsingers. *ASHA* 33, 214.

Peppard, R.C. (1991). Vocal function in singers and nonsingers. A dissertation in partial fulfillment of the doctoral degree at the University of Wisconsin-Madison.

Peppard, R.C., Bless, D.M., Milenkovic, P. (1988). Comparison of young adult singers and nonsingers with vocal nodules. *J Voice*, 2, 250–260.

Philhour, C.W. (1948). An experimental study of the relationships between perception of vocal pitch in connected speech and certain measures of vocal frequency. Doctoral dissertation. Iowa City: University of Iowa.

Pronovost, W. (1942). An experimental study of methods for determining natural and habitual pitch. Speech Monogr 9, 111–123.

Ptacek, P.H., Sander, E.K. (1966). Age recognition from voice. J Speech Hear Res 9, 273–277.

Ptacek, P., Sander, E., Maloney, W., Jackson, C. (1966). Phonatory and related changes with advanced age. J Speech Hear Res 9, 353–360.

Ramig L,A., Ringel R.L. (1983). Effects of physiological aging on selected acoustic characteristics of voice. J Speech Hear Res 26, 22–50.

Ramig, L.O., Gray, S.D., Baker, K., Corbin-Lewis, K., Buder, E., Luschei, E., Coon, H., Smith, M. (2001). The aging voice: a review, treatment data and familial and genetic perspectives. Folia Phoniatr Logop 53, 252–265.

Ringel, R.L., Kluppel, D.D. (1964). Neonatal crying: A normative study. Folia Phoniatr (Basel) 16, 1–9.

Robb, M.P. (2003). Bifurcations and chaos in the cries of full-term and preterm infants. Folia Phoniatr Logop 55, 233–240.

Ryan, E.B., Capadano, H.L. III. (1978). Age perceptions and evaluative reactions toward adult speakers. J Gerontol 33, 98–102.

Ryan, W.J., Burk, K.W. (1974). Perceptual and acoustic correlates of aging in speech of males. J Commun Disord 7, 181–192.

Sato, K., Hirano, M., Nakashima, T. (2002). Age-related changes of collagenous fibers in the human vocal fold mucosa. Ann Otol Rhinol Laryngol 111, 15–20.

Sato, K., Kurita, S., Hirano, M., Kiyokawa, K. (1990). Distribution of elastic cartilage in the arytenoids and its physiologic significance. Ann Otol Rhinol Laryngol 99, 363–368.

Saxman, J.H., Burk, K.W. (1967). Speaking fundamental frequency characteristics of middle-aged females. Folia Phoniatr (Basel) 19, 167–172.

Shipp, T., Hollien, H. (1969). Perception of the aging male voice. J Speech Hear Res 12, 703–710.

Smith, M.E., Gray, S.D. (2002). Developmental laryngeal and phonatory anatomy and physiology. Perspect Voice Voice Disord 12, 47.

Soltis, J. (2004). The signal functions of early infant crying. Behav Brain Sci 27, 443–490.

Spence, K., Gillies, D., Harrison, D., Johnston, L., Nagy, S. (2005). A reliable pain assessment tool for clinical assessment in the neonatal intensive care unit. J Obstet Gynecol Neonatal Nurs 34, 80–86.

Stathopoulos, E.T. (2002). Consideration of children's voices: understanding age-related processes. Perspect Voice Voice Disord 12, 810.

Stathopoulos, E.T., Sapienza, C.M. (1997). Developmental change in laryngeal and respiratory function with variations in sound pressure level. J Speech Lang Hear Res 40, 595–614.

Sweeting, P.M., Baken, R.J. (1982). Voice onset time in normal-aged population. J Speech Hear Res 25, 129–134.

Thiery, M., Yo Le Sian, A., Vrijens, M., Janssens, D. (1973). Vagitus uterinus. J Obstet Gynaecol Br Commonw 80, 183–185.

Tucker, J.A., Tucker, G.F. (1979). A clinical perspective on the development and anatomical aspects of the infant larynx and trachea. In G.B. Healy and T.J.I. McGill (Eds.), Laryngo-tracheal problems in the pediatric patient (pp. 3–8). Springfield, IL: Charles C. Thomas.

Van Oordt, H.W.A., Drost, H.A. (1963). Development of the frequency range of the voice in children. Folia Phoniatr (Basel) 15, 289–298.

Verdonck-de Leeuw, I.M., Mahieu, H.F. (2004). Vocal aging and the impact on daily life: a longitudinal study. J Voice 18, 193–202.

Verhulst, J. (1987). Development of the larynx from birth to puberty. Rev Laryngol Otol Rhinol (Bord) 108, 269–270.

Wang, L.P., Gao, Y., Yang, J., Wang, J. (2006). Relationship between laryngeal morphology and voice changes in old people. Zhonghua Er Bi Yan Hou Tou Jing Wai Ke Za Zhi 41, 657–660.

Wasz-Höckert, O., Lind, J., Vuorenkoski, V., Partenen, T., Valanne, E. (1968). *The infant cry.* London: William Heinemann Medical Books.

Watson, B.C. (1998). Fundamental frequency during phonetically governed devoicing in normal young and aged speakers. J Acoust Soc Am 103, 3642–3647.

Wermke, K., Mende, W., Manfredi, C., Bruscaglioni, P. (2002). Developmental aspects of infant's cry melody and formants. Med Eng Phys 24, 501–514.

Whiteside, S.P. (2001). Sex-specific fundamental and formant frequency patterns in a cross-sectional study. J Acoust Soc Am 11, 464–476.

Whiteside, S.P., Hodgson, C. (2000). Some acoustic characteristics in the voices of 6-to 10-year-old children and adults: a comparative sex and developmental perspective. Logoped Phoniatr Vocol 25, 122–132.

Whiteside, S.P., Hodgson, C., Tapster, C. (2002). Vocal characteristics in preadolescent and adolescent children: a longitudinal study. Logoped Phoniatr Vocol 27, 12–20.

Winkler, R., Sendlmeier, W. (2006). EGG open quotient in aging voices—changes with increasing chronological age and its perception. Logoped Phoniatr Vocol 31, 51–56.

Woisard, V., Percodani, J., Serrano, E., Pessey, J.J. (1996). The voice of the child, morphological evolution of the larynx and its acoustic consequences in French. Rev Laryngol Otol Rhinol (Bord) 117, 313–317.

Xue, S.A., Hao, J.G. (2006). Normative standards for vocaltract dimensions by race as measured by acoustic pharyngometry. J Voice 20, 391–400.

Young, G., Décarie, T.G. (1977). An ethology-based catalogue of facial /vocal behavior in infancy. Anim Behav 25, 95–107.

Additional Reading

Ferreri, G. (1959). Senescence of the larynx. Ital Gen Rev Otorhinolaryng 1, 640–709.

Hollien, H., Hollien, P.A., de Jong, G. (1997). Effects of three parameters on speaking fundamental frequency. J Acoust Soc Am 102, 2984–2992. (This well-written article is instructive about issues related to obtaining fundamental frequency measures.)

Kent, R.D., Vorperian, H.K. (1995). *Development of the craniofacial-oral-laryngeal anatomy.* San Diego: Singular Publishing. (This book is a must-read for students wishing to read a superb summary of human growth patterns impacting voice from birth to adulthood.)

Nishimura, T. (2003). Comparative morphology of the hyo-laryngeal complex in anthropoids: two steps in the evolution of the descent of the larynx. Primates 44, 41–49.

Nishimura, T., Mikami, A., Suzuki, J., Matsuzawa, T. (2003). Descent of the larynx in chimpanzee infants. Proc Natl Acad Sci U S A 100, 6930–6933. (The two preceding articles explain the descent of the hyoid and its importance to voice and swallow functions.)

Lind, J., (Ed.). (1965). Newborn infant cry. Acta Paediatr Scand 163(Suppl.), 1–128. (A collection of four excellent articles on cry sounds and cry motions in normal infants and in those who have craniofacial anomalies.)

Menard, L., Schwartz, J.L., Boe, L.J. (2004). Role of vocal tract morphology in speech development: perceptual targets and sensorimotor maps for synthesized French vowels from birth to adulthood. J Speech Lang Hear Res 47, 109–180. (Students completing this reading will improve their understanding of how the development of speech/voice from infancy to adulthood results from the interaction of neurocognitive, physical, and motor control abilities.)

Ramig, L.O. (1986). Aging speech: physiological and sociological aspects. Lang Commun 6, 25–34; Folia Phoniatr Logop 2001;53:252–265. (A comprehensive and classic reading on aging.)

Sato, K., Hirano, M., Nakashima, T. (2002). Age-related changes of collagenous fibers in the human vocal fold mucosa. Ann Otol Rhinol Laryngol 111, 15–20.

Sato, K., Kurita, S., Hirano, M., Kiyokawa, K. (1990). Distribution of elastic cartilage in the arytenoids and its physiologic significance. Ann Otol Rhinol Laryngol 99, 363–368. (The two preceding articles describe the age-related changes in the histoarchitecture and cartilaginous framework.)

Wilson, K. (1979). *Voice problems of children.* Baltimore: Williams & Wilkins Co. (See pp. 71–74 for an excellent review of the literature on fundamental frequency characteristics of school-age children.)

Young, G., Décarie, T.G. (1977). An ethology-based catalogue of facial/vocal behavior in infancy. Anim Behav 25, 95–107. (This unusual article will broaden the student's horizons, showing how voice is linked with emotional response and facial expression as early as infancy, suggesting that intonation later in life has reflex, inborn roots.)

Chapter 3

Voice Disorders of Structural Origin

♦ Voice Disorders Due to Structural Changes in Childhood

Structural changes of the vocal folds at any age produce one or more of the following pathologic changes:

♦ increase or decrease the mass or bulk of the vocal folds or immediately surrounding tissues

♦ alter their shape

♦ restrict their mobility

♦ change their tension

♦ modify the size or shape, or both, of the glottic, supraglottic, or infraglottic airway

♦ prevent the vocal folds from approximating partially or completely along the vibratory edge

♦ result in excessive tightness or irregularity of approximation

♦ result in irregular chaotic vibration

Laryngeal problems of a structural nature may be either congenital or acquired. In either case, they result in a disorder of pitch, loudness, or quality. One of the most unusual and rare structural voice disorders that affects pitch, loudness, and quality is that of cri du chat, or cat cry.

Cri du Chat

Infants who are ill or who have structural differences in the larynx cry differently from normal infants, and although certain types of cries are associated with specific illnesses in the newborn, nonspecific distress cries are often produced at higher than normal fundamental frequency (Mallard and Daniloff, 1973).

The syndrome of cri du chat in neonates and children was so named because the voice has a distinctive, high-pitched, plaintive wail resembling the cry of a cat, which is immediately recognizable as different from other infants. For example, the attendants in a newborn nursery had nicknamed a child "kitten" because of her weak, high-pitched mewing cry (Ward, Engel, and Nance, 1968). Similarly, a telephone repairman, not seeing the crying child, remarked to the foster mother that she had "an awfully angry cat" (Dumars, Gaskill, and Kitzmiller, 1964). This voice signature of the syndrome is a prime example of the diagnostic usefulness of voice. Three cases of cri du chat were first reported by Lejeune et al. (1963), a professor of genetics at the University of Paris. More recently, Mainardi, Pastore, Castronovo, et al. (2006) reported on the genetic characteristics of 220 patients diagnosed with cri-du-chat syndrome, which is a contiguous gene syndrome that results from a deletion of the short arm of chromosome 5 (5p) as illustrated in **Fig. 3.1.** Molecular-cytogenetic investigation (flourescent in-situ hybridization, FISH) showed a variety of aberrations including interstitial deletions, short terminal deletions, and other rare rearrangements of 5p. Cytogenetic and clinical variability in this population are the rule rather than the exception. The cat-like cry and peculiar timbre of voice were the most typical signs of the syndrome, not only at birth but also later, and these were the only signs that suggested the diagnosis in patients with small deletions and a mild clinical picture. The unusual voice, however, was only one of many genetic defects associated with this rare syndrome. In addition to abnormal laryngeal development, sucking and feeding difficulties, and respiratory infections, the syndrome presents with micrognathia, a bird- or beak-like profile, microcephaly, hypotonia, hypertelorism, downward-slanting palpebral fissures, developmental disabilities, low-set ears, strabismus, midline oral clefts, and failure to thrive. Cardiac, cerebral, renal, and gastrointestinal malformations were more frequent in the patients with unbalanced translocations resulting in 5p deletions. Mainardi and colleagues also reported intubation difficulties linked to larynx anomalies and delayed psychomotor

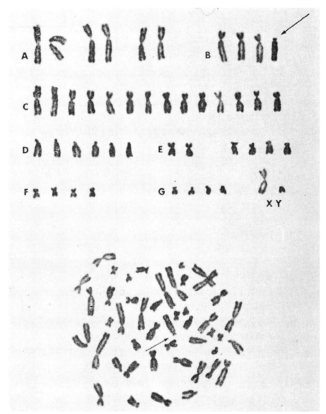

Figure 3.1   Defective B-group chromosome in patient with cri-du-chat syndrome. *Arrows* show the partial short-arm deletion of a B-group chromosome. (From Ward, P.H., Enel, E., Nance, W.E. [1968]. The larynx in the cri du chat [cat cry] syndrome. Am Acad Ophthalmol 72, 90–102.)

development related in severity to deletion size and type as well as other genetic and environmental factors. The distinctive voice characteristics resulting from the structurally small larynx and resonance chambers and the neurologic differences follow:

♦ overall fundamental frequency invariably higher (X = 860 Hz) than for pain (X = 530 Hz) and hunger (X = 500 Hz) cries of normal infants

♦ cry durations characteristically longer than normal (X = 2.6 seconds) and similar to normal pain cries

♦ flat or rising melody patterns

♦ strained quality rarely containing glottal plosives

♦ crying on inhalation with inhalatory stridor (rare in normal infants). Noteworthy is the observation that listeners had difficulty in determining whether the cry at a particular moment was occurring on inhalation or on exhalation, with the inhalatory-exhalatory cry signals failing to demonstrate the normal "on-off" phenomenon.

Congenital Laryngeal Stridor

Stridor means involuntary sound made during inhalation or exhalation. Stridor can occur from any laryngeal disease (not just laryngomalacia) that produces partial obstruction of the airway either subglottally, glottally, or supraglottally. Although obstruction can occur at any age, detection of stridor is especially critical in the newborn because it signals impending asphyxiation. Abnormal anatomic development, laryngeal masses, inflammation, and paralysis are its most common causes. Different-sounding types of stridor Rohde, M. and Banner, J. (2006). Respiratory tract malacia: possible cause of sudden death in infancy and early childhood. Acta Paediatrica 95: 867–870.

Laryngomalacia

In laryngomalacia, the laryngeal cartilages are soft and underdeveloped. Morphologically, cartilage rings are shorter and softer than normal, causing collapse, especially during forced expirations. The etiology of laryngomalacia is uncertain. The voices on exhalation, during crying, and during other types of phonation may sound normal, but on forced exhalation and inhalation there is a low-pitched vibratory fluttering or a high-pitched crowing, more often intermittent than constant. Other symptoms may include wheezing, barking cough, frequent respiratory infections, and cyanotic episodes (Rohde and Banner, 2006). The stridor is more common when the infant is supine than prone. It often goes unnoticed at birth but becomes apparent a few weeks after discharge from the hospital.

Following is the physical appearance of the larynx in laryngomalacia on examination:

♦ The epiglottis is low and narrow and has curled edges (omega-shaped).

♦ The aryepiglottic folds are approximated, obscuring the glottis; sucked into the glottis on inhalation; and blown out on exhalation.

♦ The mucosa over the arytenoid cartilages appears redundant.

All these features, it should be pointed out, can be found in the normal infant larynx, the difference between the normal larynx and laryngomalacia being one of degree. Prognosis for the disappearance of laryngomalacia within a few months to 1 year is good. Nevertheless, Rohde and Banner have cautioned, "Laryngo-tracheo-bronchomalacia (LTBM)...may be an unrecognized cause of sudden death in infancy and early childhood, and should be considered, especially in cases where there is a history of respiratory distress."

Congenital Subglottic Stenosis

Arrested embryonic development of the conus elasticus or maldevelopment of the cricoid cartilage will produce an obstructive narrowing of the airway from the level of the vocal folds down to the cricoid area, the point of maximum obstruction being 2 to 3 mm below the glottis. The voice will be stridorous from birth, but sometimes this will be noted only during respiratory infections. The voice during crying is usually normal (Ferguson, 1970).

Although the cause of the arrested development is unknown, Tateya, Tateya, Surles et al. (2006) have presented some intriguing data on malformed tracheal and laryngeal cartilages in vitamin A–deficient rats. In rats, they have shown that pups of a vitamin A–deficient mother have maldevelopment of the cricoid cartilage among other laryngeal deformities such as laryngotracheal clefts.

Laryngotracheal Cleft

Embryonic failure of fusion of the dorsal cricoid lamina leaves an interarytenoid cleft and an open larynx posteriorly. Few cases have been described, and correct identification of the defect is reportedly difficult. The cry is weak, feeble, or aphonic. Feeding difficulties and survival initially overshadow the voice disorder.

Congenital Laryngeal Web

A web of tissue covering part or all of the glottis may be present at birth because of its failure to separate during the 10th week of embryonic laryngeal development. Infants may present with various types of laryngeal webs congenitally, secondary to infection, or traumatically from intubation (Liu, Luo, Zhong, et al. 2006). The distinction is important because of the association of congenital webs with velocardiofacial syndrome (chromosome 22q11.2 deletion). Miyamoto, Cotton, Rope, et al. (2004) reported that 11 of their 17 patients with anterior glottic webs, or 65%, were positive for chromosome 22q11.2 deletion. Of these 11 patients, 5 showed subtle clinical manifestations of velocardiofacial syndrome and underwent genetic testing due only to the presence of a web. All 11 patients were diagnosed with velocardiofacial syndrome.

The extent and severity of webs vary widely. If the web is complete, asphyxiation and death are imminent unless the web is recognized and surgically divided. **Figure 3.2** shows an extensive laryngeal web, but the configuration varies;

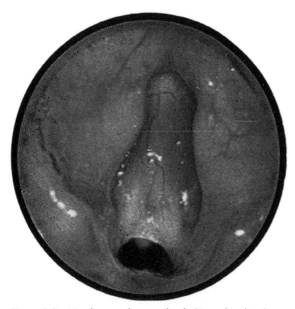

Figure 3.2   Membranous laryngeal web. (See color plate.)

some are concave posteriorly (illustrated), others are thick, and still others are so thin and transparent that vocal fold movement can be seen underneath. A small microweb near the anterior commissure may go unrecognized for years. Microwebs have been implicated as an etiologic factor in vocal nodules resistant to behavioral management (Bouchayer and Cornut, 2000). These authors suggest that in shortening the vibratory length of the vocal folds, the microweb results in greater impact stress in the midmembranous portion of the vocal fold thus making the speaker more vulnerable to vocal fold trauma. Approximately 75% of laryngeal webs occur at the level of the vocal folds, the remainder being equally distributed in the supraglottic and infraglottic larynx. The voices of infants and children who have laryngeal webs vary depending upon the location and extent of the latter. When the web is sufficient to impinge on vibration, the cry and the speaking voice are abnormal, ranging from hoarseness to aphonia. During quiet breathing, inhalatory stridor will be heard in cases of near-glottal occlusion. With lesser webs, stridor and breath impairment may be limited to periods when the child engages in vigorous physical activity.

Because webs are associated with a broad spectrum of symptoms, they require an equally broad spectrum of treatment ranging from observation alone to complex open airway surgery (Milczuk, 2000). Most critical in management decision-making is to ensure a safe airway while maximizing conservation of respiratory, phonatory, and swallowing abilities.

Congenital Cysts and Sulcus Vocalis

Sessile, nonpedunculated, fluid-filled cysts can arise from any of the laryngeal soft tissues; however, they almost always arise from the laryngeal ventricle, displacing the true and false vocal folds and causing glottic and supraglottic obstruction. The voice or cry will be feeble or aphonic but differentially diagnostic from other obstructions. These lesions are potentially remediable. Often, they are not noticed until the child develops speech. Bouchayer and Cornut (2000) have suggested that congenital cysts may rupture and leave longitudinal scars or pits (vocal sulci) or mucosal bridges that disrupt the propagation of the mucosal wave resulting in a dysphonia difficult to remediate through either surgery or behavioral management.

Papilloma

Laryngeal papillomas are common, benign neoplasms in children, have a tendency to recur despite repeated surgical removal, and inevitably produce an abnormal voice. Conventional wisdom suggests they often regress with age, disappearing during puberty, but in a description of the clinical course of 95 patients with recurrent respiratory papilloma (RRP) Maknke, Frohlich, Lippit, et al. (1996) state that puberty had no effect on the clinical course. The etiology is unknown but thought to be viral caused by the human papilloma virus (HPV) group. Different types of HPV, particularly types 6 and 11, have been implicated, which may explain differential response to treatment (Rahiknen, Aaltonen, Syrajanen, 1993). Morphologically, papillomas are tumor-like, frond-shaped

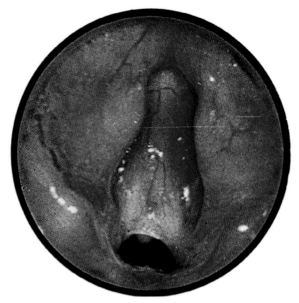

Figure 3.2   Membranous laryngeal web.

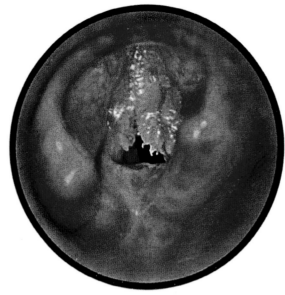

Figure 3.3   Papilloma of the larynx.

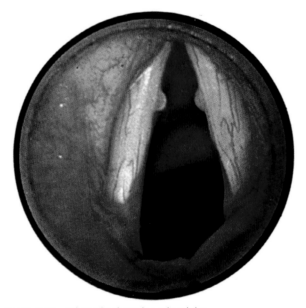

Figure 3.4a   Bilateral polypoid vocal nodules.

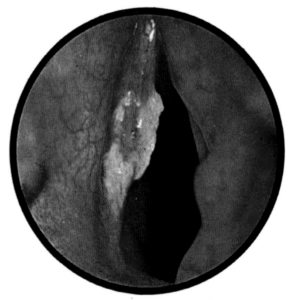

Figure 3.6   Carcinoma of the larynx.

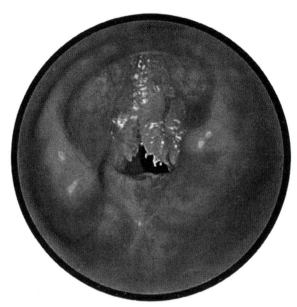

Figure 3.3 Papilloma of the larynx. (See color plate.)

proliferations of squamous cell epithelia, are exophytic, and may have a cauliflower or raspberry appearance (**Fig. 3.3**). These growths frequently extend to include the laryngeal ventricles as well as the true vocal folds. When the lesions are soft, the vocal folds remain mobile though the mucosal wave is likely to be impaired resulting in the dysphonic voice. Lesions may spread to the supraglottic and subglottic regions and even into the trachea and bronchi. If untreated, they can produce asphyxiation and death (Sone and Sato, 2006). Moreover, Mahnke, Frohlich, Lippert, et al. (1996) observed that 4 of 95 RRP patients exhibited malignancy degeneration.

Voice signs and symptoms are severe hoarseness, abnormal cry, abnormal pith, weak loudness, aphonia, and/or wheezy respiratory stridor.

The RRP lesions may be present at birth but are most often detected between the first and eighth years of life, with the most common identification occurring between ages 4 and 6 years when the child has sufficient speech and physical activities that the signs and symptoms are exacerbated.

Because of the recurring nature of this virus, treatment is difficult, and to date no single treatment has emerged as a reliable solution. Rosen and his colleagues have reported on a series of surgical and adjunct medical treatments for papillomatosis (Bryson Rosen, and Osborne, 2002; Rosen and Bryson, 2004; Lee and Rosen, 2004). They reported that whereas surgery debulks the tumors, juvenile laryngeal papilloma is resistant to cure; the growth generally recurs, which may require multiple surgeries and lead to proliferation of scarring and or webs. Holland, Koufman, Postma, et al. (2002) have proposed that prophylactic treatment of laryngoesophageal reflux may reduce the laryngeal soft tissue complications encountered in surgery for RRP patients. Nevertheless, tracheostomy may be required as a temporary measure to preserve the airway and, because of this respiratory restriction occurring in the young child, delayed speech

and expressive language development can be one of its sequelae. Adjunctive medical treatments, directed at controlling the virus and growth of the tumor including cidofovir, indole-3-carbinol (13-C), interferon, photodynamic therapy, and vaccines hold considerable promise. Rosen and colleagues have demonstrated some success with both 13-C and cidofovir but suggest further study regarding long-term follow-up, side effects, and efficacy in pediatric patients. According to Zietels (Akst, Broadhurst, Burns, et al., 2007), phonomicrosurgical microflap resection techniques can eradicate adult glottal RRP and appear to be preferable to conventional debulking or ablation techniques. Whether or not similar success occurs in children is unknown.

Inflammation

An extensive group of inflammatory reactions of the vocal folds and surrounding tissues can cause aphonia or dysphonia.

Acute Laryngitis

Hoarseness, cough, and sore throats are common signs of acute laryngitis caused by viruses, bacteria, or chemical irritants. Pharyngeal and laryngeal erythema are found on examination. When the inflammatory process is sufficient to cause increased stiffness, the vocal folds do not vibrate well resulting in aphonia or dysphonia of a few days' duration. Laryngitis lasting longer than 10 to 14 days is not normal and needs medical attention.

Croup

Several inflammatory laryngeal conditions produce a triad of hoarseness, barking cough, and inhalatory stridor called *croup*. Acute laryngotracheobronchitis, also known as viral croup, is the most common form. Acute epiglottitis, which has a similar triad of signs, occurs abruptly and is most often caused by *Haemophilus influenzae*. Diphtheritic croup, although now rare, is still another type. Each of these can progress to respiratory obstruction and death unless an adequate airway is maintained.

In contrast with those with acute laryngitis, croup patients have systemic malaise in addition to dysphonia and stridor. Acute laryngotracheobronchitis, epiglottitis, and diphtheria all cause fever and dysphagia. In diphtheria, the initial respiratory and phonatory difficulties are caused by the appearance of a thick, adherent necrotic membrane. Patients who survive this stage often develop a toxic neurologic syndrome of vocal fold and soft palate paralysis due to vagus nerve involvement. Even if the glottic obstruction is overcome, the paralysis can extend to the respiratory musculature, requiring ventilatory support to avoid a fatal outcome.

Malnutrition

The cries of malnourished infants strongly resemble those of infants with central nervous system disease (see Chapter 9) according to Lester (1976), who described the cries of 12 malnourished infants to be of high pitch, low intensity, and excessively long duration, with an abnormally long latency between the first and second cry.

Down Syndrome

Down syndrome is one of the most frequently occurring chromosomal disorders (Moura, Cunha, Vilarinho, et al. 2006). The cry of infants with Down syndrome has a flat melody, lower than normal pitch, and a tense or strident, harsh, rough, pressed, howling, and guttural quality. The tenseness or stridency has been attributed to hyperadduction of the ventricular as well as true vocal folds during phonation (Novák, 1972; Wasz-Höckert, Lind, Vuorenkoski, et al. 1968).

The majority of descriptions of the vocal characteristics of individuals with Down syndrome have come from perceptual and acoustic studies. Limited information has been reported from visualization of the larynx or vocal tract shape necessitating that inferences be made about the etiology of the vocal differences. In their study of 66 children with Down syndrome, Moura et al. (2008) noted the phenotypic characteristics of Down syndrome children include general hypotonia and maxillary hypoplasia with relative macroglossia and that these contribute to particular acoustic alterations, which they identified as a lower fundamental frequency, F(0), with elevated dispersion. The conjunction of frequencies for formants, F(1) and F(2), revealed a decreased distinction between the vowels, reflecting the loss of articulatory processing. Pentz (1987) also reported that the speakers with Down syndrome had formant amplitude intensity levels that were significantly lower than those of a similar group of nonretarded speakers. Interestingly, an earlier study done by Moran (1986) comparing perceptual and acoustic characteristics of adults with Down syndrome to adults without developmental disabilities revealed that listeners perceived hypernasality as one of the distinctive characteristics, but when voices were quantified, there was no significant difference in formant frequencies or acoustic indications of resonance differences.

The acoustic features that repeatedly have been reported as significantly different are frequency perturbation measures and spectral noise-to-harmonic component ratios (Beckman, Wold, and Montague, 1983; Moran and Gilbert, 1983; Pentz and Gilbert, 1982). Pentz and Gilbert also reported that there were significant correlations between judges' severity ratings and frequency perturbation levels, amplitude perturbation levels, and the spectral noise-to-harmonic component ratios. It is likely that the vocal tract shape differences (Beckman et al, 1983; Moura et al, 2006) coupled with motor control problems and differences in sidewall reflections from general hypotonia contribute to these distinguishing characteristic voice patterns.

With few exceptions, the majority of voice data come from studies of children over 8 years of age and adults. Studies of premeaningful vocalizations produced by normally developing infants and infants with Down syndrome by Smith and Oller (1981) demonstrate that both groups began to produce canonical, reduplicated babbling at 8 to 8½ months of age, and trends regarding consonantal and vocalic development for the two groups were very similar during approximately the first 15 months of life: a time when one could argue that hypotonia of the two groups might be more similar than in later life.

Trauma

The larynges of neonates and infants are susceptible to external and internal trauma of the blunt and penetration variety, as well as that caused by caustic substances inhaled or ingested.

◆ Voice Disorders Due to Structural Changes in Adulthood

Chronic Nonspecific Laryngitis

Dysphonia, vocal fatigue, and cough are produced by chronic laryngitis consisting of vasodilation and edema of the vocal folds. Persistent epithelial tissue changes occur in which the mucosal glands atrophy. The resulting dryness of the mucosa is called laryngitis sicca. Laryngologists believe that cigarette smoking, air pollution, alcohol, and vocal abuse are contributory factors.

Sjögren's Syndrome

Dryness of the larynx may also result from Sjögren's syndrome (Ogut, Midillik, Oder, et al. 2005). Sjögren's syndrome is an autoimmune disease affecting 4 million Americans, most commonly women in their late forties (Sjögren's Syndrome Foundation, Inc., 2007). Dry eyes, dry mouth, and dryness in other organs such as the larynx, lungs, and CNS result from the body's immune system attacking its own moisture-producing glands. The appearance of the larynx of women with Sjögren's syndrome can range from vocal folds that lack luster to vocal folds covered with a thick, tenacious, dry covering of mucus. The impact of a dry larynx on voice can be severe because it inhibits regular vocal fold vibration, decreases vocal efficiency, requiring the speaker to increase effort, which may account for the increase in vocal pathologies in this population. As example, Ogut and colleagues reported significant changes in the Reflux Finding Score (RFS) and the Reflux Symptom Index (RSI), the objective voice quality using Jitter (JITT), Pitch Period Perturbation Quotient (PPQ), Shimmer (Shim), Amplitude Perturbation Quotient (APQ), and Noise-to-Harmonic Ratio (NHR), and the presence of a variety of laryngeal pathologies in this population.

Chronic Hypertrophic Laryngitis

Hypertrophy of the laryngeal mucosa is a common result of excess smoking and alcohol. Leukoplakia, a thickening of the epithelial and subepithelial layer, is characterized by the appearance of white patches on the vocal folds, which can be premalignant. Simple chronic laryngitis is manifested by hoarseness, an urge to clear the throat, diffusely red or pink mucosa, rounded rather than sharp vocal fold margins, and strands of mucus bridging the glottis from one vocal fold to the other. Submucosal edema eventually destroys the histoarchitecture of the basement membrane separating the epithelium from the underlying structure. The superficial layer of the lamina propria, normally a somewhat amorphous space, becomes engorged with fluid; this change is called polypoid degeneration, or Reinke's edema.

Reinke's edema is often difficult to differentiate from other benign lesions arising from the superficial layer of the lamina propria because these so-called mass lesions all exhibit fluid accumulation in Reinke's space and are believed to originate from excess internal (smoking, alcohol, reflux) or external (vocal abuse or misuse) trauma.

Current measures of phenotypic expression do not always differentiate pathologies arising from the superficial layer of the lamina propria. This makes accurate diagnosis difficult and may contribute to why some patients with the "same pathology" respond differently to the same treatment. Because phenotypic markers typically used in the clinic are insufficient to differentiate disorders of the lamina propria, Gray and Thibeault have suggested using genotypic analyses.

The rationale for genetic analyses is that genetic information is used by the cells to make proteins. These proteins are then used to perform cellular and tissue functions. These cellular and tissue functions, in turn, determine the structure and its biomechanical properties. Gene expression studies of vocal lesions such as those done by Gray and Thibeault underscore the nature of its importance in increasing our understanding of vocal fold dynamics and how it is affected by the disease. They have also demonstrated in several small studies the role of microarray analysis to find genes of interest and that it is of paramount importance to increasing our understanding of the vocal fold and its diseases. The use of DNA microarray technology analysis of global patterns of gene expression can reveal unexpected networks of coordinated regulation in the extra cellular matrix (ECM) of the lamina propria. Thibeault, Hirschi, and Gray (2003) demonstrated the feasibility of using DNA microarray technology to establish transcriptional gene expression patterns for vocal fold polyp and vocal fold granulomas. Although in their initial report they only had one of each pathology to compare with one normal, they identified different gene expression in these tissues representing inflammation and wound healing.

It is well known that gene expression may be influenced by various environmental factors. This interaction between environment and genes is constantly manifested in vocal characteristics and disorders. Thus, Duflo, Thibeault, Li, et al (2006) used complementary DNA (cDNA) microarray analysis to establish distinct gene expression profiles for Reinke's edema and polyps, two phenotypically similar vocal fold lesions. They analyzed 11 Reinke's edema and 17 polyp specimens with microarray analysis for 8745 genes and further microarray analysis profiling within groups to identify molecular markers for reflux exposure and smoking. Sixty-five genes were found to differentiate Reinke's edema and polyps. In Reinke's edema, 19 genes differentiated for reflux exposure, but no genes were found to differentiate smokers

from nonsmokers. For polyps, no genes were found to differentiate for reflux or smoking. Categorization of unclassified lesions was possible with a minimum of 13 genes demonstrating not only the feasibility of benign lesion classification based on microarray analysis but also its usefulness for improving diagnosis potentially generating prognostic indicators and targets for therapy.

Thibeault, Gray, Li, et al. (2002) related gene expression in benign vocal lesions to phenotypic marker of stiffness determined from perceptual judgments of stroboscopic images. They determined there was a clear relationship between genotypic expression found in polyps and Reinke's edema. Polyps, characterized by stiffer mucosal waves, had higher levels of gene expression, whereas stiffer mucosal wave scores for Reinke's edema were associated with lower gene activity levels.

Authorities are not in total agreement about the etiology and differences in appearance of vocal nodules (**Fig. 3.4**) and vocal fold polyps (**Fig. 3.5**). Both are mass lesions with fluid accumulation in Reinke's space. Nodules are generally bilateral and symmetric, whereas polyps are more often unilateral but may cause irritation on the contralateral fold creating an appearance similar to that of nodules. Because differences are often difficult to determine from indirect or stroboscopic examination, Rosen and colleagues have suggested the term *podule*. Thibeault (2006) has demonstrated that while phenotypically they may appear similar, nodules and polyps are genetically dissimilar.

Critical to normal vocal fold vibration is the composition of the extracellular matrix of the lamina propria. Understanding the underlying molecular and genetic regulation and homeostasis of the ECM are essential to development of new clinical interventions meant to restore normal vibratory properties (Thibeault, 2005). Moreover, because the end result of the gene-environmental interaction is the production of cellular and tissue proteins, the field of proteomics holds considerable promise for helping us understand etiology of voice disorders and developing improved treatment (Gray and Thibeault, 2002).

Cricoarytenoid Arthritis

Rheumatoid arthritis (RA) is a systemic disease of connective tissue that affects joints lined with synovial membrane. According to Tarnowska, Amernik, Matyja, et al. (2004), cricoarytenoid joint involvement is found in 27 to 78% suffering from RA. Hoarseness and stridor, as well as throat pain during phonation, during swallowing, and from medial compression of the thyroid cartilage radiation to the ears, can be signs of RA. In the acute phase of the disease, patients complain of burning and foreign body sensation in the throat, hoarseness, pain on speaking, voice fatigability, and problems with swallowing. Laryngoscopy shows edema or redness, or both, of the mucosa surrounding the cricoarytenoid joints, and reduced or absent cricoarytenoid joint and vocal fold motion unilaterally or bilaterally. Patients with RA or ankylosing spondylitis and cricoarytenoid arthritis can become dyspneic because of vocal fold fixation and can require tracheostomy and arytenoidectomy. At least one such patient experienced a relief of

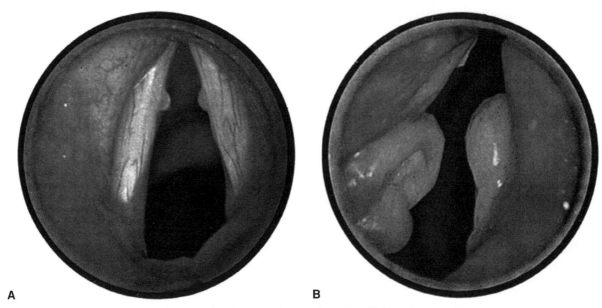

A   B

Figure 3.4 (**A**) Bilateral vocal nodules. (See color plate.) (**B**) Bilateral polypoid vocal folds and contact ulcer on left vocal process.

symptoms after corticosteroid therapy (Bienenstock and Lanyi, 1977).

Laryngeal involvement in RA is not uncommon and may include cricoarytenoid arthritis or vocal fold lesions such as vocal fold rheumatoid nodules or bamboo nodes (Speyer, Speyer, and Heijnen, 2006). These investigators used quality-of-life questionnaires to study the prevalence and the relative risk of dysphonia when suffering from RA compared with that of healthy subjects in 166 subjects with rheumatic arthritis and 148 healthy control subjects. RA patients had statistically significant higher prevalence and

relative risk of dysphonia; RA patients varied between 12% and 27%, and the healthy subjects showed prevalence data varying from ~3 to 8%.

Malignant Tumors

According to English (1976), ~80% of all laryngeal tumors are malignant (although this estimate may be low), occur most often between ages 50 and 70, are more common in men than in women, and are causally linked to cigarette smoking, alcohol, and other sources of chronic laryngeal tissue irritation. The most common malignant lesion by far is squamous cell carcinoma (**Fig. 3.6**). Adenocarcinoma, the next most common malignancy, is rare. The relative frequency of squamous cell carcinoma according to site of lesion is shown in **Fig. 3.7**. Approximately 50% originate on the true vocal folds and spread to structures beyond. Within the vocal folds themselves, 75% originate from the anterior half of the true vocal fold, or near the anterior commissure. Hoarseness is initially the only sign of laryngeal cancer when it involves the true vocal folds. Lesions in the ventricle or supraglottal area may not present with hoarseness. A lump or pain in the throat may indicate spread. Inhalatory stridor from obstruction of the airway is most often a very late sign. Throat pain, shortness of breath, difficulty in swallowing, a mass in the neck, weight loss, ear pain, cough, and fetid breath also occur, depending on the growth pattern of the tumor.

Early detection of laryngeal carcinoma cannot be overemphasized. Because hoarseness is its only early sign, its presence for more than 6 weeks should arouse suspicion of cancer until proved otherwise. If discovered early, the cancer may be kept from invading surrounding tissues supplied by the lymphatic system and thereby metastasizing to other organs.

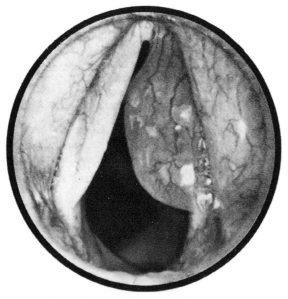

Figure 3.5 Sessile polyp of the vocal fold.

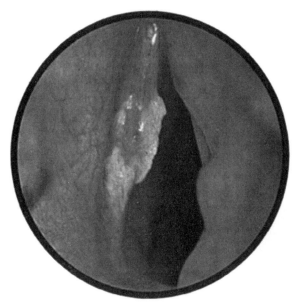

Figure 3.6 Carcinoma of the larynx. (See color plate.)

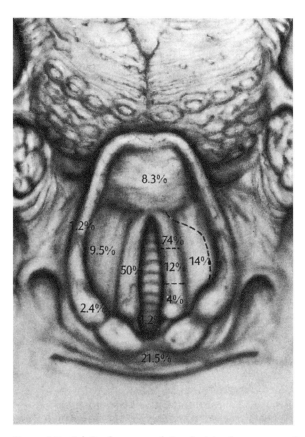

Figure 3.7 Relative frequency of site of origin of squamous cell carcinoma of the larynx. (From English, G.M. [1976]. Malignant neoplasms of the larynx. In English, G.M. [Ed.], Otolaryngology. New York: Harper & Row.)

Endocrine Disorders

Hypothyroidism

Hypothyroidism is caused by insufficient secretion of thyroxin by the thyroid gland. The term *hypothyroidism* is used in reference to the hormonal deficit when the disease is mild and *myxedema* in reference to the physical changes that appear when the disease is severe. Its onset in adults is insidious, taking months or years to develop; because of this delay, missed diagnosis is common. Lethargy, intolerance to cold, puffiness around the eyes, dryness of the skin, and loss of frontal hair are classic physical signs. In more severe hypothyroidism, the central nervous system may be affected, particularly the cerebellum, resulting in ataxia and ataxic dysarthria. As hypothyroidism becomes severe, the clinician may find intellectual, language, and personality changes. As a consequence, such patients are occasionally mistaken as demented from primary central nervous system disease.

The dysphonia of hypothyroidism is characteristically hoarse, sometimes described as coarse or gravelly, and of excessively low pitch. These voice signs are typical effects of mass loading of the vocal folds by their infiltration with myxomatous material. The importance of the dysphonia in the detection and diagnosis of hypothyroidism is illustrated by the following histories.

Case Study 3.1

A 67-year-old widow from Chicago asked her orthopedic surgeon if she could see someone about her voice. She had last been examined 6 months previously after hip joint surgery. One of her complaints was that she felt tired and fatigued and her voice had become hoarse or husky. Her vocal folds and remaining laryngologic examination were normal, and a diagnosis of "functional" voice disorder was made.

Interview with the patient about her voice revealed that it was hoarse most of the time and worse when tired. On voice evaluation, she was mildly hoarse and the pitch of her voice low, even after her age was taken into consideration. She volunteered that she found herself sleeping more than usual—3 or 4 hours a day—in addition to 8 hours at night, was chilly much of the time in her apartment, and was keeping her thermostat high. She complained that her skin was dry. A neurologist tested her Achilles' reflexes and found that her muscles were slow in returning to a relaxed state. He ordered an evaluation of her total serum thyroxine level and found that it was abnormally low. He made a diagnosis of hypothyroidism and instituted thyroid hormone replacement therapy.

Case Study 3.2

After surgery for rectal carcinoma, a 57-year-old male elementary teacher complained of cold intolerance in his feet and hands, loss of sensation in his feet—as if there were "pads" under his soles—and weakness of the lower extremities. These symptoms progressed over a 13-year period from the time of his surgery. He complained of difficulty in climbing stairs and arising from a squatting position and inability to lift modest weights. Although the weakness varied from day to day, there was no daily fluctuation, and the weakness was not related to amount of physical exertion. He had an unsteadiness of gait–a tendency to stagger more to the left than to the right–and noted loss of hair over his lower extremities, loss of sweating, and impotency.

Neurologic examination showed minimal distal sensory loss with moderate proximal weakness. Deep tendon reflexes were mildly decreased and were slow. There was a slowing and an irregularity of rapid alternating movements and a mild unsteadiness of gait. Nerve conduction studies confirmed mild sensorimotor neuropathy and mild proximal myopathy.

General physical examination revealed dry coarse skin, sparse hair, and puffy facies. He had periorbital edema, dry skin, scaling, and decreased deep tendon reflexes with a slow return phase.

Although the patient and family were not aware of any change in the patient's speech, the pitch of his voice was hoarse and deep, particularly when he was asked to sing down to the bottom of his pitch range. Articulation was performed with irregular articulatory imprecision brought out by alternate motion rate testing of /p^/, /t^/, and /k^/. The tip and blade of his tongue protruded between the teeth for the production of /s/ and /z/ sounds. The patient was facetious throughout the examination, making jokes about questions put to him concerning his illness, particularly his speech, which he said was a source of humor in the classroom.

On laryngologic examination, his vocal folds were myxedematous.

A diagnosis of advanced myxedema with myxedematous dysphonia, associated ataxic dysarthria, and lingual articulatory imprecision due to edema of the tongue was made.

In addition to the more typical myxedematous dysphonia, the clinician needs to be alert to distortions of articulation, particularly anterior lingual sounds due to increased tongue size caused by accumulation of myxomatous material in the tongue, and to ataxic dysarthria.

Hyperthyroidism

The dysphonia associated with hyperthyroidism has not been carefully described. Breathy voice quality and reduced loudness have been noted, presumably due to weakness of the respiratory and phonatory musculature. Associated with the dysphonia are anxiety, irritability, and fatigability.

Hyperpituitarism

A tumor in the region of the pituitary gland can cause oversecretion of the pituitary growth hormone somatotropin, producing an untimely enlargement of bone, cartilage, and soft tissue. The result is a condition known as acromegaly. When the condition begins in childhood, before epiphyseal fusion, gigantism results, in which the patient grows to an abnormally great height.

The dysphonia of acromegaly is an excessively low pitch and hoarseness, the consequences of enlargement of the vocal folds and laryngeal cartilage. The reduced fundamental frequency of the voice is augmented by enlarged pharyngeal and oral cavities. Because the tongue becomes enlarged and the mandible prognathic, articulation defects are common.

Amyloidosis

Systemic amyloidosis is an uncommon disease in which an abnormal fibrous protein, amyloid, infiltrates the extracellular compartments of connective tissue. The larynx is an occasional site for the localized expression of the disease. Laryngeal amyloidosis occurs as an atypical laryngeal nodule or subglottic stenosis. It is usually misdiagnosed as a vocal nodule or idiopathic subglottic stenosis. Patients with laryngeal amyloidosis have breathy, strained breathy, or hoarse voices (Aronson, Burroughs, Duffy, et al., 1991).

Virilization

Virilization refers to the development of male sex characteristics in females. For example, in the condition known as *perverse mutation*, the larynx grows to a larger-than-normal size during sexual maturation in the female because of excess secretion of the androgenic hormones. The voice is of abnormally low pitch. Females treated for menopausal symptoms with drug preparations containing androgen often develop virilization and low voice pitch and hoarseness in addition to facial hair. Damsté (1967) also noticed falsetto pitch breaks. Like myxedema, the dysphonia of virilization can develop insidiously and remain unnoticed. Estrogen or testosterone can produce laryngeal edema, causing reduced pitch (Gould, 1972).

Because the conditions are relatively rare, most of what we have learned about virilization comes from case histories. Kim, Kim, Kim, et al. (2006) reported on a 14-year-old girl and her younger sister, who presented with primary amenorrhea, deepening of the voice, and clitoromegaly. Through genetic analysis, they were able to determine the girls had 5 alpha-reductase deficiency. There was no evidence of genetic abnormality in the eight screened exons of the androgen receptor gene. Holt, Medbak, Kirk, et al. (2005) presented a case of a 28-year-old woman with virilization occurring in two successive pregnancies. In her case, differential diagnoses included ovarian disease and fetal aromatase deficiency. She presented during the third trimester of her first pregnancy with rapid onset of hirsutism, increased musculature, and deepening voice. A blood hormone profile revealed significant hyperandrogenism (testosterone, 72.4 nmol/L; normal range, 0.5 to 3.0). She delivered a normal boy, and maternal androgen concentrations returned rapidly to normal. She presented 2 years later, during her second pregnancy, with similar symptoms and biochemistry. Again, she delivered a healthy normal boy, and androgens returned immediately to normal.

A case of virilizing adrenocortical adenoma with Cushing's syndrome, thyroid papillary carcinoma, and hypergastrinemia in a middle-aged Japanese woman was reported by Fukushima, Okada, Tanikawa, et al. (XXX). This 45-year-old woman had a 10-year history of amenorrhea, hypertension, and diabetes. Physical examination showed a masculinized woman with severe hirsutism, male-like baldness, deep voice, acne in the precordia, and clitorism. After resection of the adrenocortical adenoma, preoperative high testosterone and cortisol levels decreased to the normal range.

An opposite change is desired in anthropometry with testosterone therapy in females with gender identity disorder as detailed in a case study by Yamasaki, Douchi, and Nagata (2003). They report on a 31-year-old, regularly menstruating Japanese female diagnosed as having gender identity disorder. Treated with 125 mg testosterone enanthate, intramuscularly, every 2 weeks for 4 months, her serum testosterone levels increased to the normal male value (from 28 to 432 ng/dL) and her voice became lower despite the fact that her menstrual cycle remained regular.

Use of anabolic steroids may also have a virilization side effect as reported from interview data collected from ten women athletes by Straus, Liggett, and Lanese (1985). The women perceived that their cyclical use of anabolic steroids resulted in increased muscle size and strength, deepening of the voice, increased facial hair and aggressiveness, clitoral enlargement, and menstrual irregularities. According to Strauss, Liggett, and Lanese these female athletes were willing to tolerate these side effects, though they recognized the side effects might be unacceptable to other women.

Feminization

Case studies have also enlightened us about voice disorders associated with hormonal problems in males. Akcam, Bolu, Merati, et al. (2004) described the voice characteristics of 24 males with isolated hypogonadotropic hypogonadism (IHH) before and after androgen therapy. Prior to therapy, the mean fundamental frequency (Fo) was 229 ± 41 Hz, which after treatment decreased to 173 ± 30 Hz approaching the normal male Fo. Males with IHH fail to undergo normal sexual development, including the lack of masculinization of the voice, with testosterone treatment the voice lowers to near normal male values.

Hormones and Menstrual Cycle

Several studies indicate that voice may be affected by the menstrual cycle; hoarseness and reduced pitch may be caused by vocal fold edema (Smith, 1962). Singers and actresses claim to be severely affected by these periodic episodes of dysphonia, which interfere with their performances. Minor changes in voice production, such as voice onset time (VOT), may be no less significant. Differences in VOT, frequency perturbations, vocal loading, and laryngeal appearance during different phases of the menstrual cycle have been the focus of recent studies. Recognizing that VOT may be sensitive to changes in hormones, which may affect the neuromuscular systems involved in speech production, Whiteside, Hanson, and Cowell (2004) documented effects of menstrual cycle phase on VOT characteristics in naturally timed speech using whole words. Their findings document that ovarian hormones play some role in shaping some temporal components of speech. Abitbol (2004) has suggested it is imperative that clinicians know where females with vocal

fold lesions are in their menstrual cycle when making management decisions because he has documented that the appearance of lesions change in predictable manners in concert with the menstrual cycle. This notion is supported by a study of classical singers examined before and outside menses. Chernobelsky (2002) made two clinically important conclusions: (1) premenstrual hyperchanges were a result of combined abuse-and menses-related influence on the larynx, and (2) laryngeal examinations before menstruation might be a useful test for the presence of physiologically correct singing.

In their scholarly review of hormone influence on voice Amir and Biron-Shental (2004) state that, "Sex hormone fluctuations were shown to affect female vocal folds and laryngeal function. Laryngeal changes are evident throughout the span of life, starting at puberty with the arousal of the hormonal system, fluctuating systematically during the reproductive years with the menstrual cycle, and then changing again with the decline of hormonal activity at menopause. Early studies that explored this relation were based merely on subjective impressions of voice quality, recent studies have used more objective tools for examining this relation, including histologic observations, stroboscope, electroglottography (EGG), and computerized acoustic analyses. In these studies, the larynx was shown to be a hormonal target organ and, as such, sex hormones affect its morphology, histology, and function, similar to their effect on the genitals and other organs. Examining the relation between sex hormones and the larynx could assist in understanding the mechanisms of voice production, and it could provide the clinician with supplemental diagnostic information on different medical conditions."

Because endocrine fluctuations impact voice, the possibility that use of the contraceptive pill might stabilize vocal quality by "dampening" hormonal fluctuations has recently been studied in nonprofessional voice users and in classically trained voices. In a series of studies conducted by Amir and colleagues (Amir and Kishon-Rabin, 2004; Amir, Biron-Shental, Muchnik, and Kishon-Rabin, 2003; Amir, Kishon-Rabin, and Muchnik, 2002), it has been clearly demonstrated that oral contraceptives have no adverse effect on voice quality, but, in effect, most acoustic measures show improved voice quality among women who used the birth control pill. They postulate that the differences in the noise indices between groups may also shed light on the nature of the effect of sex hormones on vocal fold activity. They further suggest that hormonal fluctuations may have more of an effect on vocal fold regulation of vibration than on glottal adduction. As example, Amir, Biron-Shental, and Shabtai (2006) reported two studies of nonprofessional voice users using birth control pills. In the first study, the researchers obtained voice samples from 30 women with no history of voice training, who used pills with different progestins (drospirenone, desogestrel, gestodene), and 10 women who did not use the pill. Comparison of recordings did not reveal acoustic differences in sustained phonation of vowels across the pill groups and controls. In the second study, the authors conducted a meta-analysis using results from their first study jointly with results from three studies reported in the literature, which used similar methodologies.

Results of this meta-analysis indicated that pill users exhibited lower jitter and shimmer values on sustained vowels, whereas no difference of fundamental frequency was observed among women who use the pill. These results support the notion that not only is there no adverse effect on voice with new-generation monophasic birth control pills, but also the acoustic properties of the voice, which are reflected in perturbation measures in sustained vowels, actually may be improved among women who use the pill.

A parallel approach recording voice acoustics of 24 professional voice users using oral contraceptive pills was taken by Van Lierde, Claeys, De Bodt, et al. (2006). Objective (e.g. Aerodynamic, voice range profile, acoustic, Dysphonia Severity index [DSI], and nasometry) and Subjective (e.g. Perceptual evaluation of voice and nasal resonance) were assessed when hormonal levels reached a steady state (between 10th and 17th day following gestation of pill) and when hormonal levels were minimized. They found no significant differences and concluded that oral contraceptive pills do not have an impact on the objective and subjective voice or resonance parameters in young professional voice users, at least as measured in this study. Analogous findings were reported in the first double-blind, randomized, placebo-controlled trial of professional classically trained singers by (2006). In fact, results from La, Ledger, Davidson, Howard and Jones (2007) double blind, randomized placebo controlled trial, designed to assess the effects of the contraceptive pill on patterns of vibration, suggest a positive effect on performance of Western classical singing repertoire. Use of the contraceptive pill, drospirenone (Yasmin, Schering AG, West Sussex, UK) with antiandrogenic and antimineralocorticoid properties, reduced the irregularity of the vibratory pattern in highly trained classical singers.

The picture appears to change when premenstrual syndrome is taken into account. Chae, Choi, Kang, (2001) evaluated the relationship between voice change and premenstrual syndrome (PMS) in positive PMS and negative PMS groups. There were no significant differences during menses phases in the negative PMS group, but perturbation measures were increased during the premenstrual phase compared with the follicular phase in the positive PMS group suggesting more careful voice habituation is required during the premenstrual phase in this group.

Trauma

Diffuse laryngeal trauma causes dysphonia or aphonia when the vocal folds and surrounding area are damaged by (1) blunt or penetrating injuries from neck injuries such as when being choked or in automobile accidents in which the victim is thrown forward, striking the larynx against the dashboard of the car and causing compression fracture; (2) penetrating wounds of the larynx from gunshot wounds or stabbings; (3) striking of the neck against wires and cables during skiing, snowmobiling, motorcycling, and water-skiing accidents; (4) biomechanical vibratory trauma; or (5) laryngeal esophageal reflux. Edema, hematoma, fractures, dislocations, lacerations, and paralysis are simultaneous tissue reactions to the first three of these injuries. The laryngeal surgeon attempts to restore damaged tissue to its normal configuration to allow

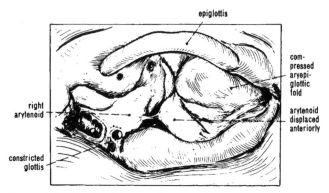

Figure 3.8 Sketch of laryngeal trauma showing anteroposterior laryngeal compression of cartilages and soft tissues.

phonation, but the initial consideration is maintaining a patent airway. Once out of danger, the patient's deglutition and voice become of concern. The voice, swallowing, and airway compete for whatever degree of functional-structural restoration is possible.

Laryngeal lesions due to trauma can be classified into supraglottic, glottic, and subglottic types. The glottic form most often results in dysphonia or aphonia, because in this type thyroid cartilage fracture in the anterior commissure area displaces fragments of cartilage posteriorly, lacerating the vocal folds and causing edema (**Fig. 3.8**).

Trauma and vocal fold paralysis can occur from laryngeal intubation for ventilatory support during surgeries especially if the endotracheal tube is too large for the patient's airway (**Fig. 3.9**) or if the patient has predisposing conditions of laryngeal esophageal reflux, vocal abuse, or a disproportioned airway space to the arytenoid cartilage. Mucosal ulceration may lead to granuloma. Edema, mucosal laceration, and abrasion are temporary. Granulomas may be self-remediated or stubbornly resist treatment and tend to recur even after surgical removal or steroid injection. Glottal strictures can result from untreated granulation. Dislocation of the arytenoid

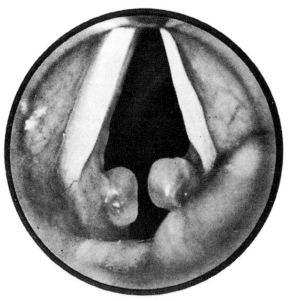

Figure 3.9 Postendotracheal anesthesia granulomas from trauma.

cartilages may also result from laryngeal intubation. Dysphonia or aphonia are inevitable in such cases, depending upon the severity of the trauma. Posterior cricoarytenoid injury can result from nasogastric intubation and can mimic recurrent laryngeal nerve palsy. Differential diagnosis is most often made through laryngeal electromyography (EMG).

Prolonged endotracheal intubation can produce serious disorders of phonation due to traumatic irritation, edema, compressive effects, inflammation, ischemia, and loss of vocal fold mass. Scarring, granulomas, ulcerations, macerations, formation of membranous fibrous tissue on the arytenoid cartilage or within the interarytenoid space, cricoarytenoid subluxation, ankylosis, vocal fold paralysis, and subglottal stenosis can be produced by excessive endotracheal tube size, tube tip irritation, cuff pressure, and the natural curvature of the endotracheal tube. In a study of 17 patients, ages 17 to 85 years, who had been intubated for periods ranging from 10 hours to 4 weeks, Gallivan, Dawson, and Robbins (1989) found a total of 31 lesions in 16 of the 17 patients, 77% involving the vocal folds, 13% the arytenoid cartilage, and 10% the interarytenoid notch and lumen between the vocal folds. Phonation, respiration, and coughing were compromised in these patients; voice impairment was virtually universal.

Endotracheal intubation also can cause vocal fold paralysis (Ellis and Pallister, 1975; Hahn, Martin, and Lillie, 1970; Holley and Gildea, 1971; Yamashita, Harada, Ueda, et al., 1965). Lim, Chia, and Ng (1987), in a report of three patients who developed right vocal fold paralysis after endotracheal intubation during surgery unrelated to the neck, found severe hoarseness and the right vocal fold paralyzed in the paramedian position up to 6 weeks after surgery in two patients, and only slight voice improvement 2 months after intubation in a third patient. In all three patients, voice improvement was due to compensation by the unimpaired vocal fold. It is speculated that the cause of vocal cord paralysis occurs from pressure arising from an overinflated cuff of the endotracheal tube compressing the peripheral anterior branches of the recurrent laryngeal nerve.

Caustic substances swallowed by children (and often by adults who attempt suicide) that cause grave damage to the larynx and esophagus are lye, ammonia, sodium hypochlorite (Clorox), and orthophenylphenol (Lysol). Thermal traumas are caused by ingestion of hot liquids or solids or inhalation of hot gasses. Irradiation burns of the larynx occur as a side effect of the treatment of malignancies of the neck. Technically, vocal nodule and contact ulcer might be included, for they too are lesions secondary to trauma and caused by vocal abuse; however, they are discussed in separate sections.

Esophageal Reflux and Granulomas

Esophageal reflux, or gastroesophageal reflux (GER), the regurgitation of hydrochloric acid from the stomach, is an internal caustic substance that has been implicated in vocal fold irritation, contact ulcers, and dysphonia. Inquiry into daytime and nocturnal acid reflux is an important component of the voice disorder history in patients with or without observed contact ulcer or contact ulcer granuloma. In a study of 32 patients suspected of having esophageal reflux, Koufman, Winer, Wu, et al. (1988) found either intermittent or chromic dysphonia in 65.6% of the patients. In one subgroup of five patients who presented with chronic hoarseness, examinations revealed erythema and edema of the posterior larynx, laryngeal granulomas, and bouts of hoarseness related to reflux history.

Laryngeal granulomas, as discussed elsewhere in this text, are presumed to be related to four predisposing factors: vocal abuse, esophageal reflux, orotracheal intubation, and morphologic structure (Pontes, DeBiase, Kyrilos, et al., 2001). Knowledge of the presence of acid reflux in a majority of chronic hoarseness is not new (Wiener, Koufman, Wu, et al, 1989). Because it it common and symptoms differ gastroesophageal reflux (GER), hoarseness treatment should include some focus on managing reflux (Toohill, Kuhn, 1997; deLima-Pontes, De Biase, Gadelha, 1999; Emami, Morrison, Rammage, et al., 1999; Havas, Priestly, Lowinger, 1999; Cohen, Back, Postma, et al., 2002), in combination with behavioral management of the voice disorder.

Because granulomas tend to recur after surgical removal, Havas and colleagues have stated that, "the only indications for laryngeal surgery are to resolve diagnostic doubt or to treat airway compromise." Alternatives to surgical intervention of granulomas are treatment with application of topical inhalant steroids (Row, Goh, Chon, et al., 1999) or treatment with intralaryngeal injection of botulinum toxin (Orloff and Goldman, 1999). Treatment with Botox (botulinum toxin) causes a temporary paresis of the vocal folds providing for a window of time during which the vocal process can heal and the granulomas resolve because it is not exposed to ongoing intermittent contact and friction with the opposing arytenoid.

Bowing of the Vocal Folds

Bowing of the vocal folds is a term that describes an elliptical glottal shape during phonation due to failure of adequate anteroposterior tension of the vocal folds, laryngeal scarring as in vocal sulci, or to loss of tissue mass. Instead of the membranous portions of the folds adducting with straight vocal edges, they are curved. The intercartilaginous portions or the vocal folds are adducted; only the membranous portions fail to adduct. Causes of bowing are (1) atrophy of the thyroarytenoid muscle owing to denervation; (2) bilateral cricothyroid muscle weakness due to superior laryngeal nerve lesions resulting in failure of anteroposterior stretching of the vocal folds; (3) loss of vocal fold tissue in the aging larynx; (4) iatrogenic lesions; (5) idiopathic lesions; and (6) infraglottic edema extending from the anterior commissure to the posterior larynx creating a pseudosulcus and bowed appearance.

Not all vocal fold bowing is due to structural changes; it can occur in patients with psychogenic voice disorders and has been observed in the hypokinetic dysarthria of Parkinson's disease (Hanson, Gerratt, and Ward, 1984) and in the flaccid dysphonia of myasthenia gravis (Neiman, Mountjoy, and Allen, 1975).

Regardless of the etiology, the associated dysphonia is breathiness and, in extreme cases, aphonia (LeJeune, Guist, Samuels, 1983; Kahane, 1987; Koufman, 1986; Tucker, 1985). Bowing of the vocal folds has also been observed in the hypokinetic dysarthria of Parkinson's disease (Hanson, Gerratt, and Ward, 1984) and in the flaccid dysphonia of myasthenia gravis (Neiman, Mountjoy, and Allen, 1975).

♦ Summary

♦ Voice disorders caused by structural changes in infants arise from congenital laryngeal malformations, neoplasms, inflammation, trauma, or malnutrition.

♦ Voice disorders caused by mass lesions in children and adults stem from inflammation, neoplasms, endocrine disease, or trauma.

♦ To understand the pathophysiology and develop new biological treatments, it is necessary to gain knowledge of the molecular genetic structure of the vocal fold.

♦ Treatment for structural changes includes behavioral management, treatment of reflux, medical management, and surgical treatment.

References

Abitbol, J. Presentation at 9th international workshop: laser, voice surgery and voice care. April 16–17, 2004, Paris, France.

Akcam, T., Bolu, E., Merati, A.L., Durmus, C., Gerek, M., Ozkaptan, Y. (2004). Voice changes after androgen therapy for hypogonadotrophic hypogonadism. Laryngoscope, 114(9), 1587–1591.

Akst, L.M., Broadhurst, M.S., Burns, J.A. Zeitels, S.M. (2007). Microflap laryngoplasty for treating an anterior-commissure web with papillomatosis. Laryngoscope. 117(8), 1496–1499.

Amir, O., Biron-She ntal, T. (2004). The impact of hormonal fluctuations on femal vocal folds. Curr Opin Otol Head Neck Surg, 12(3), 180–184.

Amir, O., Biron-She ntal, T., Muchnik, C., Kishon-Rabin, L. (2003). Do oral contraceptives improve vocal quality? Limited trial on low-dose formulations. Obstet Gynecol, 101(4),773–777.

Amir, O., Biron-Shental, T., Shabtai, E. (2006). Birth control pills and nonprofessional voice: acoustic analyses. J Speech Lang Hear Res, 49(5), 1114–1126.

Amir, O., Kishon-rabin, L. (2004). Association between birth control pills and voice quality. Laryngoscope. 114(6), 1021–1026.

Amir, O., Kishon-rabin, L., Muchnik, C. (2003). The effect of superior auditory skills on vocal accuracy. J Acoust Soc Am, 113(2): 1102–1108.

Aronson, A.E., Burroughs, E.I., Duffy, J.R., Kyle, R.A. (1991). Speech disorders in systemic amyloidosis. Br J Disord Commun 26, 201–206.

Beckman, D.A., Wold, D.C., Montague, J.C. (1983). A noninvasive acoustic method using frequency perturbations and computer-generated vocaltract shapes. J Speech Hear Res. 26(2), 304–314.

Bienenstock, H., Lanyi, V.F. (1977). Cricoarytenoid arthritis in a patient with ankylosing spondylitis. Arch Otolaryngol 103, 738–739.

Bouchayer, M., Cornut, G. (2000). Instrumental microscopy of benign lesions of the vocals. In C.N. Force, D.M. Bless (Eds.). Phonosurgery. A assessment and surgical management of voice disorders. New York: Raven Press, 1991, 25–41.

Bryson, P.C., Rosen, C.A., Osborne, J.T. (2004). Indole-3-carbinol for recurrent repiratory papillomatosis: long term results. J Voice, 18(2), 248–253.

Chae, S.W., Choi, G., Kang, H.J., Choi, J.O., Jin, S.M. (2001). Clinical analysis of voice change as a parameter of premenstrual syndrome. J Voice, 15(2), 278–283.

Chernobelsky, S.L. (2002). A study of menses-related changes to the larynx in singers with voice abuse. Folia Phoniatr Logop, 54(1), 2–7.

Cohen, J.T., Back, K.K., Postma, G.N., Koufman, J.A. (2002). Clinical manifestations of laryngopharyngeal reflux. Ear Nose Throad J, 81(9 Suppl 2), 19–23.

Damsté, P.H. (1967). Voice change in adult women caused by virilizing agents. J Speech Hear Disord 32, 126–132.

de Lima Pontes, P.A., De Biase, N.G., Gadelha, E.C. (1999). Clinical evolution of laryngeal granulomas: treatment and prognosis. Laryngoscope. 109(2 Pt 1), 289–294.

Dufflo, S.M., Thibeault, S.L., Li, W., Smith, M.E., Schade, G., Hess, M.M. (2006). Differential gene expression profiling of vocal fold polyps and Reinke's edema by complementary DNA microarray. Ann Otol Rhinol Laryngol 115(9), 703–714.

Dumars, K.W., Jr., Gaskill, C., Kitzmiller, N. (1964). Le cri du chat (crying cat) syndrome. Am J Dis Child 108, 533–537.

Ellis, P.D.M., Pallister, W.K. (1975). Recurrent laryngeal nerve palsy and endotracheal intubation. J Laryngol Otol 89, 823–826.

Emami, A.J., Morrison, M., Rammage, L., Bosch, D. (1999). Treatment of laryngeal contact ulcers and granulomas: a 12-year retrospective analysis. J Voice, 13(4), 176–180.

English, G.M. (1976). Malignant neoplasms of the larynx. In G.M. English (Ed.), Otolaryngology. New York: Harper and Row.

Ferguson, C.F. (1970). Congential abnormalities of the infant larynx. Otol Clin North Am 3, 185–200.

Fukushima, A., Okada, Y., Tanikaw, T., Kawahara, C., Misawa, H., Kanda, K., Morita, E., Sasano, H., Tanaka, Y. (2003). Virilizing adrenocortical adenoma with Cushing's syndrome, thyroid papillary carcinoma and hypergastrinemia in a middle-aged woman. Endocr J, 50(2), 179–187.

Gallivan, G.J., Dawson, J.A., Robbins, L.D. (1989). Videolaryngoscopy after endotracheal intubation: implications for voice. J Voice 3, 76–80.

Gould, W.J. (1972). Vocal cords can speak of hormonal dysfunction. Consultant 12, 101–102.

Gray, S.D., Thibeault, S.L. (2002). Diversity in voice characteristics-interaction between genes and environment, use of microarray analysis. J Commun Disord, 35(4), 347–354.

Hahn, F.W., Martin, J.T., Lillie, J.C. (1970). Vocal cord paralysis with endtracheal intubation. Arch Otolaryngol 92, 226–229.

Hanson, D.G., Gerratt, B.R., Ward, P.H. (1984). Cinegraphic observations of laryngeal function in Parkinson's disease. Laryngoscope 94, 348–353.

Havas, T.E., Priestly, J. Lowinger, D.S. (1999). A management strategy for vocal process granulomas. Laryngoscope. 109(2 Pt 1), 301–306.

Holland, B., Koufman, J.A., Postma, G.N., McGurt, W.F. (2002). Laryngopharyngeal reflux and laryngeal web formation in patients with pediatric recurrent respiratory papillomas. Laryngoscope. 112(11), 1926–1929.

Holt, H.B., Medbak, S., Kirk, D., Guirgis, R., Hughes, I., Cummings, M.H., Meeking, D.R. (2005). Recurrent severe hyperandrogenism during pregnancy: a case report. J Clin Pathol, 58(4), 439–442.

Holley, H.S., Gildia, J.E. (1971). Vocal cord paralysis after tracheal intubation. JAMA 215, 281–284.

Kahane, J.C. (1987). Connective tissue changes in the larynx and their effects on voice. J Voice 1, 27–30.

Kim, S.H., Kim, K.S., Kim, G.H., Kang, B.M., Yoo, H.W. (2006). A novel frameshift mutation in the 5alpha-reductase type 2 gene in Korean sisters with male pseudohermaphroditism. Fertil Steril, 85(3), 750–759.

Koufman, J.A., Winer, G.J., Wu, W.C., Castell, D.O. (1988). Reflux laryngitis and its sequelae: The diagnostic role of ambulatory 24-hour pH monitoring. J Voice 2, 78–89.

La, F.M., Ledger, W.L., Davidson, J.W., Howard, D.M., Jones, G.L. (2007). The effects of third generation combined oral contraceptive pill on the classical singing voice. J Voice. 21(6), 754–761.

Lee, R., Rosen, C.A. (2004). Efficacy of Cidofovir injection for the treatment of recurrent respiratory papillomatosis. J Voice, 18(4), 551–556.

LeJeune, F.E., Jr., Guist, C.E., Samuels, P.M. (1983). Early ezperiences with vocal ligament tightening. Ann Otol Rhinol Laryngol 92, 475–477.

Lejeune, J., Lafourcade, J., Berger, R., Vialatte, J., Boeswillwald, M., Seringe, P., Turpin, R. (1963). Trois cas de délétion partielle du bras court d'un chromosome-5. C R Acad Sci Paris 257L, 3098–3102.

Lester, B.M. (1976). Spectrum analysis of the cry sounds of well-nourished and malnourshied infants. Child Dev 47, 237–241.

Lim, E.K., Chia, K.S., Ng, B.K. (1987). Recurrent laryngeal nerve palsy following endotracheal intubation. Anaesth Intensive Care 15, 342–345.

Liu, R.Z., Luo, J.W. Zhong, Z.Y. Huang, Q., Chen, L.F., Zhou, H. (2006). Diagnosis and treatment of laryngeal web in infants. Zhonghua er Bi Yan Hou Tou Jing Wai Ke Za Zhi. Feb; 41(2): 120–122.

Mahnke, C.G., Frohlich, O., Lippert, B.M., Werner, J.A. (1996). Recurrent laryngeal pipillomatosis. Retrospective analysis of 95 patients and review of the literature. Otol Pol, 50(6): 567–578L

Mallard, A.R., Daniloff, R.G. (1973). Glottal cues for parent judgment of emotional aspects of infant vocalizations. J Speech Hear Res 16, 592–596.

Mainardi, P.C., Pastore, G., Castronovo, C., Godi, M., Guala, A., Tamiazzo, S., et al. (2006). The natural history of cri du chat syndrome: A report from the Italian Register. Eur J Med Genet 49, 362–383.

Mandell, D.L., Arjmand, E.M., Kay, D.J., Casselbrant, M.L. Rosen, C.A. (2004). Intralesional cidofovir for pediatric recurrent respiratory papillomatosis. Arch Otol Head Neck Surg, 130(11): 1319–1323.

Milczuk, H.A., Smith, J.D., Everts, E.C. (2000). Congenital laryngeal webs: surgical management and clinical embryology. Int J Pediatr Otorhinolaryngol, 52(1): 1–9.

Miyamoto, R.C., Cotton, R.T., Rope, A.F., Hopkin, R.J., Aliza, P., Cohen, A.P., Shott, S.R. (2004). Association of anterior glottis webs with velocardiofacial syndrome (chromosome 22q11.2 deletion). Otol Head Neck Surg, 130: 450–452.

Moran, M.J. (1986). Identification of Down's syndrome adults from prolonged vowel samples. J Commun Disord, 19(5): 387–394.

Moran, M.J., Gilbert, H.R. (1982). Selected acoustic characteristics and listener judgments of the voice of Down syndrome adults. Am J Ment Defic, 86(5): 553–556.

Moura, C.P., Cunha, L.M., Vilarinho, H., Cunha, M.J., Freitas, D., Palha, M., Pueschel, S.M., Pais-Clemente, M. (2008). Voice parameters in children with Down syndrome. J Voice, 22(1): 34–42.

Neiman, R.F., Mountjoy, J.R., Allen, E.L. (1975). Myasthenia gravis focal t the larynx. Arch Otolaryngol 101, 569–570.

Novak, A. (1972). The voice of children with Down's syndrome. In J. Hirschberg, Gy. Szépe, E. Vass-Kovács, E. (Eds.), Papers in interdisciplinary speeh research (pp. 197–200). Budapest: Akadémiai Keadó.

Ogut, F., Midilli, R., Oder, G., Engin, E.Z., Karci, B., Kabasakal, Y. (2005). Laryngeal findings and voice quality in Sjogren's syndrome. Auris Nasus Larynx, 32(4), 375–380.

Orloff, L.A., Goldman, S.N. (1999). Vocal fold granuloma: successful treatment with botulinumtoxin. Otol Head Neck Surg, 121(4), 410–413.

Pachigolla, R., Deskin, R. (1998). Stridor in neonates, infants, and children's source. Department of Otolaryngology, University of Texas Medical Branch, Grand Rounds, April 15, 1998. In F.B. Quinn (Ed.), Dr. Quinn's online textbook on otolaryngology. Grand Round Archive, 1999–present. http://www.utmb.edu/otoref/Grnds/Stridor-infants-980415.html.

Pentz, A.L., Gilbert, H.R. (1983). Relation of selected acoustical parameters and perceptual ratings to voice quality of Down syndrome children. Am J Men Defic, 88(2), 304–314.

Pontes, P., De Biase, N., Kyrillos, L., Pontes, A. (2001). Imkportance of glottis configuration in the development of posterior laryngeal granuloma. Ann Otol Rhinol Laryngol, 110(8), 765–769.

Rihkanen, H., Aaltonen, L.M., Syrajanen, S.M. (1993). Human papillomavirus in thelaryngeal papillomas and in adjacent normal epithelium. Clin Otol Allied Sci, 18(6), 470–474.

Roh, H.J., Goh, E.K., Chon, K.M., Wang, S.G. (1999). Topical inhalant steroid (budesonide, Pulmicort nasal) therapy in intubation granuloma. J Laryngol Otol, 113(5), 427–432.

Rohde, M., Banner, J. (2006). Respiratory tract malacia: possible cause of sudden death in infancy and early childhood. Acta Paediatrica. 95, 867–870.

Rosen, C.A., Bryson, P.C. (2004). Indole-3-carbinol for recurrent respiratory papillomatosis: long-term results. J Voice, 18(2), 248–253.

Sjogren's Syndrome Foundation, 6707 Democracy Boulevard Suite 325, Bethesda, MD 20817. http://www.sjogrens.org/contact.html.

Smith, B.L., Oller, D.K., (1981). A comparative study of pre-meaningful vocalizations produced by normally developing and Down's syndrome infants. J Speech Hear Disord, 46(1), 46–51.

Smith, F.M. (1962). Hoarseness–a symptom of premenstrual tension. Arch Otol, 75, 66–68.

Sone, M., Sato, E., Hayashi, H., Fujimoto, Y., Nakashima, T. (2006). Vascular evaluation in laryngeal diseases: comparisons between contact endoscopy and laser Doppler flowmetry. Arch Otol Head Neck Surg, 132(12), 1371–1374.

Speyer, R., Speyer, I., Heijnen, M.A. (2008). Prevalence and relative risk of dysphonia in rheumatoid arthritis. J Voice, 22(2), 232–237.

Strauss, R.H., Liggett, M.T., Lanese, R.R. (1985). Anabolic steroid use and perceived effects in ten weight-trained women athletes. JAMA 17; 253(19), 2871–2873.

Tarnowskia, C., Amernik, K., Matyja, G., Brzosko, I., Grzelec, H., Burak, M. (2004). Fixation of the crico-arytenoid joints in rheumatoid arthritis–preliminary report. Otol Pol, 58(4), 834–839.

Tateya, I., Tateya, T., Surles, R.L., Tanumihardjo, S., Bless, D.M. (2007). Prenatal vitamin A deficiency causes laryngeal malformation in rats. Ann Otol Rhinol Laryngol Oct: 116(10), 785–792.

Thibeault, S.L. (2005). Advances in our understanding of the Reinke space. Curr Opin Otol Head Neck Surg, 13(3), 148–151.

Thibeault, S.L., Gray, S.D., Li, W., Ford, C.N., Smith, M.E., Davis, R.K. (2002). Genotypic and phenotypic expression of vocal fold polyps and Reinke's demea: a preliminary study. Ann Otol Rhinol Laryngol, 111(4), 302–309.

Thibeault, S.L., Hirschi, S.D., Gray, S.D. (2003). DNA microarray gene expression analysis of a vocal fold polyp and granuloma. J Speech Lang Hear Res, 46(2), 491–502.

Toohill, R.J., Kuhn, J.C. (1997). Role of refluxed acid in pathogenesis of laryngeal disorders. Am. J. Med. 103(5A), 100S–106S.

Tucker, H.M. (1985). Anterior commissure laryngoplasty for adjustment of vocal fold tension. Ann Otol Rhinol Laryngol 94, 547–549.

Van Lierde, K.M., Claeys, S., De Bodt, M., Van Cauwenberge, P. (2006). Response of the femal vocal quality and resonance in professional voice users taking oral contraceptive pills: a multiparameter approach. Laryngoscope 116(10), 1894–1898.

Ward, P.H., Engel, E., Nance, W.E. (1968). The larynx in the cri du chat (cat cry) syndrome. Trans Am Acad Ophthalmol Otolaryngol 72, 90–102.

Wasz-Höckert, O., Lind, J., Vuorenkoski, V., Partenen, T., Valanni, E. (1968). The infant cry. London: William Heinemann Medical Book.

Whiteside, S.P., Hanson, A. Cowell, P.E. (2004). Hormones and temporal components of speech; sex differences and effects of menstrual cyclicity on speech. Neurosci Lett, 26:356(1), 44–47.

Wiener, G.J., Koufman, J.A., Wu, W.C., Cooper, J.B., Richter, J.E., Castell, D.O. (1989). Chronic hoarseness secondary to gastroesophageal reflux disease: documentation with 24-h ambulatory pH monitoring. Am J Gastroenterol, 84(12), 1503–1508.

Yamasaki, H., Douchi, T., Nagata, Y. (2003). Changes in anthropometry with testosterone therapy in a female with gender identity disorder. Endocr J. 50(6), 729–731.

Yamashita, T., Harada, Y., Ueda, N., Tashiro, T., Kanebayashi, H. (1965). Recurrent laryngeal nerve paralysis associated with endotracheal anesthesia. Nippon Jibiinkoka Gakkai Kaiho 68, 1452–1459.

Additional Reading

Becker, W. (Ed.). (1969). *Atlas of otorhinolaryngology and bronchoesophagology.* Philadelphia: W.B. Saunders Co. (Probably the best color photos of laryngeal diseases.)

Cohen, S.R., Thompson, J.W., Geller, K.A., Birns, J.W. (1983). Voice change in the pediatric patient: a differential diagnosis. Ann Otol Rhinol Laryngol 92, 437–443. (This article should be read for its extensive coverage of voice changes from organic disease in pediatric patients. Neurologic dysfunctions, congenital and chromosomal defects, tumors, infections, trauma, and metabolic and endocrine diseases are discussed, and several tables are given containing many diseases within these general categories.)

English, G.M. (Ed.) (1976). *Otolaryngology.* New York: Harper & Row. (This comprehensive, readable book can serve as a reference for greater depth of reading into the entire realm of organic laryngeal disease.)

Lane, R.W., Weider, D.J., Steinem, C., Marin-Padilla, M. (1984). Laryngomalacia. Arch Otolaryngol 110, 546–551. (An excellent review of a little-known voice disorder in infants accompanied by a case study of surgical treatment of this condition.)

Chapter 4

Nasal Resonatory Disorders

For when we wish to emit voice or breath through the mouth only, which may happen in the pronunciation of the letters which I shall name explosives, we shut the passage of the nostrils, as with a valve.

—Amman, 1700

♦ The Velopharynx in Life

The isthmus between the oral and nasal cavities must be closed during swallowing and speech or else food will be regurgitated out the nares, vowels will be excessively resonated in the nasal chambers, pressure consonants will lose their characteristic explosive and friction noises, and air will be audibly emitted through the nares. In Chapter 1, we noted that phonation was a phylogenetically recent acquisition among vertebrates and that the vital functions of the larynx were respiratory and protective of the airway. Much the same can be said about velopharyngeal function. The velopharyngeal port was not designed primarily as a means of coupling or uncoupling the oral and nasal cavities for speech. Rather, velopharyngeal closure exists primarily to:

1. Seal off the nasal from the oral cavities to isolate the oropharyngolaryngeal tract from atmospheric pressure during deglutition, producing a partial vacuum to facilitate compression of the food bolus by the tongue, cheeks, and pharynx, and thereby forcing it into the esophagus

2. Open the eustachian tube during swallowing to ventilate the middle ear

In only three phonemes of English, the nasal semivowels, is it permissible for the velopharyngeal valve to remain completely open, coupling the oral with the nasal cavities: /m/, /n/, and /ŋ/ (as in *sing*). The remainder of English phonemes are correctly produced with the velopharyngeal port closed, meaning all vowels and most consonants. If the port is left too open, voiced consonants will be excessively resonated in the nasal cavities, and intraoral air pressure for plosives, fricatives, and affricates will be reduced. In an attempt to produce them, air escapes through the nares and results in a weak, nasally distorted production of the target sound. It should also be mentioned that a certain amount of nasal resonation of vowels is both normal and desirable. The borderline between normal and pathologic hypernasality often is a matter of perceptual preference. This is most notable in different regional dialects some of which have increased nasal resonance as one of the distinguishing characteristics. Moreover, resonance balance is the focus of many voice therapy techniques designed to improve vocal quality and reduce laryngeal tension.

What must be remembered is that the nasal resonatory defect of hypernasality is not the only one produced by velopharyngeal insufficiency. Hypernasality may be the primary one. Secondary or associated defects are excess nasal airflow, nasal emission articulatory distortions owing to loss of intraoral air pressure stolen by the nasal air leak, compensatory articulatory and phonatory substitutions many of which are nonphonemic, articulatory distortions due to dental and palatal defects, and even dysphonia from compensatory vocal abuse.

In medical and speech-language pathology practice, hypernasality and nasal air emission and hyponasality have similar diagnostic medical implications as dysphonia from laryngeal disease. That is, they signify structural, neurologic, or psychiatric pathologic conditions and therefore are essential to medical differential diagnosis, as well as having developmental, educational, social, psychologic, and occupational handicaps that require treatment. The following transcript of a deposition illustrates these many factors involved in velopharyngeal insufficiency.

Case Study 4.1

Attorney: "Have you ever given a deposition before?"

Clinician: "No, this is my first."

A: "Let me explain that a deposition is an official transcript of testimony in place of your appearance in court. We are the attorneys for Ms. Alquist, who is suing the surgeon who removed her tonsils and adenoids. She claims as a result of that surgery her speech was so impaired that she was placed on indefinite leave of absence without pay from her teaching position. She also claims that when she swallows, fluids leak out her nose. So, we are taking testimony from specialists who have independently investigated Ms. Alquist's complaints. I understand you are the speech pathologist who evaluated Ms. Alquist's speech, and that the plastic surgeon and otolaryngologist who also saw her will be following you. This is the official stenographer who will take down your testimony. You will have a chance to read the transcript and make corrections before it is put into final form. Some of the questions I will ask may seem oversimplified, but remember, this testimony will go before a jury of lay individuals who have no technical knowledge of the subject. You have already stated your full name and address. What is your occupation?"

C: "I am a speech-language pathologist."

A: "I notice you are addressed as 'doctor.' Are you a medical doctor?"

C: "No. I hold a Ph.D. in speech-language pathology."

A: "Are you licensed to practice speech pathology?"

C: "In this state there are no licensure laws for speech pathologists."

A: "Will you tell the court what a speech pathologist is and does?"

C: "We identify, describe, diagnose, and treat people who have disorders of communication, that is, voice, speech, and language disturbances from organic or psychiatric illnesses. Where I work, speech pathologists consult to physicians of all specialties."

A: "Thank you. Now, do you know the plaintiff, and if so on what occasion have you conferred with her?"

C: "I evaluated Ms. Alquist's speech on May 21 of last year. That evaluation took approximately one and one-half hours."

A: "Are these the clinical notes that you wrote as a result of your evaluation?"

C: "Yes, they are."

A: "Are these the audiotape and videotape recordings you made of the patient during your evaluation?"

C: "Yes, they are."

A: "When you evaluate a patient's speech, doctor, what exactly do you do?"

C: "I ask the patient to perform different tasks that will provide me with an adequate sample of the patient's speech. I usually tape record the speech for more detailed analysis later. I might also make certain laboratory tests, such as aerodynamic and spectrographic assessment, that is, acoustic recordings of the patient's speech and recordings of how she uses air from her lungs for speech."

A: "Based on your analysis of Ms. Alquist's speech, would you say her speech was abnormal?"

C: "Yes, I would."

A: "In what way, specifically?"

C: "She had hypernasality and nasal emission."

A: "Would you please explain the meaning of these words for the court."

C: "Hypernasality refers to excess resonation of speech sounds within the nasal chambers because of partial or complete failure of the soft palate to close off the nasal from the oral cavities, or from incomplete closure of the hard palate."

A: "You mean like cleft palate?"

C: "Yes. But she did not have a cleft palate."

A: "Doctor, please point out on this chart the parts of the speech mechanism you are talking about."

C: "This is a side view of the head and neck. This plate of bone separates the oral from the nasal cavity. It is called the hard palate. This flap of tissue is called the soft palate or velum. It can lift upward and backward to contact the back wall of the throat. When it does, it seals off the oral from the nasal cavity."

A: "And, what if it doesn't?"

C: "As I explained before, then speech will be abnormally resonated in the nasal cavities. I would add that consonants will be heard as weak or absent if the opening is very large. People would then have trouble understanding what the speaker was saying."

A: "We will return to what you found out about the plaintiff's speech mechanism, but at this point, I would like you to explain more fully the implications of Ms. Alquist's speech defect."

C: "As I said, she was hypernasal and had nasal emission of the airstream as she spoke. If I may, I would like to play a videotape of the patient so that you can hear and see what I'm talking about. As you can hear from the tape, her speech has a noticeable and distracting nasal quality, and some of her words are difficult to understand. We call this reduced intelligibility. Also, you can see she has a tendency to narrow her nostrils and wrinkle her forehead on many consonant sounds. This is a kind of compensation people with palatal insufficiencies develop. It is an attempt to constrict the nostrils so that less air will pass out through them."

A: "How would this disorder interfere with the patient's everyday life?"

C: "A speech defect is a personal matter. Two people with defects of the same type and severity often react differently, depending upon their personality and the importance of speech in their daily lives."

A: "And, how would you characterize the effect of Ms. Alquist's defect on her?"

C: "Based on the psychologic and social history portion of my examination, Ms. Alquist was devastated by her speech disorder."

A: "What is your evidence for that statement?"

C: "She broke down several times during the examination, especially during discussions of the effects of her disorder on her professional activities. She said her speech had always been important to her; that she used her speech to favorable advantage in the classroom, that she knew she had a good voice, would often dramatize segments of the curriculum through plays and story-telling, and that she taught singing. Outside of the class-room, she was active in teachers' organizations and was known as a good public speaker and debater."

A: "Has this changed as a result of her disorder?"

C: "It has, according to what she told me, turned her life around completely. Her students, she said, became inat-tentive. She began to notice derisive facial expressions of students and colleagues as she would speak. Some of the children made fun of her. Speaking tired her out—she had to exert much more effort to make herself understood."

A: "Has her speech disorder affected her in any other ways?"

C: "According to Ms. Alquist, she was called into the prin-cipal's office and told that she would have to take a leave of absence until something was done about her speech. That was a year ago. She has not worked since. She says she has become withdrawn, has a fear of using the telephone, and has been seeing a psychiatrist for depression."

A: "Have any attempts been made to correct, treat, or rehabilitate her speech?"

C: "Not to my knowledge. No one recommended speech therapy in her locality."

A: "Doctor, let's get back to the physical examination of the plaintiff. What, in your opinion, was the reason she developed this disorder at this time in her life? Why would anyone whose speech had been not only normal, but who was in fact a skilled speaker, suddenly acquire this kind of defect?"

C: "I would feel more comfortable if you asked the plas-tic surgeon and otolaryngologist that question, although I think we agree, having discussed the case in private, on the cause of the disorder."

A: "Nonetheless, the court is interested in your opinion; as an expert witness in your field, you are justified in com-menting on the physical aspects of the case."

C: "Well, we have photographs of the patient's mouth and x-ray motion pictures of her soft palate during speech. These lateral motion picture studies clearly show that, although the soft palate is able to lift up, it is too short to make closure contact against the back wall of the throat; it elevates, but there is a considerable gap left between it and the posterior pharyngeal wall. During our examination, although the hard and soft palate looked all right when the patient opened her mouth, when we explored her hard palate we felt a notch at the back where the soft and hard palate join. This notch is called a submu-cous cleft. We also noticed, and we almost missed this because it was so subtle, that the little pendulum of tissue that hangs down from the middle of the soft palate, the uvula, was almost invisibly split; you could separate it with a tongue depressor, but most of the time the two halves stuck together so that it looked like solid tissue. You can see the split on this photograph."

A: "Would you give us the implications of all this?"

C: "We think Ms. Alquist has had a lifelong condition of submucous cleft palate, a cleft in the bone and muscular tissue that is hidden under the mucosal tissue. In her case, a speech disorder was not evident because she was able to attain adequate closure by contacting her soft palate against her adenoids. In other words, the adenoids were serving as an anatomic structure on the back wall of the throat and were helping to effect complete closure; when they were removed, the space created was too great for her soft palate to bridge. The adenoid removal unmasked the submucous cleft."

A: "Is this condition remediable?"

C: "A prosthetic device called a palatal lift would par-tially close the gap. More permanent would be a surgical procedure, a pharyngeal flap operation, in which a flap of tissue raised from the pharyngeal wall is sutured to the soft palate, or a sphincter pharyngoplasty."

A: "We want to thank you for your testimony. If we have any further questions, we'll arrange another appointment through your secretary."

As this testimony illustrates, although hypernasality and nasal emission are only aesthetically displeasing when mild, when excessive, they diminish or even destroy intelligibility, producing serious occupational and psychologic distur-bances. When hard palate or velopharyngeal port defects are left untreated in infancy or early childhood, they may impede speech and language production development and negatively influence the self-concept. Even when they occur for the first time in adulthood, as in the case just presented, they can pro-duce profound psychologic and occupational maladjust-ments. One might ask, "Which would be more devastating: aphonia (whispered speech) from laryngeal disease or severe hypernasality and nasal emission from velopharyngeal or palatal insufficiencies?" Our first impulse might be to answer that the aphonia would have more profound consequences. In actual fact, loss of normal velopharyngeal closure can be much more serious, because without adequate intraoral pres-sure, most consonants lose their identity. This fact is amply illustrated in isolated paralyses of the soft palate; respiration, phonation, and articulation are normal, yet, speech is unin-telligible solely on the basis of diminished resonance balance. When there is a leak of air into the nasal cavity, it is difficult to build up intraoral pressure and to maintain speech motor coordination necessary for intelligible speech.

◆ Nasal Resonatory Disorders

Classification and Definition of Nasal Resonatory Disorders

Nasal resonatory disorders can be classified into four main auditory-perceptual types:

1. *Hypernasality and nasal air emission*

   a. *Hypernasality* Synonyms are rhinolalia aperta, hyper-rhinolalia, and open nasality. Defined as excess reso-nance of vowels and voiced consonants within the nasal cavities. The anatomic-physiologic basis is open coupling between the oral and nasal cavities due to incomplete closure of the hard palate and/or velopharyngeal sphincter.

b. *Nasal air emission*   Defined as abnormal flow of air from the nares during the production of high-pressure consonants, it is measurable biophysically via airflow (aerodynamic) techniques. It is heard as friction noise accompanying or replacing the target consonant and may have a "gurgling" quality if there is coexisting nasal congestion. It is sometimes referred to as a nasal rustle.

c. *Nasal and/or facial grimacing*   Defined as occlusion of the nares by contracting the alae of the nose, with associated wrinkling of the forehead, during consonant production, a compensatory action in an attempt to restrict the nasal flow of air.

2. *Hyponasality*   Synonyms are denasality, rhinolalia clausa, and closed nasality. Defined as diminution or absence of normal nasal resonance of the nasal semivowels /m/, /n/, /ŋ/ and loss of normal assimilation nasality. Its physical basis is over closure of the portal or obstruction between the oral and nasal cavities owing to space-occupying lesions within the nasopharynx or nasal cavities. Two subtypes are recognized:

a. *Rhinolalia clausa, posterior*   A type of closed nasality in which the nasal semivowels lose their normal resonance because of an obstruction in the posterior region of the nasal cavities or the nasopharynx. The nasal phonemes /m/, /n/, and /ŋ/ are heard as oral stops /b/, /d/, and /g/.

b. *Rhinolalia clausa, anterior*   A type of closed nasality in which all the vowels and nasals are produced with a hollow-sounding resonance owing to obstruction in the anterior region of the nasal cavities. It is also called cul-de-sac resonation.

3. *Mixed nasality*   A synonym is rhinolalia mixta. Defined as simultaneous velopharyngeal insufficiency and nasal obstruction resulting in a hollow resonation of all vowels and voiced consonants.

4. *Resonance imbalance*   Resonance imbalance is most often exhibited in persons with hyperfunctional voice disorders. Perceptually, they may sound neither hypr-o-nor hypernasal. Voice quality is most likely to sound throaty, tight, and thin. Stroboscopic recordings of the vocal folds often reveal a long, closed phase and considerable medial or anteroposterior (A-P) constrictions of the larynx.

Etiology of Nasal Resonatory Disorders

The etiologies of nasal resonatory disorders are outlined in **Table 4.1**. Their causes can be subdivided into organic and psychogenic. Organic causes of hypernasality and nasal emission are anatomic defects, such as clefts of the hard and soft palate, obstructive tonsils, nasal structural deviations; iatrogenic from surgical removal of some portion of the palate; and neurologic disease producing paresis or paralysis of the velopharyngeal musculature. Nonorganic causes of hypernasality and nasal emission are conversion reaction, immature personality development, poor motivation, and

Table 4.1   Etiology of Nasal Resonatory Disorders

Hypernasality and nasal emission
Organic
Anatomic
Overt cleft palate with or without cleft lip
Submucous cleft palate
Congenitally short soft palate or large nasopharynx
Traumatic structural damage
Neurologic (dysarthria)
Lower motor neuron (flaccid)
Unilateral upper motor neuron ("flaccid")
Bilateral upper motor neuron (spastic)
Mixed lower-upper motor neuron (flaccid-spastic)
Hyperkinetic (dystonic-choreic)
Psychogenic
Conversion reaction
Immature personality
Poor motivation
Imitative
Hyponasality
Organic
Hypertrophied adenoids
Tumors
Inflammations
Postsurgical repair
Patulous eustachian tube
Nasal deformity
Mixed nasality
Combinations of organic etiologies of hypernasality and hyponasality

imitation. Hypernasality is also common in persons with severe, congenital sensorineural hearing loss owing to poor auditory feedback. Velopharyngeal incompetence is associated with genetic conditions and identifiable syndromes (Shprintzen, 2000a, b). Thus, velopharyngeal incompetence may result from an isolated cause or may be multifactorial in origin resulting from learning, reduced sensory feedback, poor motor control, and/or morphologic deviations in the speech structures.

Causes of hyponasality are primarily organic: space-occupying lesions, such as tumors, inflammations, nasal polyps, and hypertrophied adenoid tissue, and structural deformities, such as deviated nasal septum.

Mixed nasality is caused by coexisting velopharyngeal insufficiency and obstruction of the nasal passageways.

♦ Anatomy and Physiology of the Velopharyngeal Mechanism

Surface Anatomy

The anatomy that pertains to normal and abnormal nasal resonatory functions consists of the oral, nasal, and pharyngeal cavities bounded by muscles and their bony attachments. The x-ray in **Fig. 4.1** illustrates the separation of the oral from the nasal chambers by the bony hard palate. Suspended from its posterior edge is the resting soft palate, or velum.

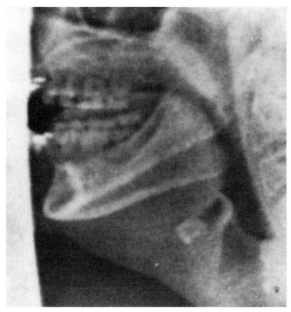

Figure 4.1 Lateral radiograph showing the hard and soft palate.

Because a lateral view of the velopharyngeal port only affords a two-dimensional appreciation of this valve, vertical and anteroposterior views are needed, shown in **Fig. 4.2**. The port is bounded anteriorly by the velum and laterally and posteriorly by the lateral and posterior pharyngeal walls. Its elliptical-shaped opening hints at its pattern of closure, which is often sphincteric, similar to a drawstring or camera aperture.

Another view of the hard and soft palate is through the open mouth, although this approach affords limited information in comparison with x-rays or nasal endoscopy. Clinicians using intraoral examination alone may make erroneous decisions about the competency of the structures because they are unable to see how adenoid pads or posterior pharyngeal wall and velum work together to achieve closure. Also, a wide-open mouth may artificially change the tension of the oral structures and subsequent movement patterns used to produce normal resonance. **Figure 4.3** shows the soft palate with its two symmetric arches. Suspended from its midline is the uvula. Running down from the arches on either side of the soft palate are two folds of tissue. The one closer to the front of the mouth is the anterior pillar of the fauces and the one

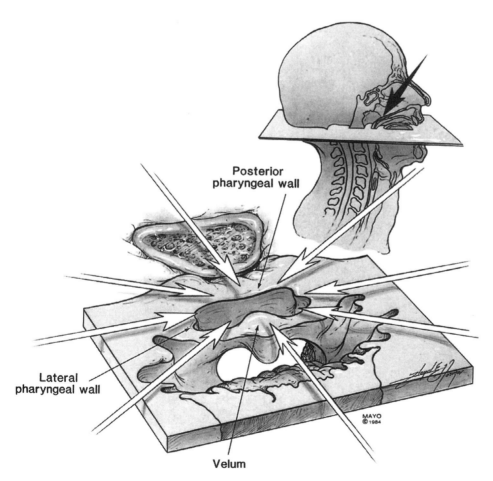

Posterior pharyngeal wall

Lateral pharyngeal wall

Velum

MAYO © 1984

Figure 4.2 Three-dimensional view of a section through the velopharyngeal port.

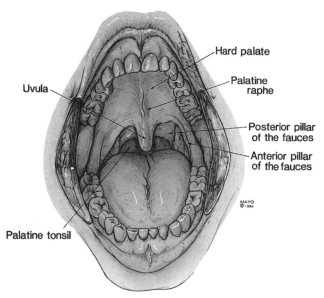

Figure 4.3 The soft palate and surrounding structures as seen on peroral examination.

toward the rear is the posterior pillar of the fauces. Nestled between them are the palatine tonsils.

The roof of the mouth is bordered by the upper dental arch and is covered by ridged mucosal tissue under which lies a thick periosteal tissue covering. The anterior two thirds of the roof consist of the hard palate and the posterior one third the soft palate. It is difficult to see where one ends and the other begins, but their junction is easy to feel by running the index finger along the midline of the hard palate from front to back until the finger sinks into soft tissue marking the border between the hard and soft palate.

Bones

The velopharyngeal musculature is suspended from three bones: the hard palate, the sphenoid bone, and the temporal bone.

Hard Palate

The hard palate is formed by the palatine processes of the maxillae and the horizontal plates of the palatine bones (**Fig. 4.4**). It is covered by a dense periosteum surfaced by mucous membrane. When stripped to the bone, the hard palate reveals that it is divided by sutures. The palatomaxillary suture divides the more anterior, larger palatine process of the maxilla from the smaller, more posterior horizontal plate of the palatine bone. Its posterior margin serves as the attachment of the soft palate. At its midline is a sharp spicule of bone called the posterior nasal spine.

The two halves of the palatine processes of the maxilla are joined in the midline at the intermaxillary suture. The two halves of the horizontal plates of the palatine bone are joined in the midline at the interpalatine suture. The opening in the anterior hard palate is the incisive fossa and in the lateral portions of the palatine bone the greater palatine foramina. Medial and posterior to these are the lesser palatine foramina.

Sphenoid Bone

The sphenoid bone lies at the base of the skull in front of the temporal bones and the basilar part of the occipital bone (**Fig. 4.5**). The lateral pterygoid plate and especially the medial pterygoid plate with its pterygoid hamulus are portions of the sphenoid bone directly concerned with the soft palate musculature.

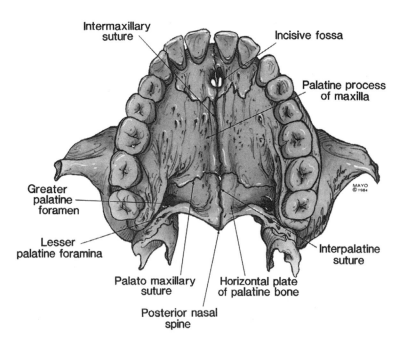

Figure 4.4 The hard palate; inferior view.

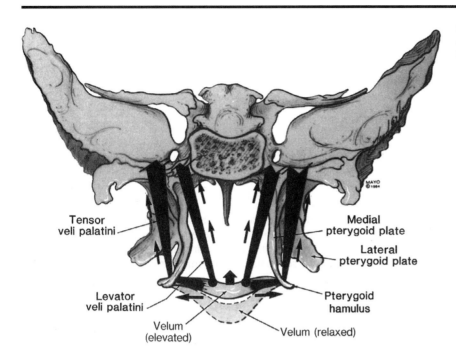

Figure 4.5 The sphenoid bone and schematic drawing of levator and tensor veli palatini muscles; posterior view.

Temporal Bone

The temporal bones form the sides and base of the skull, the latter of which is a point of attachment for the soft palate musculature.

Blood Supply

The blood supply of the hard and soft palate comes from different vascular vessels, and their vascular architectures have their own character (Zhong, Zhang, and Wang, 2001). The greater palatine artery provides the major supply to the hard palate and the ascending palatine artery is the principal source for the soft palate. The two anastomose at the junction of the hard and soft palate putting it at risk during palate repair. The greater palatine artery emerges on the oral surface of the palate through the greater palatine foramina, runs forward in a groove near the alveolar border of the hard palate through the incisive canal, and, linking up with the sphenopalatine artery, is distributed to the gums, palatine glands, and mucous membrane of the roof of the mouth. The branches of the greater palatine artery form rich anastomoses with neighboring vessels. The artery branches are arranged in lines with a tree-like appearance. The capillary network is loosely packed. In contrast, the arteries in the soft palate are crooked, exhibit directional changes, and the capillary network is densely packed.

Muscles

Levator Veli Palatini

This muscle arises from the base of the skull anterior to the carotid canal and descends anteromedially along the posteroinferior border of the eustachian tube. It inserts into the palatine aponeurosis of the middle third of the soft palate. Its fibers fan out and interweave with its mate of the opposite side and with the remaining muscles of the soft palate. Immediately prior to entering the velum, the levator divides into two parts. The smaller bundle of muscle fibers (anterolateral part) runs anteriorly, close to the lateral pharyngeal wall, and inserts into the palatine aponeurosis through several fine tendons creating a tendinous insertion. The main part of the muscle runs medially into the velum, where it fans out and forms the levator sling with the contralateral levator. Inadequate release of the tendinous insertions at the time of palate repair may tether the levator anteriorly and compromise muscle retropositioning or may split the levator rendering only part of it retropositioned.

Tensor Veli Palatini

This flat, triangular-shaped muscle originates from the base of the skull between the spine of the sphenoid bone, the root of the pterygoid process, and the eustachian tube. The muscle ends in a tendon that makes a right-angle turn around the pterygoid hamulus and then runs horizontally into the palatine aponeurosis along with the other muscles of the soft palate. Secondary insertions are present on the maxillary tuber and/or in the submucosal tissue near the palatoglossal arch. It appears to act as the dilator tubae (Abe, Murakami, Noguchi, et al., 2004). The length of the tensor veli palatine muscle attachment and its ratio to the length of the eustachian tube, particularly the cartilaginous portion, increases with age from infancy to adulthood, and decreases with age from young adulthood to later life and helps explain its functions relative to the eustachian tube (Suzuki, Sando, Balaban, et al., 2003). The tensor tympani and tensor veli palatine muscles make a functional unit (Kierner, Mayer, and Kirschhofer, 2002).

Palatoglossus

The palatoglossus forms the anterior pillars of the fauces. It is a small, thin muscle that arises from the palatine aponeurosis and descends to insert into the lateral border of the tongue, infiltrating its transverse muscle fibers.

Palatopharyngeus

This muscle forms the posterior pillars of the fauces. It is larger than the palatoglossus muscle. It has three components of pharyngeal origins and two heads of velar insertions that provide the continuity between the velum and laryngeal pharyngeal wall. It originates from the back and side walls of the pharynx and from the thyroid cartilage and ascends to the posterior and lateral portions of the soft palate. Some of its fibers insert into the tip of the medial cartilaginous wall of the eustachian tube and are considered by some anatomists to compose a separate muscle, the salpingopharyngeus. However, the bulk of the fibers extend to the posterior tonsillar pillars. This suggests that the palatopharyngeus is not only a major musculature of lateral pharyngeal wall motion but also plays an important role in velar function (Cheng and Zhang, 2004).

Constrictor Pharyngis Superior

The superior pharyngeal constrictor forms the lateral and posterior walls of the velopharyngeal port. It attaches to the pterygoid process, the pterygomandibular raphe, the mandible, and the tongue. Its most cranial portion, which attaches to the medial pterygoid plate and to the pterygoid hamulus, is most directly active in velopharyngeal closure.

Musculus Uvulae

Each bundle of the paired uvulae muscle originates lateral to the midline from the tendinous palatal aponeurosis posterior to the hard palate and just anterior to the insertion of the levator veli palatine. The paired muscles converge in an area overlying the sling of the levator muscle and course along the dorsum of the soft palate terminating as two separate bundles that subdivide and insert between the mucous glands of the uvula proper into the connective tissue and basement membrane of the mucosa (Azzam and Kuehn, 1977).

Velopharyngeal Biomechanics

Velopharyngeal closure is produced by contracting the levator veli palatini, tensor veli palatini, and superior pharyngeal constrictor muscles, actions shown in the schema of **Fig. 4.5**. The levator is the most important muscle of velopharyngeal closure during speech. It elevates the midportion of the soft palate in a superior-posterior direction. The tensor does not contribute directly to velar elevation and retraction during speech, although upon being pulled taut it may raise the velum to the level of the hard palate. It is alleged that it also depresses the anterior velum opening the eustachian tube during swallowing. The superior pharyngeal constrictor narrows the port further by moving its walls medially and anteriorly.

Contraction of the superior pharyngeal constrictor sometimes produces a slight bulge or transverse fold in the posterior pharyngeal wall that is crescent-shaped or shelf-like in appearance. It is called Passavant's ridge, first described in 1869 by Passavant as a discrete bar or protuberance that forms on the posterior pharyngeal wall during speech only and consists of pharyngeal mucous and/or pharyngeal superficial muscles. Nasopharyngoscopic and multiview videofluoroscopic studies have revealed two types of forward movement of the posterior pharyngeal wall: one is movement of Passavant's ridge and the other less sharply outlined is movement of the posterior pharyngeal wall created by contraction of a flexor muscle of the head (Yamawaki, 2003). Regardless of which type of forward movement, this prominence occurs in many normal speakers, in whom it may be of little importance, and in a much higher number of those who have velopharyngeal incompetence with and without cleft palate, in whom it probably contributes toward closure.

Velopharyngeal opening is not completely passive and due only to muscular relaxation and gravity. It is not known for sure, but the soft palate may have an active antagonist, the palatoglossus, which pulls the soft palate downward and forward. This movement may be related, at least in part, to the palatoglossus' role in respiratory activity and response to negative upper airway pressure. The negative pressure and depressed palate assists inward flow of air into the lungs. Gravitational forces on the palatoglossus differ little between the upright and supine position. However, the levator veli palatine has reduced peak activation levels in the supine body posture where gravitational effects work in the same direction toward closure (Moon and Canady, 1995).

Although contraction of the musculus uvulae shortens the uvula, the importance of its contribution to swallowing or speech is in question. On the one hand, many normal people are missing the uvula for congenital or surgical reasons without any untoward effects, but on the other hand, some individuals who have had uvulectomy surgery to reduce snoring have developed secondary velopharyngeal incompetence. Because of its location and size, it appears that contraction of the musculus uvulae adds bulk to the dorsal surface of the elevated soft palate aiding in occlusion of the velopharyngeal port during both speech and deglutition for some individuals (Azzam and Kuehn, 1977). Thus, congenital deficiency of the bulk of this muscle may be responsible for minor velopharyngeal insufficiency. Its capacity for tension production and the anaerobic metabolic activity of the muscle uvulae may also contribute to sleep apnea (Series et al, 1995, 1996, 1999).

Videofluoroscopic Studies

Static x-ray tomograms or radiographs cannot do justice to the ceaseless undulations of the soft palate as it opens and closes the port during contextual speech that alternates between nasal and non-nasal phonemes. But such photographs can allow for the beginning of understanding of the closure mechanism. In **Fig. 4.6**, an x-ray tomogram of a normal person just beginning to produce the vowel /i/, the soft palate is beginning to rise. Below, the soft palate is elevated

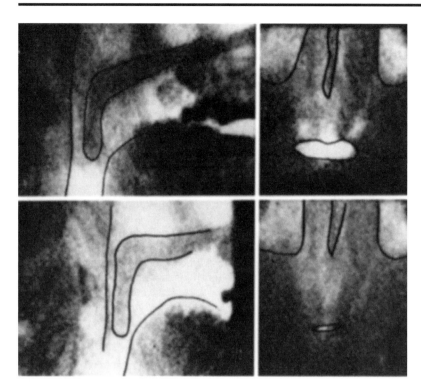

Figure 4.6 Videofluoroscopic frames showing lateral and base views of normal velopharyngeal closure. (From Skolnick, M.L. [1970]. Videofluoroscopic examination of the velopharyngeal portal during phonation in lateral and base projections. Cleft Palate J 7, 803–816.)

and retracted against the posterior pharyngeal wall. A basal view of this action shows the sphincteric configuration of this closure. From their multiview radiographic classic studies, Skolnick and colleagues (1969, 1970, 1973) have immeasurably enriched our understanding of velopharyngeal closure and concluded:

> We believe that concepts which view velopharyngeal closure as resulting from a combination of velar (flap valve) and lateral pharyngeal wall movement are only partially correct. It appears that the mechanism is really a sphincteric one poorly appreciated because of the difficulty in visualizing the velopharyngeal portal in the manner necessary to show the sphincteric movements.

Rather than conceptualizing soft palate and lateral and posterior pharyngeal wall movements as separate during closure, Skolnick showed radiographically that all move as a single, functional unit, and there is no precise demarcation between the lateral aspects of the velum and the beginnings of the pharyngeal wall. Although a lateral view is useful for demonstrating the vertical extent of the pharyngeal contribution to the sphincter, it is the basal view that permits a view of the port *en face* and gives us a true appreciation for the sphincteric concept of velopharyngeal closure.

Since this time, a variety of visualization techniques have been used to further our understanding of this mechanism. We now know that there is variable contribution to velopharyngeal closure from the velum, the lateral pharyngeal walls, and posterior pharyngeal wall from person to person and that these closure patterns change within individuals across the life span (Siegel-Sadewitz and Shprintzen, 1986).

Nasal Endoscopy

Nasal endoscopy has become a routine clinical measure to determine sphincteric closure. Using a flexible fiberoptic bundle connected to a light source and camera, clinicians are able to observe and record velar function from a superior position during a variety of speech contexts. Many argue that you can get the same information with nasal endoscopy that you can obtain from videofluoroscopy without radiation exposure. Others suggest that videofluoroscopy is preferable. Havstam, Lohmander, Persson, Dotevall, Lith, and Lilja (2005) investigated how different visual assessment information influences the recommended treatment for velopharyngeal insufficiency (VPI). They compared recommendations made from videofluoroscopy, videofluoroscopy combined with nasal endoscopy, and nasal endoscopy alone. They reported that treatment recommendations were the same for 68% regardless of the type of visual information but that the percent agreement was higher with videofluoroscopy in the lateral projection (84%) and when the lateral was combined with nasoendoscopy. They concluded that lateral projection videofluoroscopy should be the first step in visualizing VPI and nasoendoscopy should be a second step when additional information is needed. Others have suggested that nasoendoscopy should be the first step because it has the potential to determine not only if there is velopharyngeal incompetence but also the type of surgery needed. For example, a study by Armour, Fischback, Klaiman, and Fisher (2005) related speech outcomes to velopharyngeal closure pattern and type of pharyngoplasty. They concluded that pharyngeal flap pharyngoplasty was more effective in treating velopharyngeal insufficiency in patients with circular or sagittal velopharyngeal closure and less effective in treating coronal closure pattern. Coronal pattern velopharyngeal insufficiency was more appropriate for sphincter pharyngoplasty. Because these closure patterns are easily visualized with nasoendoscopy, it supports the notion of its routine use with this population.

Two additional arguments for using nasoendoscopy in cases of velopharyngeal competence come from observations of the velocardiofacial syndrome (also known as DiGeorge sequence and 22q11.2 deletion syndrome). This syndrome, or sequence, is now recognized as the most common syndrome associated with cleft palate and VPI. It is associated with cleft palate (69%), heart defects (74%), and characteristic facial deformities and learning difficulties (70 to 90%). There is phenotypic overlap with DiGeorge syndrome and velocardiofacial syndrome. It occurs because chromosome 22, particularly band 22q11.2, is predisposed to rearrangements because of misalignments of low-copy repeats (LCRs). The size and size of the deletion in many velocardiofacial syndrome and DeGeorge syndrome patients do not differ (Luerssen, 2004). This syndrome also has been associated with microwebs and with medially positioned internal carotid arteries that may be associated with posterior pharyngeal pulsations and both of which can be seen on endoscopy. Thus, an important role of endoscopy in preoperative assessment of children for palatopharyngoplasty is observation of posterior pharyngeal wall pulsations that should alert clinicians to the diagnosis of 22q11.2 deletion. Knowledge of this deviation could be useful for preventing risk of damage to carotid arteries during velopharyngeal surgery.

Similarly, Miyamoto et al (2004) have shown an association between anterior glottic webs and velocardiofacial syndrome (chromosome 22111.2 deletion). In 17 patients endoscopically diagnosed with anterior glottic web, 65% were positive for chromosome 22q11.2 deletion, and of those 11 patients only 5 showed subtle clinical manifestations of velocardiofacial syndrome, though with the aid of genetic testing all 11 were diagnosed with velocardiofacial syndrome.

Dynamic Magnetic Resonance Imaging

Dynamic magnetic resonance imaging (MRI) recordings with near-real-time temporal resolution (real-time MRI) using a turbo spin-echo (TSE) sequence (TR = 170 milliseconds, TE = 21 milliseconds, slice thickness = 6 mm, six images per second) has also been used for analyzing velopharyngeal closure during phonation. It compares favorably with multiview videofluoroscopy. It appears to have the potential to depict the pattern of velopharyngeal closure in close correlation with videofluoroscopy and may deliver additional information in selected cases (Beer et al, 2004).

Electromyographic Studies

Another approach to the study of normal velopharyngeal closure is by electromyography (EMG). Studies do not fully agree on the extent to which each of the velopharyngeal muscles participates during closure (Bell-Berti, 1976; Benguerel, Hirose, Sawashima, and Ushijima, 1977; Cooper, 1965; Li and Lundervold, 1958; Lubker, 1968; Lubker and Curtis, 1966; Seaver, 1979). This lack of agreement may be due to differences between subjects and the protocol used. A representative study of closure in normal subjects was done by Fritzell (1969), who placed EMG electrodes in the velopharyngeal musculature and measured their potentials during speech. A sample of recordings from different muscles is shown in **Fig. 4.7**. From his study he found:

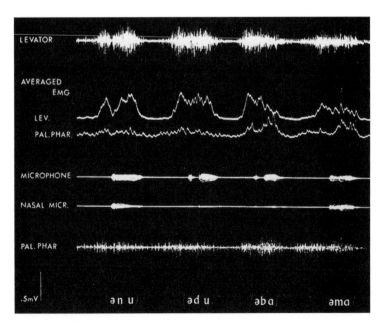

Figure 4.7 Electromyographic recording of the levator veli palatini and palatopharyngeus muscles during speech. (From Fritzell, B. [1969]. The velopharyngeal muscles in speech. Acta Otolaryngol 250 [Suppl], 13.)

1. The levator veli palatini was continuously active during speech.

   a. Activity began before onset of sound.

   b. Activity ceased before termination of phonation.

   c. Degree of activity fluctuated during speech.

   d. Little or no activity occurred during nasal semivowels.

2. The tensor veli palatini behaved with considerable inter-subject variability and in many cases with little or no activity.

3. Superior pharyngeal constrictor muscle activity was similar to levator (i.e., active during all except the nasal sounds).

4. The palatoglossus produced bursts of activity preceding nasal semivowels but was weak or inactive for oral sounds. However, there is conflicting opinion on the validity of this finding.

5. The palatopharyngeus varied considerably among subjects; it always showed some activity but of low intensity.

Fritzell drew the following conclusions from his study:

1. The levator is the most important muscle of closure during speech.

2. The tensor is nearly silent and has no typical relationship to speech.

3. The superior constrictor has patterns similar to the levator.

4. The palatoglossus actively pulls down the velum; lowering is not due only to gravity.

5. The palatopharyngeus has little activity during speech.

6. A high positive correlation (0.76) exists between extent of EMG levator activity and extent of velar displacement.

7. Velar movement begins within 40 milliseconds after onset of EMG levator activity and speech follows ~300 milliseconds later, varying widely, depending upon the initial phoneme and speaking situation.

More recently, Velepic et al (1999) used EMG to investigate the velopharyngeal sphincter structures in 75 patients. They added an additional observation to those of Fritzell suggesting EMG was useful for diagnosing the exact causes of velopharyngeal insufficiency and for choosing the best approach for treatment.

Nasal Airflow Studies

The extent of nasal airflow can be measured by a variety of instruments. Most frequently, instrumental assessments use a pneumotachograph, which consists of a flowmeter and a differential pressure transducer. Airflow from the nose passes across a wire mesh screen. The resulting pressure drop is linearly related to the volume rate of airflow and is converted by a pressure transducer into an electrical voltage that is recorded and visualized on a computer monitor.

Pressure flow studies summarized 40 years ago by Warren (1964) have yielded the following important data:

♦ Normal intraoral pressure for pressure consonants is between 3 and 7 cm H_2O.

♦ Normal consonant intraoral pressure cannot be maintained if the velopharyngeal portal is open more than 0.02 cm^2 (**Fig. 4.8**).

♦ Audible nasal emission and hypernasality occur when openings are between 0.1 and 0.2 cm^2.

♦ Influencing the amount of nasal airflow are extent of oral airway opening, amount of nasal airway obstruction, and volume of the oral cavity.

♦ Normal speakers have imperceptibly small amounts of nasal airflow during production of non-nasal phonemes.

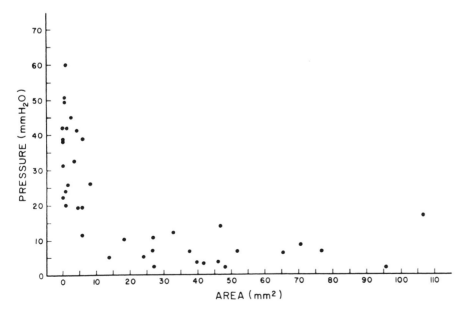

Figure 4.8 Relationship between velopharyngeal orifice size and intraoral pressure during consonant productions. (From Warren, D.W. [1964]. Velopharyngeal orifice size and upper pharyngeal pressure-flow patterns in normal speech. Plast Reconstr Surg 33, 148–162.)

♦ Speakers vary in the duration of portal opening during production of nasal phonemes.

Subsequent work by Warren and others has led clinicians to incorporate aerodynamic studies into their velopharyngeal assessment clinical protocols. A combination of simultaneously recorded nasal airflow and intraoral pressure during a variety of speech contexts appears to give the most valuable information. Clinicians are able to calculate nasal resistance and to determine how phonetic contexts, increased orality, and change in volume and pitch impact velopharyngeal valving. Several investigators have suggested that aerodynamic measures change with age (Smith et al., 2003, 2004). Pressure drops with age and nasal flow increases as do orifice areas. Variability in pressure decreases and variability in nasal airflow increases. Smith, Patil, Guyetle et al., (2004) have shown that by age 14, children tend to exhibit pressures and flows similar to those of young adults.

Acoustic Studies

Hypernasality arises from coupling between the oral and nasal cavities. Acoustic studies of hypernasalized vowels produced by normal speakers show the following spectral distortions (Dickson, 1962; House and Stevens, 1956; Peterson and Barney, 1952; Smith, 1951):

♦ reduced intensity of the first vowel formant

♦ one or more loci of antiresonance; that is, a sharp drop in the intensity of a portion of the spectrum

♦ extra resonances, contributed by the nasal cavities; that is, reinforced harmonics at frequencies at which energy is not normally expected

♦ a shift in the center frequencies of the formants

Even patients with marginal velopharyngeal closure show changes in the acoustic signal (Zhu, Sun, and Wang, 1998); there are extra formants or strong nasal formants; spike and stop gap in stops and affricatives may be absent; there is increased noise in the lowest frequency; and the acoustic features differ for the same vowel produced in isolation compared with that produced in connected speech.

Knowledge of the acoustic changes that occur with velopharyngeal incompetence has led to the development of several instruments designed to provide both quantitative and qualitative information on nasalance. One such commonly used device is the nasometer. The Nasometer II (Key Elemetries, Lincoln Park, NJ) is a noninvasive device that provides relative quantification of nasalance and visual feedback of the magnitude. A sensing device is placed under the nose and above the upper lip. The amount of nasalance relative to oral emission is expressed in percentage and imaged on a computer screen relative to a zero baseline. Data from this instrument have been reported for populations around the world. From these studies, several generalizations can be made about the clinical use of normative nasalance values (Tachimura, Mori, Hirata, et al., 2000; Van Lierde, Wuyts, De Bodt, et al., 2001; Whitehill, 2001):

♦ They should be based on speakers of the same language and geographic dialect.

♦ They are gender specific with females generally having less nasalance.

♦ They are context specific.

♦ They are age dependent.

♦ They are influenced by vocal intensity and orality.

Perceptual Analysis of Speech

Equally important as the instrumental assessment is the perceptual analysis of speech. For example, velopharyngeal gap size may be predicted from speech assessment alone. Nasal rustle suggests a small gap size and moderate to severe hypernasality a large opening (Kummer, Briggs, and Lee, 2003). In the Kummer study, perceptual characteristics of speech correctly predicted gap size for 121 of 173 subjects (70%). The specific speech characteristics to listen for are explained elsewhere in this chapter. The point we want to underscore here is that from the first utterance produced by the patient, the clinician is making perceptual judgments of communication competence, observing and gathering valuable information of both a quantitative and qualitative nature. Instrumental measures augment these observations but don't replace them.

♦ Organic and Nonorganic Hypernasality and Nasal Air Emission

Cleft Lip and Palate

Clefts of the hard and soft palate are one of the most common and serious of all causes of hypernasality and nasal emission. Because full coverage of this subject is not possible here, we especially recommend the selected readings at the end of this chapter.

Definition and Classification

Cleft lip and palate represent a failure of the lip and hard and soft palate segments to join during those stages of embryonic development when closure should have occurred. An infant with cleft palate at birth has a direct communication between the oral and nasal cavities. The air stream during speech passes, unchecked, into the nasal cavities and out of the nares. The speech effects are (1) hypernasality of vowels and voice consonants; (2) nasal emission of the air stream; and (3) weak pressure consonants due to loss of intraoral pressure. Communication may be further compromised by delayed articulatory and language development, hearing loss, and reactive psychologic and educational disturbances. In the not too distant past, this sequelae was a common occurrence in individuals with clefts. However, improved surgical procedures that can be done at an earlier age have dramatically reduced the number and severity of communication

Table 4.2 American Cleft Palate Association Classification of Cleft Lip and Palate

Clefts of Prepalate		
Cleft lip	Unilateral	Right, left
		Extent in thirds
	Bilateral	Right, left
		Extent in thirds
	Median	Extent in thirds
	Prolabium	Small, medium, large
	Congenital scar	Right, left, median
		Extent in thirds
Cleft of alveolar	Unilateral	Right, left
		Extent in thirds
	Bilateral	Right, left
		Extent in thirds
	Median	Extent in thirds
		Submucous right, left, median
Cleft of prepalate		Any combination of foregoing types
		Prepalate protrusion
		Prepalate rotation
		Prepalate arrest (median cleft)
Clefts of Palate		
Cleft of soft palate	Extent	Posteroanterior in thirds
		Width (maximum in millimeters)
	Palatal shortness	None, slight, moderate, marked
	Submucous cleft	Extent in thirds
Cleft hard palate	Extent	Posteroanterior in thirds
		Width (maximum in millimeters)
	Vomer attachment	Right, left, absent
	Submucous cleft	Extent in thirds
Cleft of soft and hard palate	Clefts of prepalate and palate	Any combination of clefts described under clefts of prepalate and clefts of palate

problems related to clefting. Despite these advances, however, the majority of preschoolers with cleft palate continue to require direct speech therapy (Hardin-Jones and Jones, 2005).

Several classifications of cleft lip and palate have been proposed. The most comprehensive is the American Cleft Palate Association's classification found in **Table 4.2**.

Embryology

The embryologic sequence of face and palate development is illustrated in **Fig. 4.9** and is described as follows:

1. *Face*

   a. *Fourth week (early)* Facial primordia begin to appear surrounding the primitive mouth or stomodeum.

      (1) Frontonasal prominence. Forms the upper boundary of the stomodeum. Originates from proliferation of mesenchyme ventral to the brain

      (2) Maxillary prominences. Form the lateral boundaries of the stomodeum. Originate from first branchial arch

      (3) Mandibular prominences. Form the lower boundary of the stomodeum. Originate from the first branchial arch

      (4) Mandibular prominences. Form the lower boundary of the stomodeum. Originate from the first branchial arch

   b. *Fourth week (late)*

      (1) Nasal placodes. Bilateral, oval-shaped thickenings develop from surface ectoderm in the lower part of each frontonasal prominence.

      (2) Medial and lateral nasal prominences. Horseshoe-shaped prominences at margins of nasal placodes develop from mesenchyme.

      (3) Nasal pits. Depressions in the nasal placodes

      (4) Maxillary prominences. Grow toward each other and toward medial nasal prominences

      (5) Nasolacrimal groove. Cleft or furrow separating lateral nasal prominence from maxillary prominences

   c. *Sixth and seventh weeks*

      (1) Intermaxillary segment of upper jaw. Formed by merging of medial nasal prominences. This segment gives rise to:

         (a) Philtrum: the middle portion of upper lip

         (b) Middle portion of upper jaw and gum

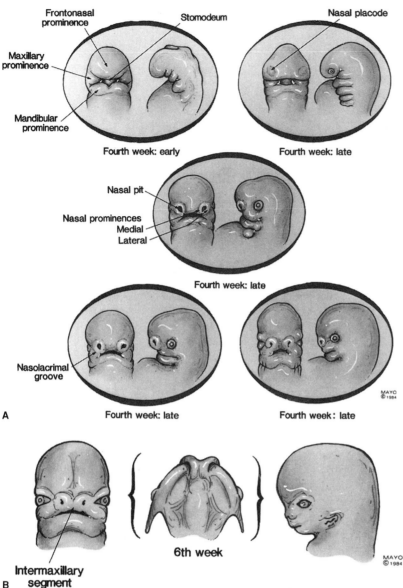

Figure 4.9 (A–B) Embryonic and fetal development of the face and palate.

(c) Primary palate

(2) Maxillary prominences. Formed by lateral parts of upper lip, upper jaw, and secondary palate. Merge laterally with mandibular prominences reducing size of mouth

(3) Primitive lips and cheeks. Invaded by second branchial arch mesenchyme, giving rise to facial muscles

(4) Frontonasal prominence. Forms forehead and dorsum and apex of nose. Sides of nose (alae) derive from lateral nasal prominences

(5) Final development of face

   (a) Nose changes from flat to more mature form

   (b) Mandible more prominent

   (c) Forehead more prominent

   (d) Eyes move medially

   (e) Ears rise

2. *Palate*   The palate develops from two parts, the primary and secondary palate, between the fifth and the twelfth weeks.

   a. *Fifth week (late)*

      (1) Primary palate (median palatine process). From the innermost part of the intermaxillary segment of the upper jaw formed by merging of medial nasal prominences. Forms a wedge-shaped mass of mesoderm between maxillary prominences and developing upper jaw

Figure 4.9 (C–D) (*Continued*) Embryonic and fetal development of the face and palate.

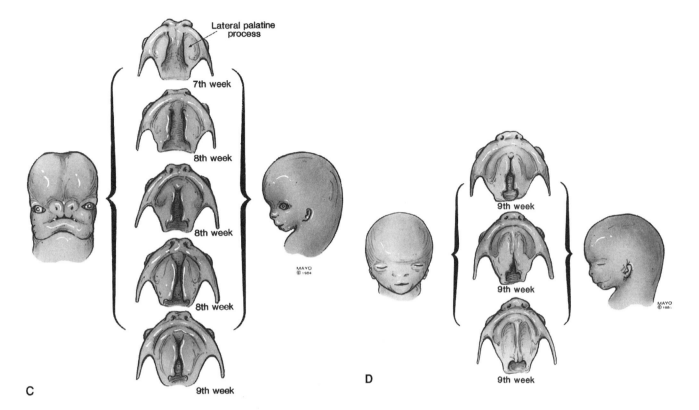

C

D

(2) Secondary palate. Formed by two horizontal projections of mesoderm from the inner surfaces of the maxillary prominences called lateral palatine processes

(a) Initially project downward on each side of tongue

(b) Later, grow toward each other and fuse

(c) Also fuse with primary palate and nasal septum

(d) Fusion begins anteriorly during ninth week and is completed posteriorly by the twelfth week

Cleft Lip

Cleft lip is not a cause of hypernasality and nasal emission, but it is associated with clefts of the palate. They can range from a small notch in the vermillion border of the upper lip to a complete cleft into the floor of the nostril and through the upper alveolar ridge (**Fig. 4.10**):

♦ *Unilateral cleft lip* Unilateral cleft lip represents a failure of the maxillary prominence on the affected side to fuse with the medial nasal prominence.

♦ *Bilateral cleft lip* Bilateral cleft lip results from failure of the maxillary prominences to fuse with the medial nasal

prominence. The clefts on both sides may be similar or have different degrees of defect.

♦ *Median cleft lip* Median cleft of the upper lip is rare and represents a partial or complete failure of the medial nasal prominences to fuse and form the intermaxillary segment. Median cleft of the lower lip is also rare and represents a partial failure of the mandibular prominences to fuse.

Cleft Palate

Cleft palate represents failure of the lateral palatine processes to fuse with each other, with the nasal septum, and/or with the posterior margin of the median palatine process or primary palate (**Fig. 4.11**).

Palatal clefts may be of the uvula only, or they may extend through the soft and hard palates, and through the alveolar process and lip bilaterally. They may be overt or submucous:

♦ *Clefts of the anterior (primary) palate* These are clefts anterior to the incisive foramen.

♦ *Clefts of the anterior and posterior palate* These are clefts that involve both the primary and secondary palate.

♦ *Clefts of the posterior or secondary palate* These are clefts posterior to the incisive foramen.

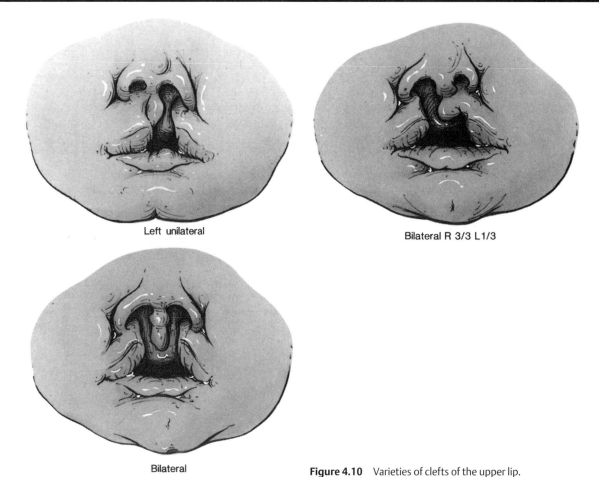

Left unilateral

Bilateral R 3/3 L1/3

Bilateral

Figure 4.10   Varieties of clefts of the upper lip.

Incidence

The worldwide incidence of cleft lip and palate is ~1 in 700 and varies according to race, sex, geographic area, and source of statistical reports (Olasoji, Ukiri, and Yahaya, 2005). Ross and Johnston (Cooper, Harding, Krogman, Mazahari, and Millard, 1979), after reviewing many surveys and selecting only those that they believed were adequately performed, showed a distinct gradient in the incidence of cleft lip and cleft palate among various racial groups:

♦ The lowest incidence was among black African Americans, ranging from 0.21 to 0.41 per 1000 live births.

♦ The highest was among Asians, with a range of 1.14 to 2.13 per 1000 live births.

♦ In the intermediate group were American and Western European Caucasians, with an incidence between 0.77 and 1.40 per 1000 births.

Associated Anomalies

Individuals with clefts show an increased incidence of associated malformations, the most common being cardiac problems, positional foot defects, extremity malformation, circulatory defects, and malformed ears, micrognathia, hypertelorism, exophthalmia, and microcephaly. Clefts of the palate are common in several syndromes, among which are the velocardiofacial syndrome, also known as DiGeorge sequence and 22q11.2 deletion syndrome (previously described), and Goldenhar, robin sequence, and Van der Woude syndromes. Because velopharyngeal incompetence is associated with genetic conditions and identifiable syndromes and because knowledge of the problems associated with the syndromes may impact management decisions, it is essential that the syndromes and comorbid conditions associated with clefting be identified. (For a comprehensive picture of syndromes associated with clefting and their influence on communication, see the Suggestions for Additional Reading at the end of this chapter.)

Etiology

Both genetic and environmental factors have been implicated in the etiology of both cleft lip with or without cleft palate and isolated cleft palate. Although its multifactorial nature is puzzling, scientists have made significant breakthroughs with respect to breaking the code related to the genetics of these conditions, in particular, characterization of the underlying gene defects associated with several important clefting syndromes (Cobourne, 2004). Cobourne suggests of particular significance is the identification of mutations in the interferon regulatory factor-6 (IRF6) gene as the cause of van der Woude syndrome and the poliovirus receptor

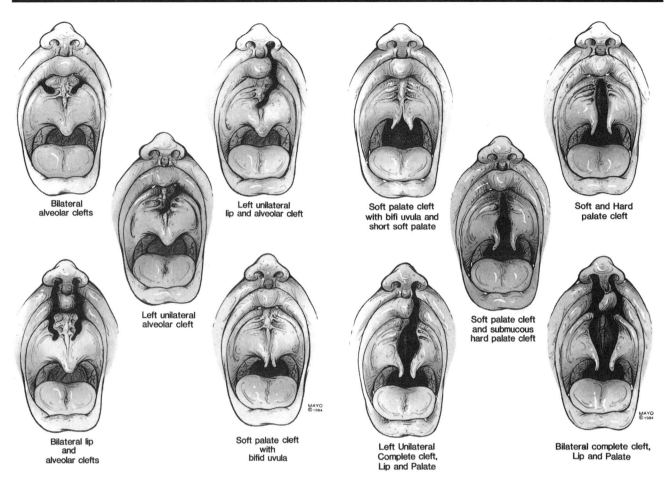

Bilateral
alveolar clefts

Left unilateral
lip and alveolar cleft

Soft palate cleft
with bifi uvula and
short soft palate

Soft and Hard
palate cleft

Left unilateral
alveolar cleft

Bilateral lip
and
alveolar clefts

Soft palate cleft
with
bifid uvula

Soft palate cleft
and submucous
hard palate cleft

Left Unilateral
Complete cleft,
Lip and Palate

Bilateral complete cleft,
Lip and Palate

Figure 4.11   Varieties of clefts of the alveolar processes and hard and soft palates.

related-1 (PVRL1) gene as being responsible for an autosomal recessive ectodermal dysplasia syndrome associated with clefting. Although no specific disease-causing gene mutations have been identified in nonsyndrome clefting, several candidate genes have been isolated through both linkage and association studies. Cobourne continues to say that although no specific disease-causing gene mutations have been identified in nonsyndromic clefting, several candidate genes have been isolated through both linkage and associated studies. And whereas it seems clear that environmental factors also play a role, the interactions that occur between candidate genes and environmental factors during embryonic development remain unknown.

Heredity   Although heredity does not even account for 50% of occurrences of cleft lip and/or palate, it is one of the most important causes of cleft lip and palate to understand because of the role of the speech-language pathologist in counseling. Two identified genetic groups are (1) cleft lip alone and (2) cleft lip and cleft palate. Both are more common in males. They have a positive family history in ~40% of cases. Cleft palate alone is more common in females. There is a positive family history in ~20% of cases (Edwards and Watson, 1980). Genetic counseling can identify high-risk families.

The mechanism of inheritance is not always clear. Cleft lip and palate pedigrees tend to show a recessive mode, although dominance does occur. Cleft palate alone shows simple dominance.

As yet, there is no way of predicting with accuracy whether a subsequent member of a family will have a cleft lip or cleft palate. The only exception to this is when a specific syndrome is recognized that lends itself to simpler patterns of inheritance. However, statistical tables for risk rates are available:

Risk rates for cleft lip (with or without cleft palate) (Fogh-Andersen, 1942) are as follows:

♦ For siblings, one child affected, parents normal, 4%.

♦ For siblings, one child affected, one parent affected, 14%.

♦ For offspring, one parent affected, 2%.

Risk-rate for cleft palate alone (Fogh-Andersen, 1942) is as follows:

♦ For siblings, one child affected, parents normal, 2%.

♦ For siblings, one child affected, one parent affected, 17%.

♦ For offspring, one parent affected, 7%.

Cleft palate (Fraser, 1970) rates are as follows:

♦ When one parent has a cleft palate, each child has roughly 1 chance in 16 of being affected.

♦ If the parents are unaffected but have a near relative with a cleft palate, the chances that these parents' future children would be affected is ~1 in 15.

♦ If the parents of a cleft palate baby are unaffected and do not have an affected near relative, the chance that they will have another child with a cleft palate is ~1 in 50.

♦ If an affected parent has an affected child, then the risk for future children goes up to ~1 in 6.

In cleft lip with or without cleft palate, if two offspring are affected, the risk goes up for subsequent offspring from 4 to 9%. There is no change in risk with cleft palate alone.

Environment   Sixty percent of cleft lip cases alone, or cleft lip and cleft palate, and 80% of cleft palate cases alone appear to be solitary occurrences with no family histories of clefts. Although intrauterine causes, for example, anatomic and physiologic variations of the uterus, metabolic alterations, infections, insufficient folic acid, drugs, diet, smoking, and x-radiation are suspected, no compelling evidence for exogenous causes in these solitary cases has been found. Incomplete family histories may account for some in this group, who really belong in the hereditary category. Others may be part of a syndrome that has not been identified.

Speech and Language Defects

No two patients with cleft palate, with or without cleft lip, have the same type and degree of communicative disorder. The end product of these palatal defects depends upon several factors: extent and location of the palatal defect; dental abnormalities; hearing loss; intelligence; cultural environment; emotional stability; prior medical and surgical therapies. Speech and language defects that can occur include but are not limited to:

♦ hypernasality of vowels and voiced consonants

♦ nasal emission on pressure consonants

♦ weak pressure consonants

♦ nonstandard laryngeal, pharyngeal, and lingual sound substitutions for standard consonants (i.e., compensatory articulations)

♦ delayed articulatory and language development

♦ articulatory defects secondary to dental defects

♦ articulatory defects secondary to hearing loss

♦ dysphonia

♦ nasal and facial grimacing associated with speaking

Articulatory Defects   Because of surgical advancements, articulatory defects are no longer inevitable in children with cleft lip and palate but still commonly occur. Rarely does cleft lip alone produce defects of articulation unless its repair produces an exceptionally short, tight upper lip that prevents the lower one from reaching it for the bilabial sounds /p/, /b/, and /m/. Perceptually acceptable, although cosmetically distracting, are the child's compensatory attempts to approximate the upper incisors with the lower lip to make bilabial sounds, called labiodentalization.

The remaining articulatory defects in children with cleft lip and palate are from the following causes described under the next six subheads.

Reduced Intraoral Pressure   Even when articulatory placements are correct, reduced intraoral pressure secondary to nasal air escape will cause consonant distortion. The greater the nasal air escape, the less intraoral air available for pressure consonants. Somewhere along the intraoral pressure deficiency continuum, intelligibility begins to deteriorate, ending in unintelligibility.

Minor velopharyngeal insufficiency producing intraoral pressure loss that results in mildly weak consonants presents a different set of problems than do large openings with correspondingly poor consonant precision. The mild or borderline insufficiencies cause more decision-making problems. Clinicians find themselves asking, "Is he hypernasal or isn't he? Are the consonants weak or aren't they? Yesterday she sounded hypernasal, today she doesn't. She's hypernasal only when she's tired or talks fast. If she puts forth considerable exhalatory pressure she is less hypernasal." What these statements reveal is that the patient has mild and inconsistent velopharyngeal insufficiency. In some instances, the slightest drop in effort during exhalation or velopharyngeal closure elicits the audible effects of the borderline velopharyngeal status. In many instances, this type of problem is easily corrected with speech therapy. In other cases, the patient is working maximally to correct the valving problem and a loss in adenoid tissue and head growth may put her over the edge and require surgical management. Another possible contributing factor is muscle fatigue. Tachimura and Nohara (2004) have shown that the velopharyngeal port mechanism appears to fatigue faster in children with velopharyngeal incompetence.

A secondary consequence of nasal emission is audible noises from air passing through the nares, distorting and masking consonants and distracting the listener.

Compensatory Articulatory and Phonatory Substitutions   Remarkably, children born with palatopharyngeal insufficiencies seem intuitively to grasp early in life the pressure physiology of their own speech mechanisms. Without instruction, they discover they can produce nonstandard sounds with the larynx, pharynx, velum, and tongue that simulate the manner of production of standard consonants, which they cannot make. The correct place of production is, however, often sacrificed. Those who acquire velopharyngeal insufficiency later in life have much less tendency to develop compensatory errors. The drawings in **Fig. 4.12** correspond with the following substitutions, derived from Trost's (1981) radiographic studies.

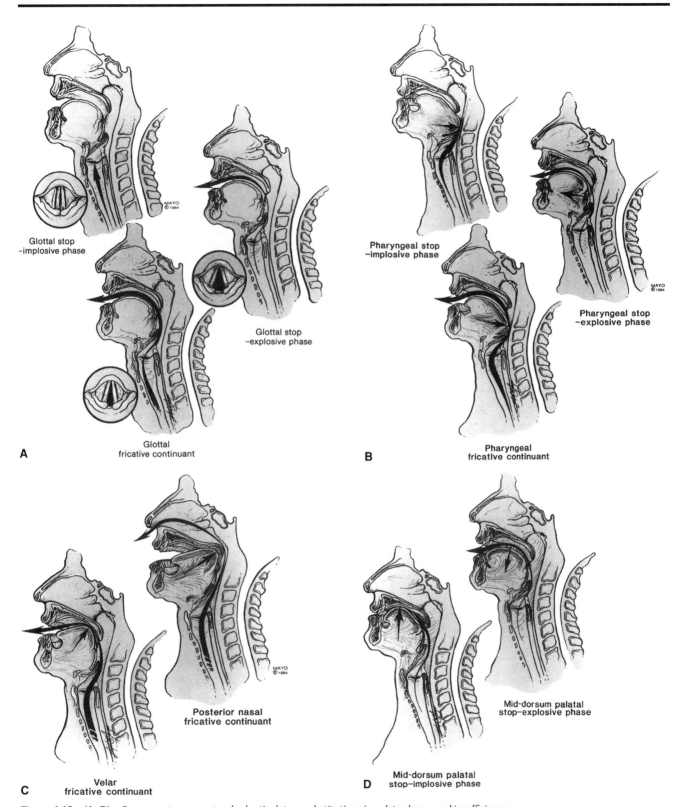

Figure 4.12 (**A–D**) Compensatory, nonstandard articulatory substitutions in palatopharyngeal insufficiency.

1. *The glottal stop* An explosive-like grunt or glottal coup /ʔ/, made by tightly adducting the vocal folds, building up infraglottal air pressure, and suddenly releasing it by abducting the vocal folds. Glottal stop substitutions are used in place of the standard stop consonants /p/, /b/, /t/, /d/, /k/, and /g/. The glottal stop is often produced simultaneously with the correct articulatory placement for the sound (coarticulation).

2. *The glottal fricative* A continuous friction noise made by approximating, but not fully adducting, the vocal folds. It is used as substitution for the standard fricative continuants /ʃ/, /z/, /f/, and /ʒ/.

3. *The pharyngeal stop* A linguapharyngeal stop consonant substitution for /k/ and /g/. It can be simulated by first walking the tongue backward from the /k/ position downward against the posterior pharyngeal wall and then suddenly releasing air that has been built up below the level of the tongue.

4. *The pharyngeal fricative* A continuous friction noise substituted in place of standard fricative-continuants, formed by retraction of the tongue against the back wall of the pharynx.

5. *Velar fricative* A continuous friction noise substituted in place of standard fricative-continuants, formed by retraction of the tongue against the posterior palate.

6. *The posterior nasal fricative* A velopharyngeal fricative produced by airway constriction as the soft palate approximates the pharyngeal wall, but which does not close the port. The air is then nasally released. The movement is sometimes aided by posterior posturing of the tongue. The sound is heard as an audible friction noise associated with nasal air escape. Radiographically, this velar articulation is seen as a blurring of movement called velar flutter. The posterior nasal fricative is used as a substitution for /ʃ/, /z/, /f/, and /ʒ/.

7. *The mid-dorsum palatal stop* A linguapalatal stop made by placing the tongue in the approximate position for the glide /j/. It is used as a replacement for /t/, d/, /k/, and /g/.

The tendency for children with cleft palate to posteriorize lingual placements has been known for a long time. The tongue can exert an upward force on whatever soft palate tissue remains in an effort to seal off the port and, at the same time, impound air behind the tongue at this presumably more advantageous location. Compensatory coarticulations or atypical simultaneous articulatory maneuvers have also been observed; for example, a glottal stop substitution for /b/ while at the same time approximating and separating the lips even though the air is released at the glottal and not at the bilabial level (Trost, 1981).

Bzoch (1979) made a useful comparison between the articulation errors of 120 children aged 3 to 6 without clefts who were considered "normal" in their articulatory development for their age range and 60 matched children with cleft palate. **Table 4.3**, which contains normative information on mastery of articulatory skills reported in now classic studies by Templin (1957) and Poole (1934), shows the differences between the normal and cleft palate children. Note the rampant glottal stop and laryngeal and pharyngeal fricative sub-

Table 4.3   Comparison of Articulatory Errors Most Often Found in Preschool Children with or without Cleft Palate

Speech Sound Element Tested	Templin Norm	Pool Norm	Errors of Control Subjects (N = 120, 3 to 6 Years)	Errors of Cleft Palate Subjects in Order of Frequency of Occurrence (N = 60, 3 to 6 Years)
/p/	3	3.5	None	ʔ/p, PF
/b/	4	3.5	p/b	m/b, ʔ/b
/t/	6	4.5	d/t	ʔ/t, PF, k/t
/d/	4	4.5	t/d	ʔ/d, PF, n/d
/k/	4	4.5	t/k	ʔ/k, PF, t/k
/g/	4	4.5	k/g, d/g	ʔ/g, d/g, PF
/f/	3	5.5	p/f, b/f, s/f	ʔ/f, PF, p/f
/v/	6	6.5	b/v, f/v	b/v, ʔ/v, m/v
/θ/	6	7.5	t/θ, s/θ, f/θ	ʔ/θ, PF, t/θ
/ð/	7	6.5	d/ð	d/ð, ʔ/ð, PF
/s/	4.5	7.5	θ/s, t/s	PF, ʔ/s, t/s
/z/	7	7.5	s/z, θ/z, d/z	PF, ʔ/z, s/z
/ʃ/	4.5	6.5	s/ʃ, t/ʃ	PF, ʔ/ʃ
/tʃ/	4.5	–	ʃ/tʃ, s/tʃ, t/tʃ	PF, ʔ/tʃ, ʃ/tʃ
/d3/	7	–	tʃ/d3, d/d3, 3/d3	PF, ʔ/d3, 3/d3
/l/	6	6.5	w/l	w/l, ʔ/l
/j/	3.5	4.5	ʔ/j	ʔ/j, w/j, l/j
/r/	4	7.5	w/r	w/r, j/r, PF
/w/	3	3.5	j/w	ʔ/w, l/w
/m/	3	3.5	b/m	PF, ʔ/m
/n/	3	4.5	m/n	ʔ/n, j/n
/ŋ/	3	4.5	n/ŋ	n/ŋ

Source: From Bzoch, K.R. (1979). Communicative disorders related to cleft lip and palate. Boston: Little Brown, p. 166.

PF, either pharyngeal or velar fricative substitution.

stitutions in the cleft palate population. Because of improved surgery, there are fewer children with clefts exhibiting the articulatory errors recorded over 50 years ago, but when the errors are present they are similar to those described.

Dental Abnormalities　Most people with cleft palate have a defect of the dental and maxillary-mandibular relationship; missing teeth; malposed teeth; malocclusions; narrow, highly arched palates; scarred palates. Articulatory distortions arise from aberrant friction noise, or absence of friction noise, on sound requiring that the air stream be deflected off of the anterior teeth. The anterior lingual consonants most affected are /t/, /d/, /s/, /z/, /ʃ/, /ʒ/, /t/, and /d/. Interdentalization of these sound is also common when the maxilla is abnormally small compared with the mandible, inducing a forward tongue carriage.

Conductive Hearing Loss　Serous otitis media producing conductive hearing loss is practically universal in the cleft palate population because of defective aeration and equilibration with atmospheric pressure of the middle ear. The cause is failure of the eustachian tube to open during swallowing due to defective velar musculature. If hearing loss is severe, it may interfere with expressive language and articulatory development or, if mild, can produce phonemic distortions.

Delayed Speech and Language Development　When research findings on articulatory and language development in children with cleft palate are collated, they provide convincing evidence that, evidence that, as a group, these children are delayed compared to typically developing children. Differences in tests used and research methodology, failures to recognize children with syndromes, and breadth of semantic assessments require that the following summary statements be interpreted cautiously,

♦ Articulatory development is slower (Bzoch, 1956; Counihan, 1960).

♦ First words are later (Bzoch, 1956).

♦ Sentences are-shorter and less complex (Spriestrsbach, Darley, and Morris, 1958).

♦ Language comprehension and usage is delayed (Philips and Harrison, 1969).

♦ Expressive language development is delayed (Smith and MeWilliams, 1968).

♦ Children with compensatory articulation disorders have abnormal language development that is greater in situational context compared to semantic or discourse (Pamplona, Ysunza, Gonzalez, Ramirez, Patino (2000).

Studies by Bzoch, Morley, Fex, et al. (1973) pointed to an even more definitive picture of expressive language delay. In 23 of 25 infants, mean age 18 months, they found an almost consistent and significant delay in expressive language but, interestingly, not in receptive, despite histories of widespread conductive hearing loss. Swanson (1973) reported similar findings in 37 infants as did Morris and Ozanne (2003) in 10 or 20 children with clefts. Morris and Ozanne selected children who had been identified at 2 years of age as either at age level or significantly delayed in

expressive abilities and repeated the tests at 3 years. The group with delayed early expressive language abilities at 2 years continued to have expressive language problems at 3 years of age and had poorer speech development compared with the nondelayed group. They concluded that there is a cleft palate subgroup that exhibits delays either because of structural/anatomic deficits, cognitive/linguistic delay, or a language/phonological disorder. Snyder and Scherer (2004) suggest that assessment of early play gestures may assist clinicians in identifying children with clefts who are at risk for later language impairment so that early intervention can be initiated.

Voice Disorders　It has been established that both children and adults with cleft palate and associated hypernasality and nasal emission have disorders of phonation often associated with hyperplasia and hyperemia of the vocal folds (Brooks and Shelton, 1963; McDonald and Baker, 1951).

Breathy, husky voice quality commonly observed in children who have cleft palate has been attributed to an attempt to compensate for the loss of intraoral pressure (Bzoch, 1964) or to compensate for an undetected laryngeal web (Luerssen, Proggmayer,Ptock, 2004) by overdriving the vocal folds to overcome reduced intelligibility of speech. McWilliams et al. (1969, 1973) found that 27 of 32 children with cleft palate were chronically hoarse and later developed bilateral vocal fold nodules. Again, compensatory laryngeal valving, overdriving the vocal folds, was blamed for these vocal abuse disorders. Bronsted, Liisberg, Orsted, et al. (1984) showed that more than half of the patients with cleft palate and velopharyngeal insufficiency were dysphonic. The incidence of structural changes of the vocal folds from hyperemia to vocal nodules is not difficult to understand in light of the fact that the use of glottal stops as compensatory plosives produces pressure, friction, and blunt trauma to the vocal folds and to the fact that those children with velocardiofacial syndrome, or 22q11 deletion often have laryngeal webs.

Leder and Lerman (1985) hypothesized that adults, like children, with cleft palate and hypernasality also hyperadduct their vocal folds to produce a constriction below the velopharyngeal portal in an attempt to decrease nasal air leak. Based on acoustic spectrographic analyses, the authors concluded that the vocal folds were inappropriately hyperadducted to provide a constriction in place of the inadequately functioning velopharyngeal portal in an effort to eliminate nasal air leak, a causal factor for increased vocal nodules in the cleft palate population.

Congenitally Short Palate and Large Nasopharynx

Velopharyngeal insufficiency can exist without overt clefts of the hard or soft palate. The suspected causes are congenital short soft palate, large nasopharynx, or both, but in many cases neither can be anatomically established and the velopharyngeal insufficiency must be considered idiopathic. These conditions often remain undetected until adenoidectomy deprives the patient of tissue mass in the nasopharynx and veloadenoidal closure (Gibb, 1958; Green, 1957; Maryn, Van Lierde, De Bodt, and Van Cauwenberge, 2004; Neiman and Simpson, 1975; Ren, Isberg, and Henningsson, 1995; Finkelstein et al., 1996, 2002). A functionally short soft palate

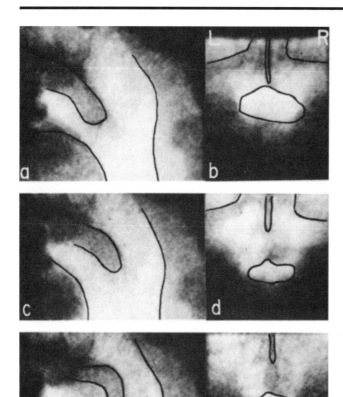

Figure 4.13 Video fluoroscopic frames showing congenital velopharyngeal insufficiency in a 6-year-old child at rest in lateral (a) and base (b) views; during nasal speech in lateral (c) and base (d) views; and during non nasal speech in lateral (e) and base (f) views. (From Skolnick, M.L. [1970]. Cleft Palate J 7, 803–816.)

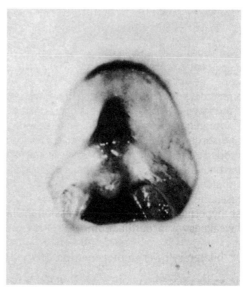

Figure 4.14 Congenital submucous cleft. (From Luchsinger, K., Arnold, G.E. [1965]. Voice speech language. Belmont, CA: Wadsworth Publishing.)

♦ surgical removal of portions of the hard and soft palate for benign and malignant tumors

♦ damage to the velopharyngeal musculature during tonsillectomy and adenoidectomy, producing scarring and stiffness of the muscles and restricting full sphincter motion

♦ sequelae to surgical removal of adenoids, unmasking submucous occult velopharyngeal insufficiency

♦ traumatic accidents, such as falling on hard or sharp objects in the mouth and other lacerations or penetrating wounds of the palate

will often look normal on routine oral examination and may elevate well, but it does not contact the posterior pharyngeal wall (**Fig. 4.13**). According to Ren, Isberg, and Henningsson (1995), enlarged tonsils may also cause hypernasality after adenoidectomy. The enlarged tonsils restrict palatal elevation and in so doing result in abnormal coupling of the nasal cavity.

Two anatomic defects sometimes associated with a functionally incompetent soft palate are submucous cleft and bifid uvula (**Fig. 4.14**). A submucous cleft can vary from a slight notch into the posterior border of the hard palate to a large, U-shaped absence of bone. Bifid uvula, partial or total, may be a clue to occult embryologic palatal defects (**Fig. 4.15**). The presence of a submucous cleft should raise the question of whether or not a genetic examination is in order. If it co-occurs with middle ear and cardiac defects, it may be indicative of velocardiofacial syndrome (Luerssen, Proggmayer, and Ptok, 2004).

Injuries

Hypernasality and nasal emission can result from traumatic damage to the palatal or velopharyngeal anatomy:

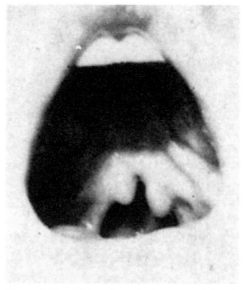

Figure 4.15 Bifid uvula and submucous cleft. (From Massengill, R. [1972]. Hypernasality. Springfield, IL: Charles C. Thomas.)

Neurologic Disease

Neurologic disease can cause hypernasality and nasal emission by producing weakness (paresis or paralysis) or incoordination of the velopharyngeal muscles. A concept already stated about neurologic voice disorders is also true of nasal resonatory disorders: Hypernasality and nasal emission due to neurologic velopharyngeal insufficiency are components and signs of a more generalized dysarthria, and, although such resonatory disorders can occur in isolation, they are most often embedded in a complex of associated respiratory, phonatory, and articulatory dysarthric signs. Hypernasality and nasal air emission can be among the first indicators of neurologic disease. The following types of dysarthria commonly manifest hypernasality and nasal emission from velopharyngeal weakness or incoordination:

♦ Unilateral or bilateral lower motor neuron (flaccid) dysarthria

♦ Unilateral upper motor neuron ("flaccid") dysarthria

♦ Bilateral upper motor neuron (spastic) dysarthria

♦ Mixed lower-upper motor neuron (flaccid-spastic) dysarthria

♦ Hyperkinetic (choreic-dystonic) dysarthria

In Chapter 5, the velopharyngeal insufficiency component of the dysarthrias is discussed. Unlike phonatory and articulatory dysarthric signs, which have individual characteristics depending upon site of lesion, thereby giving a clue to location of the lesion, there is nothing perceptually distinctive about the hypernasality and nasal emission of one dysarthria compared with another. An exception may relate to constancy or intermittency of hypernasality, depending upon whether the dysarthria is of the continuous or fluctuating type, a distinction that will be made shortly. It is, however, important for the diagnostician to know which dysarthric types produce hypernasality and which do not. For example, a patient suspected of Parkinson's disease who has hypernasality and nasal emission in addition to a hypokinetic dysarthria should be suspected of harboring a lesion in another area of the nervous system in addition to the basal ganglia, because pure hypokinetic dysarthria does not include velopharyngeal insufficiency.

Flaccid Hypernasality and Nasal Emission

Tenth (Vagus) Nerve Lesions The muscles of velopharyngeal closure for speech are innervated by cranial nerves V, IX, X, and XI. Specifically:

1. The levator veli palatini by the pharyngeal branch of the tenth (vagus) nerve

2. The tensor veli palatini, which contribution to closure is uncertain, by the motor division of the fifth (trigeminal) nerve

3. The pharyngeal muscles by the ninth, tenth, and eleventh cranial nerves (pharyngeal plexus)

In Chapter 5, **Fig. 5.3** and **Table 5.1** show that damage to the pharyngeal branch of cranial nerve X, or above that level, up to the nucleus ambiguus in the medulla, produces unilateral or bilateral flaccid paralysis of the soft palate. **Figure 5.3** shows how a right unilateral lesion of the vagal nucleus produces weakness of the soft palate on the same side of the lesion. Key points concerning this locus of lesion are:

♦ The paralyzed right side rests lower in the mouth than the normal side.

♦ On phonation or upon stimulation of the gag reflex, the soft palate pulls upward toward the normal side.

The same figure shows the effects of a bilateral lesion of the vagal nucleus:

♦ Both sides of the soft palate rest low in the mouth.

♦ On phonation or stimulation of the gag reflex, both sides move sluggishly or not at all.

Absence or reduction of a gag reflex, also called a hypoactive gag reflex, is exclusively a sign of flaccid lower motor neuron paralysis. However, it is, infrequently, also a psychogenic sign.

Neurologic diseases that commonly damage the nucleus ambiguus or the tenth nerves as they exit the base of the skull are tumors, vascular diseases, cerebrovascular accident, infectious diseases, bony malformations of the base of the skull, and degenerative diseases. Myasthenia gravis, when of the bulbar type, can affect the pharyngeal branch of the vagus nerve at the myoneural junction (Chapter 5). Hypernasality and nasal emission are prominent signs of this disease.

Unilateral Upper Motor Neuron Lesions A unilateral cortical or subcortical lesion of the pyramidal tract (upper motor neuron) often produces unilateral paralysis of the soft palate on the side opposite the lesion. The classic case is the patient who sustains a left frontal cerebral hemisphere lesion and becomes hemiparetic, dysarthric, and apraxic. These patients typically have a unilateral upper motor neuron dysarthria that consists of mild articulatory imprecision from unilateral facial and tongue weakness on the side opposite the lesion. The effects of the unilateral soft palate paresis may not be heard because of its mildness, but it can be seen on oral examination. Evidently the tongue, lower face, and soft palate are not as well endowed with ipsilateral corticobulbar fibers as the larynx, which has no such unilateral paresis from unilateral corticobulbar tract lesions.

The asymmetric appearance of a unilateral upper motor neuron paresis of the soft palate at rest is indistinguishable from a unilateral lower motor neuron paresis; in both, phonation and stimulation of the gag reflex cause the soft palate to pull up toward the normal side.

Spastic (Pseudobulbar) Hypernasality and Nasal Emission

Bilateral Upper Motor Neuron Lesions Typically, hypernasality and nasal emission are components of spastic dysarthria. However, the muscular physiology is not one of paralysis, as in flaccid dysarthria, but slowness of velopharyngeal movement due to disinhibition of antagonist muscles producing dyssynchronous movements and incomplete closure. Attesting to the intactness of its innervation is either a normal or hyperactive gag reflex; upon stroking the faucial arches or back wall of the pharynx with a tongue depressor, the gag is easily elicited; the soft palate thrusts upward bilaterally, and the pharyngeal walls briskly move medially.

Mixed Flaccid-Spastic Hypernasality and Nasal Emission

Lower Plus Upper Motor Neuron Lesions The most severe cases of neurologic-based hypernasality and nasal emission are found in patients with mixed flaccid-spastic dysarthria owing to their cumulative effects. The classic example is amyotrophic lateral sclerosis (ALS). However, any lesion that can affect both upper and lower motor neurons simultaneously can produce this same form of velopharyngeal insufficiency. In ALS, the most common disease seen in clinical practice producing this mixed dysarthria, hypernasality and nasal emission are mild in the early stages. As the dysarthria progresses, hypernasality and nasal emission worsen until there is virtually no movement of the velopharyngeal muscles. The soft palate hangs low in the mouth, immersed in ropey saliva, and remains immobile during phonation or stimulation of the gag reflex. The paralysis is not always symmetric; even though both sides of the soft palate can become paralyzed, one side may be more than the other.

Hyperkinetic (Choreic-Dystonic) Hypernasality and Nasal Emission

Basal Ganglia Lesions Fluctuating during the course of contextual speech are the hypernasality and nasal emission of the choreic and dystonic movement disorder dysarthrias. The dysarthrias of dystonia, choreoathetosis, and chorea all have periodic velopharyngeal insufficiency, whether the movement disorder is the congenital or early acquired "cerebral palsy" or of later onset. Common to all are spontaneous, uncontrolled velopharyngeal movements, more prominent in the dystonias than the choreas because of the slowness of the dystonias and longer duration of velopharyngeal opening.

Palatopharyngolaryngeal Myoclonus

Discussion of the slow (1 to 4 Hz), rhythmic, myoclonic-like movements of the soft palate and lateral pharyngeal walls in palatopharyngolaryngeal myoclonus is somewhat paradoxical here, because these movements rarely produce hypernasality or hyponasality even though each time the soft palate elevates myoclonically, it touches the posterior pharyngeal wall, and, when it pulls away, it opens the velopharyngeal port. The moment of closure is so brief that its perceptual effects escape the ear. For clinical purposes, then, palatal myoclonus is a visual not an auditory sign. But, its importance in neurologic diagnosis cannot be overstated. It is easily overlooked because of its subtle movements, yet its presence indicates a brain-stem lesion.

Psychogenic Factors

The incidence of nonorganic hypernasality and nasal emission in clinical practice is low, but a group of patients comprise what is sometimes called "functional" hypernasality. These are children and adults who sound hypernasal but who have normal palatal structure and function as demonstrated on the oral examination and videofluoroscopy. The etiologies of nonorganic "velopharyngeal insufficiencies" are:

♦ conversion reaction

♦ reduced effort to produce normally vigorous speech owing to poor self-image, sometimes combined with borderline organic velopharyngeal insufficiency

♦ reduced speaking effort as a sign of "path of least resistance" in physically ill, debilitated patients

♦ imitation of relatives or friends with whom the person strongly identifies

♦ Organic Hyponasality

Hyponasality, or denasality, is the opposite of hypernasality. It is the reduction or absence of nasal resonation on the normal nasal semivowels and during normal assimilation nasality. It is due to velopharyngeal overclosure or to obstruction. In common everyday terms, it is called *adenoid speech,* or speaking with a "stuffy nose." Curiously, many professional people in medicine and allied health fields confuse hypernasality and hyponasality; when they hear hyponasality, sometimes they not only use the term *hypernasality* or *nasal speech* instead, but they also infer velopharyngeal insufficiency instead of nasal or nasopharyngeal obstruction. It is an easy mistake to make by the untrained listener, because both types are so closely associated with the nasal cavities and perceptual changes in resistance. Official terminology for disorders of nasal resonance from nasal cavity obstruction follows:

♦ *Rhinolalia clausa* (closed nasality)

♦ *Rhinolalia clausa, posterior* A perceptually distinctive type of hyponasality from obstruction of the posterior nasal cavities or nasopharynx.

♦ *Rhinolalia clausa, anterior* A perceptually distinctive type of hyponasality from obstruction of the anterior nasal cavities.

The normal speaker can simulate both types. Posterior: Say a sentence having nasal semivowels with the velopharynx continuously closed. For example, "Many men marched and sang at night." Note that the only phonemes adversely affected are the nasals /m/, /ŋ/, and / ŋ /, which shift toward /b/, /d/, and /g/. Patients who have hypertrophied adenoids, tumors, or polyps in the nasopharynx are, in effect, speaking as if in a state of continuous velopharyngeal closure. *Anterior*: Say the same sentence with normal velopharyngeal action but while pinching the nares closed, producing the effect of an anterior nasal cavity obstruction. Now a hollow, muffled resonation on the nasal semivowels is heard for the reason that, although the nasal cavities resonate the sound, the far end is closed, a condition called cul-de-sac resonation.

A secondary effect of nasal obstruction is mouth breathing. If nasal airflow during inhalation is reduced, the only way of maintaining adequate oxygen intake is orally. The child or adult whose mouth is always open and who has hyponasal speech is likely to have nasal obstruction and ought to alert the clinician to the need for investigation of its cause. Nasal obstructions are most often due to inflammations of the nasal turbinates from upper respiratory infections or allergies, benign and malignant tumors, enlarged tonsils that can push the velum against the pharyngeal walls, deviated nasal septums, and surgical overclosure of the velopharyngeal port secondary to pharyngoplasty for velopharyngeal insufficiency. Because such operations, exemplified by the pharyngeal flap, cannot be "fine tuned," often the flap is made too wide for the nasopharynx. The patient enters surgery hypernasal and emerges hyponasal. Often, this is just temporary from edema that disappears, leaving an adequate nasal airway, but sometimes it is persistent because the flap is too wide. If this obstruction, like any obstruction not modified, is complete or nearly so, the following complications may occur:

- habitual mouth breathing
- snoring
- reduced sense of smell with loss of appreciation for food
- halitosis from susceptibility to microorganisms in the nasal cavities and drying of the oral mucosa
- drying of gingival tissues around the anterior teeth, which, according to some dentists, can lead to periodontal disease
- danger of choking on food
- elongation of the bony structures of the face resulting in adenoidal faces

The only recourse is to modify the obstruction surgically.

A pharyngoplasty procedure when a child or adult becomes hypernasal after tonsillectomy and adenoidectomy (T and A) can be premature. Many people with normal velopharyngeal function who become hypernasal, sometimes for a few months, after T and A, if left alone, will spontaneously adapt to loss of adenoid tissue and will recover normal velopharyngeal closure. Others respond quickly to behavioral modification techniques. Thinking that the hypernasality is a sign of permanent organic velopharyngeal insufficiency, surgery is sometimes performed, and then complete function of the musculature returns, with the effect of overclosure and consequent hyponasal speech and secondary obstructive effects.

Patulous Eustachian Tube (PET)

A most unusual and little-discussed cause of hyponasality is a syndrome called patulous eustachian tube (PET). It is worthy of discussion because it is easily missed and misdiagnosed. Its symptoms are:

- a roaring sound in the ears synchronous with respiration, known as autophony
- a feeling of fullness in the ears
- irritability, depression, anxiety, and preoccupation with the symptoms
- a change in speech, as if the person were talking with a cold in the nose (i.e., hyponasality)
- disappearance of symptoms when lowering the head between the knees or when lying down

The reason for patency of the eustachian tube is the loss of tissue mass surrounding its orifice or from a change in velopharyngeal muscular tonicity.

Although the etiology is unclear, loss of weight, dehydration, pregnancy, radiation therapy to the nasopharynx, fatigue, excessive estrogen, otitis media, and fibrosis of the eustachian tube mucosa secondary to inflammation have all been suggested as causative factors (Tsuji, Yamaguchi, and Moriyama, 2003).

The subjective sensation of voice amplification is due to the fact that the voice is resonated in the middle ear cavity, having traveled up the open eustachian tube, which is supposed to remain closed except upon swallowing. Autophony may have been first described by Johannes Miller, who wrote in his *Handbook of Physiology* that he could produce a snapping sound in his ears when he contracted his palatine muscles and elevated his soft palate. He said: "If immediately afterwards I emit a humming vocal tone while my mouth is either closed or slightly open, this tone has an extraordinary resonance" (Perlman, 1939).

Hyponasality as a sign and symptom of this syndrome (Landes, 1967) has an interesting purpose, chiefly protective; the patient keeps the velopharyngeal port closed to prevent the voice from reaching the eustachian tube, which opening lies above the level of the velopharyngeal sphincter. The reason the symptoms disappear with the head lowered or when the patient is lying down is that venous engorgement of the area surrounding the opening closes the eustachian tube.

Treatment consists of (1) patient education as to the causes of the disorder, (2) weight gain, or (3) injection of Teflon or autologous fat at the orifice of the tube to close it. Anxiety, depression, and the general impression of psychoneurosis improve noticeably in patients treated with augmentation procedures. Crary, Wexler, and Berliner (1979) found that 9 of 10 patients so treated said that they felt much better, had improved concentration, had increased enjoyment of life, and on the Minnesota Multiphasic Personality Inventory showed a decrease in the neurotic triad of hypochondriasis, depression, and hysteria. Doherty and Slattery (2003) successfully treated refractory PET in patients with autologous fat graft plugging of the eustachian tube at its nasopharyngeal orifice in combination with myringotomy and ventilation tube placement. Nevertheless, PET presents a challenging management problem because many methods are ineffective, and successful treatment methods are often temporary.

♦ Mixed Nasality

Mixed nasality, also called rhinolalia mixta, may seem paradoxical: simultaneous velopharyngeal insufficiency and nasal obstruction without one cancelling out the other. A mixture of hyponasality of nasals and hypernasality of vowels nevertheless does occur in patients who have coexisting obstruction in the anterior or posterior nasal cavities simultaneous with organic or nonorganic velopharyngeal insufficiencies.

♦ Clinical Examination

The following primary questions need to be answered about the patient suspected of a nasal resonatory disorder:

1. Does a nasal resonatory disorder, in fact, exist? If so:

   ♦ What type is it? (hypernasality, hyponasality?)

   ♦ How severe is it?

   ♦ What is its cause?

   ♦ How should it be treated?

2. With what physical, psychologic, and educational deficiencies is the resonatory disorder associated and what are their interactions? Are these combinations of factors indicative of need for genetic assessment?

3. How can they be reduced or eliminated?

   To answer these questions, the following data are necessary:

1. History of the primary and associated disorders

2. Perceptual examination as to presence, type, and extent of the nasal resonatory disorder

3. Examination of the speech anatomy and physiology via direct observation and indirect biophysical measurement

4. Articulation analysis

5. Language evaluation

6. Psychometric and psychologic evaluation

7. Social work evaluation

8. Hearing evaluation

9. Allied health specialists such as surgical, dental, and genetic consultative evaluations and recommendations

Perceptual Examination

Judgment as to the presence and severity of a nasal resonatory disorder lies within the ear and mind of the speech pathologist and not a mechanical or electronic instrument, although such devices can support the clinical impression.

Contextual Speech Impression

Have the patient simulate everyday speech as closely as possible. Depending upon age and cooperativeness, two kinds of connected speech samples can be obtained: conversational speech and oral reading. Simultaneous video and audio recordings may be made for confirmational analysis later. As the patient speaks, the clinician should try to answer the following questions:

1. Do I hear normal, excess, or insufficient nasal resonation?

2. How distracting is the resonatory disorder as I try to grasp the content of the patient's speech?

3. Are consonant pressures low so that the sounds are difficult or impossible to identify?

4. Are vowels hypernasal?

5. Are nasal semivowels hyponasal?

6. Do I hear nonstandard sound substitutions?

7. Do I hear standard sound substitutions?

8. What is the level of overall speech intelligibility?

9. Does language development sound delayed?

10. Is a voice (laryngeal) disorder also present, and if so, what are its perceptual features?

11. Does the patient's behavior suggest a hearing loss?

12. Does general behavior suggest intellectual, personality, or emotional disturbances?

13. What is the impression given by the patient's physical appearance?

14. Do facial grimaces or other habit patterns accompany contextual speech?

15. Does the speech pattern change with different rates of production, orality, or differences in contextual material?

Semiobjective Tests for Hypernasality and Hyponasality
Suppose, after listening to contextual speech, the clinician suspects hypernasality, nasal emission, or hyponasality. In the absence of aerodynamic or acoustic instrumentation, additional arguments for or against their presence can be obtained by means of the following informal observations or practical tests:

1. *Mirror-clouding test*

   a. *Hypernasality and nasal emission*

      (1) Place a hand mirror or cold shiny metal object such as a serving spoon under the patient's nares.

      (2) Ask the patient to repeat a sentence that is free of all nasal semivowels (e.g., "We see three geese" or "The big black dog caught the stick"). People who have normal palatal and velopharyngeal closure should not leak air out the nose during such phrases. Fogging of the metal under one or both nares indicates velopharyngeal insufficiency.

b. *Hyponasality*

(1) Ask the patient to repeat a sentence containing ample nasal semivowels (e.g., "Many men sang at noon").

(2) People with normal velopharyngeal opening should leak air out the nares during the nasal sounds, fogging the mirror. Little or no fogging indicates nasal obstruction.

2. *Nasal vibration test*

a. *Hypernasality and nasal emission*

(1) While the patient repeats a sentence free of nasal sounds, such as "We see three geese," with thumb and index finger lightly straddle the cartilaginous portion of the nose: if vibration can be felt, nasal resonation is likely.

(2) Have the patient repeat the sentence, but this time pinch the nares shut: if cul-de-sac resonation can be heard, excess nasal resonation is likely.

b. *Hyponasality*

(1) While the patient repeats a sentence rich in nasal sounds, such as "Many men sang at noon," straddle the nose with thumb and index finger: if vibration cannot be felt, suspect nasal obstruction. If pinching the nares during the production of nasal sounds does not produce cul-de-sac resonation, also suspect nasal obstruction.

3. *Consonant differential pressure test for hypernasality and nasal emission*

a. Have the patient repeat a sentence free of nasal sounds and rich in pressure consonants, such as "The paperboy saw a baseball." The first trial should be produced while the examiner listens carefully to consonant sharpness and sentence intelligibility.

b. The second trial should be produced while the examiner pinches the nares shut and listens for any change in the consonant sharpness and intelligibility. A noticeable rise in audible consonant pressure or sharpness and intelligibility with the nares pinched indicates grossly the extent of the insufficiency. It also provides an impression of what the patient's speech could be like with successful surgical or prosthetic treatment of the insufficiency.

4. *Nares occlusion test of exhalatory efficiency*

a. With nares open, ask the patient to inhale as deeply as possible and then on exhalation count to as high a number as possible until all breath is exhausted. (First demonstrate a rate of about two numbers per second.) Repeat this 3 times and take the average maximum number attained on the three trials.

b. While the examiner pinches the nares shut, the patient repeats the same three trials of counting, again taking the average of the three trials. Patients who have normal velopharyngeal closure produce little or no differences between the maximum number attained on

counting with nares open versus nares occluded. Patients who have hypernasality and nasal emission will produce a noticeably lower maximum number with the nares open versus closed, giving evidence of the extent of nasal air wastage.

These practical tests can be done in the office without special equipment. Quantification of nasal airflow and intraoral pressures by electronic instruments can yield similar results. Whereas they may not be essential for experienced clinicians, neophyte clinicians who are unsure of their ability to detect differences in nasal resonance often benefit from instrumental analysis.

Examination of the Speech Anatomy

Once the clinician has identified a nasal resonatory disorder by the methods just discussed, the next step is to find a physical explanation for the hypernasality and nasal emission or hyponasality. For this portion of the examination, the following equipment is required:

1. A quiet room

2. A chair for the patient that will enable the examiner to look into the patient's mouth at different angles; a dental chair is ideal.

3. An excellent source of light. Although a good flashlight will suffice, natural lighting, dental or surgical lighting, or light reflected from a head mirror are even better.

4. Tongue depressors

5. Dental mirror

6. Endoscopic equipment

The physical examination begins by asking the patient to sit upright, relaxed and comfortable.

1. While the patient is breathing quietly, the clinician should be thinking of the following questions:

a. Are there friction noises that suggest nasal or oral obstruction?

b. Is the patient a mouth breather?

c. Are there unilateral, bilateral, or midline clefts of the upper lip?

d. Is there evidence of surgical repair of clefts of the lip?

e. Does the upper lip appear thin or contracted?

f. Does one or both sides of the nose appear flattened or distorted?

g. Does the maxilla appear abnormally small?

h. Does the mandible appear incongruously large, protruding beyond the maxilla?

i. Does the mandible appear incongruously small in comparison with the maxilla?

2. Voluntary lip movements

   a. Does the patient have difficulty approximating the upper and lower lips?

   b. Does the patient have difficulty rounding, retracting, and protruding the lips?

3. Voluntary mandibular movements

   a. Does the patient have difficulty depressing, lateralizing, protruding, or elevating the mandible?

   b. On occluding the teeth, does the mandible protrude beyond the maxilla?

4. Dental configuration

   a. Are teeth missing in the upper or lower dental arch?

   b. Are teeth improperly formed or positioned within the dental arch?

   c. Is there malocclusion between the upper and lower teeth?

   d. Do extra teeth (supernumerary) crowd the dental arch?

5. Hard palate configuration

   a. Is there a unilateral or bilateral cleft of the hard palate?

   b. Is there an alveolar cleft?

   c. Is there a notch in the posterior hard palate on palpation?

   d. Is there a palatal fistula present?

   e. Is the hard palate abnormally high and narrow?

   f. Is the hard palate scarred from previous surgeries?

   g. Have teeth erupted from the hard palate?

6. Soft palate configuration

   a. Does the soft palate appear abnormally short at rest?

   b. Is the soft palate asymmetric at rest?

   c. Is the soft palate scarred?

   d. Are the palatine tonsils enlarged?

   e. Is the uvula absent?

   f. Is the uvula bifid or split?

   g. Is the soft palate thin and translucent?

   h. Does the soft palate elevate asymmetrically on phonation of /a/?

   i. Does the soft palate fail to elevate bilaterally on phonation?

   j. Does the soft palate fail to elevate bilaterally on stimulation of the gag reflex?

   k. On cineradiographic, videofluoroscopic, endoscopic, or nasal endoscopic examination:

      (1) Does the soft palate fail to contact the posterior pharyngeal wall on non-nasal sounds?

      (2) Does the soft palate appear short?

      (3) Does the soft palate fail to show a knee-angle during phonation?

      (4) Does the soft palate contact a Passavant's ridge on phonation?

      (5) Does the presence of adenoids provide a point of contact by the soft palate on non-nasal sounds?

      (6) Does the velopharyngeal sphincter fail to close?

      (7) Is there a reduction or absence of medial pharyngeal wall movement?

      (8) What is the pattern of closure?

Articulation Analysis

Articulatory analysis is done for three reasons in patients with palatopharyngeal insufficiency: to determine the presence or extent of deviant articulatory development; to identify distortions secondary to orofacial and dental anomalies; and to identify compensatory, nonstandard articulatory substitutions and distortions. These objectives are separate and distinct. It is important to objectify the presence of impaired articulatory development, which may or may not be caused by the palatopharyngeal insufficiency. It may be due to mental retardation, hearing loss, environmental deprivation, or any other factor that affects speech production. The second and third reasons for articulation testing are that cleft palate and other palatopharyngeal insufficiencies produce their own special articulatory defects. For example, dental, maxillary, and mandibular anomalies markedly interfere with normal articulation, and, because no two individuals have the same anatomic abnormalities, their articulatory acoustics are never identical. Hence, no standard nomenclature or precise phonetic symbols exist to indicate the peculiarity of a given individual's distortions caused by anomalous oral architecture. The same can be said for the compensatory glottal, pharyngeal, and lingual stops and fricatives so common in children and adults with cleft palate. In short, the ordinary developmental or descriptive articulation test for assessing general articulatory development needs to be supplemented to document the articulatory defects in this population that extend beyond delayed development.

Addressing the special needs of the cleft palate population, Bzoch (1979) designed an Error Pattern Diagnostic Articulation Test (**Fig. 4.16**). In addition to simple substitutions, omissions, and distortions, this test adds recording space for gross substitutions, such as glottal stops, and pharyngeal fricatives, and for nasal emissions of sounds. The clinician should also describe in detail the location of the error, particularly the nonstandard distortions and substitutions produced by atypical labial, dental, lingual, pharyngeal, or laryngeal movements.

Language Evaluation

Children with cleft lip and palate are known for their delayed expressive language in addition to delayed articulatory development. Confronting the clinician is the need to establish

BZOCH ERROR PATTERN DIAGNOSTIC ARTICULATION TESTS   1978-A

Name _____   Birth _____   Age ____ Sex ____ No. _____

Examiner _____   Date _____   Stimulus _____

C = correct.   T̃ = indistinct from nasal emission alone.   D = distortion (.5 error).   SS = simple substitution (1.0 error).
GS = gross substitution (1.5 error).   O = omission (2.0 error).

Columns: C T̃ D SS GS O (repeated three times)

PLOSIVES
/p/	Pencil	aPPle	cuP
/b/	Ball	baBy	tuB
/t/	Table	mounTain	boaT
/d/	Dog	canDy	beD
/k/	Cat	chiCKen	booK
/g/	Gun	waGon	piG

FRICATIVES
/f/	Fork	elePHant	kniFE
/v/	Vase	shoVel	stoVE
/θ/	THumb	tooTHbrush	mouTH
/ð/	THis	feaTHer	baTHE
/s/	Sun	bicyCLe	houSE
/z/	Zipper	sciSSors	noSE
/ʃ/	SHoe	diSHes	fiSH
/ʒ/	XXXXX	televiSion	garaGE

AFFRICATIVES
| /tʃ/ | CHair | maTCHes | waTCH |
| /dʒ/ | Juice | briDGes | oranGE |

ASPIRATES
| /h/ | Horse | grassHopper | XXXXXX |

GLIDES
/w/	Window	sandWich	XXXXXX
/l/	Lion	baLLoons	doLL
/y/	Yarn	onIOns	XXXXXX
/r/	Rabbit	aRRow	caR

NASALS
/m/	Man	haMMer	druM
/n/	Nail	baNana	traiN
/ŋ/	XXXXXX	haNGer	swiNG

BLENDS
SPider	STar	neST
STRawberries	SKirt	boX
SLide	SMoke	SNake
PLiers	BLock	beLT
worLD	CLown	FLag
PResent	BRoom	TRuck
DRess	heaRT	swoRD
CRy	GRapes	coRK
FRog	THRead	aRM
JropPED	inseCT	siFT
WHeel	teNT	haND

Figure 4.16 Error pattern diagnostic articulation test. (From Bzoch, K.R. [1979]. Communicative disorders related to cleft lip and palate. Boston: Little, Brown, p. 169.)

whether language is delayed and why, a more than usually complicated question within the context of cleft palate, for such delay often has multiple causes. Consequently, evaluation must consider not only documentation of language developmental milestones but also audiologic, familial, surgical, medical, social, and psychologic history as well. The clinician who works with children with craniofacial anomalies needs to be aware of the physical, environmental, and psychologic disturbances that can contribute to delayed language development.

For example:

1. The cleft itself. Inability to generate intraoral pressures within the first 2 or even 3 years of life, a period having implications for pressure-consonant development, in itself probably delays not only articulation but also intelligibility.

2. Dental anomalies. Missing and malpositioned teeth and malocclusions have the same effect of depriving the child of normal anatomy for speech development.

3. Trauma. Oropharyngeal pain from surgical procedure

4. Emotional deprivation. Rejection by parents and sibling

5. Language deprivation. Reduced language stimulation because of hospitalizations and family disruption

6. Hearing loss. From serous otitis media and middle ear infection

7. Developmental disabilities. As an associated disorder not stemming from environmental factors per se

8. Self-consciousness. Reduced willingness to speak to minimize conspicuousness

Therapy for nasal resonatory disorders and cleft palate rehabilitation have not been included in this chapter owing to their extensiveness and complexity. This subject is covered in the references listed in the suggestions for Additional Reading section at the end of this chapter.

◆ Summary

◆ Hypernasality and nasal emission interfere with the aesthetics of speech and can seriously compromise intelligibility, producing serious psychologic, educational, and occupational consequences.

◆ Hypernasality and nasal emission are caused by cleft palate, congenitally short palate or large nasopharynx, nasopharyngeal trauma, and by neurologic diseases that cause weakness and dyssynchronous movements of the velopharyngeal sphincter.

◆ Hyponasality, or denasality, is caused by obstruction of the nasopharynx or nasal passages.

◆ Normal velopharyngeal closure is produced primarily by sphincteric action of the levator veli palatini and the superior pharyngeal constrictor muscles and not solely by elevation and retraction of the soft palate.

◆ Clefts of the palate involve the primary (lip and alvaolus) palate only, the secondary palate only, or primary and secondary palates combined.

◆ Communication problems associated with cleft palate are hypernasality and nasal emission, weak pressure consonants, nonstandard substitutions of laryngeal, pharyngeal, and lingual sounds, deviant and/or delayed articulatory and language development, articulatory problems due to dental defects and to hearing loss, and dysphonia.

◆ Neurologic velopharyngeal insufficiencies are associated primarily with flaccid, spastic, and hyperkinetic dysarthrias.

◆ In a small percentage of cases, hypernasality and nasal emission can be psychogenic.

◆ Clinical examination should answer questions as to type, severity, and cause of the resonatory disorder. Associated psychoeducational, physical, physiologic, articulatory, voice, and language functions also require investigation.

References

Abe, M., Murakami, G., Noguchi, M., Kitamura, S., Shimada, K., Kohama, G.I. (2004). Variations in the tensor veli palatine muscle with special reference to its origin and insertion. Cleft Palate Craniofac J 41, 474–484.

Armour, A., Fischback, S., Klaiman, P., Fisher, D.M. (2005). Does velopharyngeal closure pattern affect the success of pharyngeal flap pharyngoplasty? Plast Reconstr Surg 115, 45–52.

Azzam, N.A., Kuehn, D.P. (1977). The morphology of musculus uvulae. Cleft Palate J 14, 78–87.

Beer, A.J., Hellerhoff, P., Zimmermann, A., Mady, K., Sader, R., Rummeny, E.J., Hannig, C. (2004). Dynamic near-real-time magnetic resonance imaging for analyzing the velopharyngeal closure in comparison with videofluoroscopy. J Magn Reson Imaging 20, 791–797.

Bell-Berti, F. (1976). An electromyographic study of velopharyngeal function in speech. J Speech Hear Res 19, 225–240.

Benguerel, A.P., Hirose, H., Sawashima, M., Ushijima, T. (1977). Velar coarticulation in French: An electromyographic study. J. Phonet 5, 149–158.

Bronsted, K., Liisberg, W.B., Orsted, Å., Prytz, S., Fogh-Andersen, P. (1984). Surgical and speech results following palatopharyngoplasty operations in Denmark, 1959–1977. Cleft Palate J 21, 170–179.

Brooks, A., Shelton, R. (1963). Incidence of voice disorders other than nasality in cleft palate children. Cleft Palate Bull 13, 63–64.

Bzoch, K. (1964). The effects of a specific pharyngeal flap operation upon the speech of 40 cleft palate persons. J Speech Hear Disord 29, 111–120.

Bzoch, K.R. (1956). An investigation of the speech of pre-school cleft palate children. Ph.D. dissertation. Evanston, IL: Northwestern University.

Bzoch, K.R. (1979). Communicative disorders related to cleft lip and palate. Boston: Little, Brown.

Bzoch, K.R., Morley, M., Fex, S., Laxman, J., Heller, J. (1973). Development of speech and language in cleft palate children. Paper presented at second International Congress on Cleft Palate, 26–31, August, 1973. Copenhagen, Denmark. Summary published by office of Naval Research, London, by Connole, P.W.

Cheng, N.X., Zhang, K.Q. (2004). The applied anatomic study of palatopharyngeus muscle. Zhonghua Zheng Xing Wai Ke Za Zhi 20, 384–387.

Cobourne, M.T. (2004). The complex genetics of cleft lip and palate. Eur J Orthod 26, 7–16.

Cooper F.S. (1965). Research techniques and instrumentation: EMG. In Proceedings of the conference on communicative problems in cleft palate (ASHA Repots 1). Rockville, MD: American Speech-Language-Hearing Association, 1965, pp. 153–168.

Cooper, H.K., Sr., Harding, R.L., Krogman, W.M., Mazahari, M., Millard, R.T. (Eds.). (1979). Cleft palate and cleft lip. Philadelphia: W.B. Saunders Co.

Counihan, D.T. (1960) Articulation skills of adolescents and adults with cleft palates. J Speech Hear Disord 25, 181–187.

Crary, W.G., Wexler, M., Berliner, K. (1979). The abnormally patent eustachian tube. Arch Otolaryngol 105, 21–23.

Dickson, D.R. (1962). An acoustic study of nasality. J Speech Hear Res 5, 103–111.

Doherty, J.K., Slattery, W.H. (2003). Autologous fat grafting for the refractory patulous eustachian tube. Otolaryngol Head Neck Surg 128, 88–91.

Edwards, M., Watson, A.C.H. (1980). Advances in the management of cleft palate. Edinburgh: Churchill Livingstone.

Ensenauer, R.E., Adeyinka, A., Flynn, H.C., Michels, V.V., Lindor, N.M., Dawson, D.B., et al. (2003). Microduplication 22q11.2, an emerging syndrome: clinical, cytogenetic, and molecular analysis of thirteen patients. Am J Hum Genet 73, 1027–1040.

Finkelstein, Y., Berger, G., Nachmani, A., Ophir, D. (1996). The functional role of the adenoids in speech. Int J Pediatr Otorhinolaryngol 34, 61–74.

Finkelstein, Y., Wexler, D.B., Nachmani, A., Ophir, D. (2002). Endoscopic partial adenoidectomy for children with submucous cleft palate. Cleft Palate Craniofac J 39, 479–486.

Fogh-Andersen, P. (1942). Inheritance of cleft lip and palate. Copenhagen: Nordisk Forlag, Arnold Busck.

Fraser, F.C. (1970). The genetics of cleft lip and palate. Am J Hum Genet 22, 336–352.

Fritzell, B. (1969). The velopharyngeal muscles in speech: an electromyographic and cineradiographic study. Acta Otolaryngol 250, 1(Suppl)1–78.

Gibb, A.G. (1958). Hypernasality (rhinolalia aperta) following tonsil and adenoid removal. J Laryngol Otol 72, 443–451.

Gorlin, R.J., Cohen, M.M. (2001). Syndromes of the head and neck. 4th ed. Oxford: Oxford University Press.

Greene, M.C. (1957). Speech of children before and after removal of adenoids. J Speech Hear Disord 22, 361–370.

Hardin-Jones, M.A., Jones, D.L. (2005). Speech production of preschoolers with cleft palate. Cleft Palate Craniofac J 42, 7–13.

Havstam, C., Lohmander, A., Persson, C., Dotevall, H., Lith, A., Lilja, J. (2005). Evaluation of VPI-assessment with videofluoroscopy and nasoendoscopy. Br J Plast Surg 58, 922–931.

House, A.S., Stevens, K.N. (1956). Analog studies of the nasalization of vowels. J Speech Hear Disord 21, 218–232.

Kierner, A.C., Mayer, R., Kirschhofer, K. (2002). Do the tensor tympani and tensor veli palatine muscles of man form a functional unit? A histochemical investigation of their putative connections. Hear Res 165, 48–52.

Kummer, A.W., Briggs, M., Lee, L. (2003). The relationship between the characteristics of speech and velopharyngeal gap size. Cleft Palate Craniofac J 40, 590–596.

Landes, B.A. (1967). Hyporhinolalia associated with eustachian tube dysfunction. Laryngoscope 77, 244–246.

Leder, S.B., Lerman, J.W. (1985). Some acoustic evidence for vocal abuse in adult speakers with repaired cleft palate. Laryngoscope 95, 837–840.

Li, C.L., Lundervold, A. (1958). Electromyographic study of cleft palate. Plast Reconstr Surg 21, 427–432.

Lubker, J.F. (1968). An electromyographic-cineradiographic investigation of velar function during normal speech production. Cleft Palate J 5, 1–18.

Lubker, J.F., Curtis, J.F. (1966). Electromyographic-cinefluorographic investigation of velar function during speech production. J Acoust Soc Am 40, 1272.

Luerssen, K., Proggmayer, M., Ptok, M. (2004). Small deletion-large effect. HNO 52, 258–260.

Maryn, Y., Van Lierde, K., De Bodt, M., Van Cauwenberge, P. (2004). The effects of adenoidectomy and tonsillectomy on speech and nasal resonance. Folia Phoniatr Logop 56, 182–191.

McDonald, E., Baker, H.K. (1951). Cleft palate speech: an integration of research and clinical observation. J Speech Hear Disord 16, 9–20.

McWilliams, B.J., Bluestone, C.D., Musgrave, R.H. (1969). Diagnostic implications of vocal cord nodules in children with cleft palate. Laryngoscope 79, 2072–2080.

McWilliams, B.J., Lavarto, A.S., Bluestone, C.D. (1973). Vocal cord abnormalities in children with velopharyngeal valving problems. Laryngoscope 83, 1745–1753.

Mehendale, F.V. (2004). Surgical anatomy of the levator veli palatine: a previously undescribed tendinous insertion of the anterolateral fibers. Plast Reconstr Surg 114, 307–315.

Miyamoto, R.C., Cotton, R.T., Rope, A.F., Hopkin, R.J., Cohen, A.P., Shott, S.R., and Rutter, M.J. (2004). Association of anterior glottic webs with velocardiofacial syndrome (chromosome 22q11.2 deletion). Otolaryngol Head Neck Surg 130, 415–417.

Moon, J.B., Canady, J.W. (1995). Effects of gravity on velopharyngeal muscle activity during speech. Cleft Palate Craniofac J 32, 371–375.

Morris, H., Ozanne, A. (2003). Phonetic, phonological and language skills of chidren with a cleft palate. Cleft Palate Craniofac J 40, 460–470.

Muller, R., Beleites, T., Hloucal, U., Kuhn, M. (2000). Objective measurement of normal nasality in the Saxony dialect. HNO 48, 937–942.

Neiman, G.S., Simpson, R.K. (1975). A roentgencephalometric investigation of the effect of adenoid removal upon selected measures of velopharyngeal function. Cleft Palate J 12, 377–389.

Perlman, H.B. (1939). The eustachian tube: abnormal patency and normal physiologic state. Arch Otolaryngol 30, 212–238.

Peterson, G.E., Barney, H.L. (1952). Control methods used in a study of the vowels. J Acoustic Soc Am 24, 175.

Philips, B.J., Harrison, R.J. (1969). Language skills in preschool cleft palate children. Cleft Palate J 6, 108–119.

Poole, I. (1934). Genetic development in articulation of consonant sounds in speech. Elementary English Rev 2, 159–161.

Ren, Y.F., Isberg, A., Henningsson, G. (1995). Velopharyngeal incompetence and persistent hypernasality after adenoidectomy in children without palatal defect. Cleft Palate Craniofac J 32, 476–482.

Seaver, E.J. (1979). A cinefluorographic and electromyographic investigation of velar movement during speech. Ph.D. dissertation. Iowa City: University of Iowa.

Series, F., Cote, C., Simoneau, J.A., Gelinas, Y., St Pierre, S., Leclere, J., Ferland, R., Marc, I. (1995). Physiologic, metabolic, and muscle fiber type characteristics of musculus uvulae in sleep apnea hyponea syndrome and in snorers. J Clin Invest 95, 20–25.

Series, F., Cote, C., Simoneau, J.A., St. Pierre, S., Marc, I. (1996). Upper airway collapsibility, and contractile and metabolic characteristics of musculus uvulae. FASEB J 10, 897–904.

Series, F., Cote, C., St. Pierre, S. (1999). Dysfunctional mechanical coupling of upper airway tissues in sleep apnea syndrome. Am J Respir Crit Care Med 159(5 Pt 1), 1551–1555.

Shprintzen, R.J. (2000a). Syndrome identification for speech-language pathologists: an illustrated pocket guide. San Diego: Singular.

Shprintzen, R.J. (2000b). Genetics, syndromes, and communication disorders. San Diego: Singular.

Siegel-Sadewitz, V.L., Shprintzen, R.J. (1986). Changes in velopharyngeal valving with age. Int J Pediatr Otorhinolaryngol 11, 171–182.

Skolnick, M.L. (1969). Videopharyngography in patients with nasal speech, with emphasis on lateral pharyngeal motion in velopharyngeal closure. Radiology 93, 747–755.

Skolnick, M.L. (1970). Videofluoroscopic examination of the velopharyngeal portal during phonation in lateral and base projections-a new technique for studying the mechanics of closure. Cleft Palate J 7, 803–816.

Skolnick, M.L., McCall, G.N., Barnes, M. (1973). The sphincteric mechanism of velopharyngeal closure. Cleft Palate J 10, 286–305.

Smith, B.E., Patil, Y., Guyette, T.W., Brannan, T.S. (2003). Pressure-flow measurements for selected nasal sound segments produced by normal children and adolescents. Cleft Palate Craniofac J 40, 158–164.

Smith, B.E., Patil, Y., Guyette, T.W., Brannan, T.S., Cohen, M. (2004). Pressure-flow measurements for selected oral sound segments produced by normal children and adolescents: a basis for clinical testing. J Craniofac Surg 15, 247–254.

Smith, R.M., McWilliams, B.J. (1968). Psycholinguistic abilities of children with clefts. Cleft Palate J 5, 238–249.

Smith, S. (1951). Vocalization and added nasal resonance. Folia Phoniatr (Basel) 3, 165–169.

Snyder, L.E., Scherer, N. (2004). The development of symbolic play and language in toddlers with cleft palate. Am J Speech Lang Pathol 13, 66–80.

Spriestersbach, D.C., Darley, F., Morris, H. (1958). Language skills in children with cleft palates. J Speech Hear Res 1, 279–285.

Suzuki, C., Sando, I., Balaban, C.D., Kitagawa, M., Takasaki, K. (2003). Difference in attachment of the tensor veli palatine muscle to the Eustachian tube cartilage with age. Ann Otol Rhinol Laryngol 112, 439–443.

Swanson, J.F. (1973). Language-development in young cleft palate children. M.A. thesis. Gainsville: University of Florida.

Tachimura, T., Mori, C., Hirata, S.I., Wada, T. (2000). Nasalance score variation in normal adult Japanese speakers of Mid-West Japanese dialect. Cleft Palate Craniofac J 37, 463–467.

Templin, M.C. (1957). Certain language skills in children, their development and interrelationships. Institute of Child Welfare, Monograph. Series 26. Minneapolis: University of Minnesota Press.

Trost, J.E. (1981). Articulatory additions to the classical description of the speech of persons with cleft palate. Cleft Palate J 18, 193–203.

Tsuji, T., Yamaguchi, N., Moriyama, H. (2003). Patulous eustachian tube following otitis media. Nippon Jibiinkoka Gakkai Kaiho 106, 1023–1029.

Van Lierde, K.M., Wuyts, F.L., De Bodt, M., Van Cauwenberge, P. (2001). Nasometric values for normal nasal resonance in the speech of young Flemish adults. Cleft Palate Craniofac J 38, 112–118.

Velepic, M., Bonifacic, M., Lustica, I., Sasso, A., Cvjetkovic, N. (1999). The role of electromyography in the diagnosis of velopharyngeal insufficiency: our experiences. Acta Med Okayama 53, 127–131.

Warren, D.W. (1964). Velopharyngeal orifice size and upper pharyngeal pressure-flow patterns in normal speech. Plast Reconstr Surg 33, 148–162.

Whitehill, T.L. (2001). Nasalance measures in Cantonese-speaking women. Cleft Palate Craniofac J 38, 112–118.

Yamawaki, Y. (2003). Forward movement of posterior pharyngeal wall on phonation. Am J Otolaryngol 24, 400–404.

Ysunza, A., Pamplona, M., Silva-Rojas, A., Mazon, J.J., Ramirez, E., Canun, S., Sierra Mdel, C., Cervantes, A. (2004). Sensitivity and specificity of endoscopy for the detection of velocardiofacial syndrome. Rev Invest Clin 56, 454–459.

Zhong, W., Zhang, K., Wang, F. (2001). Applied anatomical study of blood supply in human palate. Zhonghua Kou Qiang Yi Xue Za Zhi 36, 136–138.

Zhu, H., Sun, Y., Wang, G. (1998). The study of acoustic-phonetic features of marginal velopharyngeal closure. Zhonghua Kou Qiang Yi Xue Za Zhi 33, 178–180.

Additional Reading

Clark, H.M. (2003). Neuromuscular treatments for speech and swallowing: a tutorial. Am J Speech Lang Pathol 12, 400–415.

Cooper, H.R., Sr., Harding, R.L., Krogman, W.H., Mazahari, M., Millard, R.T. (Eds.), Cleft palate and cleft lip. Philadelphia: W.B. Saunders Co. (A comprehensive textbook covering all aspects of cleft lip and palate.)

Fritzell, B. (1969). The velopharyngeal muscles in speech: an electromyographic and cineradiographic study. Acta Otolaryngol 250, 1(Suppl). (A comprehensive electromyographic study that shows the timing and extent of velopharyngeal muscle activity in closing and opening of the velopharyngeal portal during speech.)

Golding-Kushner, K.J. (2001). *Therapy techniques for cleft palate speech and related disorder.* San Diego: Singular. (A guide to different treatment techniques thought to be successful in treating communication problems related to velopharyngeal insufficiency.)

Hirschberg, J. (1986). Velopharyngeal insufficiency. Folia Phoniatr (Basel) 38, 221–276. (This extensive article should be read for its historical and technical review of the entire subject of velopharyngeal insufficiency from Hippocrates to the present, including the anatomy and physiology of velopharyngeal closure, etiologic classification of velopharyngeal insufficiency, diagnosis, physiologic measurement, surgery, and speech therapy.)

Kummer, A.W. (2001). *Cleft palate and craniofacial anomalies: effects on speech and resonance.* San Diego: Singular. (An excellent summary of the communication problems resulting from craniofacial anomalies.)

McWilliams, B.J., Morris, H.L., Shelton, R.L. (1984). *Cleft palate speech.* Philadelphia: B.C. Decker. (A classic in the field.)

Moore, K.L. (1977). *The developing human.* Philadelphia: W.B. Saunders. (A lucid depiction of the embryology of the maxillofacial anatomy.)

Pulec, J.L., Hahn, F.W. (1970). The abnormally patulous eustachian tube. Otolaryngol Clin North Am 3, 131–140. (An excellent review of a highly uncommon cause of hyponasality that will elude the unwary clinician.)

Ross, R.B., Johnson, M.C. (1972). *Cleft lip and palate.* Baltimore: Williams & Wilkins. (A detailed discussion of the incidence, etiology, and genetics of cleft lip and palate; especially suitable for the researcher.)

Ruscello, D.M. (1982). A selected review of palatal training procedures. Cleft Palate J 19, 181–193.

Ruscello, D.M. (1994). A motor skill learning treatment program for sound system disorders. Semin Speech Lang 14, 106–118.

Shprintzen, R.J. (2000). *Genetics, syndromes, and communication disorders.* San Diego: Singular. (This should be a required reading for any clinician working with individuals with velopharyngeal incompetence. It presents a comprehensive compendium of genetics, syndromes, and communication disorders.)

Skolnick, M.L. (1969). Videopharyngography in patients with nasal speech, with emphasis on lateral pharyngeal motion in velopharyngeal closure. Radiology 93, 747–755.

Skolnick, M.L. (1970). Videofluoroscopic examination of the velopharyngeal portal during phonation in lateral and base projections—a new technique for studying the mechanics of closure. Cleft Palate J 7, 803–816.

Skolnick, M.L., McCall, G.N., Barnes, M. (1973). The sphincteric mechanism of velopharyngeal closure. Cleft Palate J 10, 286–305. (The preceding three references represent pioneering radiologic work that has changed our conception of velopharyngeal closure from a two-dimensional to a three-dimensional one.)

Trost, J.E. (1981). Articulatory additions to the classical description of the speech of persons with cleft palate. Cleft Palate J 18, 193–203. (A radiographic study that clarifies the anatomy of the articulatory compensations made by cleft palate speakers.)

Trost, J.E. (1981). Differential diagnosis of velopharyngeal disorders. In L.J. Bradford and R.T. Wertz (Eds.), *Communicative disorders, an audio journal for continuing education.* New York: Grune & Stratton. (An instructive tape-recorded lecture on velopharyngeal disorders with illustrative examples of the effects of velopharyngeal insufficiencies on speech.)

Chapter 5

Neurologic Voice Disorders

Highly integrated neurophysiologic control is necessary for normal phonation. The vocal folds must be adducted to the midline and kept there with balanced and bilaterally symmetric adductor-abductor muscle tonus. Thyroarytenoid and cricothyroid muscle tension must be optimum. Glottal opening and closing has to be precisely timed, the folds adducted at the exact moment for onset of voiced consonants and vowels and abducted for voiceless. Should they adduct too soon, voiceless sounds would be voiced; too late, voiced sounds would be voiceless. Yet they must not overadduct, for then they would obstruct the exhaled air stream and produce strained voice or voice arrest. Should they fail to adduct or suddenly abduct, voicing would become breathy or whispered. The extrinsic muscles of the larynx must be able to elevate and depress the larynx in the neck, otherwise pitch variation will be restricted. On the other hand, if fluctuations are excessive, pitch will change unexpectedly and inappropriately. Exhalatory airflow must be forced from the lungs under constant pressure from moment to moment, for a sudden increase or decrease in such pressure may adversely produce irregular pitch and loudness changes. Air must be forced from the lungs with adequate pressure, otherwise the voice will be insufficiently loud, and at other times air must escape under low pressure for low loudness levels.

When vascular, infectious, traumatic, neoplastic, and degenerative diseases damage regions of the nervous system that contain nerve cells responsible for phonation, abnormal voice is inevitable. Previous research has identified acoustically different dysarthrias and their associated dysphonias caused by damage to specific regions of the nervous system (Darley, Aronson, and Brown, 1969a,b). Flaccid, spastic, ataxic, hypokinetic, and hyperkinetic dysarthrias sound different because physiologically and anatomically dissimilar regions of the nervous system are damaged in each type, producing different muscular pathophysiology. Neurologic voice disorders exhibit the same relationship between anatomic location of lesion and acoustic effect as the dysarthrias. In fact, neurologic voice disorders, technically, are dysarthrias; although they can occur in isolation, most often they are embedded in a more widespread complex of respiratory, resonatory, and articulatory dysarthric signs. Dysphonia can be the first sign of neurologic disease, the remainder of the dysarthria following as the disease progresses. Such capricious and discrepant patterns of neurologic disease onset are common.

There are, then, as many types of neurologic voice disorders as there are dysarthrias:

1. Flaccid (lower motor neuron) dysphonia

2. Spastic (upper motor neuron) (pseudobulbar) (supranuclear, corticobulbar tract) dysphonia

3. Mixed flaccid-spastic pseudobulbar dysphonia

4. Hypokinetic (basal ganglia) (parkinsonian) dysphonia

5. Ataxic (cerebellar) dysphonia

6. Choreic (basal ganglia) dysphonia

7. Dystonic (basal ganglia) dysphonia

8. Dysphonia of palatopharyngolaryngeal myoclonus (brain stem)

9. Dysphonia of organic (essential) tremor (brain stem)

10. Dysphonia of Gilles de la Tourette's syndrome

11. Apraxia of phonation

12. Akinetic mutism

13. Foreign accent syndrome

The voices of these neurologic voice disorders tend toward either constancy or variability of phonation depending upon whether or not the pathophysiology of the disease produces relatively steady or relatively fluctuating abnormal laryngeal or respiratory muscle movements. Neurologic voice disorders are subdivided into the

Table 5.1   Effect of Lesions of the Vagus Nerve on Phonation and Resonation

Level of Lesion	Effect on Vocal Folds		Effect on Phonation		Effect on Soft Palate		Effect on Nasal Resonation	Associated Signs
	Unilateral Lesion	Bilateral Lesion	Unilateral Lesion	Bilateral Lesion	Unilateral Lesion	Bilateral Lesion		
I. (**Fig. 5.3A**) Above origin of pharyngeal, superior laryngeal, and recurrent laryngeal nerves	One vocal fold fixed in abducted position	Both vocal folds fixed in abducted position	Breathy, moderate, reduced loudness and pitch	Extremely breathy to whispered (aphonia)	One side low, immobile	Both sides low, immobile	Hypernasality, nasal emission	Glottal coup and cough absent, weak, or mushy; difficulty in swallowing; nasal regurgitation of food; aspiration of secretions; pharyngeal paralysis
II. (**Fig. 5.3B**) Above origin of superior laryngeal and recurrent laryngeal nerves but below origin of pharyngeal nerve	Same as above	Same as above	Same as above	Same as above	None	None	None	Same as above, except no pharyngeal paralysis or difficulty in swallowing
III. (**Fig. 5.3C**) Superior laryngeal nerve	Both vocal folds able to adduct, affected vocal fold shorter, asymmetric shift of epiglottis and anterior larynx toward intact side on phonation	Absence of tilt of thyroid on cricoid cartilage, inability to view full length of vocal folds because of epiglottic over-hang, vocal folds bowed	Breathy, hoarse	Breathy, hoarse, reduced loud-ness, restricted pitch range	None	None	None	None
IV. (**Fig. 5.3D**) Recurrent laryngeal nerve	One vocal fold fixed in paramedian position	Both vocal folds fixed in paramedian position	Breathy, hoarse, reduced loudness, diplophonia (not in all cases)	Breathy, hoarse, reduced loudness	None	None	None	Unilateral: Marginal airway, weak cough. Bilateral: Severe difficulty on inhaling for life purposes, inhalatory stridor, tracheostomy often necessary.
V. (**Fig. 5.3E**) Myoneural junction (myasthenia gravis)	Not applicable	Restriction of adductor-abductor movements	Not applicable	Breathy, hoarse, reduced loud-ness; symptoms worsen with sustained speaking	Not applicable	Both sides low, immobile	Hypernasality, nasal emission; symptoms worsen with sustained speaking	Difficulty in swallo-wing, nasal regurgitation of food, inhalatory stridor, articulation defects

Source: Abstracted from Rontal, M., Tontal E. (1977). Lesions of the vagus nerve: Diagnosis, treatment and rehabilitation. Laryngoscope 87, 72–86; and from Ward, P.H., Berci, G., Calcaterra, J.C. (1977). Superior laryngeal nerve paralysis: An often overlooked entity. Trans Am Acad Ophthalmol Otolaryngol 84, 78–79.

following general categories, under which are subsumed specific neurologic dysphonias and aphonias (**Table 5.1**):

1. *Relatively constant neurologic voice disorders* Abnormal voice quality, loudness, or pitch deviations are relatively constant or consistent during contextual speech and vowel prolongation. Fluctuations may be major or minor. This category includes flaccid, spastic (pseudobulbar), mixed flaccid-spastic, and hypokinetic (parkinsonian) dysphonias.

2. *Arrhythmically fluctuating, neurologic voice disorders* Abnormal muscular physiology produces unpredictable and irregular quality, loudness, and pitch fluctuations from moment to moment during contextual speech, which are especially prominent during vowel prolongation. Included are ataxic, choreic, and dystonic dysphonias.

3. *Rhythmically fluctuating, neurologic voice disorders* Abnormal voice fluctuates relatively rhythmically from moment to moment and is particularly noticeable during vowel prolongation. In this group are included the dysphonias of palatopharyngolaryngeal myoclonus and organic (essential) (heredofamilial) voice tremor.

4. *Paroxysmal neurologic voice disorders* Relatively infrequent, sudden bursts of aberrant voice are exemplified in Gilles de la Tourette's syndrome.

5. *Neurologic voice disorders associated with loss of volitional phonation* The following neurologic voice disorders are not classifiable as dysarthrias but fall under the umbrella of (a) apraxia of speech, including apraxia of phonation (no loss of muscle strength or coordination but loss of volitional control over laryngeal and respiratory movements); (b) akinetic mutism; (c) foreign accent syndrome; and (d) frontal lobe syndrome.

◆ Neurologic Voice Disorders in Infants

Infant neurologic voice disorders cannot be classified according to the above schema because of limited knowledge of the relationship between abnormal voice and the neuroanatomic location of lesions in this age group. In general, however, newborn infants with central nervous system (CNS) lesions of unspecified location cry in an excessively high-pitched, shrill, weak, and unsustained voice. They require more intense and frequent pain stimuli to induce crying, and their cries are of abnormally short duration. For example, Karelitz and Fisichelli (1962) found that only 54% of neurologically impaired infants met the 1-minute cry duration criterion, in comparison with 92% of normal infants. Such infants produced statistically significantly fewer total sounds. Some were hypernasal (Fisichelli, 1966). Cyanotic infants cried with delayed latencies (Karelitz and Fisichelli, 1962), had fundamental frequencies twice as high as normal infants, and cried longer than normal infants (Lind, Wasz-Höeckert, Vuorenkoski, et al., 1965). The infants of drug-addicted mothers cried at abnor-

mally high fundamental frequencies (Blinick, Tavolga, and Antopol, 1971).

Infants born with unilateral or bilateral vocal fold paralyses due to cranial nerve X (vagus) lesions also cry abnormally. Such injury is caused by twisting the neck during breech presentations, infections, vascular diseases, and cranial malformations. The left recurrent laryngeal branch of the vagus nerve is more frequently damaged than the right because of its longer course in the chest and, therefore, greater exposure to disease or damage from an enlarged heart, tumors, mediastinal cysts, and tracheobronchial tree malformations. The dysphonia may be solitary or one of several cranial nerve signs. The cries of infants with unilateral adductor vocal fold paralysis are either weak or absent. In bilateral abductor paralysis, the voice and cry may be paradoxically normal because of adequate approximation of the vocal folds, but such infants produce inhalatory stridor during crying because their vocal folds are too weak to abduct during inhalation.

◆ Neurologic Voice Disorders in Children and Adults

Relatively Constant Neurologic Voice Disorders

Flaccid Dysphonia: Tenth Cranial Nerve (Vagus) Lesions

Cell bodies of the vagus nerves, which supply the larynx and pharynx, are found deep within the reticular formation of the medulla in the nucleus ambiguous. Experimental evidence in monkeys indicates that the superior third of the nucleus ambiguus is responsible for the pharynx and esophagus; caudal to it is a center for cricothyroid muscle function; and caudal to that is a center for abductor laryngeal muscle function. The most caudal region is responsible for adductor muscle function. A cluster of cells ~2 cm long contains the cell bodies of cranial nerves IX, X, and XI. The vagus nerve emerges from the lateral surface of the medulla between the inferior cerebellar peduncle and the inferior olive. A series of discrete roots converge into a single trunk intracranially. Each vagus nerve trunk passes through paired openings, the jugular foramina, at the base of the skull, along with cranial nerves IX and XI (**Fig. 5.1**). Near its exit from the skull, each vagus nerve divides into three branches:

1. *Pharyngeal nerve* The pharyngeal branch becomes identifiable as it emerges from the upper part of the inferior (nodos) ganglion of the vagus nerve and descends between the external and internal carotid arteries to the left of the middle pharyngeal constrictor muscles. At that point, it again divides into numerous filaments that join with branches from the sympathetic trunk and the glossopharyngeal and external laryngeal nerves to form the pharyngeal plexus. From there, nerve fibers are distributed to the pharynx and to all the muscles of the soft palate except the tensor veli palatini, which is supplied by the motor division of cranial nerve V (trigeminal).

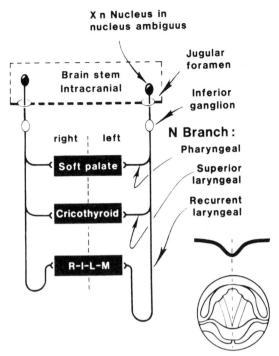

Figure 5.1 Pathway of the vagus nerve from brain stem to larynx. R-I-L-M, remaining intrinsic laryngeal muscles.

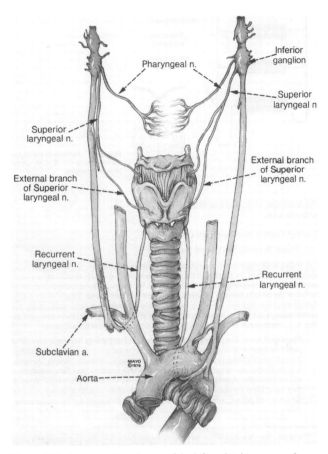

Figure 5.2 Asymmetric pathways of the left and right recurrent laryngeal nerves.

2. *Superior laryngeal nerve* This branch of the vagus nerve emerges from the inferior ganglion and descends alongside the pharynx, first posterior to the internal carotid artery and then medial to it. About 2 cm below the inferior ganglion, it divides into two additional branches: the internal and external laryngeal nerves.

   a. *Internal laryngeal nerve* This branch of the superior laryngeal nerve descends to the level of the thyrohyoid membrane and, piercing and entering it, further divides into two additional branches. Both contain afferent or sensory fibers from mucous membrane that lines the larynx above the level of the vocal folds. They also contain fibers from muscle spindles and other stretch receptors in the larynx. The upper branch of the internal laryngeal nerve supplies the mucous membrane of the epiglottis, the vallecula, and the vestibule of the larynx. The lower branch supplies the mucous membrane of the aryepiglottic folds and the dorsum of the arytenoid cartilages.

   b. *External laryngeal nerve* This efferent or motor branch of the superior laryngeal nerve descends posterior to the sternothyroid muscle and innervates the cricothyroid muscle. It also branches to the inferior pharyngeal constrictor.

3. *Recurrent laryngeal nerve* The term *recurrent* refers to the anatomic course of this nerve, which first descends to the lower neck and into the chest and then courses superiorly again. This nerve pair, unlike the rest that supply the larynx, is not bilaterally symmetric (**Fig. 5.2**).

The right recurrent laryngeal nerve arises from the vagal trunk, it ascends alongside the trachea behind the common carotid artery and, higher up, in or near the groove between the trachea and esophagus, entering the larynx behind the articulation between the inferior horn of the thyroid and the cricoid cartilage. In 70 to 80% of cases, the nerve divides into two or more branches before entering the larynx. The left recurrent laryngeal nerve splits off from the trunk of the vagus to the left of the arch of the aorta, winding under it from front to back. Ascending lateral to the trachea, it then pierces and enters the larynx, as on the right side. Both right and left recurrent laryngeal nerves supply all intrinsic muscles of the larynx except the cricothyroid. They also supply sensory filaments to the mucous membrane lining the larynx below the level of the vocal folds, and they carry afferent fibers from stretch receptors to the intrinsic laryngeal muscles.

The extrinsic laryngeal musculature is also implicated in lower motor neuron disease, although to a much lesser extent than the intrinsic muscles. Of the suprahyoid muscles, the anterior belly of the digastric is innervated by the mylohyoid branch of the inferior alveolar nerve; the posterior belly by cranial nerve VII; the stylohyoid by cranial nerve VII; the mylohyoid by the mylohyoid branch of the inferior alveolar nerve; and the geniohyoid by the first cervical spinal nerve (C1) via the hypoglossal nerve. The infrahyoid muscles—the sternohyoid, sternothyroid, and omohyoid—are all innervated by the ansa cervicalis, and the thyrohyoid is innervated by fibers from C1 via the hypoglossal nerve.

The autonomic nerve supply to the larynx originates in the dorsal motor nuclei of the vagus as parasympathetic fibers that synapse in the inferior ganglion and accompany the somatic motor nerves to the larynx. Sympathetic nerve fibers enter the motor nerves through connections with the superior cervical ganglion. Autonomic nerve fibers have chiefly secretory and vasomotor functions and maintain muscle tonus.

Effects of Tenth Cranial Nerve Lesions on Vocal Fold Movement and Phonation Lesions of the tenth cranial nerve at any point along its pathway from the nucleus ambiguus in the brain stem to the musculature cause flaccid paresis (weakness) or paralysis (immobility) of laryngeal muscles as well as dysphonia or aphonia. The extent of weakness, the position of vocal fold fixation, the unilaterality or bilaterality of the weakness, and the degree of voice impairment depend upon the location of the lesion along the pathway of the nerve and whether one or both nerves of the pair have been damaged. Refer to **Fig. 5.3** and **Table 5.1** for the following discussion.

1. Intramedullary and extramedullary lesions affecting all branches of the vagus nerve to the larynx (**Fig. 5.3A**).

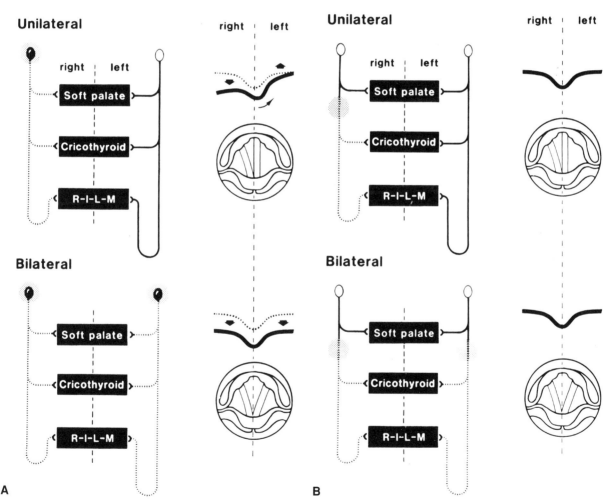

A   **B**

Figure 5.3 (**A**) Effects of unilateral and bilateral vagus nerve lesions at different locations on vocal fold and soft palate functions. Stippled line indicates lesions. (See **Table 5.1** for corresponding information.) Top: Unilateral lesion of vagus nerve (nucleus), above origin of pharyngeal, superior laryngeal, and recurrent laryngeal nerves. The right vocal fold is fixed in an abducted position, whereas the left adducts to the midline on phonation. The soft palate is paralyzed on the right, is resting, and pulls to the left on phonation. Bottom: Bilateral lesion. Both vocal folds are fixed in an abducted position on phonation. The soft palate is bilaterally paralyzed, is resting low, and does not move on phonation. R-I-L-M, remaining intrinsic laryngeal musculature. (**B**) Top: Unilateral lesion of vagus nerve above origin of superior laryngeal and recurrent laryngeal nerves but below bifurcation of pharyngeal nerve. Same effect on vocal folds as (**A**; top), but soft palate functions normally. Bottom: Bilateral lesion. Same effects on vocal folds as (**A**; bottom), but soft palate functions normally. *(Continued on page 74)*

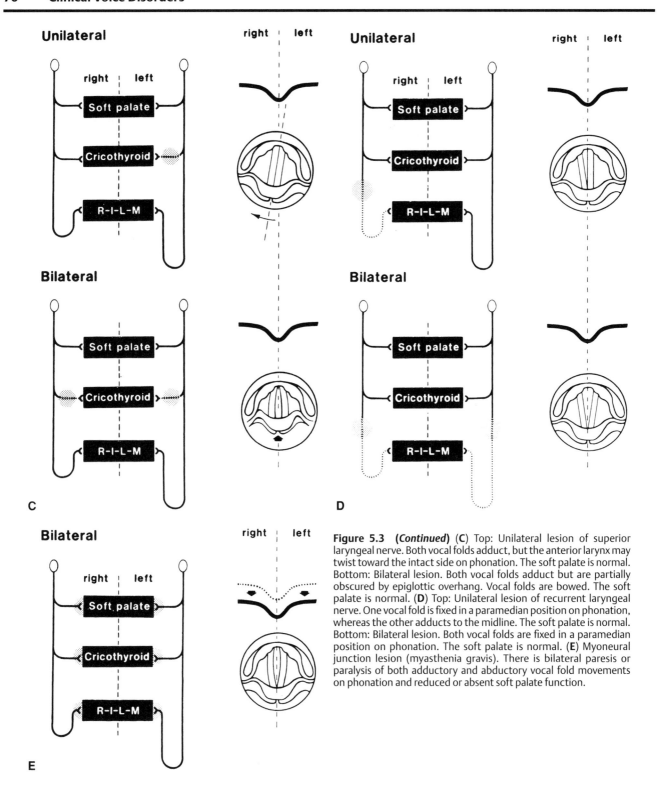

Figure 5.3 (*Continued*) (**C**) Top: Unilateral lesion of superior laryngeal nerve. Both vocal folds adduct, but the anterior larynx may twist toward the intact side on phonation. The soft palate is normal. Bottom: Bilateral lesion. Both vocal folds adduct but are partially obscured by epiglottic overhang. Vocal folds are bowed. The soft palate is normal. (**D**) Top: Unilateral lesion of recurrent laryngeal nerve. One vocal fold is fixed in a paramedian position on phonation, whereas the other adducts to the midline. The soft palate is normal. Bottom: Bilateral lesion. Both vocal folds are fixed in a paramedian position on phonation. The soft palate is normal. (**E**) Myoneural junction lesion (myasthenia gravis). There is bilateral paresis or paralysis of both adductory and abductory vocal fold movements on phonation and reduced or absent soft palate function.

Lesions that damage vagal nuclei within the brain stem are called intramedullary. When the nerve trunk just outside the brain stem but still within the cranial cavity is damaged, the lesion is called extramedullary. If the lesion affects the nerve after it exits from the skull, it is called extracranial. Lesions at any of these three levels damage the vagus nerve above the separation of its pharyngeal, superior laryngeal, and recurrent laryngeal branches. Therefore, all muscles supplied by those branches of the vagus nerve below the level of the lesion will be weak or paralyzed. Affected muscles then will be one of three types: (1) those supplied by the pharyngeal branch of the vagus nerve. Consequently, the levator muscle of the soft palate, the levator veli-palatini, will be weak or paralyzed on the same side as the lesion. (2) Because the superior laryngeal branch also lies below the level of the lesion, the cricothyroid muscle will be weak or paralyzed on the side of the lesion. (3) Because the recurrent laryngeal branch lies below the level of the lesion, the remaining intrinsic muscles of the larynx will be weak or paralyzed on the side of the lesion. The vocal folds will be paralyzed and fixed in the abducted position unilaterally or bilaterally. At rest and during phonation, the soft palate will hang lower on the paralyzed side, the nonparalyzed side will elevate, pulling the uvula and the midline of the soft palate toward the normal side. In bilateral lesions, the soft palate will rest at a lower than normal position and on phonation will elevate minimally or not at all bilaterally.

Unilateral lesions above the bifurcation of the pharyngeal branch of the vagus nerve causing unilateral vocal fold paralysis will produce severe breathiness to whispered voice and diplophonia and, in some instances, a flutter or rapid tremor on vowel prolongation. There will be reduced loudness and pitch and possibly falsetto pitch breaks.

In bilateral vocal folds paralysis where both folds are abducted, the voice will be virtually whispered, owing to the wider glottal chink than is found in unilateral paralysis and markedly reduced loudness. Unilateral soft palate paralysis will produce mild-to-moderate hypernasality and nasal emission, which will be much more severe if the paralysis is bilateral.

Associated signs will be a weak, mushy, or absent glottal coup or cough, dysphagia, and nasal regurgitation on swallowing liquids and solids. Pharyngeal paralysis results in a reduced or absent gag reflex and aspiration of secretions, which, if severe, may require tracheostomy. Diseases that cause tenth cranial nerve lesions at this level are of several types: vascular, such as brain-stem hemorrhage, thrombosis, and arteriovenous malformation; traumatic; primary or metastatic neoplastic; congenital defects of bone, such as Arnold-Chiari malformation; inflammatory, such as poliomyelitis and Guillain-Barré syndrome; degenerative, such as amyotrophic lateral sclerosis (ALS); metabolic, exemplified by myasthenia gravis; toxic, such as metal (arsenic) or organic (botulism) poisoning; and others such as multiple sclerosis, diphtheria, and tetany.

2. Extracranial lesions of the superior and recurrent laryngeal nerves, but not the pharyngeal nerve (**Fig. 5.3B**). Extracranial lesions high in the neck can spare the pharyngeal branch of the vagus but damage the nerve above the origin of the superior and recurrent laryngeal nerves. Because the pharyngeal nerve lies above the level of the lesion, the muscles of the soft palate and pharynx will be normal. However, because the superior and recurrent laryngeal branches lie below the level of the lesion, the cricothyroid and remaining intrinsic muscles of the larynx will be paralyzed, having the same effects on the vocal folds and voice as described in the previous section.

Causes of lesions below the bifurcation of the pharyngeal nerve but above the superior laryngeal include surgical trauma and infectious and idiopathic disease. The latter are discussed in greater detail later in this chapter.

3. Extracranial lesions of the superior laryngeal nerve but not the pharyngeal and recurrent laryngeal nerves (**Fig. 5.3C**). A lesion of the superior laryngeal nerve causes weakness or paralysis of the cricothyroid muscle. Because the pharyngeal and recurrent laryngeal branches are spared, the soft palate and remaining intrinsic laryngeal muscles are normal. On laryngoscopic examination, the vocal folds appear deceptively normal. Consequently, dysphonia due to cricothyroid muscle weakness is often either missed or misdiagnosed as "functional." In unilateral cricothyroid muscle paralysis, both vocal folds appear to abduct normally on phonation, but on closer scrutiny the vocal fold on the affected side may appear shorter, and an asymmetric lateral shift of the epiglottis and anterior larynx toward the intact side may be noted. The notion that unilateral cricothyroid paralysis always causes an observable twisting has recently come into question suggesting this movement pattern is not always present. In bilateral cricothyroid paralysis, there will be an absence of tilt of the thyroid cartilage on the cricoid cartilage during phonation, the vocal folds will appear shorter than normal, the epiglottis will overhang and obscure the anterior portion of the vocal folds, and there will be bowing of the vocal folds (**Fig. 5.4**). The soft palate will be normal because the pharyngeal branch of the vagus nerve has been spared. Unilateral cricothyroid muscle paralysis produces mild breathiness or hoarseness, normal or mildly reduced loudness, and mild inability to alter pitch, interfering with singing in the upper part of the range and vocal projection. In bilateral cricothyroid muscle paralysis, breathiness and hoarseness will be mild to moderate, loudness will be reduced, and ability to alter pitch will be moderately to severely impaired, causing serious interference with singing. The cause of cricothyroid muscle paralysis is usually surgery, other trauma, or infection.

4. Extracranial lesions of the recurrent laryngeal nerve but not the pharyngeal and superior laryngeal nerves (**Fig. 5.3D**). All muscles supplied by the recurrent laryngeal nerve are paralyzed, whereas those supplied by the remaining branches of the vagus, namely, the cricothyroid muscle and soft palate, are spared. The vocal folds are fixed in the paramedian position unilaterally or bilaterally. It is important to understand why the vocal folds are not paralyzed in the abducted position, as in the case of a lesion above the bifurcation of the superior laryngeal branch: the intact cricothyroid muscle, still capable of stretching the vocal fold anteroposteriorly, acts as an adductor, thereby pulling the vocal fold closer to the midline. Lesions above the level of the superior laryngeal nerve result in fixation of the vocal fold more laterally, in the abducted position (causing virtual aphonia), because the cricothyroid muscle as well as the remaining intrinsic muscles is paralyzed and unable to exert its abducting influence. In bilateral paralysis of the vocal folds due to

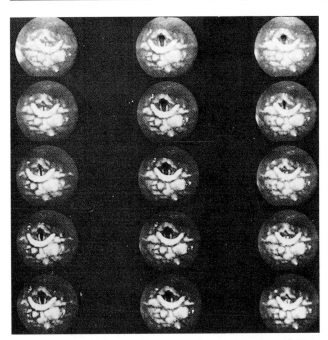

Figure 5.4 Frames from motion picture photographs of vocal folds in bilateral cricothyroid muscle paralysis due to superior laryngeal nerve lesions. Absence of anterior tilt failing to lengthen and tense the vocal folds is noted by failure of anterior movement of the epiglottis, making it difficult to visualize the anterior commissure. Also visible is failure of complete vocal fold approximation on adduction due to bowing. (From Ward, P.H., Berci, G., Calcaterra, T.C. [1977]. Superior laryngeal nerve paralysis: an often over-looked entity. Trans Am Acad Ophthalmol Otolaryngol 84, 78–89.)

recurrent laryngeal nerve lesions only, the vocal fold rests so close to the midline that phonation is virtually normal. Paralysis of the abductors prevents widening of the glottis on inhalation, however, resulting in inhalatory stridor and compromising the airway. Breathy-hoarse quality, reduced loudness, and in some cases diplophonia and falsetto pitch breaks are heard in unilateral vocal fold paralysis from recurrent laryngeal nerve lesions. Associated signs of unilateral vocal fold paralysis are a marginal airway and a weak cough or glottal coup. In bilateral paralysis, the airway is severely compromised, resulting in respiratory distress often requiring tracheostomy.

Conditions that cause recurrent laryngeal nerve lesions include trauma due to surgery, tumors of the nerve itself or impinging upon the nerve, vascular disease, infection, metabolic diseases, and idiopathic disorders.

Occasionally, inhalatory stridor can be mistaken for abductor vocal fold paralysis or an asthmatic attack when, in fact, these events, in all probability, are psychogenic (Appelblatt and Baker, 1981; Cormier, Camus, and Desmeules, 1980; Kellman and Leopold, 1982; Patterson, Schatz, and Horton, 1974; Rogers, 1980; Rogers and Stell, 1978) or paradoxical vocal cord dysfunction. Christopher, Wood, Eckert, et al. (1983) reported on five patients who had dramatic episodes of wheezing and who had been diagnosed as having uncontrolled asthma, symptoms that continued despite aggressive pharmacologic therapy.

Laryngologic, psychiatric, and speech pathology studies, however, proved that these patients had a nonorganic disorder of the larynx that mimicked bronchial asthma. Indirect laryngoscopy disclosed that the asthmatic-like sounds were coming not from the lungs but from an unusual mode of glottic closure on inhalation and exhalation during tidal breathing. Psychiatric examinations indicated that all of the patients were unaware of their upper airway obstruction and thought that they were having bronchial asthmatic attacks. They were unable to reproduce the abnormal sound voluntarily. In all patients, treatment by a speech pathologist was effective, and after 3 to 21 months of follow-up, these patients were asymptomatic. This problem described by Christopher and colleagues is what we now recognize as vocal cord dysfunction, or VCD. It is considered to have many etiologies including redundant tissue, anxiety, and damage to the brain stem. What must be borne in mind, however, is that patients with extrapyramidal movement disorders also can produce laryngeal stridor at rest during tidal breathing because of adventitious adduction of the vocal folds as a component of their movement disorder. Moreover, sudden paroxysmal inhalation often accompanies these stridorous inhalations.

5. Myoneural junction disease: myasthenia gravis (**Fig. 5.3E**). The reduced availability of acetylcholine at the myoneural junction in myasthenia gravis causes progressive flaccid weakness or paralysis with strenuous muscular effort, as in prolonged voice use. Sometimes, muscles supplied by the vagus nerve are the first to be affected by this disease. When it is confined to the larynx and soft palate, the signs often erroneously lead the examiner into nonorganic avenues of diagnostic thinking. Because myasthenia gravis causes bilateral weakness of the intrinsic laryngeal muscles, the vocal folds abduct incompletely, sometimes bowing during phonation. Because abduction may be incomplete as well, inhalatory stridor occurs in more severe cases. The soft palate elevates minimally or not at all on phonation, resulting in hypernasality and nasal emission. The voice of patients with myasthenia gravis is breathy, sometimes hoarse, and flutter or tremor-like fluctuations on vowel prolongation may be heard. Loudness is usually reduced, and there is a restriction of pitch range. All defects become progressively worse with protracted speaking.

Most often, myasthenia gravis produces the full complement of flaccid dysarthria: consonant imprecision, breathiness, hypernasality, and nasal emission due to associated velar, tongue, lip, mandibular, and respiratory muscle weakness. The cough and glottal coup are weak or mushy, depending on the severity of the disease at the time of examination. The etiology of myasthenia gravis has been described as a defect in the neurochemistry at the myoneural junction, specifically a failure of acetylcholine production. However, recent research gives evidence of an autoimmune mechanism responsible for the disorder.

6. Disease of muscle. Muscular dystrophies or myopathies can cause flaccid dysphonia. The three types of muscular dystrophies are the pseudohypertrophic (Duchenne), the limb-girdle, and the facioscapulohumeral (Landouzy-Dejerine).

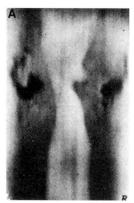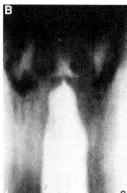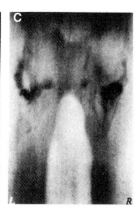

Figure 5.5   X-ray tomograms (posteroanterior) showing right vocal fold paralysis during quiet breathing, phonation, and effort closure. (**A**) Quiet breathing. The paralyzed vocal fold projects into the airway. The smoothly contoured side is the normal side. (**B**) Prolongation of the vowel /i/. The normal vocal fold adducts to meet the paralyzed one, giving a deceptively normal appearance, but there are asymmetric contours of the subglottic walls. (**C**) Bearing down producing effort closure, illustrating the retained capacity for gross glottic closure activity. (From Ardran, G.M., Kemp, F.H., Marland, P.M. [1954]. Laryngeal palsy. Br J Radiol 27, 201–209.)

Their general features are a family history of disease, early age of onset, and atrophy or dystrophy of muscle. A heredofamilial type of myopathy is myotonic dystrophy, in which there is selective atrophy of muscles, including the speech musculature, resulting in flaccid dysarthria, including dysphonia. The masticatory and facial muscles may be especially involved. The disease is progressive and appears for the first time in adulthood, between the ages of 20 and 30 years.

7. Idiopathic vocal fold paralysis. Some vocal fold paralyses defy diagnosis; that is, a specific etiology cannot be discovered despite thorough investigation. These are called *idiopathic*[1] vocal fold paralyses. Williams (1959) reviewed the records of patients with vocal fold paralysis over a 6-year period; 66 of 181, or 36%, had an idiopathic disorder, consistent with the 33% found by New and Childrey (1932). The average duration was ~5 months, after which spontaneous recovery occurred, although the dysphonia averaged 1 month longer than the vocal fold paralysis. The left vocal fold was paralyzed in 43 patients (65.2%), the right in 19 (28.7%), and 4 (6.1%) had bilateral paralyses. Blau and Kapadia (1972) consider idiopathic unilateral vocal fold paralysis to be one of the cranial mononeuropathies: a benign condition in which individual cranial nerve function is partially or totally impaired, the site of involvement undetermined and the etiology unknown, and which has a high rate of spontaneous recovery within a period of 9 months, as in the case of idiopathic tenth cranial nerve interference.

Pathophysiology of Flaccid Dysphonia   The basis of the abnormally breathy and weak voice of flaccid vocal fold paralysis is an increased volume velocity of airflow through the glottis and a failure of complete vocal fold vibration because of its flaccidity and improper position within the airway. The perceived breathiness is produced by air turbulence as air flows through the glottis, which remains open throughout the glottic cycle. Posteroanterior tomograms of normal and paralyzed vocal folds are shown in **Fig. 5.5**. In

Fig. 5–5A, the tomogram is of a patient with right unilateral vocal fold paralysis in which the fold projects out into the glottis during quiet breathing. The following points are also notable.

1. The vocal fold on the normal left side is turned upward, its free edge close to the lower surface of the ventricular fold. The laryngeal ventricle is barely visible.

2. On the paralyzed side, the vocal fold projects across the glottis, its edge close to the midline. The laryngeal ventricle is wide and the ventricular fold is prominent and nearer to the midline than is the normal side.

3. The lateral wall of the subglottic space on the normal side is flattened or slightly convex and on the paralyzed side it is concave. The airway is consequently narrowed, and its central axis is deviated toward the normal side.

In **Fig. 5.5B**, the same patient is prolonging the vowel /i/. This illustration shows:

◆ The normal vocal fold on the left approximates the paralyzed fold on the right and is aligned more horizontally with a thickened free edge.

◆ On the paralyzed side, the vocal fold is tilted slightly upward and its free edge is "tongue-shaped."

◆ The laryngeal ventricle is larger on the paralyzed side.

◆ The glottal slit appears to be displaced toward the paralyzed side.

◆ The ventricular fold appears to be more prominent on the paralyzed side.

The tomogram of **Fig. 5.5C** is of the patient during effort closure while bearing down. Despite the paralysis, effort closure is complete, demonstrating the compensatory ability of the sphincter-like closure mechanism, although in some patients the location of closure differs.

Posteroanterior tomograms of a patient with bilateral vocal fold paralysis are shown in **Fig. 5.6**. The tomogram of **Fig. 5.6A** illustrates quiet breathing, showing the vocal folds resting toward the midline, creating a narrower than normal glottis. On prolongation of the vowel /i/ (**Fig. 5.6B**), there is

[1]As defined by *Dorland's Illustrated Medical Dictionary*, a morbid state of unknown causation or of spontaneous origin.

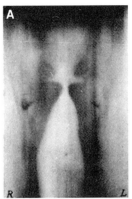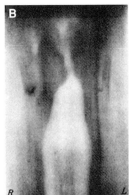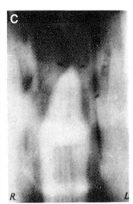

Figure 5.6 X-ray tomograms (posteroanterior) showing bilateral vocal fold paralysis during quiet breathing, phonation, and effort closure. (**A**) Quiet breathing. Both vocal folds project into the airway. (**B**) Prolongation of the vowel /i/. Incomplete adduction of true vocal folds and lack of demarcation between true and false folds are seen. (**C**) Bearing down producing effort closure, illustrating the retained capacity for gross glottic closure activity. (From Ardran, G.M., Kemp, F.H., Marland, P.M. [1954]. Laryngeal palsy. Br J Radiol 27, 201–209.)

no demarcation between the true and false vocal folds, contrary to what is expected in the normal larynx. The axis of the vocal tract is asymmetric, and there is a wide glottal channel even during voice production. The tomogram of **Fig. 5.6C** shows the same patient bearing down, again illustrating the reserve sphincter power of the larynx despite a bilateral vocal fold paralysis and inadequacy of phonation. In fact, all 15 patients examined by Ardran, Kemp, and Marland (1954), despite their dysphonias and aphonia, were able to adduct the vocal folds during gross sphincteric effort closure.

Breathy voice quality and reduced loudness in unilateral and bilateral vocal fold paralysis, fewer syllables per exhalation, and more frequent inhalation during speech result from increased airflow through the glottis.

Hirano, Koike, and von Leden (1968) obtained maximum phonation times, mean flow rates, and phonation quotients of patients who had vocal fold paralyses (**Table 5.2**). In 10 of 13 patients, maximum phonation time was shorter than normal, the product of excess expenditure of air. Mean flow rates in 8 of 13 patients were greater than normal, and in 7 of 11 patients the phonation quotients were greater than normal. In 3 patients whose vocal folds had been injected with Teflon, clinical improvement was confirmed by an increase in maximum phonation time and a decrease in mean flow rate and phonation quotient. Ultraspeed motion picture studies of unilateral vocal fold paralyses show marked pitch and amplitude perturbations caused by the different rates of vibration of each vocal fold (**Fig. 5.7**).

Table 5.2 Maximum Phonation Time, Mean Flow Rate, and Phonation Quotient in Cases of Vocal Cord Paralysis*

Case	Sex	Age (Years)	Maximum Phonation Time (Seconds)	Mean Flow Rate (cm³/s)	Phonation Quotient (cm³/s)	
43	M	39	14.4	205	331	Left, paramedian
44	M	45	3.9	382	1254	Left, intermediate,
		45	18.7	125	261	with atrophy. After Teflon injection
45	M	59	5.8	484	559	Left, intermediate,
		59	15.6	201	208	with atrophy. After Teflon injection
46	M	32	6.8	621	706	Left, intermediate, with atrophy
47	M	71	9.9	270	310	Left, intermediate.
		71	24.1	117	128	After injection
48	M	78	21.6	99	141	Left compensated
49	M	42	36.0	53	126	Right compensated
50	F	29	7.6	280	*	Bilateral paramedian
51	F	40	7.4	378	*	Bilateral paramedian
52	F	67	18.8	92	160	Bilateral paramedian
53	F	69	12.8	105	189	Bilateral paramedian
54	F	64	8.1	309	316	Bilateral paramedian
55	F	47	9.5	315	346	Right, intermediate.
		47	20.6	145	160	Restricted abduction

Source: From Hirano, M., Koike, Y., von Leden, H. (1968). Maximum phonation time and air usage during phonation. Folia Phoniatr 20, 158–201.

* Respiratory tests inadequate.

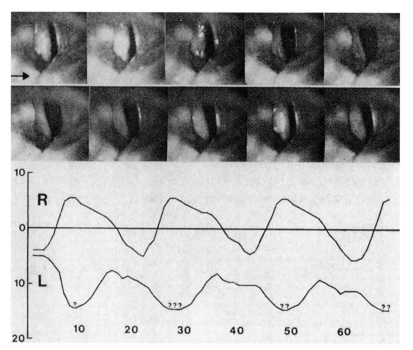

Figure 5.7 Frames from ultraspeed photography of unilateral vocal fold paralysis. Male larynx with paralysis of the left vocal fold. The sequence of photographs progresses from left to right in the top row followed by the same order in the second row. The graph illustrates the motions of the approximate anteroposterior midpoints of the glottal borders and demonstrates the absence of glottal closure, the crossing of an arbitrary median sagittal plane by the healthy vocal fold reaches its medial limit, and vibrations of both folds at the same frequency. (From Moore, G.P. [1976]. Observations on laryngeal disease, laryngeal behavior and voice. Ann Otol Rhinol Laryngol 85, 553–564.)

Diplophonia, the simultaneous perception of two different pitches, is common in unilateral vocal fold paralysis. It is presumably caused by each vocal fold vibrating at a different frequency, owing to differences in their tensions. Triplophonia, three pitches being heard simultaneously, has also occurred.

Etiology of Vocal Fold Paralyses Producing Flaccid Dysphonia In a study of 633 cases of vocal fold paralysis, Huppler, Schmidt, Devine, et al. (1955) found that the largest number, 272 patients (43%), was caused by thyroidectomy. The female to male ratio was 6:1, and in half the group, the vocal fold paralysis was bilateral. Treatment has changed since the 1950s, and the percent of paralysis cases caused by thyroidectomy has decreased. Cancer of the breast, thyroid gland, lung, tongue, mouth, pharynx, or larynx, as well as other primary and metastatic cancers of the neck was the reason for surgery in these cases. Cardiovascular disease produced paralysis on the left side in all cases. The specific causes of heart disease were mitral stenosis, syphilitic aortitis and aneurysm, nonsyphilitic aneurysm, cardiomegaly, and congenital heart disease. Other causes of paralysis included specific neurologic diseases such as syringobulbia, poliomyelitis, and multiple sclerosis; trauma caused by automobile accidents, gunshot wounds, falls and blows to the neck, endotracheal intubation, bronchoscopy ingested foreign body; infection; diphtheria; granuloma and empyema. It is important to remember that 184 (29%) were idiopathic as previously discussed. This figure, too, has changed over the years because of improved diagnostic abilities.

Vocal fold paralysis and flaccid dysphonia can occur as one of several signs in certain neurologic disease syndromes. In the jugular foramen syndrome, a lesion, usually a tumor, within or adjacent to the jugular foramen compresses cranial nerves IX, X, and XI, causing ipsilateral weakness of the pharyngeal, laryngeal, trapezius, and sternocleidomastoid muscles. Another syndrome is caused by posterior inferior cerebellar artery occlusion, producing infarction of the lateral medulla. Known as Wallenberg's syndrome, it is marked by dysarthria and dysphagia, ipsilateral impairment of pain and temperature sensation on the face, and contralateral loss of pain and temperature in the trunk and extremities. Because the nucleus ambiguus undergoes destruction, unilateral vocal fold paralysis and flaccid dysphonia occur. In general, any vascular or space-occupying lesion within the posterior fossa is capable of damaging one or both tenth cranial nerve nuclei or their nerve trunks, causing unilateral or bilateral vocal fold paralysis and dysphonia.

Special Considerations in the Diagnosis of Flaccid Dysphonia: Myasthenia Gravis

1. Breathy voice and reduced loudness, even though the laryngologic examination is normal, ought to alert the clinician to the possibility of flaccid dysphonia due to lower motor neuron disease.

2. Worsening of breathiness and weakness as a consequence of sustained effortful speaking ought to alert the clinician to the specific flaccid dysphonia of myasthenia gravis. The fewer pathologic changes seen laryngologically, the more important is clinical listening. Bilateral, minimal weakness of the vocal folds is the most common reason for the failure to identify flaccid dysphonia laryngoscopically and is the reason such patients are often misdiagnosed as having functional or psychogenic voice disorders. On videostroboscopic examination, the vocal folds generally appear intact, but the closed phase is extremely short, and aperiodicity may be increased. It is important to remember that flaccid dysphonia can be the sign of an encroaching neurologic

disease of the peripheral nervous system. The dysphonia of myasthenia gravis is a classic example of a frequently misdiagnosed voice sign. Most of the time, it produces a complete dysarthria involving phonation, resonation, and articulation and is not difficult to identify. (See **Table 5.3** for a complete description of the dysarthria.) The changes of identification become considerably poorer when only one of the components of the peripheral speech mechanism is affected; the larynx is such a component. Several cases of monosymptomatic dysarthria in myasthenia gravis have been reported, as for example hypernasality (Wolski, 1967). Myasthenia gravis focal to the larynx producing breathiness and weakness without accompanying hypernasality of articulatory defect has also been reported (Neiman, Mountjoy, and Allen, 1975). In an article on early motor unit disease misdiagnosed as psychogenic dysphonia, Aronson (1971) reported the following case study.

Case Study 5.1

A 20-year-old secretary returned from vacation, and her parents noted that she had a weak voice. Two laryngologists and one internist diagnosed her voice change as "functional (nonorganic) dysphonia." Yet psychiatric examination was unable to find a plausible psychologic explanation for her voice disorder. The following edited transcript of the intake interview shows the importance of history-taking in the diagnosis of voice disorders and how small clues can help the clinician think deductively about possible causes.

Clinician: When did all this speech business begin?
Patient: I was never one for speaking, because I was always quiet, but I suppose this summer I've noticed, uh, well, its been called to my attention that I slur words.
C: What were you doing this summer when your voice disorder began?
P: Oh, I don't know. Like, I'd be sitting at the supper table and my words would seem all jumbled together. I think my parents were the first ones that called this to my attention. Ever since then I've caught myself.
C: Were you feeling well otherwise?
P: Yes. I had gone on vacation in May. I went down to the Bahamas about two weeks.
C: When you came back from vacation, did you go right back to work?
P: Yes, like, I'd be on the phone a lot. My voice, first my throat, like my words wouldn't come out right, like they'd have to shove their way through.
C: Did you have any funny feelings in your throat?
P: Yeah, I've had difficulty swallowing. I mean, it doesn't hurt, or anything. It's just that it feels like a narrow passage—either when I am talking or swallowing.
C: Have you had any occasion to notice fluids coming through your nose as you swallowed?
P: Wait, like when I'm drinking like when it seems to go right up my nose?
C: Yes, how often?
P: Quite a bit of the time when I drink.

Table 5.3 Laryngeal-Phonatory Characteristics in the Flaccid Dysarthria of Myasthenia Gravis

	Findings
Perceptual	
Phonation	Breathy voice quality, weak intensity. Deterioration of phonation during stressful counting or other prolonged speaking activities; reduced sharpness of cough after stressful speaking. Can exist in the absence of remaining signs of dysarthria
Resonation	Initially normal; hypernasality develops after stressful speaking
Articulation	Initially normal; articulatory imprecision develops after stressful speaking
Language	Normal
Physical	
Larynx	In milder cases, vocal folds may appear normal in structure and function despite dysphonia; absence of positive laryngologic findings does not exclude presence of milder degrees of bilateral adductor weakness of vocal folds. In more severe cases, folds may fail to adduct and abduct completely, bilaterally. Bowing may be present.
Velopharynx	Initially normal; velopharyngeal insufficiency after stressful speaking. Hypoactive gag reflex
Tongue	Initially normal; tongue weakness after stressful speaking
Lips	Initially normal; lip weakness after stressful speaking; lateral smile
Teeth	Normal
Hard palate	Normal
Mandible	Initially normal; mandibular muscle weakness after stressful speaking
General Medical	Patient may complain of general fatigue, particularly after exercise. Findings can be nonspecific, leading to erroneous diagnosis of functional illness
Other Neurologic Signs	
Peripheral nervous system	Weakness of bulbar musculature; positive Tensilon test
Central nervous system	Normal
Psychiatric/ Psychologic	Patient may complain of fatigue, loss of energy, or loss of interest, which may be erroneously diagnosed as signs of primary depression. Patients may become secondarily depressed about lack of energy.

C: And that is something new?
P: Yes, it didn't happen before this summer. And, my mouth was always really dry. You know, like when you wake up in the morning? It feels like that all day.
C: Tell me, any emotional problems lately? Depressed at all? That kind of thing?

P: Hmm, nothing exciting's happened, but I don't think I've been really depressed.

C: Your speech, you know, gives the impression of a certain lack of vitality. Not very vivacious. Are you that type of person?

P: No, when I was at college I was a cheerleader, and I was loud then.

C: You were loud then! (C. surprised at this description because of their extremely flat, lethargic affect.)

P: Yes, I mean, I could really belt it out, hours on end; but now, it's like I get tired inside, or something.

C: And that, again, has been true just since last summer?

P: Yes, I slowly noticed it.

C: How do you get along with your family at home?

P: Fine.

C: No problems especially around June? How about your love life? Anything developing there? Any disappointments?

P: I would like to get married next fall.

C: And, how long have you been going with this person?

P: About a year and a half.

C: Has this been a satisfactory relationship?

P: Uh huh.

C: I want to be sure that there isn't something that's really disappointing you, or something that you're keeping back, because if there is, we'd like to know about it.

P: No. Truthfully, I can't say that there is any one thing that I've been depressed about.

C: When you say that there isn't any one thing, does that mean there are many things?

P: No (long pause) I don't know, I get nervous fast.

C: Tell me about that.

P: There's not much to say. I don't tolerate much. I know I should, but I just, I'm short-tempered, and little things irritate me.

C: Like what, for example?

P: For example, like last week when I was here and we flew home and we flew over Chicago for an hour and a half, I was madder than a wet hen. And then they flew us back to Madison and we had to take the bus. [Laughs] I was just so nervous and uptight because of that. I was just so, I didn't want to talk to anybody.

C: Have you found this to be more apparent as of late? Or is this pretty much the way you've always been?

P: Hmm, I've always been kind of short-fused.

C: So this recent thing with the airline delay, your reaction didn't surprise you, particularly.

P: No, not really.

Physical examination of her peripheral speech musculature failed to disclose any obvious asymmetries or weakness of the lips, tongue, mandible, or soft palate at rest or during voluntary movement. Her general demeanor was introverted and expressionless, undoubtedly fostered by the low volume of her voice, its breathy quality, and the absence of pitch and inflection variations. Her cough was possibly reduced in explosive power, but one could not be sure. The test for fatigue of the motor speech mechanism in which the patient is asked to count rapidly and vigorously until told to stop revealed deterioration, not only of phonation in the direction of greater breathiness but also of palatopharyngeal and articulatory functions as well by the time the patient had reached the count of 90. Then number of syllables per exhalation began to drop because of air wastage at the glottis, and by the time the patient had reached 100, hypernasality and nasal emission had become apparent; one could feel vibration on the bridge of her nose during production of non-nasal phonemes. By 150, her hypernasality and nasal emission had become clearly audible, and by 225 her articulation was markedly indistinct, the patient physically unable to continue.

The neurologic examination revealed mild but significant muscular weakness; there was slightly greater width of the left palpebral fissure than the right, mild facial weakness on the left, mild diplopia on lateral gaze, bilateral weakness of the soft palate, and on repetition of the counting test of endurance, a similarly high degree of speech deterioration.

After speech deterioration due to prolonged counting, 0.2 mL edrophonium chloride (Tensilon edrophonium chloride; ICN Pharmaceuticals Inc., Costa Mesa, CA) was administered intravenously. The patient had begun to count immediately after the injection, and ~30 seconds later, audible improvement in her speech was noted, and according to the patient, it was approaching normal. Electromyography provided evidence of defective neuromuscular transmission in all muscles tested with repetitive electrical stimulation, and the diagnosis of flaccid dysphonia, and later dysarthria, due to myasthenia gravis was made.

A common clinical diagnostic trap is the interpretation of signs and symptoms as psychogenic because the patient has a history of psychiatric illness. That the complaint can be organic in spite of such a history is illustrated in the following lesson learned by Ball and Lloyd (1971).

A slim, 16-year-old girl was admitted to the psychiatry ward after a series of arguments with her mother. She had been staying with an aunt who was a member of a religious sect in which "speaking in tongues" periodically occurred during times of religious ecstasy. Religion was continually held up to the patient as a way of salvation.

One day during an unusually emotional religious service, when the congregation was praying for the patient, she suddenly lost her voice. It returned spontaneously, but disappeared again on a similar occasion. She also complained of feeling tired and lacking energy. A few months later, she developed difficulty in swallowing food, suffered aspiration pneumonia, and had to be hospitalized. Physical examination, including neurologic studies, gave negative results, and the patient was placed under the care of a psychiatrist. It was his opinion that she was suffering from "hysteria," and a second psychiatrist described her as having severe personality disturbance with schizoid features and tending toward psychotic episodes.

In light of the previous negative physical findings, the disturbed family background, a schizophrenic mother, a premorbid history of shyness, and living with an aunt who placed great importance on "speaking in tongues," a diagnostic formulation of hysterical aphonia, dysphagia, diplopia, and fatigue in a vulnerable personality would have been understandable. Instead, the patient was closely watched. Fatigability became obvious and confirmed the suspicion that the patient had an organic disease. Subsequently, myasthenia gravis was clearly demonstrated. After treatment with pyridostigmine (Mestinon, pryridostigmine bromide, USP; valeant Pharmaceuticals International, Atiso Viejo, CA) and thymectomy, her condition improved. She became attractive and outgoing, developed a wide range of interests, and began working normally as a typist.

Equivocal and episodic physical signs in early myasthenia gravis are well-known and are often precipitated by emotional stress, accounting for the disease being commonly mistaken for a conversion disorder. This case illustrates the dangers of indiscriminate use of the "hysterical" diagnostic label, stresses the value of adequate neurologic training, and draws attention to the pitfalls resulting from reliance on preconceived ideas in diagnosis.

Occasionally, conversion dysphonia can most certainly masquerade as myasthenia gravis. Certain patients, because of knowledge of the disease gained through reading or contact with others who have had it, develop, on a conversion reaction basis, voice signs similar to those found in myasthenia gravis. By use of a control such as intravenous saline (the patient believing it to be Tensilon), the physician can establish whether, in fact, myasthenia gravis is present.

Case Study 5.2

An 82-year-old former elementary school teacher was evaluated for severely breathy dysphonia which had been diagnosed elsewhere as myasthenia gravis and for which she had been taking pyridostigmine (Mestinon). She was of the opinion that her dysphonia signified that she was being improperly treated for her disease. The neurologist began injecting normal saline solution, the patient believing that he was using Tensilon. As she began to count, by the time she had gotten to 10 her voice had become perceptively louder, and by 50 it had returned to normal. After informing the patient that she did not have myasthenia gravis, we found that dysphonia was psychogenic and related to increasing irritation with her hard-of-hearing husband, with whom she found she could no longer communicate. Her voice disorder was eventually psychiatrically diagnosed properly as a conversion disorder.

Myasthenia gravis is a neuromuscular disease manifested by weakness and fatigability of striated muscles. Although its clinical features were isolated by the beginning of the 20th century, it was much later that the mechanism of the weakness was identified: a reduction of available acetylcholine receptors at the neuromuscular junction caused by autoimmune mechanisms.

Muscle contraction is dependent upon stimulation of the motor end-plate by the neurochemical transmitter acetylcholine, which is synthesized in the motor nerve terminals and is stored in vesicles. Each vesicle, or "quantum," contains ~10,000 acetylcholine molecules. When a nerve impulse is transmitted down the axon of the lower motor neuron, the acetylcholine is released at specific sites opposite acetylcholine receptors on the postsynaptic membranes. When the acetylcholine combines with its receptors, a transient increase in membrane permeability to sodium and potassium ions results in muscle depolarization. This process is extremely swift, occurring in milliseconds, and is terminated by removal of acetylcholine by diffusion away from the myoneural junction and by the counteraction of acetylcholinesterase, which hydrolyzes the acetylcholine. The amplitude of depolarization is directly related to the number of acetylcholine molecules that stimulate receptor molecules. Any reduction of acetylcholine receptor interactions below a safely margin will result in failure of neuromuscular transmission, a principle necessary to the understanding of the decrement of muscle strength in myasthenia gravis.

Spastic (Pseudobulbar) Dysphonia: Pyramidal Corticobulbar System Lesions

The remaining neurologic dysphonias are caused by supranuclear lesions, that is, lesions above the level of the tenth cranial nerve nucleus and within the CNS. Not much is known about normal CNS control over the tenth cranial nerve, although probably corticobulbar tracts synapse with vagus nerve nuclei in the same way as they do with the other cranial nerve nuclei. However, it is also likely that vagus nerve nuclei receive a disproportionately larger share of subcortical innervation to facilitate reflex laryngeal function, owing to its important life-sustaining responsibility. Such subcortical representation is substantiated by clinical and experimental evidence that phonation is preserved despite congenital absence of cerebral tissue and massive surgical, traumatic, infectious, or degenerative destruction of the cerebral hemispheres. What is singular about CNS control over the final common pathway to the larynx is the apparent extensive neural redundancy of the system to ensure the organism's survival, and the bilaterality of its laryngeal functions. The integration of the two sides of the larynx is such that under normal conditions, a discoordinated movement between the vocal folds has never been reported; what one side of the larynx does the other does simultaneously and equally, as if both right and left halves of the larynx were under the control of a single CNS center—unlike the unilateral control of the extremities and the lower facial musculature.

The tenth cranial nerve nuclei are under the influence of both pyramidal and extrapyramidal systems. Voluntary control over the larynx is accomplished through the pyramidal system, sometimes referred to as the *direct activating system*, and neuroanatomically known as the corticobulbar tracts. **Figure 5.8** schematizes the following.

1. The corticobulbar tracts begin in the precentral gyri of both cerebral hemispheres.

2. They descend as the corona radiata, become condensed in the internal capsule, and pass through the cerebral peduncles.

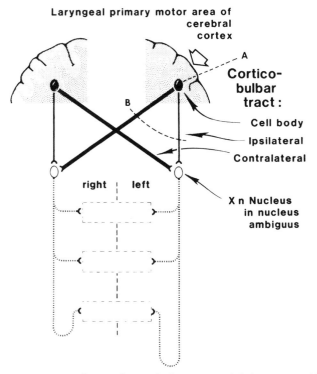

Figure 5.8 Pathways of corticobulbar tracts and their synapses with the tenth cranial nerve (vagus) nuclei. Ipsilateral as well as contralateral innervation explains why unilateral corticobulbar tract lesions do not produce unilateral vocal fold paralyses.

3. At the upper border of the medulla, some of the fibers cross over (decussate) to the other side of the brain stem, where they synapse with vagal nuclei in the nucleus ambiguus. The remainder synapse with vagal nuclei on the same (ipsilateral) side. The implication of such bilateral corticobulbar innervation is that rarely, if ever, will a unilateral cortical or corticobulbar tract lesion cause unilateral vocal fold paralysis. Such is not the case when the cell bodies or axons of the corticobulbar tracts are damaged bilaterally. Then, a characteristic and often severe dysphonia called pseudobulbar (spastic)—not to be confused with spasmodic—dysphonia is heard, the voice having a harsh, strained-strangle quality, abnormally low pitch, monopitch, monoloudness, and reduced loudness. Rarely, however, does the dysphonia occur in the absence of its accompanying dysarthria. (See **Table 5.4** for a summary of signs found in spastic [pseudobulbar] dysarthria.) Botulinum toxin vocal fold injection was used for pseudobulbar dysphonia with some success; acoustic and aerodynamic results were comparable with those reported for individuals with spasmodic dysphonia. The most marked change was an increase in airflow. Despite persistent breathiness, the participant reported great satisfaction with the result because of more appropriate loudness and less listener burden because of a more relaxed and pleasant voice quality after injection (McHenry, Whatman, and Pou, 2002). Before injection, the strained-strangled, harsh voice quality is caused by

Table 5.4 Laryngeal-Phonatory Characteristics in Pseudobulbar (Spastic) Dysarthria

	Findings
Perceptual	
Phonation	Hoarseness or harshness having a strained-strangled quality. Pitch is abnormally low. Monopitch. Loudness is reduced. Monoloudness. Almost never occurs without accompanying signs of dysarthria. Inappropriate crying or laughter may be present.
Resonation	Hypernasality
Articulation	Imprecise consonants; abnormally slow rate
Language	Normal, provided language areas are spared
Physical	
Larynx	Vocal folds appear normal in structure. Normal to hyperadduction of true and false vocal folds may occur bilaterally.
Velopharynx	Bilateral velopharyngeal insufficiency. Hyperactive gag reflex
Tongue	Topographically normal; may be smaller, more contracted than normal. Tongue weakness. Slow alternate motion rate (AMR) on lateral movements an on /tʌ/ and /kʌ/ syllable repetitions.
Lips	Weak, slow movements on AMR for /pʌ/
Teeth	Normal
Hard palate	Normal
Mandible	Slow AMR
General Medical	Nonspecific
Other Neurologic Signs	
Peripheral nervous system	Normal
Central nervous system	Signs of spasticity
Psychiatric/ Psychologic	Nonspecific. Pseudobulbar crying and laughter may give erroneous impression of emotional liability and intellectual deterioration.

hyperadduction of the true and false vocal folds (i.e., glottic constriction and resistance to the exhalatory airflow).

Pseudobulbar Crying and Laughing   Of all the different sounds that humans produce, crying and laughing are unique reflex responses that originate from multiple sources in the CNS and that become disinhibited when damaged from neurologic disease. Pyramidal and extrapyramidal tract lesions can produce compulsive crying and laughter because of a "release" of volitional control excited by an inborn mechanism that underlies these emotional responses.

Included in these CNS regions are unilateral and bilateral corticobulbar tract lesions, globus pallidus, putamen, thalamus, anterior regions of the internal capsule geniculate fascicle supranuclear pontine center, hypothalamus, floor of third ventricle, motor cortex, and temporal lobe.

Called emotional lability or emotional incontinence, these phenomena are most commonly observed in patients with the syndrome of pseudobulbar palsy and progressive supranuclear palsy that includes spasticity of the extremities and spastic dysarthria.

Seriously incapacitating, these emotional responses need to be recognized as one of the great psychologic burdens borne by these patients. This emotional lability usually occurs in response to emotionally loaded conversation between patients and others. Usually, the triggering topic is touching, sad, or sentimental. The cry emerges suddenly without antecedent frowning or the graded smile before laughter, so that these responses give the impression of being stereotyped automatic and paroxysmal. The patient may switch back and forth between the two responses, but once it has begun, it is almost impossible to stop or arrest.

The cry sometimes is associated with clinical depression secondary to the realization that the patient is suffering from a lethal illness that has a bleak future. Depressive crying is different from the compulsive neurologic crying described here; it is less abrupt, explosive, or precipitous. Aronson (1980) published an article describing his own emotional lability associated with a thromboembolic stroke that occurred during thoracic surgery. The embolus lodged in his right middle cerebral artery distribution including branches to his right internal capsule, producing a left spastic hemiplegia and dysarthria producing deep depression and grief over his inability to walk or use his left upper extremity.

During his recovery in the hospital, he would experience sudden uninhibited crying in reaction to almost all stimuli that were sad, touching, or sentimental. These episodes were embarrassing and disconcerting because of the ease with which they could be triggered and their intensity and uncontrollability. Music could easily precipitate the cry, especially violin music (he had played the violin since childhood). Now he could not even hold the violin with his left hand. The very issue would bring forth explosive sobbing accompanied by copious tears. He wrote, "I knew that clinically I was depressed for the loss of a lifelong companion, my left side."

With the cry accompanying emotional liability, you feel as if you are in the clutches of some kind of seizure. Subjectively, the cry does not feel particularly different from other crying but is unique in its sudden unpredictability and inability to arrest once it has started. It begins with a feeling of constriction or contraction in the thoracic, abdominal, laryngeal, and pharyngeal muscles then rolls into uninhibited forced exhalation and a forced sustained phonation rising in pitch and loudness. Some clinicians have said that the cry and laughing lack justification or motivation. The emotional incontinence is not considered to be an affective disorder proper like those found in psychiatric practice.

1. The degree of facial, thoracic, and abdominal muscle contraction visibly and incongruously exceeds accompanying phonatory signs of crying, laughing, or tears. One acoustic characteristic of the cry is a long wail that rises in pitch, often reaching falsetto levels. At times the crying will be produced with an unvoiced air stream, aptly labeled *mute grimacing.*

2. The patient may switch back and forth between crying and laughing without reason, giving the erroneous impression of emotional liability.

Such patients are subject to misinterpretation as being not only emotionally unstable but demented as well, a presumption not supported by a study of 60 patients who had pseudobulbar palsy. In this study, it was found that when intelligence test scores were adjusted for age and slowness of response caused by the spasticity, the patients performed as well as normal controls.

Lesions that produce pathologic laughter can be located in the corticobulbar tracts and beyond. Involuntary laughter has been reported in patients with tumors of the brain stem and hypothalamus, caused by either stimulation of the floor of the third ventricle or infarction of the temporal lobe (Achari and Colover, 1976; Haymaker and Kuhlenbeck, 1976). Other studies have implicated the internal capsule and surrounding basal ganglia.

Pseudobulbar palsy can result from any lesion of the corticobulbar tracts bilaterally: vascular and degenerative diseases involving the motor cortical areas bilaterally, vascular diseases and tumors of the internal capsule or brain stem, degenerative diseases involving the entire corticobulbar tract system, and infectious diseases. Unilateral lesions can have the same result.

Mixed Flaccid-Spastic (Pseudobulbar) Dysphonia: Tenth Cranial Nerve and Pyramidal Tract Lesions

Dysphonias in mixed dysarthria produce the voice signs of each dysarthric component simultaneously. A common example is the mixed dysarthria in flaccid-spastic paralysis as exemplified by ALS. A degenerative disease of bilateral corticobulbar tracts and lower motor neuron nuclei, spastic and flaccid paralysis and associated dysarthrias occur simultaneously, although the proportion of one over the other varies from patient to patient and within a given patient, depending upon the stage of the disease. Should the paralysis be predominately spastic, hyperadduction of the true and false vocal folds will be seen, and the effect will be a primarily spastic or pseudobulbar dysphonia. If the disease expresses itself primarily as flaccid weakness, hypoadduction of one or both vocal folds will be seen on laryngologic examination, and the dysphonia will be predominately flaccid. Pooling of saliva in the pyriform sinuses is common.

The dysphonia of mixed, flaccid-spastic dysarthria is typically a harsh, strained-strangled sound with degrees of breathiness, reduced loudness, audible inhalation, and "wet hoarseness." The "wet" or gurgly sounding voice is due to the accumulation of saliva in the pyriform sinuses and on the vocal folds resulting from the reduced frequency of swallowing. Rapid tremor or flutter on vowel prolongation, also noted in pure flaccid dysphonia, is common. Although the frequency of the flaccid "flutter" is yet to be quantified by research, Aronson and colleagues at the Mayo Clinic estimated that the range is from 9 to 12 Hz. **Figure 5.9** is a comparison between the vowel prolongation of a normal subject and that of a patient with ALS. Note the considerable

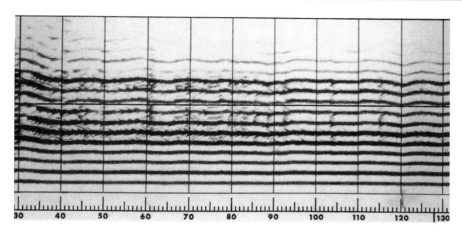

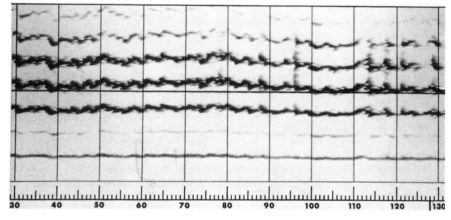

Figure 5.9 Sonogram of a normal subject's vowel prolongation (top) and that of a patient with amyotrophic lateral sclerosis (bottom). Note the relatively smooth tracing of the normal subject compared with the rapid undulations indicating the flaccid "flutter" of the patient with amyotrophic lateral sclerosis. (50 mm = 1 second.)

difference between the rapid undulations in the vowel prolongation of the patient with ALS and the relatively smooth output of the normal subject. **Table 5.5** is a summary of the mixed dysarthria of ALS.

Carrow, Rivera, Mauldin, et al. (1974) analyzed and rated the dysarthrias of seven patients, aged 20 to 65 years, who had motor neuron disease, including ALS. Speech samples were rated on a 1 to 7 scale of severity, 1 being normal and 7 severe (**Table 5.6**). Approximately 80% had harsh voice quality, 75% hypernasality, 65% breathy voice quality, 63% voice tremor, 60% strained-strangled quality, 41% audible inhalation, 38% excessively high pitch, and 8% excessively low pitch. It is apparent that dysphonia is a prominent and incapacitating characteristic of motor neuron disease.

The terms *motor neuron disease* and *ALS* are often used interchangeably, although it is preferable to use the term *ALS* only when pyramidal tract signs predominate. In patients in whom lower motor neuron signs are the most prominent, the term *progressive muscular atrophy* (PMA) is used. The peak incidence of motor neuron disease is in the fifth to seventh decades of life, with ALS occurring slightly later than PMA. The male to female sex ratio in ALS is 3:2, and in PMA it is 5:1. The disease presents with brain-stem (i.e., bulbar) palsy in 30% of cases and progresses more rapidly than the spinal form, with death usually occurring within 3 years. Fasciculations are seen more often in ALS. Speech disturbance is considered to be the earliest sign in the bulbar type, according to Rose (1977), who states that the bilabial plo-

sives are affected first owing to facial muscle weakness, the patient initially noticing difficulty in whistling. Palatal weakness causing hypernasality and nasal emission is usually, but not always, symmetric. The mandible droops, particularly in the pseudobulbar variety. The tongue is flaccid and atrophic, and it fasciculates.

The etiology of ALS is unknown. Theories include viral infection, the effect of malignancy, and in the familial form a genetic deficit of neuronal enzymes. An endemic form has been described in Guam among the Chamorro people, where the incidence is the highest in the world (57%). The most common causes of death are respiratory failure, pneumonia, and pulmonary infarction.

Hypokinetic (Parkinsonian) Dysphonia: Basal Ganglia Lesions

The basal ganglia have both subcortical and cortical connections. This portion of the extrapyramidal system modulates nerve impulses to lower motor neurons. Damage to the substantia nigra in the basal ganglia releases inhibition of nerve impulses to the lower motor neuron, causing rigidity and slowness of movements. When the speech muscles are affected, the dysarthria of parkinsonism (i.e., hypokinetic dysarthria) occurs (**Table 5.7**).

The dysphonia of parkinsonism consists of reduced loudness and monopitch (Darley, Aronson, and Brown, 1969a,b). In a study of 200 parkinsonian patients undertaken by

Table 5.5 Laryngeal-Phonatory Characteristics in the Mixed Dysarthria of Amyotrophic Lateral Sclerosis*

	Findings
Perceptual	
Phonation	Hoarseness or harshness having a strained-strangled quality; "wet" or "gurgly" component. Rapid tremor or "flutter" on vowel prolongation. Breathy if strong flaccid component; pitch is abnormally low. Monopitch. Loudness is reduced. Monoloudness. Inhalatory stridor if severe. Reduced sharpness of cough. Inappropriate crying or laughter may be present.
Resonation	Hypernasality; nasal emission
Articulation	Imprecise consonants; abnormally slow rate
Language	Normal
Physical	
Larynx	Vocal folds appear normal in structure. If major component is spastic, vocal folds appear to adduct normally or may hyperadduct, along with false vocal folds. Adduction may be bilaterally symmetric, or one vocal fold may adduct less fully than the other. If there is a major flaccid component, vocal folds may adduct and abduct with less than normal excursions.
Velopharynx	Bilateral velopharyngeal insufficiency, possibly asymmetric. Hyperactive gag reflex
Tongue	Topographically normal; furrowed and reduced in size owing to atrophy. Fasciculations. Weakness. Slow alternate motion rate (AMR) on lateral movements and on /tʌ/ and /kʌ/ syllable repetitions
Lips	Weak, slow movements on AMR for /pʌ/
Teeth	Normal
Hard palate	Normal
Mandible	Slow AMR
General Medical	Nonspecific
Other Neurologic Signs	
Peripheral nervous system	Signs of flaccid paralysis
Central nervous system	Signs of spasticity
Psychiatric/ Psychologic	Nonspecific. Pseudobulbar crying and laughter may give erroneous impression of emotional lability and intellectual deterioration

*Basically the same as in any other nervous system disease affecting both pyramidal and lower motor neuron tracts bilaterally.

Table 5.6 Abnormal Voice Dimensions in 79 Patients with Motor Neuron Disease (ALS) Exhibiting Abnormal Voice

Characteristics Dimension	Affected Percentage (%)
Harsh voice	79.95
Hypernasality	74.68
Breathy voice	64.56
Voice tremor	63.29
Strained-strangled voice	59.49
Audible inspiration	40.51
High pitch	37.97
Low pitch	7.59

Source: From Carrow, E., Rivera, V., Mauldin, M., Shamblin, L. (1974). Deviant speech characteristics in motor neuron disease. Arch Otolaryngol 100, 212–218.

larynx, that the vocal folds be stretched and loosened by cricothyroid muscle contraction and relaxation, and that infraglottal air pressure be increased and reduced. If the laryngeal and respiratory musculature is rigid, as in parkinsonism, range of motion will be diminished. Controlled changes of infraglottal air pressure, necessary for the stress and emphasis of normal prosody, appear to be lacking in parkinsonian patients, whose respirations are shallow owing to the reduced range of motion of thoracic and abdominal muscle, and whose discrete chest pulses are diminished or absent. The loss of variation in emphasis and stress in contextual speech is what gives the overall effect of flattening of prosody.

Clinicians need to be alert to reduced loudness and breathy voice quality as a sign of early hypokinetic dysarthria, even though remaining signs of the dysarthria and nonspeech signs of parkinsonism are not apparent. Such patients are frequently misdiagnosed as having "functional" dysphonia.

Case Study 5.3

A year before coming to the clinic, a 64-year-old minister had a coronary attack. He had been working exceptionally hard and had been under much stress trying to minister to a parish with insufficient funds. During the year after this attack, he noticed a diminution in the loudness of his voice and described it as "muffled." He revealed that, in his opinion, he might also have had a slight "stroke," because his left side seemed weak and his gait unsteady.

Laryngoscopic examination detected little in the way of laryngeal pathologic changes, the only finding being slightly greater than normal spaces in the interarytenoid region of the glottis during phonation. A diagnosis of functional voice disorder was made.

On closer scrutiny, however, the patient's alternate motion rates on /pʌ/, /tʌ/, and /kʌ/ appeared slightly accelerated and were produced with a less than full range of motion. The patient admitted to a slowing of his thinking during the year and a change in his handwriting.

Neurologic examination confirmed the presence of early parkinsonism. Although no single sign was convincing, when the speech, mild masking of facial expression, reduced arm swing, and cogwheeling of extremities were assembled, they argued strongly in favor of this neurologic diagnosis.

Logemann, Fisher, Boshes, et al. (1978), 178 (89%) had signs of laryngeal dysfunction; 30 (15%), had breathy voice quality; 58 (29%) had roughness; 90 (45%) had hoarseness; and 27 (13.5%) had tremulousness of voice. The characteristically monopitched voice arises from the rigidity and reduced range of motion of the intrinsic and extrinsic laryngeal muscles. Pitch change requires that the strap muscles elevate and lower the

Table 5.7 Laryngeal-Phonatory Characteristics in the Hypokinetic Dysarthria of Parkinsonism

	Findings
Perceptual	
Phonation	Monopitch; reduced stress; monoloudness; reduced loudness; harsh voice quality; breathy voice quality
Note: Reduced loudness and breathiness in the absence of other neurologic signs can indicate early parkinsonism.	
Resonation	Normal
Articulation	Imprecise consonants; short rushes of speech; accelerated rate: stuttering-like repetitions of syllables, words, or phrases (palilalia)
Language	Usually normal. Language functions may be decreased as part of overall slowing of general intellectual processes.
Physical	
Larynx	Vocal folds appear normal in structure. Adductor, abductor movements are bilaterally symmetric, but there may be incomplete closure of vocal folds, accounting for breathy voice quality.
Velopharynx	Normal
Tongue	Topographically normal; alternate motion rates (AMRs) for /tʌ/ and /kʌ/ sound rapid and are reduced in amplitude of movement
Lips	AMRs for /pʌ/ sound rapid and are reduced in amplitude of movement
Teeth	Normal
Hard palate	Normal
Mandible	Reduced range of motion during articulation
General Medical	Nonspecific
Other Neurologic Signs	
Peripheral nervous system	Normal
Central nervous system	Signs of hypokinesia elsewhere in the body *Note:* Hypokinetic dysarthria in the form of dysphonia only can be the first sign of early parkinsonism.
Psychiatric/ Psychologic	Nonspecific. Masked facies may give the erroneous impression of flatness of affect or of depression.

Motion picture studies of the vocal folds during phonation in 30 patients with Parkinson's disease disclosed a direct relationship between breathiness, and reduced loudness, and increasing amounts of glottic gap and bowing of the vocal folds (Hanson, Gerratt, and Ward, 1984).

Physical measurements of respiration in hypokinetic dysarthria prove that such patients have shallow irregular breathing, pause between respirations, and experience peri-ods of increased depth of respiration that alternate with periods of respiratory arrest. Postencephalitic parkinsonism patients have shallow respiration of twice the normal frequency; negligible differences between vegetative, deep, and speech breathing; smaller than normal vital capacities; air wastage before speaking; and exhalations repeatedly interrupted by small inhalations (Darley, Aronson, and Brown, 1975).

The results of studies of frequency and intensity of parkinsonian patients are equivocal. Canter (1963) found that parkinsonism patients read orally at a median fundamental frequency of 129 Hz, which was statistically significantly higher than the median frequency of 102 Hz found in a control group of normal subjects. A similar increase in fundamental frequency was found by Kammermeier (1969), but Schilling (cited by Darley, Aronson, and Brown, 1975), on the other hand, found pitch range to be considerably decreased. The results of studies of vocal intensity, or loudness, in parkinsonism have demonstrated that the lower-intensity levels exhibited by these patients can be significantly elevated with intensive voice treatment (Lee Silverman voice treatment LSVT) and maintained at the louder level. On average, patients treated with LSVT raised their vocal intensity level for reading 9 dB SPL and that intensity decreased by only 3 dB SPL (sound pressure level) when tested 2 years after treatment was terminated (Ramig, Sapir, Countryman, et al., 2001).

Arrhythmically Fluctuating, Neurologic Voice Disorders

Ataxic Dysphonia: Cerebellar Lesions

The cerebellum coordinates muscles and regulates skilled movements. Contained within the skull's posterior fossa, the cerebellum consists of an anterior lobe, a posterior lobe, and a flocculonodular lobe. It connects with the brain stem and structures above and below it by means of incoming and outgoing fibers that pass through the inferior, middle, and superior cerebellar peduncles to brain-stem nuclei, the dentate nucleus, the thalamus, and the cerebral cortex. Of the many functions of the cerebellum, including equilibrium, posture, and gait, the posterior lobes are particularly concerned with voluntary movements. Lesions in this area result in a loss of muscle coordination, known as dyssynergia; a loss of the ability to measure range of motion, known as dysmetria; and tremor during voluntary movement, known as intention tremor. General movements are clumsy and uncoordinated (Daube, Sandok, Reagan, et al., 1978).

Whether or not dysphonia is present may depend upon the severity of the ataxia. The dysphonia may take one of several forms: sudden bursts of loudness, irregular increases in pitch and loudness, or coarse voice tremor (**Table 5.8**).

Hyperkinetic (Choreic) Dysphonia: Basal Ganglia Lesions

Quick, jerky, irregular, and unpredictable movements caused by lesions of the basal ganglia, probably the caudate nucleus, are found in Sydenham's chorea in children and Huntington's chorea, the hereditary type, in adults. In addition to the

Table 5.8 Laryngeal-Phonatory Characteristics in Ataxic Dysarthria

	Findings
Perceptual	
Phonation	Frequently normal. Others have harsh voice quality, monopitch, monoloudness, excess, and equal stress on ordinarily unstressed words or syllables, excess loudness, bursts of loudness, and coarse voice tremor.
Resonation	Normal
Articulation	Imprecise consonants; irregular articulatory breakdown; distorted vowels; slow rate
Language	Normal
Physical	
Larynx	Vocal folds appear normal in structure and function
Velopharynx	Normal
Tongue	Topographically normal; irregular and slow alternate motion rates (AMRs) on /tʌ/ and /kʌ/ and on all lateral tongue movements
Lips	Irregular and slow AMRs for /pʌ/
Teeth	Normal
Hard palate	Normal
Mandible	Normal
General Medical	Nonspecific. *Note:* Ataxic dysarthria may be a sign of moderate to severe hypothyroidism and drug and alcohol abuse.
Other Neurologic Signs	
Peripheral nervous system	Normal
Central nervous system	Signs of ataxia
Psychiatric/ Psychologic	Nonspecific

Table 5.9 Laryngeal-Phonatory Characteristics in the Hyperkinetic Dysarthria of Chorea

	Findings
Perceptual	
Phonation	Intermittently harsh, strained-strangled voice quality; transient breathiness; distorted vowels; monopitch; excess loudness variations; monoloudness; excess, equal stress on ordinarily unstressed words or syllables; reduced stress; sudden forced inspiration/ expiration
Resonation	Intermittent hypernasality
Articulation	Imprecise consonants; distorted vowels, prolonged intervals between syllables and words; variable rate; inappropriate silences; prolonged phonemes; short phrases; irregular articulatory breakdown
Language	Normal; defective in patients who have undergone intellectual deterioration
Physical	
Larynx	Vocal folds appear normal in structure, intermittent hyperadduction
Velopharynx	Normal in appearance
Tongue	Topographically normal; quick unpatterned movements at rest and during alternate motion rates (AMRs) for /tʌ/ and /kʌ/, which are irregular
Lips	Quick and unpatterned movements at rest and during AMRs for /pʌ/
Teeth	Normal
Hard palate	Normal
Mandible	Quick asymmetric movements at rest and during speech
General Medical	Nonspecific
Other Neurologic Signs	
Peripheral nervous system	Normal
Central nervous system	Choreic movements elsewhere in the body
Psychiatric/ Psychologic	Intellectual and behavior changes associated with dementia, if present

sudden uncontrolled movements of the lips, tongue, and mandible, movements of the respiratory and laryngeal musculature produce irregular pitch fluctuations and voice arrests, giving speech a jerky quality. In a study done by Darley, Aronson, and Brown (1969a,b), the following phonatory aberrations were found: sudden forced inspiration or expiration; harsh voice quality; excess loudness variations; strained-strangled phonation; monopitch; monoloudness; reduced stress; transient breathiness; and voice arrests. **Table 5.9** summarizes the hyperkinetic dysarthria of chorea.

Hyperkinetic (Dystonic) Dysphonia: Basal Ganglia Lesions

A slower form of hyperkinesia known as *dyskinesia* or *dystonia* is manifested by repetitive, slow, twisting, writhing, or flexing movements of the musculature. When only the speech musculature is affected, the terms *orofacial dyskinesia* or *focal mouth dystonia* are employed. In addition to vascular, degenerative, or mass lesions, this movement disorder can result from prolonged use of psychotropic and antiparkinsonian drugs. In cases caused by drug therapy, the

dyskinesia does not appear until after prolonged use, and so the term *tardive dyskinesia* is used in reference to the late (tardy) appearance of the dyskinesia (Portnoy, 1979).

In addition to rounding, pursing, protruding, and lateralizing lip movements and tongue protrusions, rotation, and lateralization, similarly uncontrolled adductor and abductor laryngeal spasms cause strained hoarseness and breathiness, and sometimes paroxysmal inhalatory stridor. A form of dystonia involving the entire body is dystonia musculorum deformans. This disorder can produce profound laryngeal spasms that cause a highly strained or groaning dysphonia of a waxing and waning character.

Athetosis, also a slow hyperkinesia that is commonly seen as one form of cerebral palsy, produces similar strained hoarseness and breathiness in addition to the writhing movements of the head, neck, torso, and extremities. In a study done by Darley, Aronson, and Brown (1969a,b), patients who had dystonia gave evidence of harsh, strained-strangled voice; excess loudness variations; voice arrests; short phrases; monopitch, monoloudness; reduced stress; inappropriate silences; and excess and equal stress on all syllables of words. **Table 5.10** summarizes the hyperkinetic dysarthria of dystonia.

Rhythmically Fluctuating, Neurologic Voice Disorders

Organic (Essential) Voice Tremor

Voice tremor is a component of the essential tremor syndrome, called *benign heredofamilial tremor* when familial. The voice tremor can be monosymptomatic without evidence of tremor

Table 5.10 Laryngeal-Phonatory Characteristics in the Hyperkinetic Dysarthria of Dystonia

	Findings
Perceptual	
Phonation	Slow, continuous changes in strained-hoarse quality; breathiness; excess; loudness variations; voice arrests; monopitch; monoloudness; reduced stress; excess and equal stress on ordinarily unstressed syllables and words
Resonation	Normal
Articulation	Imprecise consonants; distorted vowels, short phrases; inappropriate silences
Language	Normal. May be defective if dysarthria is associated with focal language disorders of diffuse intellectual disorders
Physical	
Larynx	Vocal folds appear normal in structure and function; intermittent hyperadduction
Velopharynx	Normal
Tongue	Topographically normal; slow, unpatterned protrusive, lateral, and rotatory movements at rest and during speech. Alternate motion rates (AMRs) on /tʌ/ and /kʌ/ are slow and highly irregular.
Lips	Slow unpatterned lip rounding and spreading. AMRs for /pʌ/ are slow and highly irregular.
Teeth	Normal
Hard palate	Normal
Mandible	Slow unpatterned depression, lateralization, and elevation
General Medical	Nonspecific
Other Neurologic Signs	
Peripheral nervous system	Normal
Central nervous system	Signs of dystonia may be confined to larynx or may occur elsewhere in the body
Psychiatric/ Psychologic	Nonspecific. Intellectual and behavioral aberrations present if diffuse central nurvous system disease is present

elsewhere in the body or can accompany the full syndrome of tremor of the upper limbs, head, face, or neck musculature. The rate of the tremor ranges most often from 4 to 7 Hz, and this tremor must be distinguished from those associated with parkinsonism, cerebellar disease, thyrotoxicosis, and anxiety. Normal humans have small tremor amplitudes of 6 to 12 Hz at rest and during intentional movements (Brumlik, 1962). Normal physiologic tremor has been reported in children at 5 or 6 Hz and in young adults at 10 Hz, the change in rate taking place during puberty (Marshall, 1962). After about age 40 years, the tremor begins to decline from 10 to 6 Hz.

No uniform location of the lesion in the nervous system has been found in organic voice tremor. In his wide-sweeping review of the literature, Critchley (1949) documented many brain-stem lesions causing tremor; caudate nucleus, putamen; loss of cells in the cerebellum and dentate nuclei; and loss of cells within the triangle connecting the red nucleus, dentate nucleus, and inferior olive. Essential tremor can produce three kinds of effects on voice:

1. If the alternating contractions of the adductors and abductors of the vocal folds are of equal strength, typical organic voice tremor will occur.

2. If the adductor movements are disproportionately stronger than abductor, the vocal folds will meet momentarily in the midline causing voice arrests, producing adductor spasmodic dysphonia of essential tremor (see Chapter 6).

3. If the abductor movements are disproportionately stronger than adductor, the vocal folds will overabduct causing breathy air release, producing abductor spasmodic dysphonia of essential tremor (see Chapter 6).

The onset of organic voice tremor can be gradual or sudden. Brown and Simonson (1963) found that 5 of 27 patients had rapid onset of voice tremor: one while reciting the Lord's Prayer, a second while singing in church, and a third while talking at a board meeting. The other two noted abrupt onset of hoarseness and a strained feeling in the throat while talking, and, as these symptoms cleared, the voice tremor appeared. That these patients were older than the age of 50 years led the researchers to conclude that the rapid onset was due to occlusive vascular disease.

The voice of an individual with an organic tremor has a characteristically quavering intonation because of tremor of the laryngeal muscles and often of the articulatory and respiratory muscles as well. Severe cases have a staccato abruptness of voice heard as rhythmic voice arrests. The tongue also moves in a rhythmic tremor both at rest and on protrusion.

Clinicians should remember that voice tremor can occur without associated tremors elsewhere in the body. Brown and Simonson (1963) found voice tremor to be the only tremor in 6 of 23 patients. For the entire group, the voice tremor ranged from 4 to 8 Hz, although in 16 to 23 cases, the tremor frequency was concentrated in the 5- to 6-Hz range.

The voice tremor in organic tremor is best demonstrated during vowel prolongation. The tremor can be smooth or interrupted by the previously noted voice stoppages or vocal arrests. These voice arrests are caused by momentary obstruction of the exhaled air stream due to complete glottic closure simultaneous with vertical movements of the larynx.

A mild organic voice tremor is often masked by contextual speech. As Brown and Simonson noted in their study of 31 patients with this disorder, short-duration vowels were uttered without perceptible impairment, but the tremor became obvious during production of sounds of longer duration. It is of clinical importance to know that the severity of the tremor is greater during emotional stress and fatigue. Patients show little in the way of psychoneuroses, but many cases have occurred after acute emotional stress. **Table 5.11** is a summary of the dysarthria of organic voice tremor.

Palatopharyngolaryngeal Myoclonus

Palatopharyngolaryngeal myoclonus refers to rhythmic or semirhythmic movements of the soft palate, pharyngeal walls, laryngeal musculature, eyeballs, diaphragm, and tongue. Technically, it is a slow form of tremor; myoclonus may be a misnomer. These signs may exist in isolation or in various combinations. When the soft palate is involved, abrupt, rhythmic, anteroposterior, and vertical movements are present during speech and at rest. Pharyngeal muscle contractions can open and shut the eustachian tube, producing a bruit or clicking sound transmitted by the tympanic membrane and sometimes heard by others at a fair distance at the same rate and rhythm of the myoclonic contractions.

Case Study 5.4

A 51-year-old male came to the clinic because of spasmodic blinking of his eyelids and right arm clumsiness after attacks of influenza. He noted a clicking sensation in his larynx that seemed to obstruct his breathing, and he complained of episodes of aphonia, breathy dysphonia, and a sensation of spasm in the larynx. At times he would gasp for air on inhalation. He had frequent contractions of the orbicularis oculi. He had slight bilateral sensory and motor paralysis of the pharyngeal muscles. Also, although he had some adductor weakness of the vocal folds, the outstanding feature noted on laryngoscopic examination was constant, involuntary, rhythmic bilateral adductor movements of the vocal folds that occurred 60 to 80 times per minute and frequently interfered with inspiration by producing complete adduction before inhalation had been completed. He also had myoclonic twitching of the facial muscles synchronous with movements of the vocal folds. The pharyngeal muscles and soft palate did not participate in these movements. The disorder was diagnosed as postencephalitic myoclonic movements of the larynx and pharynx (Childrey and Parker, 1931).

Rhythmic adductor movements of the vocal folds, and gross upward and downward movements of the larynx, cause momentary, rhythmic, phonatory interruptions. However, because each myoclonic movement is brief, voice interruptions are rarely audible during contextual speech though they can be easily seen on kymographic and high-speed

Table 5.11   Laryngeal-Phonatory Characteristics in the Hyperkinetic Dysarthria of Organic (Essential) Tremor

	Findings
Perceptual	
Phonation	Quavering or intermittent voice arrests during contextual speech. Rhythmic tremor and/or voice arrests on vowel prolongation ranging from ~4 to 7 Hz. *Note:* In severe organic voice tremor, the voice arrests take the form of severe larygospasm that may be mistaken for the syndrome of spastic (spasmodic) dysphonia. Patients with voice arrest will show a smoothing out of these arrests into ordinary tremor when sustaining a vowel at a high pitch level. Fluctuating strained-hoarseness along with tremor in more severe cases
Resonation	Normal
Articulation	Normal. May have irregular articulatory breakdowns reminiscent of ataxic dysarthria
Language	Normal
Physical	
Larynx	Vocal folds appear normal in structure. On vowel prolongation, adductor-abductor oscillations synchronous with voice tremor can be seen as well as pharyngeal wall movements. Tremor movements of the larynx can be seen under skin of neck, with the larynx oscillating vertically. Voice arrests occur at the maximum laryngeal height of each oscillation.
Velopharynx	Normal. Soft palate may move synchronously with laryngeal tremor
Tongue	Topographically normal; on vowel prolongation, tremor movements of tongue may be seen synchronously with laryngeal tremor.
Lips	Normal, may be tremorous
Teeth	Normal
Hard palate	Normal
Mandible	Normal, may be tremorous
General Medical	Nonspecific
Other Neurologic Signs	
Peripheral nervous system	Normal
Central nervous system	Head and hand tremor, unilateral or bilateral, may be present *Note:* Organic voice tremor may occur as an isolated sign, which is prone to misinterpretation as being psychogenic.
Psychiatric/ Psychologic	Many patients report onset of voice, head, or hand tremor after an emotionally stressful life event. There is a danger of interpreting such events as proof that the tremor is psychogenic.

images. They become perceptually apparent, however, during vowel prolongation, when one hears momentary voice arrests ranging among patients from 60 to 240 beats per minute. In rare instances, the laryngeal myoclonus can be so severe that abrupt, strained voice arrests are produced giving the impression of adductor spasmodic dysphonia.

It is easy to miss this disorder by failing to test for it by means of vowel prolongation, because the voice arrests are usually masked by contextual speech. Also, oral examination of the pharyngeal and palatal musculature at rest is imperative to detect the myoclonic movements. Scrutiny of the external surfaces of the neck is important to note subcutaneous laryngeal movements. Subjective signs of the syndrome are a clicking sensation in the larynx and a sensation of laryngeal spasm. Myoclonic movements can be unilateral or bilateral.

Although the syndrome is found in people of all ages, it is most common in those older than the age of 50, and it is most often of vascular origin. In an unpublished study of 28 Mayo Clinic patients, 13 had brain-stem or cerebellar infarction, 8 had a tumor of the cerebellum or fourth ventricle, 5 had head trauma producing posterior fossa damage, and 2 had degenerative CNS disease, including cerebellar atrophy in 1. The site of the lesion varies, although the general region is the brain stem, specifically the dentate nucleus, inferior olive, superior cerebellar peduncle, red nucleus, and restiform body. Additional neurologic signs of a brain-stem lesion can accompany palatopharyngolaryngeal myoclonus. **Table 5.12** summarizes the dysarthria of palatopharyngolaryngeal myoclonus.

Paroxysmal Neurologic Voice Disorders

Gilles de la Tourette's Syndrome

Georges Gilles de la Tourette (1885) first described the syndrome that bears his name in a report of nine patients with multiple tics and involuntary vocalizations that included coprolalia (the uncontrolled utterance of socially unacceptable language having to do with sexual and other bodily functions), and echolalia. Isolating the movements and sounds in this unusual disorder is difficult because they blend into appropriate cultural, environmental, and psychologic contexts involving speech and throat-clearing. A variety of involuntary movements have been observed: jumping, squatting, skipping, hitting, kicking; repetitive movements, for example, touching the floor; hesitating to pick up objects as if they were hot; and touching chin, lips, tongue, throat, and other people. Other complicated movements include startle reactions, esophageal spasm, and echopraxia.

Speech and nonspeech vocalizations include grunts, barking, coughing, throat-clearing, echolalia, and coprolalia.

In a study done by Shapiro, Shapiro, and Wayne (1973), of 34 patients, 27 male and 7 female, the average age of onset was 7.4 years, ranging from 3 to 13 years. The age of onset is difficult to determine and is probably reported considerably later than the actual date.

According to Cohen, Shaywitz, Caparulo, et al. (1978), a neurologic basis for Gilles de la Tourette's syndrome is strongly supported by the high incidence of abnormal electroencephalographic and other neurologic findings and a

Table 5.12 Laryngeal-Phonatory Characteristics in the Hyperkinetic Dysarthria of Palatopharyngolaryngeal Myoclonus*

	Findings
Perceptual	
Phonation	Momentary voice arrests during contextual speech if severe, but often undetectable under this condition. On vowel prolongation, momentary voice arrests occur rhythmically ranging from 60 to 240 beats per minute (1 to 4 Hz). *Note:* Because often undetectable during contextual speech, vowel prolongation must be tested in all suspected cases.
Resonation	Normal
Articulation	Normal. Patient may have articulatory defects or flaccid, spastic, or ataxic dysarthria.
Language	Normal
Physical	
Larynx	Vocal folds adduct rhythmically and momentarily on vowel prolongation, synchronously with voice arrests. Myoclonic movements of larynx and pharynx can be seen by observing the movements beneath skin of the neck.
Velopharynx	Soft palate elevates and falls, and lateral pharyngeal walls adduct and abduct synchronously with above structures
Tongue	Normal. May enter into myoclonic movements in synchrony with above structures
Lips	Normal
Teeth	Normal
Hard palate	Normal
Mandible	Nonspecific
General Medical	Nonspecific
Other Neurologic Signs	
Peripheral nervous system	Normal
Central nervous system	Other signs of brain-stem lesion may be present or absent
Psychiatric/Psychologic	Normal

*To detect presence of this syndrome, observation of the oral musculature while patient is quiet and holding mouth open as steadily as possible is imperative; myoclonic movements are present at rest as well as during phonation.

history of difficult birth. Although only 3 of 15 patients studied by Golden (1977) had major personality problems, 11 of 15 had difficulties with school work, 8 having learning disabilities. Only 4 of 15 had made a completely normal adjustment to school.

A 17-year-old male wrote the following letter:

I think I have that Tourette's syndrome. It's crazy. All these years I have been trying to cure it myself, trying to control all those nervous mannerisms that drove me up the wall. Like stuttering, my eye twitching, coughing, shaking, whatever. I said, "How am I ever going to become a dancer or a lawyer if I can't get up in front of a crowd?" You know what this syndrome does? It prevents people from being comfortable or being themselves so they just clam up and don't take that risk of being uncomfortable. They begin to reject themselves for what they are then. It's not like being fat or having crooked teeth, you can control those but this is something you have absolutely no control over . . . there is nowhere to run, it is inside you, with you, and you can't leave it behind.

Patients with Gilles de la Tourette's syndrome respond well to haloperidol. Abuzzahab and Anderson (1974), in their review of drug treatment of the disease, found that 89% of patients improved and 67% maintained the improvement longer than 6 months, although there was no evidence that treatment alters the eventual outcome of the disease. **Table 5.13** is a summary of the dysarthria of Gilles de la Tourette's syndrome.

Neurologic Voice Disorders Due to Loss of Control over Volitional Phonation

Apraxic Aphonia and Dysphonia

Apraxia of phonation and respiration for speech along with apraxia of articulation results from lesions of Broca's area in the dominant cerebral hemisphere. More than one type of phonatory manifestation of apraxia of phonation and respiration occur: (1) no articulatory movements or laryngeal sound, voiced or unvoiced; (2) articulation produced with an unphonated air stream (i.e., whispered speech); (3) articulatory movements without accompanying exhalatory activity, patients being unable to inhale or exhale voluntarily on command or in response to imitation, even though they are able to do so reflexly for vital purposes. They are unable to cough volitionally, showing instead confusion and trial-and-error efforts, yet they are able to cough automatically. When asked to cough, they will sometimes say the word *cough* rather then produce the cough itself. See **Table 5.14** for a summary of laryngeal-phonatory signs in apraxia of speech.

Table 5.13   Laryngeal-Phonatory Characteristics in the Hyperkinetic Dysarthria of Gilles de la Tourette's Syndrome

	Findings*
Perceptual	
Phonation	Involuntary grunting, coughing, throat-clearing, barking, squealing, shrieking, screaming, gurgling, moaning
Resonation	Snorting, sniffing
Articulation	Whistling; clicking; lip-smacking; spitting; stuttering-like repetitions of sounds
Language	Echolalia, coprolalia
Physical	
Larynx	Vocal folds appear normal in structure and function
Velopharynx	Normal
Tongue	Normal
Lips	Normal
Teeth	Normal
Hard palate	Normal
Mandible	Normal
General Medical	Nonspecific
Other Neurologic Signs	
Peripheral nervous system	Normal
Central nervous system	Jerky bodily movements
Psychiatric/Psychologic	Emotional behavioral problems secondary to adverse social effects of above

*Findings vary among patients; not all are found in a given patient.

Table 5.14   Laryngeal-Phonatory Characteristics in Apraxia of Speech

	Findings
Perceptual	
Phonation	Varies, from normal in some patients to mutism in others. Phonation may be impossible because of apparent loss of recall for integration of respiratory and laryngeal movements, resulting in trial-and-error efforts to phonate, but silent nevertheless. Aphonic (whispered) speech can occur. Inability to cough volitionally or clear throat
Resonation	Normal
Articulation	Phoneme omissions, substitutions, reversals, and additions; stuttering-like blocking
Language	May be relatively normal or aphasic
Physical	
Larynx	Vocal folds appear normal in structure and function
Velopharynx	Normal
Tongue	Topographically normal. May have associated dysarthric signs. Trial-and-error nonspeech volitional movements (oral nonverbal apraxia)
Lips	Trial-and-error nonspeech volitional movements may be present. Sequential motor rates, the rapid sequencing of sounds from /pʌ/ to /tʌ/ to /kʌ/, may be mildly to severely impaired.
Teeth	Normal
Hard palate	Normal
Mandible	Normal
General Medical	Nonspecific
Other Neurologic Signs	
Peripheral nervous system	Normal
Central nervous system	A wide variety of dysarthric, apraxic, and other abnormal signs may coexist.
Psychiatric/Psychologic	Nonspecific

Akinetic Mutism

Deep and widespread cerebral and brain-stem lesions can cause (1) muteness and failure to respond to questions or comments; though patients are alert and have eye contact, they are indifferent to the examiner. These clinical behaviors have been noted in presenile and senile dementia (Alzheimer's and Pick's diseases), hydrocephalus, frontal lobe lesions and brain-stem trauma, and after seizures in children.

The akinetically mute patient sits with eyes open, performs no or few voluntary movements, is unresponsive, looks away from the examiner, may have sucking movements, and is mute. The mutism is relative (i.e., mute except when prodded, in which case the patient will speak, usually normally, if no associated dysarthria, apraxia, or aphasia is present). A spectrum of severity must be taken into consideration; a given patient may be mute all the time early in the recovery period, may be mute only some of the time later on, and may show only vestiges of mutism during advanced stages of recovery by nothing more unusual than prolonged latency of speech response. Akinetic mutism can result from anoxia, metabolic diseases, subdural hematomas with compressions, cerebrovascular accident, or tumors, and may be seen in advanced parkinsonism and after thalamotomy.

The original description by Cairns, Oldfield, Pennybacker, et al. (1941) of the akinetically mute patient follows:

The patient sleeps more than normally, but is easily roused. In the fully developed state he makes no sound and lies inert, except that the eyes regard the observer steadily, or follow the movement of objects, and they may be diverted by sound. Despite a steady gaze, which seems to give promise to speech, the patient is quite mute, or answers in whispered monosyllables ... commands may be performed in a feeble, slow and incomplete manner, but usually there are no movements of a voluntary character, no restless movements, struggling, or evidence of negativism. Emotional movement also is almost in abeyance. A painful stimulus produces reflex withdrawal of the limb, and if the stimulation is sustained, slow, feeble voluntary movement of the limbs may occur in an attempt to remove the source of stimulation, but usually without tears, noise, or other manifestations of pain or displeasure. The patient swallows readily, but has to be fed ... fluctuations may occur in the intensity of this state. In its incomplete manifestations, the patient may respond at times, though slowly and imperfectly by speech and voluntary movement ... incontinence persists and there is little or no trace of spontaneous activity or speech.

Klee (1961), in his review of the literature, summarized the varied clinical behaviors of many patients with akinetic mutism:

Patients remained in akinetic and mute states for periods ranging from weeks to months, then gradually began to follow movements in their vicinity with their eyes but without interest ... consciousness clear, no disturbances of orientation, memory or powers of observation; always possible to make contact although required much patience ...

able to answer questions adequately but in monosyllables and apparently with difficulty ... trance-like states ... episodes during which the patient would, in the midst of household activities, suddenly become inert and unresponsive and as suddenly, about ten minutes later would resume where she had left off.

Daly and Love (1958) described a 14-year-old boy who had an astrocytoma of the upper part of the fourth ventricle, extending around the lower end of the aqueduct, with the ventricular system cephalad to the tumor being greatly dilated. After the operation, he developed a condition in which speech and movements were inhibited, although he could understand what happened around him and what was said to him. He began to speak 34 days after the operation, at first using only monosyllabic words and short sentences, and movements became gradually less inhibited during the latter part of a 2-month observation. Klee (1961) expands on the point that the degree of inhibition changes from one minute to the next and that the duration of inhibition can be minutes to months:

The patient may be almost totally immobile and mute or may have only a suggestion of hampering of speech and movement. In the most inhibited states, the appearance and movements of the eyes may be the only indication that the patient is conscious. If he speaks, it is often only after a long latent period, and then with monosyllabic words or short sentences, in a monotonous voice. Movements are slow, and they show a similar long latent period; spontaneous activity may be less hampered than the voluntary. Variations in the degree of inhibition may occur from one minute to the next, and the inhibition may last for minutes or months. The patient's experience of the inhibition of speech seems to be that they know what they wish to say but that the words cannot be said aloud. They do not appear to have a clear idea of how inhibited they actually are.

A summary of the lesions that have caused akinetic mutism follows: tumors of the third ventricle; hemangioma of the mesencephalon and in and around the third ventricle; basilar artery thrombosis; Wernicke's encephalopathy; encephalitis; and bullet wounds through the frontal lobes.

Frontal Lobe Dysphonia, Aphonia, and Mutism

Severe breathiness, aphonia, and mutism are common in patients who have had frontal lobe lesions, most commonly from traumatic head injuries, tumor, or vascular disease. It has been speculated that such disturbances in phonation are associated with affective or personality changes from damage to the limbic system and its cortical and subcortical connections, which are thought to be important in regulating affect and emotion and their vocal expression. These patients demonstrate generally reduced drive and apathy. In their review of a large number of studies of the effects of frontal lobe lesions on phonation, Sapir and Aronson (1985) concluded:

These reports argue that damage or disturbance to the limbic system and its neocortical and subcortical connections has profound effect on emotions and affect, vocal-facial expressions, and the conscious monitoring of these expressions. Specifically, such neural disturbances are said to be responsible for apathy, a "flat" affect and lack of drive, aphonic or hypophonic vocalization . . . and poor insight into the inappropriateness of one's vocal and nonvocal behaviors.

Nevertheless, there always exists the potential for a patient who has a neurologic disease to develop a psychogenic voice disorder that can be misinterpreted as neurologic by association with the neurologic disorder. In four patients who had central and peripheral nervous system disease described by Sapir and Aronson (1987), their dysphonias turned out to be psychogenic because of time-related psychosocial problems. These experiences taught the authors the importance of not automatically assuming that all dysphonias associated with neurologic disease are neurologic, and that the clinician always needs to be sensitive to the possibility of a dysphonia triggered by the anxiety or depression over the neurologic disease itself or by personal and family problems generated by illness and hospitalization.

Foreign Accent Syndrome

Foreign accent syndrome is an acquired speech disorder perceived by others as if the person is speaking his or her native language with a foreign accent or dialect. This impression is caused by segmental and suprasegmental deviations in pronunciation; these foreign accent syndrome patients develop their problem after either cerebral vascular accident or other CNS lesion. The syndrome can occur in association with dysarthria, apraxia of speech, or aphasia. The main speech changes are suprasegmental pitch, stress, and rhythm patterns. Phonetic and phonemic aberrations can be found in their speech; shortening of vowels, insertion of schwa vowels, and dentalization of lingua-alveolar consonants. Not all listeners agree on which foreign language the speaker's accent represents. Most cases are associated with left precentral gyrus lesions.

The Case of Astrid L.

On September 6, 1941, during an air raid over Oslo, Norway, a 30-year-old woman named Astrid L. was struck in the head by a shell fragment that took away her left frontal bone, exposing extruded, lacerated brain. Upon recovery of full fluency, she sounded as if she were speaking her native Norwegian with a German accent. This strange development proved embarrassing for her, as her country was at war with Germany. She complained bitterly about being taken for a German in shops, where clerks refused to sell her merchandise. Yet she had never left Norway and had had no contact with the German language or with German-speaking people at any time in her life.

That a person could, as result of a head injury, seem to be speaking in a foreign accent is difficult for serious students of communicative disorders to accept. Dialects traditionally are considered learned behavior. The pronunciation of consonants and vowels, the stress patterns placed on syllables of words,

Table 5.15 Pseudo–Foreign Dialect

Number of Cases Reported, 1907–1978			
Mayo Clinic			13
Other			12
Total			25
	Number	**Percentage (%)**	**Age (Years)**
Females	16	64	27–59
Males	9	36	29–71

and the pitch-inflectional patterns superimposed on syntax follow logical laws of learning. Astrid was decidedly an enigma to her neurologist, Monrad-Krohn (1947), who reported that she had undergone a complete change in the melody of her language. She overemphasized final pronouns, and her pitch would rise on such pronouns at places where they should fall. She failed to blend the final sounds of words with the initial sounds of succeeding words. *Dysprosody* was the term he used to describe aberrations of normal pitch stress patterns such as this, analogous to what American phoneticians refer to as intonation and stress, what the French call *chanson de parler*, and what the Germans refer to as *sprach-melodie*.

Before Monrad-Krohn's report, in 1907 Pierre Marie had described a Frenchman who began to speak in an Alsatian dialect after a cerebrovascular accident. In 1919, Arnold Pick reported a 29-year-old Czechoslovakian who began to speak in a Polish dialect, also after a cerebrovascular accident, right hemiparesis, and aphasia. A search of the literature uncovered 25 such cases noted between 1907 and 1978, 13 from Mayo Clinic files; 12 from other sources (**Table 5.15**). Sixteen (65%) were females aged 27 to 59 years, and 9 (36%) were males aged 29 to 71 years. One patient had shifted from French to Alsatian, one from Czech to Polish, one from Norwegian to German, three from British English to Welsh, and one from British English to French. From American English, four switched to German, two to Swedish, two to Norwegian, one to Spanish, two to "New England," one to Welsh, Scottish, or Irish, and three to Italian. Three were difficult to classify. It is interesting that 10 patients (40% of the group) had a shift to dialects that could be described etymologically as Germanic (German, Swedish, or Norwegian).

The onset of foreign dialect was associated with neurologic disease. Fourteen (56%) developed a dialect after a cerebrovascular accident; 6 (24%) after head trauma; and 5 (20%) had histories of seizures after cerebrovascular accident or brain trauma. An effort was made to determine the number of patients whose foreign dialect was embedded in or followed more classic dysarthria, apraxia, or aphasia. Seventeen (68%) had one or more of these neurologic speech language signs in addition to the foreign dialect. In 8 (32%) it was impossible to determine the presence of these associated signs. These unusual cases raise several questions:

♦ Are these so-called dialectal changes truly dialectal or do they only sound as if they are because the direction of defect is coincidentally the same as one finds in the learned behavior of a true dialect?

- Is the dialect a primary component of the speech disorder or is it a compensatory reactive change to a more primary one?

- What specifically is happening at the phonemic, stress, and pitch-inflectional levels that gives the impression of foreign dialect?

- Of the thousands of patients who develop speech changes due to cerebral disease, why have so few demonstrated this unusual dialectal change?

- Are the pitch changes that partially characterize the dialect a signal that those regions of the brain that subtend musical production have been impaired?

- What is the connection between the onset of foreign dialect and the high incidence of its occurrence during the recovery stages of dysarthria, apraxia, and aphasia?

If one were to submit the following speech characteristics to a specialist in neurologic communicative disorders without informing the clinician of the patient's history or clinical studies, into what classification of speech or language disorder would these signs best fit?

- Distortions and prolongation of vowels and semivowels

- Consonants produced with slightly off-target tongue and lip placements (i.e., the sound is an allophonic deviation)

- Substitution of one phoneme for another

- Blocking on initial consonants

- Equal stress placed on all syllables in words and sentences

- Prolongation of silent intervals between words

- Insertion of vowel sounds between words

- Inappropriate pitch patterns

- All the above produced inconsistently

These composite features of patients with "foreign dialect" most closely resemble the patient who has apraxia of speech; they are characteristic of neither dysarthria nor aphasia. That is to say, they are similar to apraxia in a general sense. Obviously, there is something special about the "foreign dialect" patient's specific errors that distinguishes that person from the typical apraxic. Pitch inflectional patterns may be the major factors responsible.

A search through the histories of such patients reveals a common denominator: the presence of severe dysarthria and apraxia of speech. Although some are also aphasic, in several no aphasia was present.

A 27-year-old female who had sudden onset of numbness in her right hand, right facial weakness, mild dysarthria, and no previous history of foreign language exposure eventually developed an apraxia of speech. As the hours passed, her rate of spontaneous speech again became normal. However, she spoke with a foreign accent that several independent witnesses identified as German. The "r" sound was susceptible to mispronunciation and she hesitated slightly in an apparent search for

either the right word or articulatory position, yet her speech was free, appropriate, and completely intelligible. There was no dysphasia, and when examined 1 month later and 7 weeks after onset, her speech had returned to normal in all respects. Her foreign accent had disappeared (Whitty, 1964).

A 31-year-old female, after awakening and relieving herself, became dizzy, could not get words out, and by the end of the day was able to say only one-syllable words, although she never had difficulty thinking of the right words. By the end of 3 weeks, she was talking in complete sentences, at first in a flat intonational pattern. As inflectional changes returned, they took on a Spanish-sounding accent. Another, a 46-year-old female with cerebral ischemia following clamping of the left common carotid artery and left cervical sympathectomy for left internal carotid artery aneurysm, had a "New England" dialect for the first time in her life and an oral verbal apraxia in which she groped for tongue positions and initiated words incorrectly. She was also mildly aphasic.

Of 13 Mayo Clinic histories, 8 (62%) had apraxia of speech as an antecedent to the onset of the "foreign dialect."

A 41-year-old woman developed a Germanic-sounding dialect after a gunshot wound in the right occipital and parietal bone. The patient had spent 3 years in Germany, where she had learned German while married to an Air Force pilot. She had a left hemiparesis, left homonymous hemianopsia, spasticity of the right leg, apraxia of the left leg, an ataxic gait, and an abnormal EEG indicating a focal abnormality with epileptogenic components, from the right posterior temporal regions predominately. The evolution of her dialect began with complete absence of speech and a period of dysarthria and apraxia of speech that gradually disappeared, leaving the "foreign dialect" in its wake.

Broca's area is most frequently implicated in cases of sudden onset of foreign dialect. Very few dispute this localization except Cole (1971), who wrote about a patient who developed an Eastern European dialect after a brain-stem lesion.

Summary

- Neurologic voice disorders are components of dysarthria and are classified into the same subtypes as the dysarthrias, based on the location of the lesion in the nervous system and muscular pathophysiology.

- Most neurologic voice disorders are acoustically distinctive, which contributes to their differential diagnosis.

- Neonates and infants with neurologic disease cry abnormally.

- Vocal fold paralyses due to tenth cranial nerve (vagus) lesions and their effects on voice depend upon the location of the lesion along the nerve pathway from brain stem to muscle.

- Ever present is the danger of misdiagnosis of neurologic dysphonia as being psychogenic, especially those resulting from mild neurologic diseases of the tenth cranial nerve and from early bulbar myasthenia gravis.

♦ Flaccid dysphonias caused by tenth cranial nerve or myoneural junction disease are generally breathy and reduced in loudness due to vocal fold hypoadduction.

♦ Spastic (pseudobulbar) dysphonia generally has a harsh, strained-strangled quality due to vocal fold hyperadduction.

♦ Hypokinetic (parkinsonian) dysphonia is generally characterized by monopitch and reduced loudness resulting from the rigidity of muscles.

♦ Ataxic dysphonia, when present in ataxic dysarthria, may be tremorous or may show sudden bursts of loudness due to reduced muscular feedback.

♦ Choreic dysphonia consists of sudden alterations in pitch, loudness, and quality and, often, voice arrests, resulting from uncontrolled jerking muscular movements.

♦ Dystonic dysphonia consists of slower alterations in pitch, loudness, and quality and, often, voice arrests, resulting from slower, uncontrolled muscular movements.

♦ Organic voice tremor can exist in isolation or as one of several tremors distributed throughout the body. The voice tremor, ranging from 5 to 12 Hz, when severe, contains voice arrests resulting from hyperadduction of the vocal folds.

♦ The rhythmic interruptions (60 to 240 beats per minute) on vowel prolongation in palatopharyngolaryngeal myoclonus are marked but rarely heard during contextual speech.

♦ In Gilles de la Tourette's syndrome, uncontrolled spontaneous coughing, grunting, throat-clearing, and other aberrant laryngeal behaviors occur often, although not always.

♦ Apraxia of speech can include apraxia of phonation, in which muteness or aphonia exist in place of volitional phonation, yet voice can be produced automatically, as in coughing or throat-clearing.

♦ Muteness may be complete in severe cases of the akinetic mutism syndrome and partial during later stages of recovery.

♦ Aberrations in melody, stress patterns, and articulation in patients who have suffered CNS lesions can give the impression of a foreign dialect, called foreign accent syndrome.

References

Abuzzahab, F.S., Anderson, F.O. (1974). Gilles de la Tourette's syndrome: cross-cultural analysis and treatment outcomes. Clin Neurol Neurosurg 1, 66–74.

Achari, A.N., Colover, J. (1976). Posterior fossa tumors with pathological laughter. JAMA 235, 1469–1471.

Ardran, G.M., Kemp, F.H., Marland, P.M. (1954). Laryngeal palsy. Br J Radiol, 27, 201–209.

Appelblatt, N.H., Baker, S.R. (1981). Functional airway obstruction: a new syndrome. Arch Otolaryngol 107, 305–306.

Aronson, A.E. (1971). Early motor unit disease masquerading as psychogenic breathy dysphonia: a clinical case presentation. J Speech Hear Disord 36, 115–124.

Aronson, A.E. (1998). Dysarthria, crying and laughing in pseudobulbar palsy from right middle cerebral artery CVA: overview and personal account. J Med Speech-Lang Pathol 7, 111–114.

Ball, J.R.B., Lloyd, J.H. (1971). Myasthenia gravis as hysteria. Med J Aust 1, 1018–1020.

Blau, J.N., Kapadia, R. (1972). Idiopathic palsy of the recurrent laryngeal nerve: a transient cranial mononeuropathy. BMJ 4, 259–261.

Blinick, G., Tavolga, W.N., Antopol, W. (1971). Variations in birth cries of newborn infants from narcotic-addicted and normal mothers. Am J Obstet Gynecol 110, 948–958.

Blumstein, S.E., Cooper, W., Goodglass, H., Statlender, S., Gottlieb, J. (1980). Production deficits in aphasia: a voice-onset time analysis. Brain Lang 9, 153–170.

Blumstein, S.E., Stevens, K.N. (1979). Acoustic invariance in speech production: evidence from measurements of the spectral characteristics of stop consonants. J Acoustic Soc Am 66, 1001–1017.

Brown, J.R., Simonson, J. (1963). Organic voice tremor. Neurology 13, 520–525.

Brumlik, J. (1962). On the nature of normal tremor. Neurology 12, 159–179.

Cairns, H., Oldfield, R.C., Pennybacker, J.B., Whitteridge, D. (1941). Akinetic mutism with an epidermoid cyst of the third ventricle. Brain 64, 273–290.

Canter, G.J. (1963). Speech characteristics of patients with Parkinson's disease: I. Intensity, pitch, and duration. J Speech Hear Disord 28, 221–229.

Carrow, E., Rivera, V., Mauldin, M., Shamblin, L. (1974). Deviant speech characteristics in motor neuron disease. Arch Otolaryngol 100, 212–218.

Childrey, J.H., Parker, H.L. (1931). Myoclonic movements of the larynx and pharynx. Arch Otolaryngol 14, 139–148.

Christopher, K.L., Wood, R.P., Eckert, R.C., Blager, F.B., Raney, R.A., Souhrada, J.F. (1983). Vocal cord dysfunction presenting as asthma. N Engl J Med 308, 1566–1570.

Cohen, D.J., Shaywitz, B.A., Caparulo, B., Young, G., Bowers, M.D. (1978). Chronic, multiple tics of Gilles de la Tourette's disease. Arch Gen Psychiatry 35, 245–250.

Cole, M. (1971). Dysprosody due to posterior fossa lesions. Trans Am Neurol Assoc 96, 151–154.

Cormier, Y.F., Camus, P., Desmeules, M.J. (1980). Nonorganic acute upper airway obstruction: description and a diagnostic approach. Am Rev Respir Dis 121, 147–150.

Critchley, M. (1949). Observations on essential (heredofamilial) tremor. Brain 72, 113–139.

Critchley, M. (1970). *Aphasiology and other aspects of language.* London: Edward Arnold.

Daly, D.D., Love, J.G. (1958). Akinetic mutism. Neurology 8, 238–242.

Damasio, A.R. (1989). Time-locked multiregional retroactivation: a systems-level proposal for the neural substrates of recall and recognition. Cognition 33, 25–62.

Darley, F.L., Aronson, A.E., Brown, J.R. (1969a). Differential diagnostic patterns of dysarthria. J Speech Hear Res 12, 246–269.

Darley, F.L., Aronson, A.E., Brown, J.R. (1969b). Clusters of deviant speech dimensions in the dysarthrias. J Speech Hear Res 12, 462–496.

Darley, F.L., Aronson, A.E., Brown, J.R. (1975). *Motor speech disorders.* Philadelphia: W.B. Saunders.

Daube, J.R., Sandok, B.A., Reagan, T.J., Westmoreland, B.F. (1978). *Medical neurosciences.* Boston: Little, Brown.

Fisichelli, V.R. (1966). The phonetic content of the cries of normal infants and those with brain damage. J Psychol 64, 119–126.

Gilles de la Tourette, G. (1885). Etude sur une affection nerveuse caracteries e par de l'incoordination motrice, accompagnee d'echolalie et de copro-lalie. Arch Neurol 9, 158–200.

Golden, G.S. (1977). Tourette syndrome. Am J Dis Child 131, 531–534.

Goodglass, H. (1993). *Understanding aphasia.* New York: Academic Press.

Graff-Radford, N.R., Cooper, W.E., Colsher, P.L., Damasio, A.R. (1986). An unlearned foreign 'accent' in a patient with aphasia. Brain Lang 28, 86–94.

Gurd, J.M., Bessel, N.J., Bladon, R.A.W., Bamford, J.M. (1988). A case of foreign accent syndrome. Neurophyologia 26, 237–251.

Gurd, J.M., Coleman, J.S., Costello, A., Marshall, J.C. (2001). Organic or functional? A new case of foreign accent syndrome. Cortex 37, 715–718.

Hanson, D.G., Gerratt, B.R., Ward, P.H. (1984). Cinegraphic observations of laryngeal function in Parkinson's disease. Laryngoscope 94, 348–353.

Haymaker, W., Kuhlenbeck, H. (1976). Pathologic laughter and crying. In A.B. Baker, and L.H. Baker (Eds.), *Clinical neurology.* Hagerstown, MD: Harper & Row.

Hirano, M., Koike, Y., von Leden, H. (1968). Maximum phonation time and air usage during phonation. Folia Phoniatr (Basel) 20, 185–201.

Huppler, E.G., Schmidt, H.W., Devine, K.D., Gage, R.P. (1955). Causes of vocal cord paralysis. Proc Staff Meet Mayo Clinic 30, 518–521.

Ingram, J.C.L., McCormack, P.F., Kennedy, M. (1992). Phonetic analysis of a case of foreign accent syndrome. J Phone 20, 457–474.

Kammermeirer, M.A. (1969). A comparison of phonatory phenomena among groups of neurologically impaired speakers. Ph.D. dissertation. Minneapolis: University of Minnesota.

Karelitz, S., Fisichelli, V.R. (1962). The cry thresholds of normal infants and those with brain damage. An aid in the early diagnosis of severe brain damage. J Pediatr 61, 679–685.

Kellman, R.M., Leopold, D.A. (1982). Paradoxical vocal cord motion: an important cause of stridor. Laryngoscope 92, 58–60.

Klee, A. (1961). Akinetic mutism: review of the literature and report of a case. J Nerv Ment Dis 133, 536–553.

Kreindler, A., Pruskauer-Apostal, B. (1971). Neurologic and psychopathologic aspects of compulsive crying and laughter in pseudo-bulbar palsy patients. Rev Roum Neurol 8, 125–139.

Kurowski, K.M., Blumstein, S.E., Alexander, M. (1996). The foreign accent syndrome: a reconsideration. Brain Lang 54, 1–25.

Lahiri, A., Gewirth, L., Blumstein, S.E. (1984). A reconsideration of acoustic invariance for place of articulation in diffuse stop consonants: evidence from a cross-language study. J Acoustic Soc Am 76, 391–404.

Lecours, A.R., Lhermitte, F., Bryans, B. (1983). *Aphasiology.* London: Balliere Tindall.

Lind, J., Wasz-Höeckert, O., Vuorenkoski, V., Valanne, E. (1965). The vocalization of a newborn brain-damaged child. Ann Paediatr Fenn 11, 32–37.

Logemann, J.A., Fisher, H.B., Boshes, B., Blonsky, E.R. (1978). Frequency and concurrence of vocal tract dysfunctions in the speech of a large sample of Parkinson patients. J Speech Hear Disord 42, 47–57.

Marshall, J. (1962). Observations on essential tremor. J Neurol Neurosurg Psychiatry 25, 122–125.

Monrad-Krohn, G.H. (1947). Dysprosody or altered "melody of language." Brain 70, 405–415.

McHenry, M., Whatman, J., Pou, A. (2002). The effect of botulinum toxin A on vocal symptoms of spastic dysarthria: a case study. J Voice 16, 124–143.

Moonis, M., Swearer, J.M., Blumstein, S.E., Kurowski, K., Licho, R., Kramer, P., Mitchell, A., Drachman, D. (1993). Foreign accent syndrome following a closed head injury: Perfusion deficit on SPECT with normal MRI. Neurology 43(Suppl. 2), 381.

Neiman, R.F., Mountjoy, J.R., Allen, E.L. (1975). Myasthenia gravis focal to the larynx. Arch Otolaryngol 101, 569–570.

New, G.B., Childrey, J.H. (1932). Paralysis of the vocal cords. Arch Otolaryngol 16, 143–159.

Nielsen, J.M., McKeown, M. (1961). Dysprosody. Report of two cases. Bull Los Angeles Neurol Soc 26, 157–159.

Patterson, R., Schatz, M., Horton, M. (1974). Munchausen's stridor: nonorganic laryngeal obstruction. Clin Allergy 4, 307–310.

Peterson, G., Barney, M. (1952). Control methods used in a study of the vowels. J Acoustic Soc Am 24, 175–184.

Pick, A. (1919). Uber Anderungen des Sprachcarakters als Begleiterscheinung aphasicher Storungen. Zeitschrift fur gesamte. Neurol Psychiatr (Bucur) 45, 230–241.

Portnoy, R.A. (1979). Hyperkinetic dysarthria as an early indicator of impending tardive dyskinesia. J Speech Hear Disord 44, 214–219.

Ramig, L.O., Sapir, S., Countryman, S., Pawlas, A., O'Brian, C., Hoehn, M., Thompson, (2001). Intensive voice treatment (LSVT (r)) for patients with Parkinson's disease: a 2 year follow up. J Neurol Neurosurg Psychiatry 71, 493–498.

Rogers, J.H. (1980). Functional inspiratory stridor in children. J Laryngol Otol 94, 669–670.

Rogers, J.H., Stell, P.M. (1978). Paradoxical movement of the vocal cords as a cause of stridor. J Laryngol Otol 92, 157–158.

Rose, F.C. (Ed.). (1977). *Motor neuron disease.* New York: Grune & Stratton.

Ross, E.D. (1981). The aprosodias: functional–anatomic organization of the affective components of language in the right hemisphere. Arch Neurol 38, 561–569.

Ross, E.D., Mesulam, M. (1979). Dominant language functions of the right hemisphere: prosody and emotional gesturing. Arch Neurol 36, 144–148.

Ryalls, J.H. (1984). An acoustic investigation of vowel production in aphasia. Ph.D. dissertation. Providence, RI: Brown University.

Sapir, S., Aronson, A.E. (1985). Aphonia after closed head injury: etiologic considerations. Br J Disord Commun 20, 289–296.

Sapir, S., Aronson, A.E. (1987). Coexisting psychogenic and neurogenic dysphonia: a source of diagnostic confusion. Br J Disord Commun 22, 73–80.

Schiff, H.B., Alexander, M.P., Naeser, M.A., Galaburda, A.M. (1983). Aphemia: clinical-anatomic correlations. Arch Neurol 40, 720–727.

Shapiro, A.K., Shapiro, E.S., Wayne, H.L. (1973). The symptomatology and diagnosis of Gilles de la Tourette's syndrome. J Am Acad Child Psychiatry 12, 702–723.

Stevens, K.N., Blumstein, S.E. (1978). Invariant cues for place of articulation in stop consonants. J Acoustic Soc Am 64, 1358–1368.

Takayama, Y., Sugishita, M., Kido, T., Ogawa, M., Akiguchi, I. (1993). A case of foreign accent syndrome without aphasia caused by a lesion of the left precentral gyrus. Neurology 43, 1361–1363.

Van Lancker, D.R., Bogen, J.E., Canter, J.E. (1983). A case report of pathological rule governed syllable intrusion. Brain Lang 20, 12–20.

Verhowevon, J., Marelü, P. Prosodia characteristics of a case of foreign accent syndrome.

Department of Germanic Languages Universiteitsplein 1 B-2610 Wilrjik General Hospital Middelheim Department of Neurology, Lindendreef B 2020 Antwerp. 1996, pp 1–148. Paper posted on Web at http://webh01.ua.ac.be/apil/apil100/FAS.pdf.

Von Leden, H. (1968). Objective measures of laryngeal function and phonation. Ann N Y Acad Sci 155, 56–67.

Whitaker, H.A. (1982). Levels of impairment in disorders of speech. In R.N. Malatesha and L.C. Hartlage (Eds.), Neuropsychology and cognition (pp. 168–207). Vol. 1. Nato Advanced Study Institutes Series D, No. 9. Hague Martinus Nijnoff Publishers.

Whitty, C.W.M. (1964). Cortical dysarthria and dysprosody of speech. J Neurol Neurosurg Psychiatry 27, 507–510.

Williams, R.G. (1959). Idiopathic recurrent laryngeal nerve paralysis. J Laryngol Otol 73, 161–166.

Wolski, W. (1967). Hypernasality as the presenting symptom of myasthenia gravis. J Speech Hear Disord 32, 36–38.

Zue, V.W., Laferriere, M. (1979). Acoustical study of medial /t, d/. J Acoustic Soc Am 66, 1039–1050.

Additional Reading

Adour, K.K., Schneider, G.D., Hilsinger, R.L., Jr. (1980). Acute superior laryngeal nerve palsy: analysis of 78 cases. Otolaryngol Head Neck Surg 88, 418–424. (This article should be read from a more detailed analysis of the laryngologic and voice signs and symptoms of lesions of the superior laryngeal nerve.)

Aronson, A.E. (1998). Dysarthria, crying and laughing in pseudobulbar palsy from right middle cerebral artery CVA: overview and personal account. J Med Speech-Lang Pathol 7, 111–114. (A must read.)

Faaborg-Andersen, K., Munk-Jensen, A. (1963). Unilateral paralysis of the superior laryngeal nerve. Acta Otholaryngol 57, 155–159.

Findley, L.J., Gresty, M.A. (1988). Head, facial, and voice tremor. Adv Neurol 49, 239–253. (This reference is an excellent review of the entire subject of tremor involving different parts of the body, their frequency characteristics, physical appearance, etiology, and management. It contains a well-described section of tremor of the voice.)

Gacek, R.R., Malmgren, L.T., Lyon, M.J. (1977). Localization of adductor and abductor motor nerve fibers to the larynx. Ann Otol Rhinol Laryngol 86, 771–776.

Larson, C.R. Brain mechanisms involved in the control over vocalization is considerably incomplete.

Larson, C., Garrett, J.D. (1991). Brain mechanisms in control of vocalization in phonosurgery: Assessment and surgical management of voice disorders. C.N. Ford and D.M. Bless (Eds.). New York: Raven Press. (This compact and lucid review of animal experiments and the effects of central nervous system lesions on phonation in humans identifies cortical and subcortical centers responsible for reflex and volitional vocalization.)

Ward, P.H., Berci, G., Calcaterra, T.C. (1977). Superior laryngeal nerve paralysis: an often overlooked entity. Trans Am Acad Ophthalmol Otolaryngol 84, 78–89. (This article amplifies this chapter's discussion of the effects of vagus nerve lesions on vocal fold function.)

Chapter 6

Spasmodic Dysphonia

When we approach the problem of spastic dysphonia we see so many different opinions about any of its many aspects that we come to the conclusion that one of the following two things has happened: either we are not speaking about the same thing or we look at the same thing with different eyes. And these "eyes" depend upon our culture and on the understanding that even scientific "truths" are, frequently, provisional.

—Bloch

In this chapter, we discuss a voice disorder that has a history of being the most serious, controversial, and challenging regarding its etiology and treatment of all voice disorders in our field. Once upon a time it used to be called *spastic dysphonia*. Contemporary clinicians and researchers have settled upon *spasmodic dysphonia*, originally recommended by Aronson et al. (1968a,b) because of the confusing implications of the word *spastic* (confusable with the spasticity of pseudobulbar dysphonia, which can produce *similar* voice signs and symptoms). Throughout its history, spasmodic dysphonia has had many synonyms: spastic dysphonia, lalophobia, phonatory glottic spasm, mogiphonia, psychophonastachesia, and stuttering at the glottal level.

The term *spasmodic dysphonia* is defined as voice breaks or stoppage stemming from cessation of vocal fold oscillation generally from hyperadduction of the true and/or false (ventricular) folds during attempted phonation, producing a voice that is strangled, hoarse, and effortful, which is often continuous or sustained, intermittent or choppy. In some patients, the vocal fold adductor spasms can be so intense that a patient shows engorgement of the veins of the neck, flushing of the face, or at times cyanosis accompanied by grunting, groaning, and extreme fatigue. The voice is so bizarre that it is profoundly incapacitating, disturbing to patient and listener, having profound psychiatric, social, and vocational repercussions severely compromising one's quality of life.

Historically descriptions of spasmodic dysphonia have a long history. In 1875 Jonann Schnitzler, a prominent laryngologist in Vienna, first described a condition he called "spastic dysphonia," where symptoms ranged from severe cases of vocal cord cramping preventing emission of sound, to milder cases where the voice is forced each time phonation is attempted. Subsequently, other clinicians described it and made astute observations about its characteristics, range in signs and symptoms, and possible influencing variables. A selected sample of these early observations include: a spasmodic activity of the tensors of the vocal cords that provoke a feeble, intermittent, jerky voice (Mackenzie, 1880); excessive innervation that goes beyond the voluntary occlusions (Stern, 1928); a rare illness, most of the time undiagnosed and difficult to treat, that attacks subjects who do much speaking (Nadoleczny, 1938); a disordered phonation characterized by vocal force, grunting, and inhibition; whispered voice in severe cases going to total aphonia with maximal tension. The disorder is manifested above all during communicative speech, more rarely in speaking without listeners (Berendes, 1938). A disorder of speech, grunting, can be emitted in a forced fashion with vowels often separated into two accentuations. The disorder is rare. Because its severity is often dependent upon the situation or emotional status of a patient, numerous authors classify it among the neuroses (Luchsinger, 1949); not as a clinical entity, but as being symptomatic of a larger neurologic syndrome (Robe, Brumlik, Moore 1960). From the late 1800s through the middle of the 20th century, clinicians were mixed about the etiology of this disorder.

◆ Terminology and Definitions

Spasmodic dysphonia is an example of the way in which the meanings of words change with time and the expansion of knowledge and of the confusion that accompanies such change. Early in the history of this disorder, those few clinicians who wrote about it seemed to be in reasonable agreement that spasmodic dysphonia was intended to mean a single entity, distinct from other voice disorders, which conformed to fairly narrow criteria. The original definition of adductor spastic dysphonia, reviewed by Arnold (1959), is paraphrased as follows:

♦ A voice that is variably squeezed, strained, choked, staccato, stuttering-like, jerky, grunting, groaning, effortful, pinched, grating, and has periodic breaks in phonation. It has a tendency to be monopitched and reduced in loudness, and vowels are initiated with hard glottal attacks.

♦ The abnormal voice occurs only during voluntary phonation for communication purposes and not during singing, vowel prolongation, laughing, or crying.

♦ The abnormal voice is the effect of hyperadduction of the true and false vocal folds.

♦ The disorder is caused by psychoneurosis from either occupational stress or emotional trauma, such as family conflicts, accidents, terrifying events, or accumulated frustrations.

What needs to be remembered is that this definition originated with a few otolaryngologists and psychiatrists, whose experience with patients who had this kind of strained voice was limited and whose knowledge of both the psychiatric and neurologic characteristics of their patients paralleled the relatively undeveloped state of both specialties. The first article written on the subject by Traube in 1871, setting into motion and directing subsequent thought on this disorder, described it as "a spastic form of nervous hoarseness." At least a half dozen other writers before 1900 also linked the disorder to psychoneurosis (Kiml, 1963). Their early impressions about psychogenic etiology, given at the dawn of modern psychiatry and psychology, have ultimately proved to be correct for some of the patients exhibiting this disorder. However, subsequent experience has shown—particularly during the past 20 years—that what these clinicians had failed to notice, understand, and document during the early years was that there were people whose affected voices sounded very much like the spastic dysphonia as defined originally but were caused by neurologic, not psychogenic, disorders. This, too, is understandable because the specialty of neurology at the turn of the century was in a similar state of primitive evolution, as were psychiatry and psychology.

With the passage of time, more clinicians began to witness cases of strained hoarseness of different types, many of which were eventually suspected of being of neurologic etiology, and still others for whom neither psychoneurosis nor neurologic substrates could be demonstrated. Although these patients failed to conform to the early criteria for spastic dysphonia, their disorders were called *spastic dysphonia* nevertheless, mainly because that was the way they sounded, and diagnosis is made by auditory perception.

Terminology being vitally important to clarity, we are faced today with the following dilemma: either there is only one true spasmodic dysphonia, the specific criteria for which were set down by the early writers on the subject and just listed in this chapter, or all other strained voices are not true spastic dysphonia and should either be called something else, or the term should be modified to specify etiology. We no longer use the term *spastic dysphonia*. It has been replaced by *spasmodic dysphonia* advocated by Aronson (1968a) when he wrote

We would like to advocate a change in the term used to describe the voice disorder we have been calling spastic dysphonia. In the neurologic world the term spastic is commonly used to imply disease of corticobulbar or corticospinal (pyramidal) pathways.... It is also our observation that the strained voice quality in this disorder waxes and wanes from moment to moment in a spasmodic fashion.[1] For these reasons, therefore, we propose the term spasmodic dysphonia to prevent the confusion that arises from the use of the term spastic (p. 200).

The viewpoint taken in this book is that the latter course is preferable to the former because it recognizes the everwidening recognition of the multiple origins of adductor laryngospasm. Therefore, the following definition and criteria pertaining to the voice disorder concept of spastic dysphonia are recommended, based on evidence to be presented later in this chapter:

♦ The term *adductor* should be used as a prefix to designate a class of voice characteristics produced by hyperadduction of the vocal folds.

♦ Continuing along this line of thinking, then, *adductor spasmodic dysphonia* is a perceptual term that refers to a strained, groaning, staccato, effortful voice, no different from the original definition.

♦ It varies within and among patients according to severity and detailed voice characteristics.

♦ Though generally neurologic, it may be of psychogenic, neurologic, or of unknown (idiopathic) etiology.

♦ If data lead the clinician to conclude that the laryngospasms are psychogenic beyond a reasonable doubt, then the term used should be *psychogenic adductor spasmodic dysphonia*.

♦ If data lead the clinician to conclude that the laryngospasms are neurologic beyond a reasonable doubt, then the term used should be *neurologic adductor spasmodic dysphonia*.

♦ If data fail to prove either psychogenic or neurologic etiology, then the term *idiopathic adductor spasmodic dysphonia* should be used.

In summary, a modern definition of the term *adductor spasmodic dysphonia* is that it applies to a family of strained voices produced by adductor laryngospasm that arise from different etiologies. These laryngospasms are abnormal involuntary movements that are action-induced by speaking for specific tasks as the larynx is generally normal at rest (Brin, Fahn, Blitzer, et al., 1992). To distinguish among them is not a trivial academic exercise. It has considerable importance to clinicians responsible for establishing a differential

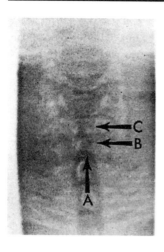
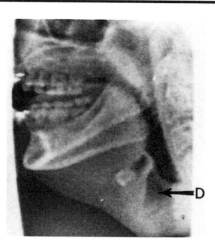

Figure 6.1 Frames from anteroposterior and lateral cineradiography of vocal folds during onset of laryngospasm in spastic dysphonia. (**A**) Glottis is open. (**B, C**) True and false vocal folds, respectively, relatively demarcated by laryngeal ventricle in between. (**D**) Hypopharynx is open, the larynx still relatively low in the neck.

diagnosis of laryngospasms in patients who along with their physicians need to know the truth about their abnormal voices and whose treatment may depend upon the type of adductor spasmodic dysphonia that they have.

♦ Adductor Spasmodic Dysphonia

Pathophysiology

The common denominator underlying all types of adductor spasmodic dysphonia is adductor laryngospasm of the vocal folds. While keeping in mind that within and among patients the degree and frequency of adductor laryngospasms vary considerably, the following kinds of laryngeal adductor, and sometimes even sphincter, actions have been observed during videofluoroscopy and videofiberoptic laryngoscopy (McCall, Skolnick, and Brewer, 1971; Parnes, Lavarato, and Myers, 1978):

♦ *Adductor spasms of the true vocal folds only*   Hyperadduction of the true vocal folds alone occurs in mild cases. Although the degree of adductor force cannot be seen readily during such spasms, the midline separation

between the ligamentous portions of the vocal folds may be obscured owing to compression of one vocal fold against the other. The vocal folds can be seen to snap shut synchronously with each voice arrest.

♦ *Adductor spasms of both the true and false vocal folds*   During moderate to severely strained voice or voice arrest, the false or ventricular vocal folds close over and obscure the true folds.

♦ *Supraglottic constriction*   Severely strained voice or voice arrests are accompanied by constriction of the hypopharynx (i.e., the inferior pharyngeal constrictor just above the level of the false vocal folds). The shape of the lumen during such closure is not an anteroposterior, elongated one, as in true and false vocal fold hyperadduction alone, but is sphincteric or circular. Moreover, the true and false folds hyperadduct along with the pharyngeal constrictors. What appears to be true, then, is that the more severe the adductor laryngospasms, the greater the vertical extent of intrinsic laryngeal muscle participation. As tightness of spasms increases, constriction progresses superiorly from the true folds to involve the ventricular folds, and, ultimately, the pharyngeal constrictors (**Figs. 6.1, 6.2**). The acoustic consequences of these constrictions are displayed in a sonogram in Figure 6.3.

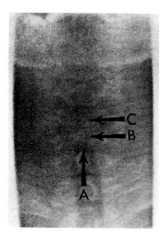
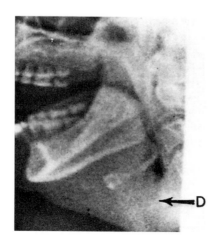

Figure 6.2 Frames from anteroposterior and lateral cineradiography of vocal folds at height of laryngospasm in spastic dysphonia. (**A**) Glottis is closed. (**B, C**) True and false vocal folds, respectively, massively adducted and poorly demarcated. Laryngeal ventricle is obliterated. Vocal fold position is elevated. (**D**) Hypopharynx obliterated owing to sphincteric closure and elevation of larynx.

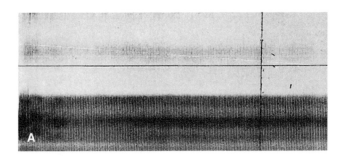

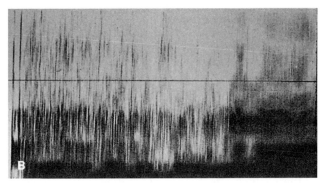

Figure 6.3 Sonogram of a prolonged vowel produced with normal voice (**A**) and a spasmodic dysphonic voice (**B**). Vertical striations (each one representing a glottal pulse) in A are equally spaced and regular, whereas in B they are irregular. In A, dark bands of energy and formats run across the length of the sonogram, but are interrupted and difficult to ascertain in the vowel prolongation in the lower figure because of voice breaks.

Although hypercontraction of the intrinsic laryngeal and pharyngeal muscles is fundamental to the adductor spasmodic dysphonias, moderate to severe laryngospasms are accompanied by synchronous movements of the entire larynx, most often in a superior (cephalad) direction, as shown in the succeeding figures. Associated laryngeal movements implicate the extrinsic laryngeal muscles as well. Such movement can also be seen through the skin of the neck. Downward and forward displacement of the larynx occurs less often. As expected, increased amplitude of electromyographic potentials in the general neck region have been recorded during such spasms (Tarrasch, 1946). It is important to realize, then, that the adductor spasmodic dysphonias are disorders not just of the true and false vocal folds but also of the supraglottic pharyngeal constrictors and the strap muscles, moving the body of the larynx. The neuroanatomic implications of these facts is that not only the tenth cranial nerve, innervating the intrinsic laryngeal muscles, but also the ninth cranial nerve to the pharynx and the cervical spinal nerves to the extrinsic laryngeal muscles may transmit nerve impulses responsible for the spasms. However, this observation is not to be misinterpreted as suggesting the problem is peripheral, because current theory suggests the muscle and nerve abnormalities reflect central remodeling rather than a peripheral disorder.

Aberrant respiratory movements often accompany the laryngospasms. The clinician can see sudden, jerky arrests and other dysrhythmic movements of the thorax and abdomen synchronous with strained voice or voice arrests. Respiratory dysfunction is most probably the secondary effect of the uncontrolled glottic closures (i.e., during adduc-

tor spasm, increased exhalatory effort is required to force air through the constricted glottis). If an adductor spasm is particularly abrupt, the exhalatory muscles react to the sudden laryngeal arrest of exhaled air by contracting more quickly and forcefully, actions that can be seen with the naked eye. The speaker, in effect, is caught in the throes of a series of involuntary effort closures or Valsalva maneuvers. The normal speaker can simulate adductor spasmodic dysphonia realistically by trying to phonate while straining or bearing down. Notice how exhalatory arrests are accompanied by sudden, visible abdominal and thoracic movements. This might lead clinicians to the incorrect conclusion that the respiratory behaviors are all secondary. This notion is dispelled by presentation of six patients reported by Brin (1992) who all exhibited respiratory adductor abnormal involuntary adduction of the vocal folds on respiration but were normal during phonation. Whether voice or respiratory in origin, severe laryngospasm produces other visible features, such as flushing of the face. Silent lip movements may occur during moments of voice arrest. Even stuttering-like articulatory repetitions during inaudible voice are common as the patient struggles, by repetition, to compensate for moments of unintelligibility. Other signs of struggle are excessive contractions of the neck muscles, shoulder girdle, and upper arms. Typically, patients with a severe, long-standing dysphonia will present with a strained facial expression consisting of frowning, squinting, and downward turning of the angles of the mouth. What is unseen by the observer is the intense physical effort and fatigue felt by the patient. So tiring is speaking that many patients elect to whisper because of the freer airflow that it provides or become recluses and avoid talking whenever possible. It should come as no surprise then that therapeutic alleviation of laryngospasm is as much a physical relief as it is a contribution to voice improvement.

Incidence

Although the incidence and prevalence of adductor spasmodic dysphonia in the general population is unknown, the National Spasmodic Dysphonia Association estimates there are between 35,000 and 50,000 Americans afflicted with this disorder. Additionally, limited data on frequency of occurrence, age, and sex in individual practices are available. The reader must bear in mind two kinds of errors in reporting: (1) Most past and even current reports do not identify the patients studied according to etiologic type. Patients are chosen almost exclusively on the basis of the sound of their voices, and the clinicians making judgments have varying knowledge and experience with the disorder. Quite likely, then, these are not homogeneous populations. More probably, they represent mixtures of psychogenic, neurologic, and idiopathic types. (2) In collecting statistical data in clinical practice, some clinicians fail to recognize the disorder when confronted by it, and others identify it erroneously when it does not exist. These sources of error must be considered, particularly the first, when critically reading studies reported here and elsewhere. Problems encountered in critically reading existing literature to determine the incidence, age of onset, or etiology are not limited to the clinical sources of error. An evidence-based literature search on all articles published on spasmodic dysphonia medical interventions between 1966 and 2000 found that whereas there were 1324 subjects included in the 24 articles meeting search criteria, the actual number of different subjects was estimated at only 395. Consequently, readers also need to recognize that a single center publishing several articles on the same, or nearly same, set of subjects can skew general impressions of a population toward whatever unique characteristics their population might appear to possess such as age of onset, concomitant health problems, or specific etiology. The following data and those later in this chapter are given with awareness of these limitations.

The consensus is that adductor spasmodic dysphonia is rare. Most clinicians who do not work in specialty clinics witness only a few cases over a lifetime, and some have never had any direct experience with such patients.

Age of Onset

Most research publications cite middle age as the time of onset. Aronson (1968a) reported distribution of age of onset in spastic dysphonia in 34 patients. The average age was 44 years (range, 28 to 69 years): 20 to 29 years, 9%; 30 to 39 years, 24%; 40 to 49 years, 29%; 50 to 59 years, 20%; and 60 to 69 years, 18%. Brodnitz (1976) reported a mean age of 50.2 years in 130 patients with the following distribution: 20 to 30 years, 10%; 31 to 40 years, 16%; 41 to 51 years, 27%; 51 to 60 years, 29%; older than 60 years, 18%. His youngest patient was 27 years, his oldest 76 years. In another study of 100 patients, Aronson (1979) found a median age of onset of 50 years.

The difficulty getting a handle on the incidence is underscored by an evidence-based literature search on medical interventions reported between 1966 and 2000 that although 1324 total subjects were reported in the 24 articles reviewed, the number probably represented a total number of 395 different subjects (Duffy and Yorkson, 2003).

Sex Ratio

The male to female ratios reported in different studies range from ~1:1 to 1:4. Because patients usually present themselves for examination, they introduce a self-selection factor that may not be a true indication of incidence in the general population.

Onset and Course

With rare exception, adductor spasmodic dysphonia begins insidiously as a nonspecific hoarseness, at first fluctuating in severity, with intervening periods of normal voice. Then, gradually, the strained adductor laryngospasms intrude into the hoarseness. The disorder may plateau or continue to worsen until phonation during speech is all but impossible. From a follow-up study of 100 patients, Aronson (1979) found that the median time necessary for spastic dysphonia to develop into its full-blown state from onset was approximately 1 year in both males and females. Although some patients consulted a specialist almost immediately after onset, others waited as long as 8 years. The median period from onset until consultation was 2 months. These patients consulted an average of four specialists, although some had gone to as many as 25 in search of help. Izdebski, Dedo, and

Boles (1984), in a survey of 200 patients, found gradual onset in 84% of patients; the remainder reported sudden onset. They found that in patients whose disorder had begun gradually, the voice declined and reached a plateau within 6 to 9 months. Patients whose voices intermittently fluctuated between abnormal and normal from onset deteriorated and reached a plateau after ~23 months. Once the disorder takes hold, remissions are rare unless the spastic dysphonia is of the conversion reaction type. In an 18-year follow-up study of 10 spastic dysphonic patients, Borenstein, Lipton, and Rupick (1978) found that in all 10 patients, the disorder had remained; four reported no change during the intervening years, two reported that their voices had worsened slightly, three had mildly improved, and one improved substantially.

Factors Affecting Severity

During the life of the disorder, patients report unexpectedly wide fluctuations in severity. Periods of emotional stress make the disorder worse. Talking on the telephone and to authority figures is especially difficult, and the voice is vulnerable to moods of anxiety and depression. Physical labor also can cause the voice to worsen. One patient reported that if he knew he needed an especially good voice for some occasion, he would refrain from lifting, pushing, or digging. The temptation is to conclude from such testimony that voluntary effort closure increases susceptibility to spasm. Yet, at other times, the spasms can be mild, prompting many patients to claim periods of nearly normal voice. These moments of relief are usually accompanied by feelings of relaxation and freedom from anxiety. For that reason, the voice is often much better while the patient is on vacation. One patient reported that while on a trip to Hawaii, her voice began to improve incrementally in proportion to the distance from the California coast, so that by the time she had reached the islands her voice was the best it had ever been. On her trip home, the closer her plane got to the mainland, the worse her voice became. By the time the plane had landed, her dysphonia was as bad as when she had left. These patients have a baffling ability to produce normal voice when surprised or taken off guard, such as when they are greeted by a passer-by or spoken to from behind. The common factor seems to be a high level of situational spontaneity in which the patient does not have time to think before speaking. The more patients concentrate on what they wish to say, the worse their voices become. Many patients report that even the affective content of their thoughts and mood fluctuations can alter severity; that when thinking pleasant thoughts their voices are better, the reverse being true for unpleasant ones. Normal voice during singing was one of the earliest observations described and contributed to early postulations that the problem was psychogenic in origin. It is logical to conclude that spasms are linked to volitional, intellectual, or executive speech functions and disappear during uninhibited, emotional, automatic, nonintellectual speech. Contemporary writings suggest symptoms of spasmodic dysphonia result from abnormal motor responses to sensory input and laryngeal feedback, possibly by disinhibition of laryngeal motor responses.

Factors Associated with Onset

The clinician's ability to uncover factors associated with onset of any disorder is contingent upon the patient's ability to remember or willingness to disclose such information. Even when patients report events antecedent to or concurrent with onset, there is a danger that the examiner will conclude they are necessarily cause and effect. Also, because the onset is often insidious and most patients do not seek help immediately, it may be difficult for them to be accurate reporters, and they, too, may be trying to associate a cause and effect.

Upper respiratory infections, as discussed elsewhere in this book, are commonly reported with the onset of all voice disorders. Asked if their disorder had occurred after a cold, sore throat, or laryngitis, 35% of patients answered in the affirmative, and 17% said it occurred after a "flu-like" illness (Aronson, 1979). Izdebski, Dedo, and Boles (1984) found that 15% of their patients reported nonspecific vocal tract illness as well as colds and viruses as being associated with onset. What remains unknown is whether these laryngeal and respiratory illnesses were true infections that had some physical bearing on the disorder or whether they were unconscious simulations of respiratory infections that provided the psychologic rationale for announcing the disorder, as is known to occur in psychogenic voice disorders as a group.

An unavoidable fact, again not necessarily indicative of cause and effect but in many cases highly suspicious and even compelling, is the co-occurrence of acute or chronic psychologic stress. It is possible that the neurochemical changes co-occurring with stress contribute to the disorder or that the stress of struggles to communicate cause stress. In their survey of stress and emotional trauma, Izdebski, Dedo, and Boles (1984) found that ~16% of patients thought that stress had caused their disorder. Brodnitz (1976) found that 40% of his patients had described what he called trigger incidents: death of a relative, severe automobile accident in which the patient was not physically harmed, witness to murder of a relative, divorce of a relative, unremitting work stress, marital conflict, and perpetually demanding responsibility. The term *trigger incident* is an apt one in any discussion of cause and effect, for later in this chapter the distinction will be made between stress as a primary psychogenic cause and stress as a trigger or precipitant of a latent neurologic disorder. Meanwhile, one should resist the temptation to conclude that cases are primarily psychogenic merely on the grounds that the disorder coincided with upsetting life circumstances.

In a study of 100 spastic dysphonia patients, Aronson (1979) found an extraordinarily high percentage of patients who had reported a close temporal relationship between stress and the onset of their voice disorder. Did spastic dysphonia occur after a sudden emotional event? Forty-five percent said it had. Had the dysphonia been accompanied by a continuous, ongoing stressful situation? Fifty-five percent answered affirmatively. One must then ask would similar percentages of persons admitting to stress occur in the normal-speaking population.

The following are samples of patient reports of acute, emotionally traumatic events shortly after which the dysphonia surfaced: "Auto accident; family death; son got divorced; angered at work over a situation I could not handle; death in family followed by marital, family, and business stress; dispute over property; daughter's marriage; unmarried daughter became pregnant; brother killed in auto accident and husband died of heart attack in close succession." On a frequency of occurrence basis, family illness and death rank high as antecedents of adductor spasmodic dysphonia.

Typical chronic stress situations reported were "hectic worried life; unemployment; hospitalizations; pushing self too hard; continuous job pressure; under tension because of husband's business; having marital difficulties; passed over for promotion; responsibility for caring for alcoholic brother; responsibility for caring for aged mother; taking care of invalid husband and his eventual death; own cancer surgery; homosexual son living at home and his objectionable friends who come to visit."

Many patients have no recollection of physical illness or emotional stress at the time of onset of their dysphonias. Whereas in some cases they have forgotten, in others they may be guarding or repressing sensitive information. In still others, no event occurred at the time of onset. An attempt will be made in the Etiology section to clarify the implications of these variations.

Psychosocial Effects

It does not matter if the etiology of adductor spasmodic dysphonia is psychogenic, neurologic, or idiopathic; the voice disorder in its own right is a dire threat to the patient's psychologic equilibrium. Self-consciousness, feelings of inadequacy, paranoid ideation, diminished interpersonal communication, social withdrawal, alcoholism, depression, and even suicidal tendencies are found in a majority of these patients to some degree. The intensity of these emotions is roughly proportional to the severity and duration of the voice disorder and to the importance of communication in the patient's daily life. Some patients are prime candidates for psychiatric and psychologic help strictly on the basis of the voice effects alone. These patients prove how considerably important normal voice is to the maintenance of a secure self-image and how alienated we become with ourselves and society when our self-image, epitomized by our voices, is threatened by our own and others' adverse reactions to it.

Spasmodic dysphonia affects the emotional, social, and occupational life of each person differently, depending upon each patient's premorbid personality and life circumstances. The extent of incapacitation depends upon the patient's reliance on speech occupationally and socially. Occupational effects can be devastating in those whose livelihood is heavily dependent upon oral communication, for example, teachers, attorneys, physicians, clergy, entertainers—any human endeavor in which the personality, ethos, or persuasiveness of the speaker is integral to that person's need to communicate. In a survey of the effects of spasmodic dysphonia on job performance, Izdebski, Dedo, and Boles (1984) found that the dysphonia seriously interfered with job performance in 93% of men and 77% of women, and, as a result, 26% of men and 37% of women were forced to change jobs or to be reclassified, usually with adverse financial and emotional consequences. Aronson (1979) found that 64% of spasmodic dysphonic patients surveyed reported having become socially withdrawn and depressed after developing the condition. Forty-one percent said it interfered with their earning a living. The following are excerpts from that survey. It is likely that if these studies were to be repeated today, the percentages affected would be even more dramatic because in the ensuing 25 years, significantly more women have entered all aspects of the professional workforce. Representative samples of occupational, emotional, and social effects reported by patients in response to Aronson's survey follow. The comments are devastatingly telling of the adverse impact of this disorder.

Occupational Effects

◆ "It caused me to retire. I could no longer work like I used to."

◆ "I had to be placed on disability pension."

◆ "In my work, the ability to communicate is essential. My voice has resulted in my passing up or not doing some things I might have done otherwise for added income, like negotiating teacher contracts."

◆ "By the time I reached retirement age I was ineffective on the telephone, inadequate in communicating with employees or in participating in management sessions. I had to quit."

◆ "I live in a secluded world and don't apply the potential I know I have. I don't work toward a better life."

◆ "I have missed several promotions due to my voice situation."

◆ "I have kept my job as a college professor by using 'self-paced' nonlecture methods of teaching. But, this requires more time, and my productivity has dropped."

◆ "Mine is a small business and I cannot find help. I have to wait on customers and communicate with them. I become very worn out and tired, angry at myself and depressed."

◆ "My job as a consultant consists of sales pitches directly, and due to my voice problem, I haven't been able to communicate properly with customers. I work on a commission basis, and sales have dropped."

◆ "How can clients have confidence in me as their attorney with a voice like this? Some of them look at me strangely, and when there is any office noise they can't hear me. Trial work is impossible, now. I let my partner do that."

Social Effects

◆ "I no longer want to go to social events or meet with people."

◆ "I try to avoid talking to people. I avoid meetings of any kind; going to people's houses or having guests at home. It's embarrassing."

◆ "I cannot speak comfortably in crowded rooms, automobiles, buses, or airplanes."

◆ "I have been hesitant and have withdrawn from taking office in several clubs and fraternal activities where use of the voice is involved."

◆ "People shy away because they cannot hear, and I, in turn, do likewise, because I am aware of their discomfort."

◆ "I am unable to carry on a conversation without straining my throat and am silent most of the time, even at home. When I am with other people I listen and seldom enter the conversation."

◆ "It's embarrassing to talk, because people stop and stare. Children and teenage boys ridicule me."

◆ "I can't visit as I would like. Sometimes my experiences have been knowledgeable, and I would like to express them, but I cannot, and it appears to others that I am stupid."

◆ "I used to sing in the church choir. Now my singing is horrid."

◆ "I'm not completely withdrawn but am more selective. I try to avoid one-on-one social events and tend more to group events. Also, I try to socialize with those who have heard me and understand my problem."

Emotional Effects

◆ "I try to talk and words won't come out. I get frustrated and feel like crying or just getting away from people. I get frustrated, then angry, but it's hard to get angry when you can't raise your voice."

◆ "I really freaked out and was put in the hospital for two weeks under sedation. After I came home it was several months before I had any interest in living. I even contemplated suicide, but I felt I couldn't do that to my family."

◆ "Lack of vocal confidence is a very emotional experience when you have talked normal all of your life and then your voice becomes less proficient; you tend to become depressed. The question 'Why?' is always present."

◆ "Certainly, any person who enjoys life and people would be depressed. It's hell not being able to communicate."

◆ "I have been depressed much of my life; always had suicidal tendencies; couldn't communicate with the world, and children especially."

◆ "Black moods. Hopelessness. Helplessness. Haplessness."

◆ "I feel like my life is being wasted and that I'm being a burden to my husband."

◆ "It's hard to put into words, but I feel shut away from the world."

◆ "My self-concept has become much more negative. I withdraw socially and become depressed when I think of how well I used to do things, like meet people and make friends. It also had an effect on my marriage. I feel it was the cause of our separation."

◆ "I began to feel very sorry for myself. I felt I was being punished for something I had done wrong in life. My marriage problems grew worse as I focused more on myself. I was very unsure of everything."

The preceding testimonies of the destructive life effects of adductor spasmodic dysphonia do not mean every patient who acquires this disorder is destined to suffer in this way. As stated earlier, this is not a homogenous disorder; many patients after a time learn to live with the disorder. They adopt a philosophic point of view, but usually these are not the more severe cases. These patients are often the more stable and self-sufficient ones who do not rely heavily on speech as a means of emotional expression or social satisfaction and who do not use speech as a primary means of earning a living.

Etiology

Adductor spasmodic dysphonia should not be regarded as a single disorder or disease entity but as a voice sign of any one of several different causes. These causes should be specified whenever possible and may be neurologic, psychogenic, or abnormal motor patterning. To specify cause, a thorough clinical study of each patient is necessary.

Psychogenic Adductor Spasmodic Dysphonia

Whether or not a sign or symptom is psychogenic is usually based on indirect, circumstantial, and impressionistic data. The credibility of evidence for psychogenicity as a primary cause of any disorder is proportional to the time devoted to the psychosocial interview; skill, wisdom, and judgment of the clinician; and the honesty, insight, and verbal ability of the patient. It is not difficult to find lives riddled with conflict, strife, disappointment, tragedy, insecurity, rage, hostility, suspiciousness, and other signs of emotional turmoil. It would be too simple, and erroneous, to assign a speech complaint to any change of job or to an argument with a spouse. However, when the following relationships can be demonstrated, a strong likelihood that a voice disorder is psychogenic must be considered:

1. The onset of the voice disorder and the stressful life event occur in reasonable proximity to one another.

2. Verbal communication is important to the patient in the conflict, however trivial it might appear to you.

3. During disclosure of delicate or confidential information to the clinician, the voice becomes appreciably improved or normal.

4. During trial symptomatic voice therapy, the voice improves appreciably or becomes normal.

5. When the conflict is moderated, or the patient takes a vacation, the voice improves considerably or becomes normal.

6. The patient reports multiple sensory complaints and somatizations.

7. Obvious psychiatric disturbances.

Because numbers 1, 3, 4, and 5 are common clinical features among neurologic dystonias (Brin, Fahn, Blitzer, et al, 1992), the clinician's diagnostic task is difficult. In fact, diagnosis of psychogenicity might not be possible until the clinician has begun trial therapy. Few people would argue against the diagnosis of psychogenic adductor spasmodic dysphonia if, during the course of the psychosocial interview or reduc-

tion of musculoskeletal tension, the voice returned to normal and remained that way for a reasonable duration. Organic, neurologic voice disorders do not fluctuate to such extremes or disappear completely though on a short-term basis non–psychogenic patients with spasmodic dysphonia may be able to modify their voices.

Adductor Spasmodic Dysphonia of Conversion Disorder
A review of the early literature indicates that the majority of clinicians perceived their patients to be psychoneurotic and thought their strained, groaning, effortful voices were directly caused by and were manifestations of such psychoneurosis. Specifically, the spastic voice was regarded as a conversion disorder (Bloch, 1965; Kiml, 1963). Contemporary experience sustains the validity of this initial etiologic conceptualization for some patients. The evidence, then and now, is based on the logical relationship between the dysphonia and certain life events surrounding its development and the ease and manner in which the dysphonia is alleviated during the verbalization of emotional conflict and by symptomatic voice therapy. A review of the theory of conversion disorder in Chapter 10 and references given there will remind the student of the strong and symbolic relationship between unresolved conflict and abnormal voice.

Spasmodic dysphonia can be a sign of conversion disorder no different from conversion aphonia or nonorganic dysphonia as of other voice descriptions. The spasmodic dysphonia serves to erect a barricade against the dangers of self-revelation. The squeezed, groaning, effortful voice communicates suppression of intense aggression and fear of verbal expression. Heaver (1959), one of a handful of psychiatrists, convincingly established the conversion type. The following study by Heaver, and other cases, can be found in Bloch (1965), and these should be read for their psychologic correlative evidence. The student should always ask in contemplating single-case and group research studies here and elsewhere, "What is the likelihood that these stories are reasonably, symbolically, and temporally related to the voice disorder? Or, to what extent are these life storms and the dysphonia merely coincidence?" The following is a synopsis of Heaver's classic case of conversion adductor spasmodic dysphonia.

Case Study 6.1

This is the case of a 56-year-old woman who is married to a pharmacist. She manifested envy for her husband's several academic degrees and was driven to engage in outside activities. Four years before admission, the patient gradually became completely aphonic. It was necessary for her daughter to learn lip reading. Her aphonia, the patient said, followed a series of "severe emotional shocks." Their son was in battle in the South Pacific, the husband for a time was thought to have throat cancer, she had a painful thrombophlebitis, and was concerned over her son's impending divorce. This last was connected very closely to her voice symptoms. When the divorce question arose she was no longer permitted to see her grandchildren. The son was doing poorly economically. Her daughter broke off two successive engagements.

The ear, nose, and throat examination showed a larynx of normal size with injected mucosa. The mobility of the congested cords appeared spastic and sphincter-like. During phonation, there was congestion of the external jugular veins. Vocal analysis revealed spastic respiration, low pitch, choked timbre, rigid inflection, hoarse quality, weak volume, a limited range, and spastic vocal attacks. It was noted that the singing voice was not affected. Diagnosis: typical spastic dysphonia with marked laryngeal sphincter action.

The initial Rorschach study revealed a personality structure characterized by much energy and strong self-will, a need to maintain control of others and to exert her influence on all about her. Marked childish narcissism was coupled with general negativism, aggression, and hostility. Strong self-doubts and concern over self-image of failing sexual attraction. In group therapy she sat apart, interrupted others with comments, and seemed to enjoy herself.

Minor degree of improvement occurred with voice therapy. She was not cooperative regarding the advice received during psychotherapy. Her voice ran into total spastic aphonia and even intermittent mutism. It was recommended that voice therapy be combined with dramatic and suggestive but non-probing psychotherapy. Gradually, her mutism returned to the previous spastic dysphonia. She expressed her underlying aggressive and hostile feelings toward her family, friends, and medical staff covertly disguised by facetious and joking attitudes. She maintained evasiveness and resistance to any effort, no matter how superficially leveled, to analyze her attitudes and voice problem. Her behavior is erratic and histrionic; her urge to dramatize her feelings is strong, as it is to attract attention. Whenever she neared discussion of emotionally charged personal material, she conjured some rationalization to discontinue her visits temporarily. Her most extended period of absence of spastic voice symptoms occurred during the second year of therapy with the second therapist. For almost three weeks, she spoke in her previous normal fashion. With her mother's death, her spastic syndrome rapidly returned. Since then, she is sometimes a little improved, sometimes notably worse, and on a few transitory occasions she was free of dysphonia.

Hostility, verging on rage, inability to verbalize aggression, and entrapment in life circumstances with no apparent means of escape, so common in the conversion reaction type of adductor spasmodic dysphonia, is further exemplified in the following case study of a 45-year-old woman who had been diagnosed as having adductor spasmodic dysphonia several years before this interview:

Case Study 6.2

Clinician: When did you first start having trouble with your voice?

Patient: Well, seven and a half years ago when I was pregnant with my little girl.

C: Had you ever had any such trouble before?

P: Yes. Nine years ago I had a little boy, he was seven months old, he is nine now, and I would just have flashes of something and . . . .

C: Similar to what you have now?

P: Yes, it was frightening whatever it was; I couldn't seem to control it. It only happened a few times and I went on a vacation and it came back.

C: Same kind of voice that you had seven and a half years ago?

P: Well, I can't really remember it.

C: But the present problem began in earnest seven and a half years ago.

P: Yes.

C: What did you notice first? Was it the same kind of voice that you have now, or was it something different?

P: Oh . . . well, I can't really remember it. It is just hard to speak. Sometimes shakiness. I had left my husband. I was living with my daughter who was going to college, and I've had a lot of trauma the last nine years.

C: Do you remember exactly or approximately when the voice trouble began? Was it while you were pregnant or after the birth of your child?

P: While I was pregnant, and then that summer all of a sudden I had gone back on the ranch and I couldn't speak at all, it didn't really happen suddenly but probably over a period of a week.

C: And has the voice trouble been present ever since?

P: More or less. Sometimes it does get better.

C: Has it ever disappeared completely?

P: No. Only three times when I drank way more than I should have. Usually drinking makes it worse.

C: Under what conditions will it be better?

P: Well, I can't really say.

C: Under what conditions will it be worse?

P: Well, when I'm under extreme stress, and talking about it makes it worse.

C: And what previous help have you sought for the problem?

P: First, seven and a half years ago, I went to a throat specialist twice. The first time he gave me cortisone and I went home and took it faithfully, and then after two days I couldn't talk at all. My husband had to call him back, so I went back and he gave me Valium, and that is the last time I ever saw him.

C: So, except for a brief episode or two about nine years ago, the voice trouble really started about seven years ago.

P: Yes.

C: Now, was that period in your life a significant change over the way it was before that time?

P: Well, I guess, because I have a troubled marriage, that got worse. It has never gotten better. I had left my husband and after my baby was born I had gone back. It was just a real bad time.

C: At the present time what would you consider the major problem in your life?

P: My marriage.

C: Would you describe that in as much detail as you can?

P: Well, it's bad. I don't see any way out, because I have these two perfectly delightful children who are happy and secure and they have a wonderful home in a small town. Their life is just ideal, and I just can't ruin it for them.

C: Why do you say that there is no way out?

P: Well, I've been married for 30 years, and now I was thinking about it last night, for the last year I think I've just had a few emotions. My love for my children and then all the rest of them are just completely negative. All hate, which I know is the worst thing that you can . . . it is very devastating.

C: What do you mean hate?

P: Well, I just don't like my husband.

C: Why not?

P: Oh, it has gone on for so long. When I was 18 I thought he was great; he is seven years older than I am, and I just kind of married him out of, just for security. I was kind of the first hippie, or I feel like I was, and I thought he was nice, but now I've grown up and I know what he is like, and I'm sure, well, we just both tried to destroy each other. I feel as though he has tried to destroy me, and I feel like I've given him way, way more, but he is very, very unyielding and completely unable to . . . I work very, very hard and have tried to suppress all kinds of emotions or feelings. The only time I really let go is in a screaming fight.

C: How is your voice during those fights?

P: Well, it comes out pretty good. That's why he says "there is nothing wrong with your voice now." Of course, it is still very forced, but sometimes I feel like my voice is a substitute for crying, because I have quit crying. I decided a long time ago that that is really useless to do. Sometimes I think it was good for me to cry, and now I can't. I had breast cancer a year ago last February and had a mastectomy, and my husband knew that I had a lump for four to six weeks. When I discovered it I knew immediately that it was bad, and I called him into the bathroom and he said, "Oh I knew you had that four to six weeks ago, and I said 'why didn't you tell me.' " And he had come up behind me and grabbed me which makes me want to kill, and I guess I elbowed him or he said, "Oh, you're so mean" or something, and now I'm really very bitter about that. I keep telling him that I can't forgive him for it, but he is the kind of person that he can't even yield enough to say, well I did make a mistake, or I don't know why I did that. He can't even do that. He just says, "Well, if you're so stupid that you can't find your own lump" more or less to that effect. Oh this is so painful.

C: It was four weeks before.

P: He said four to six weeks.

C: So when was that?

P: Well, I had my mastectomy a year ago, last February.

C: So that certainly didn't improve the situation.

P: No. Not my marital situation. I don't think it affected my voice any.

C: But it reinforced your feelings toward your husband.

P: I don't understand. I do understand him in a way, because I know the rest of his family.

C: But the marriage was in trouble before your voice trouble started, wasn't it?

P: Yes.

C: And yet you had no trouble with your voice seven years ago.

P: No. I love to talk. I used to, but, of course, now I don't.

C: Well, what do you see for yourself in the future?

P: Well, about the only solution, he says that he will go to a marriage counselor. He is such a contradictor. He has gotten totally dependent on me. He annoys me because he thinks he has to talk about everything. It's like someone thinking aloud. He just talks me to death telling me what he is going to do. If he is going to go up the hill and feed the horse he has to tell me. He feels threatened, I know, about all kinds of things.

C: Like what?

P: Well, I know that he thinks that I am independent and strong, and I'm sure that he feels threatened by that, and when I do things on my own I know that he feels threatened by that. He is terribly jealous. Terribly, and we don't like the same people, or he doesn't fit in with the people that I like. Of course, in the town I live in I don't have . . . I like where I live. I love my home, and it would be very hard to leave, but I don't really have any close friends that I relate to. I have the kind of friends that I have to use poor grammar around every once in a while, or they would think that I'm, you know, trying to be something else. I hate to say it without sounding snobbish, because I really am fond of the people that are good to me, but sometimes I'd like to go to the university and take a course in creative writing and an art course. I do a lot of painting, I do some rosemaling, and I feel deprived in that way. I really don't feel like a martyr for my children, because they are the most important thing that I have.

C: So you have said, then, that your husband has felt jealous and threatened and at the same time you'd like to go back to school and take some courses.

P: You asked me what I saw ahead. I told you what I'd like to see. This is what I do see ahead. He did say that he would see a marriage counselor. I don't know what they are like, but I know we have to work something out; we have to. We just can't go on like we have this summer. But last summer he changed. I think possibly he could have been having affairs, but that doesn't bother me all that much really, but it has been bothering me that he seems to be regressing. I feel as though he is growing old without ever growing up. He doesn't have any interests; he is not doing anything in particular. He just likes to hang around the house.

C: Is that threatening to you?

P: Well, it annoys me, because he doesn't have any, you know, I think he should have interests. The people in his family have an idea that the older you get the easier you should take it. You know, you should just sort of roll into a steady decline. And my life isn't going to be long enough for me to do all the things I want to do, and I just can't stand people like that. And he doesn't like it; he hates my reading; he doesn't like books. He is very scornful of people . . . and he never reads. He does better than he did when I first married him, because he only read comic books then. I should have realized then that a 25-year-old man that read comic books was a little bit . . . But he is intelligent.

C: Why do you say that you are not going to live long enough?

P: Well, I mean I have so many things I want to do. I don't have any idea that I'm not going to last very long, because I promised my kids that I'll live forever. No, I don't want you to think I'm making a death wish or anything. No.

C: So you and he think something needs to be done?

P: It has to be. We can't go on this way, because finally I've given up keeping a pretense by trying to move out of his bedroom. Up until a month ago I still tried to be pleasant by talking to him as much as I could, but finally he wanted to drag me to an alumni thing at his old high school, and I just couldn't face it, especially not with my voice being bad. People I don't care for and I just couldn't face it. And we had just had a disastrous trip.

C: Disastrous?

P: Well, it was just disastrous. We hated it. I hated him. We went to see my daughter, and she was having difficulties with her husband. Her husband is quite a bit older than she is, and he is the very same kind of person. They both have the very same ideas about what a woman or a wife should be and do, and what a man should be and do, and how it should be, and the two of them were buddy-buddy. So when he wanted me to go on this trip, I knew everything was going to hit the fan, and I knew it wasn't very smart of me, but I'm so tired of pretending. I just said I made up my mind when I got back that I'm not even going to ride in town with him let alone go on a weekend trip. And of course, you can guess what all that led to.

C: What?

P: Well, just terrible, terrible things that I said to him and he said to me. But we don't fight in front of the kids. No one but my closest friends know that I'm anything but Miss Mary Sunshine. My voice. This is the worst it has been, just talking about these things. It is very difficult, but usually when I go into town and buy groceries and take the kids to the swimming pool I can get by, but my whole life is a pretense except when I'm with my kids.

C: Again, your whole life is a pretense.

P: Well, I mean because I am keeping up a front, you know, you don't go around telling everybody you're not happy.

C: Have you been getting unhappier as the years have gone by?

P: Yes, well, we've hit a new low.

C: Why?

P: Because we're fighting.

C: You are fighting more this summer than ever before you think?

P: Yes.

C: Why do you think that is so?

P: Well, because I finally just told him I, well, something has happened to me, because I was always able to try and come around and say, Oh he's not such a bad guy, and I guess I'll be able to stick it out till, you know . . . .

C: Could you summarize for me what it is about him that you find so objectionable?

P: I feel that he is unyielding and he is a chauvinist. He just can't accept letting me just be.

C: What is the nature of this relationship that makes you feel as antagonistic toward him as you do? What is there about him?

C: He has a cruel streak. Very cruel.

P: What do you mean?

C: Oh, things that he says to me. Of course, I say cruel things to him, too. But I think he hits deeper than I do, I don't know. I hated my father. I just completely disassociated myself from my mother and sisters. Oh I didn't want to get into that. I don't know . . . Oh, I said I hated my father. Well he reminds me of my father.

C: Your husband has many of your father's traits?

P: Yes, in fact most of them I think. But he certainly would have been a complete opposite as far as I can see when I married him.

C: You didn't see that other side to him?

P: No. I didn't deliberately choose someone who was like my father.

C: What has the sexual part of the marriage been like for the past seven years?

P: Oh, pretty fair. Of course, there hasn't been any sex for the past probably four months. And for me I don't want him to touch me, ever.

C: Up until that time you were having a normal sexual relationship?

P: I would say that it has never been enough for him, which turns me off.

C: But, for the past four months there has been no sexual activity at all.

P: No.

C: What caused that?

P: Well, I don't know. I just plain moved out of the bedroom.

C: Why did you do that?

P: Because . . . he just repels me.

C: Why now?

P: Well, I don't like him. If you don't respect . . . you certainly have to like someone you have sex with and I don't like him.

C: Have you told him that?

P: Well, I think it is obvious to him that I don't like him.

C: What was his reaction to this move on your part?

P: Well, his idea of a confession is to, after we've had a big fight, never to admit anything but to come up and say "Can I mix you one?" "Can I get you a cup of coffee?" And that is supposed to be his wanting to make up. Everything is just supposed to be forgotten. He has made these overtures to me wanting to just forget the whole thing, and he hasn't said a word about my moving out of the bedroom. We don't even talk about sex any more. It used to be a big hassle but there, it's just, I can't give you any answers without talking for an hour on each thing. I can hardly do it. [Pause]

C: We are not completely sure that this voice disorder is caused by marital problems, but I think in this case there is a good chance that it is.

P: Except that there have been times when I've been extremely happy, at least thought I was, and relaxed and it has still been bad.

C: At any rate, before saying it is or it isn't, I think we are going to need a psychiatric opinion about this. I have a colleague in psychiatry who has been seeing patients of mine who have voice disorders for several years. And I would like him to see you if that is all right with you.

P: Yes.

C: Even if you had no voice problem, it would still be definitely indicated for you to see somebody, as I'm sure you have already concluded that yourself.

P: I know.

C: "Something has got to be done"; those are your words and there is no time like the present, in my opinion. What is yours?

P: The same. That's why I'm here. Oh, something else. Did I mention the fact that I'm sure that he has never wanted me to have, to do anything about my voice? I'm sure of that.

C: What makes you say that?

P: Well, because he has never encouraged me to, or never said, "Why don't we . . . ," he says he loves me but he has never said "Why don't we take you somewhere and see what we can do?" I had a few sessions with a speech pathologist last summer, and it kind of helped because just, temporarily, I was enjoying the idea that I was doing something about it, but he never asked me a question about it. Or he didn't say "You're better," or "How are you doing?" or "What are they doing with you?" or anything. Not one word. And when I wanted to come here my husband informed me that he wasn't going to pay for any trip. So I borrowed the money to come here.

In a study of the possible psychiatric background in patients with adductor spasmodic dysphonia, Aronson, Brown, Litin, et al. (1968a) submitted 29 of 34 patients to psychiatric interviews averaging 2 hours in duration. In 18 (62%), the psychiatrists judged the histories and personality characteristics to be indicative of psychoneurosis; 5 had significant psychiatric problems and 13 presented with equivocal psychiatric findings. Eleven patients were psychiatrically normal.

As a group, the 62% who had emotional problems of varying degrees—regardless of whether or not these problems can be considered causally related to spastic dysphonia—possessed the following traits: (1) They were compulsive and perfectionistic, not very tolerant of error in others or themselves, and had to do things "right." (2) They had a tendency to suppress their anger resulting from their relationships with other people. (3) They had lifelong tendencies toward verbal repression rather than free expression of ideas. (Not all patients had all three traits.) The psychiatrists agreed that:

Generally, these patients were rigid, conscientious people who took their responsibilities very seriously. They tended to be worriers and perfectionistic. In addition, and common to many psychiatric conditions, their means of dealing with their feelings of anger, resentment, and irritation were faulty and inefficient; instead of expressing their angry feelings in a socially acceptable way, they usually would choose to keep their anger to themselves. With disconcerting frequency, these patients described themselves as "the quiet ones" in their families, from childhood on. One or both parents or a sibling was often the dominant one as far as verbal expression was concerned and these patients had little opportunity or need to participate verbally (Aronson, Brown, Litin, et al., 1968a, p. 215).

A review of the Aronson, Brown, Litin, et al. (1968a) study shows reasonable psychogenic certainty in 5 of the 29 patients who had undergone psychiatric examination. However, 13 produced equivocal information and 11 were thought to be free of any evidence of psychiatric disorder. Only in retrospect do these discrepancies become explainable. The study had been done when its authors were just beginning to become aware of neurologic etiology. To be noted is that 71% of the patients in the study had voice tremor. Probably the authors had reported on the psychologic results of a heterogeneous group of adductor spasmodic dysphonic patients whom they had regarded as homogeneous. The neurologic patients, in other words, were mixed in with the psychogenic types.

Brodnitz (1976) describes 53 of his spastic dysphonia patients who volunteered, under careful probing during the initial interview, what they considered to be the events that triggered the development of their disorders. Examples are death of a near relative, 13 cases (five from laryngeal cancer); severe automobile accident without personal injury, eight cases; climactic marital crisis, eight cases (one starting suddenly in a divorce court after verbal abuse by the opposing attorney); laryngeal surgery for removal of benign lesions, five cases. One woman became dysphonic after her husband threatened to kill her, another after her husband was murdered, a third after her brother was shot to death in a holdup, a fourth after observing her child's first seizure.

Case Study 6.3

A young psychiatrist was told that his training in analysis was complete. A few weeks after his cutting of the analytical umbilical cord, he developed spastic dysphonia. He discussed it with his analyst who agreed to take him back for three more months. Immediately his voice became normal only to revert to the dysphonia when the analyst told him at the end of these three months that he should now be able to stand on his own two feet (Brodnitz, 1976, pp. 212–213).

Aside from these 53 patients who could pinpoint the onset of the disorder, there were 28 who exhibited many of the characteristics of severe neuroses. Eight of them had already had long periods of psychiatric treatment before they developed spastic dysphonia. This leaves only about one third of the cases reported in this paper where no obvious psychogenic background could be found. This is not an unusual situation in psychosomatic disorders, particularly in manifestations of conversion hysteria. In a summary of 562 spasmodic dysphonia patients seen at a neurological institute, Brin, Fahn, Blitzer, and Ramig (1992) report that only 17%, or 98 patients, had a secondary dystonia of some type, but they do not specify what fraction of the 17% is psychogenic. (They consider psychogenic dystonia a form of secondary dystonia because the phenomenology is dystonic and the etiology is psychiatric.) Brin and his colleagues do, however, state "We suspect that psychogenic spasmodic dysphonia is very rare, and indeed have never seen a confirmed case. . . . we suspect that we have not seen these patients because they are treated by speech language pathologists and are not referred for evaluation". "Of course, everybody who has had frequent contact with cases of spastic dysphonia has entertained the suspicion that an organic neurologic factor may be the etiological basis of the more severe forms of the disorder. Possibly, future research with more refined methods may demonstrate such a connection in some cases" (Brodnitz, 1976, p. 213). Indeed, during the past two decades, numerous histologic, neurophysiologic, magnetic resonance imaging (MRI), functional magnetic resonance imaging (fMRI), and positron emission tomography (PET) studies have been completed in an attempt to determine the neurologic locus of spasmodic dysphonia. Thus far, they have failed to locate consistent abnormalities within laryngeal nerves (Carlson, Izdebski, Dahlqvist, et al., 1987; Ravits, Aronson, Desanto, et al., 1979) or any particular brain structure or region (Aronson and Lagerlund, 1991; Devous, Pool, and, Finitzo, 1990). In their scholarly review of historical approaches to the treatment of adductor spasmodic dysphonia (ADSD), Pearson and Sapienza (2003) state that whereas ADSD is a voice disorder of uncertain origin, the origin is likely to be neurogenic and that current theory views ADSD as a problem of motor circuitry rather than a byproduct of damage to any one cortical or subcortical area.

Adductor Spasmodic Dysphonia of Musculoskeletal Tension Reaction Some patients develop the *voice* of adductor spasmodic dysphonia on the basis of a relatively simple muscle tension reaction also called vocal hyperfunction. Although these dysphonias are technically psychogenic, caused by heightened anxiety, tension, or depression, they are not the more serious conversion disorder types.

Increased musculoskeletal tension as a cause of the voice symptoms of adductor spasmodic dysphonia has been called the tension-fatigue syndrome, the components of which are hoarseness, often of the strained variety, vocal fatigue, poor respiratory support, and pain on phonation. The dysphonia of musculoskeletal tension or the tension-fatigue syndrome can have all of the earmarks of adductor spasmodic dysphonia. This category of voice disorder is highly amenable to symptomatic voice therapy (Koufman and Blalock, 1988; Roy, Ford, and Bless, 1996).

Neurologic Adductor Spasmodic Dysphonia

This section endeavors to demonstrate that strained, staccato, effortful voices within the perceptual definition of adductor spasmodic dysphonia can be caused by, and are often signs of, two major categories of neurologic disease or syndromes and their subsidiaries:

1. Organic (essential) tremor

2. Dystonia

   a. Meige's syndrome

   b. Spasmodic torticollis

   c. Mixed dystonia-tremor

The following preliminary points about these syndromes should be noted:

♦ The dysphonia perceived during contextual speech is *superficially* indistinguishable from the psychogenic forms. Unless neurologic signs in addition to the dysphonia are present, and often either they are not or they are so subtle as to go unnoticed, it is almost impossible to tell the neurologic from the psychogenic forms.

♦ The above syndromes are established organic disorders recognized by academic and clinical neurologists. Additionally, there are recognized nonlaryngeal focal dystonias that include blepharospasm, oral mandibular dystonia, and writer's cramp, which similar to spasmodic dysphonia are uncontrolled and abnormal muscle contractions (Ludlow, 2000).

♦ They are caused by a lesion or lesions within the extrapyramidal system.

♦ The motor signs of these syndromes do not express themselves identically in all patients, who differ from one another according to how much of the body is involved, the range extending from a single muscle group to the entire body; the onset of the disease, which may begin in one organ or structure and spread to others, or, the disease may remain confined to a single organ; severity, which may range from threshold to severe levels; if the disease affects the respiratory, phonatory, resonatory, and articulatory musculature, in which case the result is a hyperkinetic dysarthria of which strained, effortful, or staccato voice is but one component; and the site of the disease. When the disease expresses itself solely or predominately in the larynx, the shift of perceptual attention to the voice induces the clinician also to shift the terminology to spasmodic dysphonia. Technically, then, the adductor dysphonia of these neurologic syndromes are dysarthrias or components thereof.

♦ The unusualness and often bizarreness of the movements in these syndromes routinely lead less experienced clinicians of all specialties to diagnose them incorrectly as psychogenic and to rationalize the unusual movements, for example, tic-like contractions, facial grimaces, and blepharospasm (squinting and frequent eye blinking), as secondary psychogenic struggle reactions when, in fact, they are signs of the disease.

♦ Confusing and misleading to clinicians unless they have been forewarned is that neurologic movement disorders are often forced into the open for the first time by acute emotional trauma or chronic stress and, once in evidence, usually worsen with the pressures of daily life or fatigue and improve when the patient is relaxed. Emotional stress as the trigger of organic disease, well known in general illness, is common throughout the histories of patients who develop many different kinds of neurologic diseases. The idea that sudden shock or protracted aggravation can produce irreversible structural or neurochemical changes in the nervous system may tax credibility, but experienced neurologists who have witnessed this correlation unreservedly support this concept.

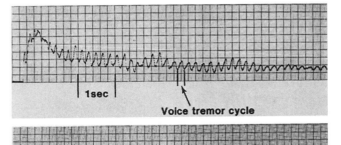

Figure 6.4 Oscillographic tracings comparing organic voice tremor without voice arrest and with voice arrests during vowel prolongation. (**A**) Organic voice tremor without voice arrests. (**B**) Adductor spasmodic dysphonia of organic voice tremor. Note the rhythmic voice arrests. (From Aronson, A.E., Hartman, D.E. [1981]. Adductor spasmodic dysphonia as a sign of essential [voice] tremor. J Speech Hear Disord 46, 52–58.)

Adductor Spasmodic Dysphonia of Organic (Essential) Voice Tremor   Noted in Chapter 9 are several important points. (1) The quavering voice called organic or essential voice tremor is often a component of the essential tremor syndrome. (2) The voice tremor can involve the larynx only. (3) The rate of the voice tremor ranges from 5 to 12 Hz. (4) Onset can be sudden or gradual. (5) The voice tremor can be best demonstrated during vowel prolongation. (6) The perceived tremor is produced by alternating adduction and abduction of the true and, often, false vocal folds, which may be synchronous with vertical oscillations of the larynx. (7) The perceived tremor may result from involuntary rhythmic movements of the intrinsic or extrinsic laryngeal muscles or pharynx. (8) The voice tremor can be smooth (**Fig. 6.4A**) or it can be interrupted by hoarse voice arrests. (9) When organic voice tremor becomes sufficiently severe, the range or amplitude of the vocal fold adduction is so extensive that they momentarily meet in the midline and seal the glottis, producing a strained or staccato voice arrest. Repeated voice arrests cause the voice to lose its qualities of tremor and take on those of adductor spasmodic dysphonia (**Fig. 6.4B**). (10) Clinically, adductor spasmodic dysphonia of organic tremor can be confirmed by rhythmic, semirhythmic, or irregular voice arrests during vowel /a/ prolongations that may or may not be separated by several cycles of voice tremor[1] or by associated tremor of the head, lips, mandible, tongue, velum, pharynx, and thorax during phonation and of the upper extremities. The differential diagnosis between spasmodic dysphonia due to essential tremor versus that due to a dystonic tremor can be difficult (Brin, et al., 1992).

The evidence linking adductor spasmodic dysphonia to essential tremor follows.

♦ Spastic dysphonia in two patients with heredofamilial tremor was reported by Critchley (1939, et al., 1949).

---

[1]In very severe cases, the compensatory spasms may be sufficiently intense to produce a continuously strained voice rather than tremor on vowel prolongation. Raising the pitch level may enable voice tremor to break through when produced on an extended vowel. However, these corroborative signs may be absent or so mild as to go unnoticed by all except those trained to recognize them.

♦ In a neurologic study of 10 spastic dysphonia patients, all 10 had scattered neurologic signs. One of the patients had heredofamilial tremor involving the head and both upper extremities (Robe, Brumlik, and Moore, 1960).

♦ A neurologic and psychiatric study of 31 patients disclosed regular voice tremor during vowel prolongation in 71% of patients. Six patients had accompanying head or hand tremor (Aronson, Brown, Litin, et al., 1968b).

♦ A videofluoroscopic study of three patients showed intermittent voice stoppages associated with complete glottic and supraglottic closure and tremor of the larynx, hypopharynx, and tongue during quiet respiration and contextual speech and were consistent with the patients' tremulous voice quality. Tremor amplitude increased markedly during intermittent voice stoppages (McCall, Skolnick, and Brewer, 1971).

♦ In a study of 21 patients with voice tremor, 10 were described as having spasmodic dysphonia. In three there was a family history of tremor. Vowel prolongations showed irregular intervals of complete voice arrest at around 6 Hz (Dordain and Dordain, 1972).

♦ In 12 patients, tremulous, quavering phonation was found in at least three and postural tremor in three. In one case, tremor elsewhere in the body appeared 5 years after onset; in another, 1 year after onset. In one patient, tremor had appeared 20 years before onset of the voice disorder (Aminoff, Dedo, and Izdebski, 1978).

♦ A study compared three groups of patients, one consisting of 14 essential tremor patients without voice arrest, a second of 16 essential tremor patients with occasional voice arrests, and a third of 22 patients suspected as having the tremor type of adductor spasmodic dysphonia. On vowel prolongation, median voice tremor frequencies of 5.7, 5.0, and 5.5 Hz. were found in the three groups, respectively. The differences were statistically insignificant. Tremors in other parts of the body were found in 93% of the first group, 81% of the second group, and 50% of the third group (Aronson and Hartman, 1981).

Though difficult, it is important to try to differentiate the regular tremor seen in benign essential voice tremor from the irregular dystonic tremors. Based on electromyographic recordings, Blitzer (1985) noted that 25% of his laryngeal focal dystonic, or spastic dysphonic, patients had irregular tremors. Unfortunately, when patients present with symptoms of essential tremor in other parts of their bodies, the clinical distinction cannot always be made (Aronson, Brin, and Ludlow cited in Brin, et al., 1992).

Emotional Stress as a Precipitant of Adductor Spasmodic Dysphonia of Organic (Essential) Voice Tremor   One would hope for the sake of simplicity that all psychogenic adductor spasmodic dysphonias showed a history of acute or chronic emotional stress and that absence of such a history would characterize the neurologic types. Regrettably, and remarkably, such is not the case, for convincing evidence from several different sources shows that both essential voice tremor and the adductor spasms of essential tremor frequently follow emotional stress. That stress can produce permanent neurologic change is based on indirect data correlating life history with onset of the neurologic disorder. However, the time and circumstantial relationship is so close in single-case and group studies as to be highly convincing. As noted elsewhere, the concept that stress can precipitate incipient neurologic disease or be a primary cause of it is accepted doctrine in medicine and is not considered to be particularly unusual. Examples of case studies reported in the literature that seem to support this notion follow:

♦ A 72-year-old woman with a 20-year history of face and hand tremor developed voice tremor shortly after the death of her husband (Ardran, Kinsbourne, and Rushworth, 1966).

♦ In three patients who had the tremor type of spasmodic dysphonia, the voice and associated tremors occurred after emotional shock several days after the traumatic event (Dordain and Dordain, 1972).

♦ Emotional stress was associated with onset in two groups of essential voice tremor patients, 29% and 25%, and in 41% of adductor spasmodic dysphonias of essential tremor (Aronson and Hartman, 1981).

The kinds of stress that precipitate adductor spasmodic dysphonia of organic voice tremor are not qualitatively different from those responsible for the psychogenic type. Death of a relative and violation of mores within the family are common themes responsible for both the psychogenic and neurologic types. However, many more neurologic than psychogenic patients give histories free of such stresses and appear to have well-adjusted personalities.

Adductor Spasmodic Dysphonia of Dystonia   Evidence strongly supports the concept that adductor spasmodic dysphonia can also be a laryngeal sign of dystonia. As noted in Chapter 9, the larynx can be involved in the hyperkinetic dysarthrias of which dystonia is one type. *Dystonia* is a general term referring to a group of isolated neurologic signs or complete syndromes. Potentially confusing are several synonyms used to describe these signs: Meige's syndrome, Brueghel's syndrome, orofacial dyskinesia, and focal dystonia. Spasmodic torticollis, athetosis, and writer's cramp also fall within the purview of the dystonias. Spasmodic torticollis as a specific type of dystonia can coexist with dyskinetic facial and lingual movements and even tremor.

Dystonia refers to patients who have relatively slow, adventitious, uncontrolled, nonrhythmic contractions of the lips, mandibular muscles, tongue, velopharyngeal muscles, larynx, thorax, or extremities. Dystonias are caused by lesions of the extrapyramidal system. The contraction of different muscle groups can occur in any combination. Often they are confined to one region of the body, such as to the head and neck musculature. They can even involve a single muscle group, especially in the early stages of the disorder if it is progressive; in many patients it is static. Laryngeal dystonias are characterized as abnormal involuntary movements that are typically action-induced by the act of speaking. Because the resultant dystonic movements are unusual and rare, dystonias are one of the most frequently misdiagnosed neurologic conditions (Nutt, Muenter, Aronson, et al, 1988) including those emanating from the larynx.

The evidence will show that adductor spasmodic dysphonia can be an example of a dystonia isolated to the larynx (i.e., a focal laryngeal dystonia) or it can be one component of a more generalized dystonia. As mentioned in the previous section on spasmodic dysphonia of organic voice tremor, when dystonia is focal to the larynx, the tendency is to describe the effect as spasmodic dysphonia. When additional speech muscles are affected, the tendency is to call the entire speech disorder hyperkinetic dysarthria.

Meige's Syndrome   Meige's syndrome, originally called medial facial spasm, is a type of dystonia that consists of symmetric dystonic spasms of the facial muscles, which may first involve the eyes, producing blepharospasm, and later the remainder of the facial muscles, producing lip retraction and uncontrolled jaw opening and closing. Day-to-day fluctuations are typical, aggravated by stress, improved by sedation, and disappearing during sleep. A similar syndrome is called Brueghel's syndrome or blepharospasm-oromandibular dystonia syndrome (Tolosa and Klawans, 1979).

Jacome and Yanez (1980) described a 49-year-old man who had typical spasmodic dysphonia for 3 years that began with blepharospasm, symmetric facial spasms, and mild jaw retraction. Symptoms improved with rest and were worse under stress. He could talk and sing normally at times. "We believe this patient has a combination of Meige's disease and spastic dysphonia,[2] with blepharospasm and medial facial spasms as described by Meige, as well as typical spastic dysphonia." Marsden and Sheehy (1982) found that the most common speech difficulty of patients with the dystonic spasms of Meige's syndrome was "having to force air through a tight throat and mouth resulting in a strained,

---

[2]They might have rephrased their statement to say Meige's disease, of which spasmodic dysphonia was a sign or component, for that is probably what they had intended.

monotonous, slurring speech, which resembled closely the classical description of spastic dysphonia. . . . Since spastic dysphonia may occur in the same syndrome, *it is quite likely that isolated spastic dysphonia itself may be a sole focal manifestation of dystonia* [emphasis mine]. Indeed, we have encountered a small number of patients with speech disturbance indistinguishable from that seen in Meige Syndrome, patients who would be classified as cases of spasmodic dysphonia but which we believe to be examples of isolated focal laryngeal dystonia."

Jankovic and Ford (1983) studied 100 patients with signs of dystonia. Twenty-one were found to have spastic dysphonia. In 15, the dysphonia was accompanied by blepharospasm, orofacial movements, and tremor. In six patients, spastic dysphonia was the only sign. In view of the previous discussion of emotional stress as a precipitating, not a causal, factor in essential tremor and the spasmodic dysphonia of essential tremor, it is important to note that the dystonic patients in this study yielded similar psychiatric signs: "Although we found no evidence to support hysterical origin of the facial movements, many patients had psychiatric problems which were preceded, followed by, or associated with the movement disorder. These include marked depressions (one-quarter of the patients), anxiety, obsessive-compulsive personality, schizoid personality, space phobia, and a variety of other psychological abnormalities."

In a study of 10 patients with Meige's syndrome during neurologic examination, Golper, Nutt, Rau, et al., (1983) documented laryngospasm in five of the patients studied. One was described as having an alternating strained/strangled voice quality and voice stoppages; a second voice stoppage on vowel prolongations; a third voice stoppage and phonation on inhalation; a fourth strained/ strangled voice; and a fifth, a question of voice tremor.

In 1875, Schnitzler (Kiml, 1963) described two patients with spastic dysphonia who had dystonic movements of the arms and legs.

In three of 12 spastic dysphonic patients studied by Aminoff, Dedo, and Izdebski (1978), one had torsion dystonia, a second had buccolingual dyskinesia, and a third had blepharospasm. The authors stated:

> *Our own findings would certainly suggest that spasmodic dysphonia should be regarded as a focal dystonia of the laryngeal musculature. . . . The high incidence of tremor among our patients with spasmodic dysphonia accords with the high incidence reported in patients with torsion dystonia . . . or related movement disorders such as spasmodic torticollis.*

Spasmodic Torticollis   Spasmodic torticollis, also once thought to be a psychiatric disorder, is now regarded by most neurologists as a dystonia caused by a lesion within the extrapyramidal system. People who acquire this disease experience an uncontrollable pulling, twisting, or tilting of the head to one side. Variations may be a retrocollis in which there is an extension of the head backward, or a procollis, in which there is flexion of the head forward. The disease often shows signs of dystonic facial movements, blepharospasm, and

dysarthria, including voice tremor. But, in addition to these classic signs, adductor laryngospasms may precede, follow, or parallel the development of spasmodic torticollis. Since Critchley's (1939) early report of a patient with spastic dysphonia who had spasmodic torticollis, the association between the dysphonia and this disease has been observed by many clinicians, particularly when the illness is in its full-blown stage. The association between torticollis, dystonia of other types, and tremor indicates the more than casual interrelationship among these various extrapyramidal syndromes. Schaefer (1983) also recognized the close connection between adductor spasmodic dysphonia and spasmodic torticollis because of the frequent occurrence of both diseases in the same patient, the association of tremor in both diseases, and the similarities in the historical controversy as to whether spasmodic torticollis was psychogenic or neurologic. Once considered to be psychogenic, few would argue against the fact that spasmodic torticollis is now well accepted as neurologic.

Looking back, what has been emerging is a picture of one form of adductor spasmodic dysphonia as a solitary or coexisting sign of any one of several extrapyramidal movement disorders. These, it should be emphasized, are syndromes of the central nervous system. During a brief period in the search for neurologic etiology, the notion was advanced that the voice disorder could arise from a peripheral nervous system lesion, specifically of the tenth cranial nerve, and was of viral origin (Bocchino and Tucker, 1978; Dedo, Izdebski, and Townsend, 1977). These clinicians based their hypotheses on the finding of what they thought were demyelinated nerve fibers in specimens taken from adductor spasmodic dysphonic patients during nerve resection. However, Ravits, Aronson, Desanto, et al. (1979) were unable to find any evidence of differences between the nerve fibers in spasmodic dysphonic and normal subjects. On other grounds, it is unlikely that such a peripheral nerve lesion could produce massive spasticity; flaccidity is usually the result of such lesions. The hypothesis also could not account for periods of normal voice in many spasmodic dysphonic patients.

Idiopathic Adductor Spasmodic Dysphonia

The term *idiopathic adductor spasmodic dysphonia* is reserved for patients in whom no convincing evidence of psychogenic or neurologic etiology can be found. Some clinicians have a tendency to infer etiology without adequate proof, interpreting the patient's dysphonia according to their own biases. To do so is not in the best interest of the patient or conducive to scientific thought. Loose diagnostic formulations given to the patient are usually taken to heart and can adversely influence the patient's self-concept.

The category of idiopathic adductor spasmodic dysphonia is not diagnostic but a means of placing the diagnosis in suspense until further data have been acquired to show a definite etiology. If the patient is suitably followed over a long period of time, a psychogenic or neurologic etiology often will reveal itself, permitting a change of classification. One example is that of a 34-year-old attorney who was referred by an otolaryngologist who cited adductor spasmodic dysphonia as the only complaint. The psychiatric history and neurologic examinations failed to disclose any evidence of cause from either discipline. Three years later, on the patient's return to the clinic, dystonic leg movements and procollis were found on neurologic examination, in addition to a worsening of his dysphonia.

Summary of Adductor Spasmodic Dysphonia

- Adductor spasmodic dysphonia is characterized by a strained, groaning, effortful, staccato voice varying in qualities of these components among different patients and also in severity.

- The strained, effortful voice is the product of hyperadduction of the true, and often false, vocal folds and accompanied by excessive extrinsic laryngeal muscle action that usually elevates the body of the larynx in synchrony with the spasms.

- The psychogenic causes of adductor spasmodic dysphonia are conversion disorder or musculoskeletal tension.

- The neurologic causes are organic (essential) tremor, orofacial dyskinesia, focal dystonia or dystonia (Meige's syndrome), and spasmodic torticollis. These extrapyramidal diseases can occur singly or in combination. Their spasmodic dysphonias can occur in isolation in the beginning, and as the disease progresses, other signs will appear. Often, the dysphonia may be the only sign or the predominant one.

- It is advocated, therefore, that the type of adductor spasmodic dysphonia be designated in any ultimate diagnostic categorization (e.g., adductor spasmodic dysphonia of essential tremor, adductor spasmodic dysphonia of dystonia). If no specific cause can be found, the term *idiopathic adductor spasmodic dysphonia* should be employed.

- In most cases, adductor spasmodic dysphonia, regardless of etiology, begins gradually in the middle years, somewhere between 40 and 50 years, although studies have shown onset in childhood. The ratio of males to females ranges from 1:1 to 1:4, depending upon studies consulted.

- For both psychogenic and neurologic types, a high percentage of patients experience onset as associated with emotional stress, causal in the former type and as a triggering of the neurologic disease in the latter.

- Regardless of cause, the disorder usually produces serious occupational, social, and emotional disturbances.

Treatment of Adductor Spasmodic Dysphonia

Any consideration of therapy for adductor spasmodic dysphonia must account for the following realities: (1) Not one, but several, different types of the disorder exist. Therefore, no single therapy can be recommended for all types. Moreover, for any single type, there may be multiple treatments or combination of treatments recommended. (2) It is notorious for its fluctuations in severity in response to mood and environment. Therefore, valid, reliable assessment of the effectiveness of therapy cannot be made on the basis of office sampling alone but needs to be based on a cross section of communicative experiences. (3) Clinicians differ among themselves in their criteria for improvement, because the results of therapy are more often partial than complete. (4) Clinicians differ from patients in their criteria for improvement owing not only to differences in their expectations but also because improvement in the amount of physical effort required to phonate can only be evaluated by the patient and cannot be judged by an observer. (5) Studies of the effectiveness of therapy are difficult to compare owing to different methodologies, for example, decision as to what constitutes adductor spasmodic dysphonia, failure to consider etiology with respect to homogeneity or heterogeneity of the patient population, method of measurement of the effects of therapy, and type and duration of follow-up.

Therapy and Diagnostic Examinations

Establishment of the different etiologic types of adductor spasmodic dysphonia has been based on after-the-fact research findings. However, in actual clinical practice, although etiology can be apparent in the evaluation, a differential diagnosis among psychogenic, neurologic, or idiopathic types may be difficult and not apparent until the patient is well into therapy. For example, dysphonias that disappear for extended periods of time in response to symptomatic voice therapy or psychotherapy are not likely to be of neurologic etiology. For this reason, in the interest of conservative patient care, it is wiser to begin with a trial of symptomatic voice therapy and to reserve more risky types of therapy for intractable patients.

What seems to be emerging through experience with voice disorders, but in particular with adductor spasmodic dysphonia, is that therapy is more often successful when it is based on a solid foundation of diagnostic examinations from an interdisciplinary team consisting of a speech-language pathologist, neurologist, otolaryngologist, and psychologist or psychiatrist. The information obtained is obviously of primarily differential diagnostic value, but not entirely. If the clinician assumes that all patients who have adductor laryngospasms are alike, the probability is high that the wrong therapy will be selected, and, because patient education is indispensable, the clinician will not be in a very comfortable position to convey sufficient or correct information. The prematurely informed, and therefore, the often misinformed patient is unusually common in cases of adductor spasmodic dysphonia. If at all possible, the following examinations should be collaborative.

Laryngologic Examination   At the earliest opportunity, the patient should be scheduled for a thorough laryngologic examination. Although the signs of adductor spasmodic dysphonia are easily identifiable through listening, the ear, nose, and throat examination is important for several reasons: (1) The patient expects, and needs to be reassured by, a physical inspection of the interior of his or her larynx. (2) The clinician cannot confidently divest patients of their commonly held beliefs that tumors or other structural lesions are causing their dysphonias unless the clinician is convinced on the basis of firsthand information that such lesions are absent. (3) A minority of adductor spasmodic dysphonic patients have vocal nodules, polyps, or contact ulcers traumatically induced by their adductor laryngospasms, which contribute to the severity of their dysphonias. (4) Rhythmic adduction of the vocal folds producing voice tremor and rhythmic hyperadduction producing voice arrest can be viewed on laryngoscopic examination and is important diagnostically.

Speech Examination   A thorough speech examination is a necessity and should include a motor speech test for dysarthria. The reason for this prescription will be apparent if it will be recalled that spastic dysphonia may be of the neurologic type, and signs, often quite subtle, of tremor or movement disorder of the oral musculature may reveal information that can be of use to the neurologist and in planning of treatment.

Of all the speech tests that are usually administered during such an examination, none is more critical than vowel prolongation structured sentence production. The reason for sustained vowel production is that irregular laryngospasms during contextual speech may become regular or rhythmic during vowel prolongation, revealing that the patient's spasmodic dysphonia is of the essential (organic) tremor type. Structured sentences contrasting words beginning with vowels with those beginning with fricatives help differentiate spasmodic dysphonia of muscle tension dysphonia from other types (Idzebski, Dedo, et al., 1985; Roy, Gouse, Mauszycki, 2005). Also of particular importance is to obtain baseline audiotape and, if possible, videotape recordings for a more detailed study of the patient and for comparison with subsequent recordings, especially during and after therapy. Recordings may be used to quantify voice breaks and tremor type, regular or irregular.

Musculoskeletal tension testing and brief efforts to reduce such tension through laryngeal manipulation, as described elsewhere in this book, is another indispensable portion of the examination. Patients who have such tension associated with psychogenic forms of the disorder will often respond with enough voice improvement for a sufficient length of time during the examination to convince the clinician, and the patient, of a nonorganic form of the disorder, thereby approximating the diagnosis and indicating the direction that therapy should most likely take.

Psychosocial Examination   No patient with the voice signs of adductor spasmodic dysphonia should be denied the benefit of an exploration of possible psychologic causes, precipitants, or effects of the voice disorder. As noted elsewhere in this book, a preliminary psychosocial history surrounding the onset and development of the dysphonia deserves careful investigation, preferably by the examining speech pathologist or by a psychiatrist, psychologist, or psychiatric social worker of known qualifications. This examiner should collaborate with the laryngologist and speech pathologist. Here, again, the patient will often reveal the etiologic diagnosis by providing psychodynamic information to help explain the

voice disorder and, during the course of such revelations, demonstrate diminution or disappearance of the spastic dysphonia.

Neurologic Examination   Referral of the patient for a neurologic examination is not routinely warranted, but if there is any doubt about the patient's neurologic status, such referral can be highly clarifying, for example, when tremor or movement disorders are suspected of being related to the spastic dysphonia.

Armed with data from these different disciplines, the speech clinician in collaboration with the other specialists can chart a plan of action to help the patient with this most incapacitating of all voice disorders. A review of the findings with the patient is always a wise decision. Information itself is therapeutic beyond question even when nothing can be done for the voice for the time being. Based on all of these data, the voice team must decide whether symptomatic voice therapy alone, psychotherapy alone administered by a qualified therapist, surgical treatment, or some combination in parallel is warranted, with the idea held in reserve that should these fail, more drastic measures may have to be considered. The complexity of these decisions has been summarized by Pearson and Sapienza (2003) in their review and tutorial of the historical approaches to treating spasmodic dysphonia (see bibliography for specific reference).

Symptomatic Voice Therapy

Symptomatic voice therapy as the first stage in attempts to alleviate the disorder should be started with all patients except those in whom a neurologic type that will not respond to behavioral management has been definitely established. However, even when behavioral management is not considered to be effective as a primary approach, Murry and Woodson (1995) have demonstrated it may enhance and/or prolong effects of phonosurgical interventions. The voices of patients who have the tremor and dystonic types do not respond well to attempts to alter their control over their spasms. Although there is no harm in trying such therapy with patients whose dysphonia is neurologically related, especially if the clinician is not sure about the etiology, expectations of improvement should be guarded. These patients often give the impression of being able to alter their voices during therapy, but their ability to sustain less spastic voice in their daily lives usually breaks down.

Musculoskeletal Tension Reduction

In patients who have nonorganic forms of adductor spasmodic dysphonia, muscle tension reduction, as described elsewhere in this book, will often yield normal, or nearly normal, voice within a brief period of time. If the muscle tension is associated with an active conversion reaction, such physical manipulation will be only partially successful or totally unsuccessful, pending resolution of the underlying emotional conflict. However, even in cases in which conflict is active, considerable voice improvement can be expected. However, such patients will also require psychologic counseling.

Voice Quality and Pitch Modification

Paradoxically, normal or nearly normal voice under certain conditions of phonation becomes apparent to most clinicians as they investigate patients who have adductor spasmodic dysphonia, except the essential tremor type. A patient may have a severely strained voice during contextual speech most of the day, but it may be normal on arising, when shouting, laughing, crying, or singing. It may also be free of spasm during vowel prolongation even though not during conversation. It may be nearly normal at higher pitch levels or when phonating with a breathy voice quality.

These conditions of improved voice often give promise of relief, suggesting to the clinician that if the patient can phonate more easily at a higher pitch or using a breathy voice during vowel prolongation, or during reading of practice material in the clinic, the patient consciously ought to be able to sustain spasm-free voice during daily conversational speech. And, in many patients, such improvement has been effected. Cooper's (1980) therapy program for adductor spasmodic dysphonia is an example of the school of thought that believes voluntary alteration of phonation, and respiration, can benefit these patients. He advocates as individual and group therapy (1) reestablishment of natural or optimum pitch and "tone focus in the mask area" using the spontaneous "um-hum" method, (2) correct breath support using gentle, abdominal breathing, and (3) "peripatetic" voice therapy during which the clinician works with the patient at the actual site and under actual speaking conditions.

One of the few data-driven reports on success of behavioral management with this population was reported by Murry and Woodson (1995). Unlike Cooper, they did not work directly on tone focus but rather facilitated reductions in voice break and vocal effort by using "easy onset" voicing, continuous airflow during phonation, and reduction in articulatory effort. This direct voice therapy was combined with Botox (Botulinum toxin, Allergan, Inc., San Francisco) injections and resulted in the positive effects from Botox lasting longer thereby decreasing the number of injections required. Dedo and Idzebski (1983a,b) also emphasize the importance of voice therapy in combination with surgery for maximum rehabilitation results. Boutsen (1992) and Pearson and Sapienza (2003) suggest that this may be a form of sensorimotor retraining. "Theory holds that muscular weakening (such as that occurring after Botox injection) effectively suppresses maladaptive sensorimotor loops, which feed dystonic symptoms. It is during this period of weakening that the patient is most able to acquire (and ideally habituate) new sensorimotor templates. In the case of ADSD, this retraining holds as its focus the production of 'easy' and continuous voicing while minimizing extraneous muscular tension" Pearson and Sapienza, 2003, p. 334).

Harrison, Davis, Troughear, et al. (1992) have suggested an alternative approach using inspiratory voicing. In theory, this treatment requires abduction of the vocal folds coincidently with activation of the inspiratory muscles and provides a counter force to the abnormal adductory muscle action and produces more fluid speech. In practice, it is difficult to habituate, rarely sounds normal, and works for a limited number of patients.

Psychotherapy

As a means of alleviating adductor spasmodic dysphonia, historically psychotherapy has been highly suspect. This attitude may have developed because of a failure to separate the neurologic from the psychogenic types. Adductor spasmodic dysphonia due to conversion reaction or to depression or anxiety often yields to the emotional catharsis and discussion and resolution of emotional conflict. Often, the spastic dysphonia, whatever the cause, produces such withdrawal and depression that psychologic help is warranted on that basis alone.

Recurrent Laryngeal Nerve Resection

The first person to perform surgery to alleviate sphincter laryngospasm responsible for spastic-like disturbances of voice was Réthi (1952), who blamed the disorder on the stylopharyngeus muscle and divided it in one such patient. Twenty years later, Hammenberg (1972) advocated injecting either the posterior wall of the pharynx or the stylopharyngeus muscle to anesthetize these sphincters, describing the effect of the injection as highly favorable, the voice recovering in quality and volume and even persisting after the Novocain (procaine hydrochloride) had worn off. Neither surgery to the stylopharyngeus muscle nor injection of the pharynx ever became popular as a therapy for adductor spasmodic dysphonia. What did was a surgical approach in which one of the recurrent laryngeal nerves in the neck is severed, paralyzing one vocal fold and thereby reducing the degree of adductor force, allowing a freer flow of air through the glottis during phonation. Called the recurrent laryngeal nerve section, the procedure was first introduced in 1976 by Dedo. After first temporarily paralyzing one vocal fold by injecting one recurrent laryngeal nerve with lidocaine and listening for improvement in the voice to determine if the patient is a good candidate, a recurrent laryngeal nerve section is done.

Under general anesthesia, a collar incision is made one finger-breadth below the cricoid cartilage. Dissection is carried down to the anterior surface of the trachea and around its right side to the tracheoesophageal groove. The recurrent nerve is identified ordinarily at the level of the inferior pole of the right thyroid gland 1 cm lateral to the trachea. Direct laryngoscopy is then performed so that the right vocal fold can be observed while an assistant crushes the presumed recurrent nerve with a hemostat. If the vocal cord contracts abruptly at the instant of crushing, the structure is presumed to be the whole recurrent nerve and is ligated . A 1-cm segment is then removed adjacent to the inferior pole of the thyroid gland ~3 to 4 cm below the cricoid (Dedo, 1976).

Since Dedo's initial description, recurrent laryngeal nerve surgical variations have included laryngeal nerve crush (Biller, Som, and Lawson, 1983), recurrent laryngeal nerve avulsion (Weed, Jewett, Rainey, et al., 1996), and selective laryngeal adductor denervation-reinnervation (Berke, Blackwell, Gerratt, et al., 1999; Smith et al, 2006). The history of the results of recurrent laryngeal nerve surgery and estimates of its value reported by different investigators require careful reading and thought because of differences in surgical procedures, philosophies and methods, and length of postsurgical follow-up. All the references on the surgery cited at the end of this chapter in the Additional Reading section ought to be carefully scrutinized. When the findings from all of these studies are weighed, they demonstrate:

♦ The immediate postsurgical effects on the voice are overwhelmingly favorable, and for the following reasons. The voice is freed of the strained, hoarse quality and the often fatiguing physical effort to produce it. Facial grimacing and other body movements associated with the spasms diminish or disappear. Patients experience a reversal of their depression and withdrawal.

♦ The voice quality during the early postsurgical period tends to be breathy, weak, and hoarse. With time, the voice becomes clearer and louder. However, only a minority of patients can be said to achieve a completely normal voice. Often some degree of breathiness or hoarseness remains in patients regarded as successful. If either of these symptoms is intolerable for the patient, secondary surgical procedures have been developed.

♦ With the passage of time, many patients experience partial or complete return of their adductor spasmodic dysphonia to presurgical levels of severity or worse. The percentage of patients who fail depends upon which studies are consulted. They range from 15 to 64% failure 3 years after surgery.

♦ Explanations for return of the spastic dysphonia are neural regrowth or "sprouting" and/or overcompensation. Overcompensation may involve hyperfunction of the contralateral true and false, or supraglottic pharyngeal constrictors or sphincteric action of the false vocal folds and inferior pharyngeal constrictor muscles. Some patients benefit from secondary procedures done to debulk the vocal folds.

♦ Females experience a higher failure rate than males for unknown reasons.

♦ There is no way of predicting who will succeed in the longer term and who will fail.

♦ Patients have a greater tendency than clinicians to rate the postsurgical voices as better (Sapir et al, 1986).

♦ To the patient, the reduction of effort and fatigue of phonation is as important as improvement in the sound of the voice.

♦ Many patients who have failed within 3 years of the surgery say they were grateful for whatever relief they had from the spastic dysphonia.

♦ Postsurgical voice therapy may help patients destined to remain improved to maintain a smoother, clearer voice but will probably not prevent recurrence of the spastic dysphonia in patients whose voices are destined to deteriorate.

♦ Side effects of the surgery are minimal. Some patients experience a temporary need to swallow fluids carefully to avoid minor dysphagia, but this is not a serious or long-term complaint.

♦ Patients who have experienced a return of the spastic dysphonia are sometimes helped by further surgery, consisting of vocal fold thinning with carbon dioxide laser.

♦ Patients whose voices have remained excessively breathy for a long period after surgery owing to an excessively wide glottis may benefit from vocal fold medialization by injection of some material into the paralyzed vocal fold or thyroplasty.

♦ An alternate surgical procedure in which the laryngeal nerve is crushed instead of severed is not recommended owing to the unusually high failure rate, greater than 85%, within 10 months, and is probably due to reinnervation of the nerve.

What can clinicians conclude about the wisdom and advisability of performing recurrent laryngeal nerve removal or sectioning on adductor spasmodic dysphonia patients? How should they counsel their patients when the subject of surgery is raised? A conservative answer is to advise them of all treatment options and of the results of studies that show a degree of risk of return of the voice, but that there should be no fear that they would be worse off from the surgery than if they had not elected it. The positive aspects of the surgery need to be presented as well; that successful patients can experience excellent voice and are grateful for the benefits of the surgery. The lidocaine block as a preliminary procedure to allow the patient, family, and clinician to evaluate the simulated effects of surgery is a highly useful way of eliminating patients who are poorly motivated or who have excessively high expectations from the surgery. Allowing prospective patients to evaluate the audiotape and videotape recordings of patients who have had the surgery is another useful way of educating the patient as to the effects of surgery. The most balanced view of the surgery would be that, whereas it is not the solution for all patients, it can afford value for others. It should be carefully offered as a temporary benefit for highly motivated patients who have severe adductor spasmodic dysphonia and who have seriously suffered psychologically and vocationally from their disorder.

Botulinum Toxin Injection

Injections of botulinum toxin (Botox) has emerged as the preeminent and preferred approach due to its high rate of success and low risk of side effects (Blitzer, Brin, Stewart, 1998). Botox is injected either unilaterally or bilaterally directly into the thyroarytenoid or lateral cricoarytenoid or a combination of both muscles, which produces partial paralysis, preventing spastic hyperadduction of the vocal folds.

Botulinum toxin is a potent neurotoxin produced by the bacteria *Clostridium botulinum* found in one form of food poisoning. Of eight known strains, the type A botulinum toxin is the most potent and may be crystallized in stable form. When injected in low doses, it binds firmly to muscle and is rapidly fixed at the terminal nerve fibers with little remaining toxin allowed to pass into the general circulation, accounting for its relative safety (Cohen and Thompson, 1987). In the rare instances when after repeated injections patients have built up sufficient antibodies that they no longer respond to type A botulinum toxin, an alternative form may be used.

Physiologically, botulinum toxin blocks the release of acetylcholine from the nerve ending, interfering with calcium metabolism and, in effect, denervating muscle fibers for months; because the motor end plate does not release acetylcholine, the muscle fibers cannot contract. When denervated, the muscle atrophies but then develops new nerve sprouts, reinnervating the muscle, reversing the weakness over a period of approximately 3 months.

The toxin is injected either percutaneously, transorally, or transnasally. Percutaneous injections are made through the cricothyroid membrane into the thyroarytenoid muscle by means of a syringe with a monopolar, Teflon-coated, hollow electromyographic recording needle. The hypodermic needle functions as an electromyographic electrode to locate the thyroarytenoid muscle before the toxin is injected into it. The alternative injection techniques were developed in an effort to increase the accuracy with which toxin could be administered and eliminate the need for electromyography (EMG) monitoring. Surgeon preference and training, individual patient needs, equipment availability, and convenience generally determine the type of injection.

The toxin has been injected in patients' vocal folds both unilaterally and bilaterally. A meta-analysis of existing literature suggests that neither bilateral nor unilateral vocal fold injection is consistently associated with better outcomes (Boutsen, Cannito, Taylor, et al., 2002). Nevertheless there are suggestions in the literature that the two techniques have different outcomes. Blitzer (1988) suggests bilateral is preferable to unilateral for the reasons that bilateral injections require considerably less toxin and that a better voice can be achieved. Bielamowicz and associates (2002) provide some evidence supporting unilateral preference to minimize side effects of persistent breathiness and increase duration of symptom relief. In a comparison of unilateral and bilateral injections, both Ludlow, Bagley, Yin, et al. (1992) and Maloney and Morrison (1994) concluded that unilateral techniques in females result in better functional results. Patients who have had a return of their spastic dysphonia after recurrent laryngeal nerve resection have also benefited from the procedure.

The toxin takes effect within 24 to 72 hours, during which the voice becomes breathy. However, patients' voices respond differently because of differences in the severity of their spastic dysphonia and because the amount of toxin needed depends on the individual patient. Laryngoscopic examination after the induced weakness of the vocal folds discloses that they are not completely paralyzed but appose each other with less than full closure, revealing a slight glottal opening during phonation. The initial breathiness disappears within days, and a smoother, nearly normal voice can last from 3 to 6 months, toward the end of which the strained voice gradually returns to its preinjection status signaling the need for reinjection.

Injections are performed on an outpatient basis with a minimum of discomfort. The degree of weakness can be controlled by the administration of low doses of the toxin in the beginning and by titrating the dose until the proper amount for producing optimum voice with minimal side effects is found.

The voice quality achieved from the botulinum toxin injection has been found to be at least as good as, and in some cases better than, the voice quality obtained from recurrent laryngeal nerve resection (Miller, Woodson, and Jankovic, 1987). In addition to the improved voice, as in recurrent laryngeal resection, patients also report reduced physical effort to phonate, corroborated quantitatively by a considerable reduction in pre- and postinjection intrathoracic pressures. For example, in a study reported by Miller, Woodson, and Jankovic (1987), in one patient the preinjection intrathoracic pressure was 22 to 23 cm H_2O and 5 cm H_2O after injection, and in a second patient, it was 75 cm H_2O preinjection and 3.5 cm H_2O postinjection.

To review, the botulinum toxin injection for adductor spasmodic dysphonia is currently the therapy of choice for intractable adductor spasmodic dysphonia that is refractory to other therapies, though it is not necessarily the ultimate answer and the search for better treatments continues. The voice quality obtained is as good or better than the recurrent laryngeal nerve resection, the injection can be given as an outpatient procedure rather than under general anesthesia, and the toxin does not produce a permanent paralysis of a vocal fold. The latter advantage is especially attractive to patients and practitioners alike who are reluctant to paralyze a vocal fold permanently if it can be avoided. Repeated injections produce similar or identical results. The main disadvantage to the procedure is that the patient needs to be reinjected within 3 to 6 months. However, highly motivated patients have reported that this is a minor inconvenience considering the relief from the laryngospasms and improvement in voice and ease of phonation. Because the long-term effects of repeated injections have not yet been determined, it is not known for how many years patients will continue to derive benefit from repeated injections or whether the immune system will eventually negate the effects of the toxin over time (Blitzer, Brin, Fahn, et al., 1988; Brin et al, 1987). Because the injections for spasmodic dysphonia are given in small amounts of toxin, particularly in contrast with other Botox treatments such as for torticollis, for which there are longer-term data, the risk of acquiring resistance to Botox is considered low.

Laryngeal framework surgery done to reduce laryngeal tension has also been reported with variable success. This midline lateralization (Isshiki type II) thyroplasty decreases vocal fold closure by increasing the lateral dimensions of the glottis. In this procedure, the thyroid cartilage is split down the middle, and shims are placed between the two to widen the space. If the mechanical advantage desired by this surgery is not initially achieved, the shims can be down- or upsized as needed in a secondary procedure (Isshiki, 1998).

Case studies using alternative treatments such as hypnosis and acupuncture have been reported with varying degrees of success (Scheer and Lee, 2001). The fact that they are case studies does not mean that they should be negated but rather used to point to directions of future inquiry.

In summary, therapy outcomes for ADSD are mixed. There is no single treatment that has consistently positive results without side effects or need for subsequent procedures.

Behavioral management coupled with various surgical procedures appears to enhance results.

◆ Abductor Spasmodic Dysphonia

Definition

As previously stated, spasmodic dysphonia is not a homogenous condition. We now turn our attention from adductor spasmodic dysphonia to abductor spasmodic dysphonia. *Abductor spasmodic dysphonia* is a term used in reference to a perceptually distinctive voice in which normal or hoarse voice is interrupted by moments of breathy or whispered (unphonated) segments (Aronson, 1973). The term *abductor spasmodic dysphonia* was chosen because it appeared as if the vocal fold physiology responsible for the voice disorder was the opposite of that which occurs in adductor spasmodic dysphonia; that is, instead of spastic or spasmodic hyperadduction of the vocal folds producing moments of strained voice or voice arrests, the vocal folds spasmodically hyperabduct, releasing bursts of unphonated air. Although the disorder has not been long recognized, evidence is beginning to show that, as with the adductor forms, abductor spasmodic dysphonia may not be due to a single cause but may have either psychogenic or neurologic substrates.

Pathophysiology

Fiberscopic viewing of the vocal folds during connected speech discloses that, with each breathy air release, a synchronous and untimely abduction of the true and false vocal folds occurs exposing an abnormally wide glottic chink. This wide glottic chink may encompass the length of the glottis or may be exhibited as a bowed configuration of the midmembranous portion of the glottis. Frequently, bowed vocal folds also may be found on laryngoscopic examination. These abductor spasms, or loss of laryngeal tone, are triggered by consonant sounds, particularly the unvoiced ones, especially when they are in the initial positions of words. For example, in some patients it is possible to inhibit the breathy release of air entirely by having the patient read material containing only voiced consonants. Conversely, it is possible to precipitate rampant bursts of breathiness by asking the patient to read passages saturated with unvoiced consonants. The duration of breathy segments evoked by initial stop consonants has been measured at 2 to 3 times normal, but the total duration of words can remain normal nevertheless; the period of aspiration intrudes into the vowel segment, depleting its energy (Zwitman, 1979).

Figure 6.5 shows spectrographs of a normal speaker and an abductor spasmodic dysphonic speaker producing the sentence: "Berries are good on bread." The abductor breathy segments can be detected by the diminished or absent voice fundamental frequency energy at the following points: (1) a prolonged interval between the /z/ ending the word *berries*

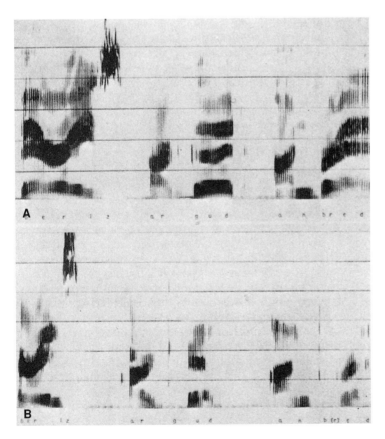

Figure 6.5 Spectrographs of (**A**) a normal speaker and (**B**) a patient with abductor spasmodic dysphonia producing the sentence: "Berries are good on bread." (From Zwitman, D.H. [1979]. Bilateral cord dysfunctions: abductor type spastic dysphonia. J Speech Hear Disord 44, 373–378.)

and the /a/ vowel beginning the word *are*; (2) between initiation of the sound /g/ and the vowel /u/ in *good* with some loss of sound energy during the vowel; (3) a prolonged interval between the final /d/ of *good* and the initial /a/ of *on*; and (4) during production of the /b/ and /r/ phonemes of the word *bread*. Aspiration time occupied 96 of 260 milliseconds, or 36.5% of the word, whereas no aspiration occurs during normal production of the word. However, sentences spoken with abductor breathiness can take longer than normally phonated ones as noted in a study of Merson and Ginsberg (1979) in which one patient required 2150 milliseconds compared with a normal control who spoke the same sentence in 1775 milliseconds, and whose mean airflow rate was 77 cm^3/s compared with the dysphonic person's airflow of 400 cm^3/s.

Onset, Course, and Factors Affecting Severity

Abductor spasmodic dysphonia usually begins insidiously, not essentially differently from onset in patients who develop adductor. The voice may begin as a nonspecific hoarseness or breathiness and over a period of days or weeks begin to show signs of intermittent breathy air release.

Severity of the dysphonia fluctuates under conditions similar to the adductor type. When the patient is relaxed and free of tension, pressure, or worry, the voice can be nearly normal. It can be better or nearly normal during conditions of anger or laughter. It is much worse when the patient is emotionally upset, when required to speak with figures of authority, or when the communicative content of speech is more than usually important. Severity can be temporarily reduced by avoiding voiceless consonants, voicing unvoiced consonants, and by phonating at higher pitch levels.

Factors Associated with Onset

Factors associated with onset are not essentially different in these patients as in those who have adductor type. The disorder can occur in the absence of any known associated event or it can follow laryngitis with sore throat or domestic or work-related emotional stress.

A history of previous dysphonias and factors associated with onset in five patients who today would be designated as having abductor spasmodic dysphonia were reported by Aronson, Peterson, and Litin (1964), who found that three had had previous episodes of pure whispered (aphonic) speech, all five had had previous hoarseness, in two the onset had been associated with cold or influenza, in all five the onset had been associated with fatigue or exhaustion, and in two the onset had been associated with feelings of tightness in the throat.

Etiology

With the continual gathering of data on these patients, a pattern appears to be emerging in which these patients, like their adductor counterparts, may be divided into psychogenic, neurologic, and idiopathic types, and in which psychologic stress may precipitate the neurologic ones. In a study by Hartman and Aronson (1981), 10 of 13 (77%) patients had a scattering of neurologic signs: deterioration in writing,

synkinetic facial movements, hyperreflexia, ataxic gait, nasal regurgitation, and dysphagia. However, more importantly, this study also uncovered a neurologic parallel to one form of adductor spasmodic dysphonia of essential tremor. In five (30%) of the 17 patients, voice tremor on vowel prolongation was documented within the range of 4.5 to 6.0 Hz, which is well within the limits of the essential tremor syndrome. On laryngoscopic examination, in some patients the abductor spasms are rhythmic, and a breathy release of air occurs on the abductor phase of each tremor cycle. In other patients, voice tremor without breathy air releases is audible on vowel prolongation (**Fig. 6.6A**). Four (31%) of the 13 patients in the study who had been given neurologic examinations had tremor of the head, face, and extremities. There may be, then, at least one definable neurologic type of abductor spasmodic dysphonia that parallels the adductor form: abductor spasmodic dysphonia of essential voice tremor.

Some patients have a mixed abductor-adductor spasmodic dysphonia; moments of breathiness occur alternately with moments of strained-harshness or voice arrest (**Fig. 6.6B**). Noting the co-occurrence of abductor and adductor laryngospasms, Cannito and Johnson (1981) advanced the reasonable proposition that, rather than adductor and abductor spasmodic dysphonia being separate disorders, they exist on a continuum, a view that is not only plausible but one that would help to explain their similarities pertaining to nature of onset, factors influencing severity, and multiple etiologies.

Convincing evidence also is accumulating to show that there is a psychogenic form of abductor spasmodic dysphonia as well as neurologic. In a psychiatric study, seven patients, who had what was then called *intermittently whispered-phonated speech* before the coining of the term *abductor spasmodic dysphonia*, had various combinations of the following: histories of chronic stress, clinical signs of hysterical personality, histories of other conversion somatic signs, marital discord, repressed anger, immaturity and dependency, neurotic life adjustments, mild to moderate depression, and the "conversion V" on the Minnesota Multiphasic Personality Inventory test (Aronson, Peterson, and Litin, 1966). Voice signs of abductor spasmodic dysphonia of conversion disorder were found in the following patients:

Case Study 6.4

A 46-year-old housewife and beauty salon operator had been under chronic stress from several sources. Her 25-year-old son had a behavior problem. She harbored unspoken hostile feelings toward her husband, who had never adequately supported the family and who was unemployed. She was perpetually irritated with her employees for their inability to measure up to her standards but was unable to express her feelings to them. She had chronic and overwhelming fatigue by early afternoon and would have to retire to her bed. Her marginal insight into her problem was evident from her statement that "I am afraid my employees think I am angry with them when I lose my voice and can't talk" (Aronson, Peterson, and Litin, 1966, p. 117).

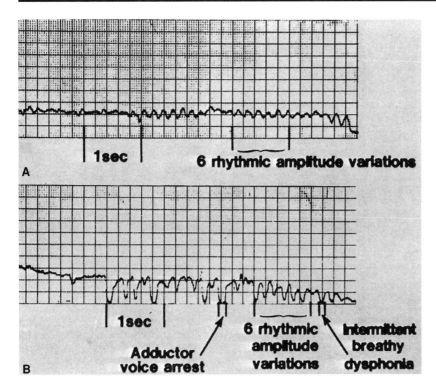

Figure 6.6 Oscillographic tracings. (**A**) Tracing of an abductor spasmodic dysphonic patient of the essential tremor type during vowel prolongation. The patient has almost continuous tremor. Patient (**B**) has mixed abductor-adductor spasmodic dysphonia of the essential tremor type. Note moments of both adductor and abductor (intermittent breathy dysphonia) spasms. (From Hartman, D.E., Aronson, A.E. [1981]. Clinical investigations of intermittent breathy dysphonia. J Speech Hear Disord 46, 428–432.)

A religious, perfectionistic woman had a long-standing disappointment in her married daughter who drank and read "unacceptable" literature. She disapproved of the way her daughter was raising her children. The patient asked if "being frustrated and never letting anyone know" could cause her to "lose" her voice. Later in the interview, she came closer to the central issue. "My only daughter annoys me constantly, but I never let her know. . . . Where did we fail with this daughter?. . . . I can't reprimand her. I can't get on her back, because it may be something I have done that's wrong. . . . I don't admire people who show anger. I think you should control it. I have been so angry that I have felt actually warm inside, but no one has known that I was angry. . . . Joy and love are emotions to be expressed, but not anger" (Aronson, Peterson, and Litin, 1966, p. 120).

A 45-year-old married woman has had intermittent moments of breathiness for the past 2 years. Laryngologic examination shows normal vocal cord structure and function. The patient's voice disorder began during an intensely troubled period of her life. Active in a women's service organization and in line for the presidency, she was defeated for this office by a false rumor that she had misused the organization's finances. When the patient learned of this plot, she was furious and resentful and was strongly tempted to express her contempt toward the membership, but decided against this course of action because she could not bring herself to express the unlady-like feelings she felt toward them.

During this time of anger, frustration, defeat, and violent arguments at meetings of the organization, she began to detect feelings of tension in her throat followed shortly thereafter by a gradual change in her voice. As the arguments grew in ferocity, her voice symptoms became increasingly disabling.

One month after the first signs of the voice change, she became involved in an extramarital affair. She recalls, "I was a sitting duck to get involved." After 1 year it was discovered by the man's wife. "She came over and called me every name in the book. I was ashamed, humiliated, furious." Her voice disorder, by now well entrenched, became progressively worse after this confrontation. At present, she feels tremendously guilty toward her husband, whom she describes as "so good and unsuspecting." She would like to tell her husband of the affair but is so "deeply in love" with the other man that she cannot give him up. As a result, she is caught in a perpetual conflict (Aronson, 1973, p. 51).

This discussion of abductor spasmodic dysphonia would not be complete without some patient example. Thus, we present a verbatim interview with a patient who came to the clinic with moderate to severe abductor spasmodic dysphonia. The etiology remains unclear from the interview and examination, and the disorder has to be considered idiopathic until the accumulation of further evidence. The interview was selected because of the patient's exceptional ability to describe the onset and course of his voice disorder, its symptoms, efforts toward therapy, and his reactions to the disorder. It is also illustrative, rather typically in many ways, of the pilgrimage many patients enter into to find a cure for their voice disorders.

Case Study 6.5

Clinician: Could you tell me now, first of all, your age.
Patient: I'm 38.
C: And what is your occupation?
P: A corporate representative.
C: Are you married?
P: Yes.
C: Do you have any children?
P: I have three children.
C: Had you ever had any voice trouble like this before as a child or as an adolescent?
P: No.
C: Tell me when this first started.
P: It first started about 6 years ago. I had a very bad cold one weekend and when the cold got a little better, I was left with laryngitis, and that was the outset of the thing. The laryngitis got a little better within about a week, but after that it was difficult to say certain words. To begin with it was just every so often and just one particular sound, which was a hard "c" like "Carol" or "cam," or a "k" sound like in "keep." It was barely noticeable, but then it seemed like each year it got a little bit worse and there would be new sounds that would prove more difficult.
C: What came next?
P: It seems like it was anything like a "p" or "t" going into vowels, and I remember most specifically "Porsche" because I was selling foreign cars then. Then it seems like maybe "s" and "h" came next.
C: How long after the laryngitis did the breathy trouble start?
P: Oh, it was the next week.
C: The laryngitis disappeared.
P: The laryngitis disappeared but the other didn't. And then it has just gotten progressively worse through the years, and it can be a great deal better one day and a great deal worse the next.
C: What kinds of things make it better or worse?
P: I think the things that make it better are almost complete relaxation. If I can get into a super relaxed position and get my voice into a real low level, then it tends to operate fairly well. Many people who might meet me in this circumstance might think that I don't really have any voice problem. Unfortunately, the world that we live in doesn't permit us necessarily to operate at this voice level.
C: Are you saying that the louder you talk . . .
P: The louder I talk the worse it gets.
C: Let's hear you count to five softly and then do it loudly. [Patient follows instructions.]
C: It does make a difference, doesn't it?
P: You were asking what makes it a little better, and I think anybody who runs into something like this makes compensatory adjustments. I know which words I'm going to have difficulty with to a large degree, so I can avoid those words. For instance, I know that I can't say the word "hard" so I don't say it. I say "difficult." I started to say "words that I can say" and it was like a trigger; you can't say that, so I didn't say "say" I said pronounce.

C: Does time of day make it better or worse?
P: Yes. Usually it is easier early in the morning and it gets, depending on what I do during the day, progressively worse.
C: If you should go on vacation or be involved in some other release from work, will it be better?
P: To a degree. Very early on the degree might have been greater when, say, I went to the lake or something and just did nothing but lay on a beach or go fishing. The degree that it gets any better is less now than it was very early.
C: Let's go back to the beginning of this voice disorder. I wish you would think about the answer to this question very carefully. Before or during the time that you had this laryngitis and developed the voice disorder, were you under any unusual stress different from what might have been under usual life circumstances?
P: I'm not giving you a quick answer, because I have thought about this a lot, because the question has been asked a lot. The only thing that I can remember as being unusual is, I knew for six months in advance of the voice trouble that I was being considered for a promotion. I know that I was pushing, because I wanted it, and the weekend that the voice disorder came on was when I got the promotion.
C: Were you looking forward to the promotion?
P: Yes, I wanted the promotion. I was not looking forward, and I have to say this in all honesty, to the prospects of having to work very closely with the owner of the company that I would be working directly with. He was a very abrasive, intimidating individual, and I knew I was going to have to work with him if I got the promotion. I'll be as honest as I can be; I am sure that gave me some apprehension, because he was a very intimidating individual.
C: Well, you've left that company since.
P: Yes, that company went out of business.
C: How long were you working for this individual before that happened?
P: Three years.
C: And during that time your voice disorder got gradually worse.
P: Yes.
C: Did the relationship between you and this man work out to be as threatening as you thought it would be?
P: No.
C: Was it as traumatic as you had anticipated?
P: No, it wasn't.
C: And so here you are another three years after parting company with this individual still with the voice disorder.
P: Right.
C: We want to be careful not to assign effects to erroneous causes.
P: Oh, I understand.
C: Two things that happened in close proximity don't necessarily mean that they are cause and effect. Did any of the psychologists or psychiatrists you had consulted attach any importance to the anticipation that you had about the promotion as it might relate to the voice disorder?

P: Not any major importance. They didn't really think there was any direct relation there.

C: And as far as you know there were no other emotionally upsetting family or business problems.

P: Not at that point. There have been since then, but not at the outset.

C: And stresses that have happened since. Have they worsened your voice?

P: Well, I don't know whether they worsened my voice or whether it would have gotten worse anyhow. There has been a fairly progressive deterioration through the years. There probably has not been any deterioration this year. Maybe the last two years it has been fairly stable.

C: How would you honestly assess the effects of the voice on your professional, domestic, and social life?

P: I don't want to use the word devastating, because that seems to be a little too much, but it has had a very dramatic effect.

C: In what way.

P: For instance, I'll talk about just little things. When I was coming over here today on the bus there was a gentleman sitting in the seat beside me. I would normally be very eager to strike up a conversation with him, but I am very reticent [sic] to do that because it is going to be embarrassing, so as a result I don't seek out people. I avoid saying anything just in day to day conversation; when you go to a restaurant and something is amusing and you want to tell somebody about it, I don't. I don't participate.

C: Why is that?

P: Because the words don't happen. The words don't come out, and it's embarrassing.

C: Have you had abnormal reactions from other people?

P: Not generally. People normally don't have anything to say about it. That is on a very basic level. On a professional level, it does affect me, particularly with new customers. I will avoid going to see people whom I should go see, customers or potential customers. Even if there were no voice problem there would be a certain amount of stress involved in going to see these people anyhow due to the nature of their business, the size of their business, the nature of the individual, or whatever. Just recently I was being considered for a promotion in my company, and my boss, quite candidly, said that I would not get it as a result of the speech disorder. He told me that as a friend as much as anything else, because the particular position would involve a great deal of sales training, which is getting in front of a group and teaching them about machinery, which I am good at. I'm as good as anybody I have ever seen at sales training, at taking a group of people and keeping them interested in what they are learning as they sit there an hour or two hours. I can do that, and I can do it well, but I can't do it under the circumstances that I am working with now. So, instead of looking for opportunities to do that, I look for ways to avoid it. In social situations if I'm at a party or something, rather than seeking out people to talk to I try to get into a corner or get where I can talk with just somebody that I know rather than getting into a threatening situation.

C: Has the total effect of the voice made you periodically or chronically depressed?

P: Periodically, yes. I would be the first to admit that.

C: How bad is it?

P: Here again, sometimes it is worse than others. The last two and a half years have added to my voice problem. I went into business, which failed. My wife became seriously ill. So, in answer to your question, do I ever get depressed, yes I do but I really make an effort not to. As a matter of fact the people in my office, the people that I talk with daily over the telephone, they say, "Golly, I've never known anyone who stays up like you do. How do you do that? You just always seem to have something nice to say." I really work at doing that because I don't want to be the other way.

C: What therapies have been tried from the very beginning to help the voice?

P: At the very beginning I went to the regular doctor, and he said I had an inflammation and then gave me penicillin, or something, which did nothing. Then I went to an ENT specialist, and he tried a couple of medicines on me, I don't remember what they were, and then he said maybe you need to try speech therapy. So I went to the Speech and Hearing Center for nine months.

C: Any benefit?

P: None. Then several months after that I went back to the ENT doctor, and he didn't really know what to do. Then I went to a regular GP, and immediately, he said "I think this is something that has an emotional base," so he set up an appointment for me to see a psychiatrist. I said, "That's great. I'll go see a psychiatrist." So I went to see a psychiatrist for about six months, and he said one day, "Mr. —, we can keep doing this, but I don't think I'm doing you any good, and I don't think there is any evidence of a hysterical reaction, or hysterical conversion. There is just nothing that leads me to believe that so I really don't think we ought to continue." So I didn't do anything there again for a bit. I went to another throat specialist, did that for several months. I ended up at another GP, and he said, "I think you ought to try hypnosis." I said, "Okay I'm open. I'll do it." So he said, "All right, let's do that." He was trained in hypnosis. I did that for about three months. He said, "It just doesn't seem to be doing any good and I don't understand it. I thought that it would." Another doctor referred me to a second speech pathologist. She is the one that first used the word "spastic dysphonia." She said, "There is really nothing that you can do for spastic dysphonia other than speech therapy, and there is a psychologist here who specializes in this with hypnotherapy, and I want you to go see him." I said, "All right, I've been through it once, but maybe I wasn't at the right place." I went to the hypnotherapist there and was there once a week for about a month, and it just didn't do anything even though my speech was a little better under hypnosis. I can do that to myself just by relaxing, so they weren't really doing anything. I went back to the ENT doctor and he said the only thing he could do was refer me for speech therapy. I had already been through it once but thought maybe I just didn't have the right person, so I went back into speech therapy for little over a year, and at the end of about a year she helped to a degree. I think she would help anybody with speech to a degree, and she did work with me on breath control and relaxation techniques and some of the compensatory techniques. For instance, like, if you can avoid attacking a word, just to roll through a word. If I were to say "trouble" then it is difficult if I just attack that word "trouble," but if I'm talking to you about "somebody-in-trouble" then it rolls right on in there. So she helped me to that degree.

C: So the learning how to attack the words helped somewhat, but it didn't really make . . .

P: No. Then another doctor said, "There is a psychologist who has treated spastic dysphonia patients. I spoke with her and she thinks she can help you with therapy." I'm off again. That was last year. I had begun to get a little bit of information that this thing may have something to do with neurology or neurologic condition.

C: Before you get onto that, you had some more psychotherapy with the psychologist. Did it benefit?

P: No. It didn't help at all.

C: How long did that go on?

P: That went on for almost a year.

C: Then you started . . .

P: Then I went to a neurologist just about when I started going to that psychologist. He was very honest. He gave me a neurologic exam. He said, "I just did not see any evidence of a neurologic condition, but I will if you are interested in doing this be happy to prescribe some medicines that are used to treat certain movement disorders, which might be of some benefit. If they do any good that is great. If they don't do any good, then we will stop and try something else."

C: There were several different kinds?

P: There were about six.

C: And after that . . .

P: And after that I haven't really been doing anything, because I really didn't know what to do. Then, about six months ago I went back to therapy a little bit, we used a voice masker, the Edinburgh Voice Masker, and that had a little positive effect when I first put it on and then after I used it for just a few minutes the effect diminished but I felt like maybe if I wear that enough that will help, so I ordered the Edinburgh Voice Masker. When I did that I got on somebody's mailing list for stuttering. I got a newsletter from — University, the stuttering center. So, I wrote, and they wrote back and said there is really nothing we can suggest other than speech therapy and I am sure there is a very good speech pathologist in your area if you'll get in touch with somebody. Then, you wrote me and here I am.

C: Did the university people talk to you on the telephone?

P: No.

C: I wonder if they didn't think you had the other kind of spastic dysphonia.

P: I would imagine that they did.

C: You understand there are two kinds and the kind that is most familiar to people is the kind in which the vocal cords come together excessively.

P: The adductor.

C: They probably thought what you meant by "spastic dysphonia" in your letter was the adductor type, but you really meant abductor.

P: Well, I didn't know that until I talked to you.

Summary of Abductor Spasmodic Dysphonia

♦ *Abductor spasmodic dysphonia* is a term that describes breathy releases of air owing to sudden hyperabduction or loss of tone of the true vocal folds.

♦ Evidence indicates that these spasms can be due either to psychogenic (conversion reaction) or neurologic (essential tremor) causes or can be idiopathic.

♦ There is a propensity for the abductor spasms to occur most strongly during the production of unvoiced consonants, to a lesser extent during voiced consonants, and least of all during vowels.

♦ Like the adductor spasmodic dysphonias, onset is gradual and often associated with psychologic stress

Treatment of Abductor Spamodic Dysphonia

Resistance to therapy is as true for abductor spasmodic dysphonia as it is for the adductor type. The approach to therapy should take a form similar to that for adductor spasmodic dysphonia.

First, it is necessary to determine if the disorder is primarily psychogenic by means of a thorough psychosocial history. As in other psychogenic voice disorders, disclosure of personal problems may be accompanied by improvement or disappearance of the dysphonia.

Symptomatic voice therapy should always be tried. For abductor spasmodic dysphonia specifically, the abductor laryngospasms and breathy air release will diminish or disappear if the clinician teaches the patient to voice all unvoiced consonants. For example, saying the phrase "coffee cream" will produce severe breathy air releases in most abductor spasmodic dysphonic patients. However, if the clinician then tells the patient to substitute the /g/ for the /k/ phoneme in "coffee cream," the breathy air releases will be diminished. In the same way, if the patient is taught to voice all of the remaining voiceless consonants, it is possible that the abductor spasmodic dysphonia will either diminish considerably or disappear completely. Telling the patient to keep the vocal cords vibrating through all of connected speech will accomplish the same objective.

Similarly, like adductor spasmodic dysphonia, some abductor spasmodic dysphonia patients have benefited from phonosurgery. Botulinum toxin injections in the cricothyroid and/or posterior cricoid arytenoid (PCA) have temporarily reduced symptoms in some patients. However, in comparison with patients with adductor spasmodic dysphonia due to dystonia, its effectiveness is less pronounced and occurs in a smaller percentage of patients (Duffy and Yorkston, 2003). Medialization by vocal fold injection or type I bilateral thyroplasties to bring the membranous vocal folds closer together have benefited others. However, there is no consistently successful surgical treatment for this population.

We close this chapter with a description of the treatment journey experienced by a patient with adductor spasmodic dysphonia. The treatise is a typical description of experiences reported by other patients and helps the beginning student comprehend the significance of the problem and of the difficulties and frustrations faced by the patient.

◆ Confessions of an Adductor Spasmodic Dysphonia Patient

Pre–Botulinum Toxin Injection

Four and one-half of the past 5 years of my life have been spent in bewilderment. "Why do I sound like this?" The last 6 months have been spent with a certain knowledge of what spasmodic dysphonia is and of a possible route that can be pursued to periodic relief.

Joshua Liebman once wrote a book titled *Peace of Mind*, in which he describes the handling of the death of a dear one as a prescribed series of stages through which one must pass.

I felt, as one with spasmodic dysphonia, that I too went through similar stages which I refer to as my plateaus.

Plateaus

These plateaus ascended and descended in no apparent order. At one extreme, the strongest, I felt rage. My Plateau of Rage. An inner rage, which at times went out of control, during which, in hopeless frustration, and a sinking capability of toleration, I, as a person who had always prided herself on some semblance, at least, of gentility and femininity, wanted to smash and destroy all that was in my way to expose my helpless anger at not being able to speak and to be understood.

As the antithesis of this plateau, I passed through my Plateau of Peaceful Acceptance during which I felt rather intelligent at being able to lead a life of newly acquired passive submission.

I called this plateau, Moving into My Silent World. I substituted a normal existence of verbal contact, physical endeavors, shopping, sociability, meetings, and so forth, with an ersatz life consisting of multihours of piano practice daily, followed by hours spent writing three different books that I assumed would, at least, be bound for family and/or friends. The fact that I learned to play piano rather well again or that I wrote 200 poems offered no consolation. I had merely filled my days with lonely creativity.

Yet, even here, lack of speech halted my efforts because I was unable to communicate with a printer regarding the finished form of these writings. At this point I stopped, and the writings remained in my desk drawer. Frustration had even entered my silent world.

The most interesting plateau was reached on August 7, 1989, when the Mayo Clinic informed me that I had a neurologic, not a psychologic, disorder. Here began my Bravado Plateau.

For a brief period of time I put to rest the agonizing. I shifted the gears of my attitudes. I had been told, at last, exactly what spasmodic dysphonia was.

No longer would I need weekly allergy shots for an allergy that I never had. No longer the meetings with speech pathologists in which I tried hopelessly to emit clear sustained sounds of which I was not capable. No longer to be told that I used this horrible strangled speech so that people would feel sorry for me. I look back, now, to such a remark as insulting; to imply I could speak clearly if I wished. How sad, when it was all beyond my physical control.

While in my Bravado Plateau my voice problem became everyone else's problem. Not mine. Others would have to learn to like my voice as it was what it was. This was, of course, my briefest, shortest lived plateau because too soon the inability to communicate on the simplest terms returned and the ball of speaking-hardship was back in my court.

Prior to the botulinum toxin injection, I struggled through the Plateau of Research and Attempted Comprehension. Once I knew that spasmodic dysphonia was a neurologic disorder, I began to read every medical abstract I could find to ascertain not only the why of spasmodic dysphonia, but why me.

I read each paper assiduously, laboriously working my way through every intricate medical word and sentence with the *Merck Manual* and the *American Medical Dictionary* close at hand. I compiled my own handwritten dictionary filled with words like central cranial dysfunction, monopolar electrode, cholinergic, and so forth, none of which I completely understood.

There is no information as harmful as too little information. This was, gratefully, my last plateau as I realized I must have faith with those who wrote the abstracts and who would soon help me.

Yet, as with all other plateaus that had been self-sought during my life with spasmodic dysphonia, this one served me in fulfilling more silent weeks alone.

Telephone Communication

It has been established in the various papers I have read that speaking on the telephone is, to say the least, difficult when one has spasmodic dysphonia. I found this to be true and I felt it was thus not only because I could not articulate without spasms but because I could not rely on any facial expression to help convey the meanings behind my spastic words.

Communication is a process of interpreting symbols. Words are symbols. In any life we misinterpret more than we should, perhaps because our deepest intentions are at odds with the messages we project. I could project nothing.

I felt the strongest reactions of pure, sheer terror at the sound of the telephone bell. An actual physical distress. As if choreographed: When the telephone rang, though someone else would answer it for me, my head would immediately, automatically, turn from side to side in panic signifying "No!" and I could not relax until I felt, with absolute certainty, that the telephone would not be handed to me.

I knew at an intellectual level this fear was not one that I admired in myself, yet the ability to act otherwise was quite beyond my control—as long as I had the voice of spasmodic dysphonia. In the last 6 months of my 5-year ordeal I devised a system for incoming calls from my husband and my daughter, both of who called me daily, they would ring 3 times, hang up, and re-ring before I would answer the telephone. What torment I felt, how filled with sorrow I was, as I stood there waiting to count the rings to see if this would be a call I was capable of answering.

All other incoming calls were recorded on the telephone's answering machine. I am at a loss to convey, and will probably find it the most difficult to ever forget, the extreme self-pity I experience as I stood frozen near the telephone and listened to a friend leave a message, realizing I was so lacking in confidence that I could only stand there in tears, unable to reach forward to pick up the telephone.

At such times I stood outside of myself and saw a pathetic woman whose continual eruptions of tears had become a daily part of living in those months before my botulinum toxin injection.

Social Life

Before I brought all social participation to a halt, I had noticed some rather interesting displays of change among our female friends. For example, at dinners, when I would be forced into silence because of my broken speech, after futile attempts at dinner chit-chat, the other women became excessively talkative. Dull personalities who previously added monosyllables to conversation became strangely loquacious, while I sat silently at the table.

Were other women more nervous than I? Was that the reason? Did my feelings of inadequacy make their talk seem more emphatic to me than perhaps it really was? Nevertheless, interestingly, it was a consistent pattern among other women in my presence. It is mentioned here because it contributed to my need to abort all social contacts.

There are many people who feel unsure when offering their arm to a blind person who might be waiting at a corner to cross a street. Perhaps, in a fashion, people also feel unsure in the company of someone with spasmodic dysphonia and its obvious audible speech disorder.

However, my female friends never abandoned me, nor did male friends. They always urged me to join them. They called about my welfare. They did not care, they said, how badly I sounded when I tried to speak. But I did.

Well-meaning friends would say, "At least you have no pain." True. No physical pain, but, ah, the mental pain and grief. The destruction of an entire thinking process added to a weary exhaustive frustration.

Religion

I have walked out of a sanctuary during religious services because I had experienced the beginning of a true physical discomfort coursing through my body as I sat there. Such a strong negative reaction in a house of God, where one seeks peace, mystified me.

I could not vocally participate in prayer services while around me hundreds of people did so with no difficulty. Women many, many years older than I responded with

forceful clear voices. When I tried to respond, people would turn to look at me. The humiliation destroyed me.

I discovered then the world is not necessarily inhabited by kind, feeling, sensitive individuals.

Stress

I never thought of stress as the primary source of my speech difficulty or of its agony, even before being informed of its neurologic origin. I thought of stress, then, as minor problems with which we all cope daily. I, on the other hand, had something that was much more serious (although I did not know what it was) than mere stress.

I became, with the passage of time, incapable of making decisions. I experienced a complete loss of assertiveness, of interest. My words were spoken in monotone. I perceived my voice as a crying, nonexpressive monotone. My speech had no nuances. My sound held no laughter.

Often I felt as if the flow of thought and the flow of speech were not meant to become as one. In normal instances, we conceive a thought and with unconscious speed we emit the words that project the thought from mind to the ears of the listener. With spasmodic dysphonia, a different "process" aborted this continuation of my thought/speech pattern. This "process" blinked out a quick message to me somewhere between thought and speech. This "process" said, "Why bother? It will not come out right. It will not be understood." I could have filled volumes with my thoughts never spoken.

I developed, quite without thinking about it, an involuntary movement with my hand. As I would begin any sentence, to a stranger or to a store clerk, for example, my hand would automatically fly to my throat with the very first word I uttered, and I would explain, "I have laryngitis." Or "I have an allergy." And, worse yet, "I'm sorry." Always an apology for the sound of my voice when I knew, full well, the other person did not know me, could not care less, had never seen me before, would possibly never see me again. But that hand flew to my throat when I tried to speak, from the moment I left my apartment until I returned.

Physical Attitude

I had always walked very straight and erect. Proud, actually, of my good posture. When I sat, as a rule, I did so most comfortably with my back seldom touching the back of a chair. I attributed this, and a self-competitive physical attitude, to 16 years of ballet training and performance.

However, with my dysphonia, although in these instances speech was not involved, I realized I had begun to slump, round shouldered, curved spine. Worse, I did not care. It didn't matter. I would shrug my shoulders to imply lack of interest.

Before the dysphonia took over my life with its cruel force, I would swim 60 laps every day. In addition I would jog 4 miles every day. I gradually became too tired to walk for only 10 minutes. To walk and to try to speak at the same time became impossible without experiencing fatigue. So then even an activity that I could have done in relative solitude was restricted to me, becoming, as the dysphonia became worse, a nonaccomplished effort. I finally submitted and gave up, thus contributing to my further helplessness and demoralization.

I had always been in competition with myself where physical endurance was concerned. If I did six of anything today, I must do eight tomorrow. This was pleasurable to me, an achievement, a satisfaction. Soon gone.

Not only the sense of competitive accomplishment was withdrawn but simple maintenance, as well, could not be achieved. Pleasures became impossible, replaced by hopelessness.

I lost the desire to strive.

Tolerance Levels

My tolerance dropped, with the passage of time, in direct proportion to the increasing frequency of spasms in my speech. All external forces became extremely objectionable. It was too noisy, too dark, too light, too long, too short, too fast, too slow.

I had to exert the effort to work at exercising patience for nearly everything, seldom succeeding. My tolerance was always in simultaneous accord with the way I perceived my spastic voice. Life was filled with irritants. I could not help myself. My dysphonia had taken me out of the bounds of ordinary daily acceptance.

Familial Significance

Some additional insight into the psyche of this patient with spasmodic dysphonia may be found in the following excerpts from a letter that I wrote to my husband. This letter had been given to him as I walked into the room for my botulinum toxin injection. In part, it reads:

"These have been the unhappiest 5 years of my life. This past month has been the worst of all. I have fought depression daily. I have done battle with it and I was able to hold myself, at least, to being merely sad, somber, and withdrawn."

"Sometimes the rage within me exploded out of my system when the frustration of living the life of a recluse became more than I could handle."

"I don't know who I am (or was) anymore. I tried to move into my 'silent world' like a lady. But it's been hard. I'm not sure if I made it, but know I tried."

"Trying to speak to you has been such an effort, so tiring. But my heart has always been filled with appreciation. I want you to know how much I have always appreciated the overwhelming patience that you have had for me through these past few years."

Through these past 5 years, from time to time, through the cheerfulness of one daughter who called me daily, I did find the only touches of humor that sustained me. She brought this gift of humor, which came to me like flashes of clear, bright light into my otherwise darkened life.

Without these brief daily moments of shared laughter, which began and ended with her contact, the years would have been still more intolerable.

I could not have struggled in a world where people did not understand me when I spoke unless a corner of my brain could send a signal to me that implied there can be some laughter along with the tears.

I am indebted to my daughter for lifting my spirits as I am to my husband for his sustained love and patience. Without each I was never quite sure that I would have endured as well.

As is obvious here, I gave myself little credit for any inborn stamina or fortitude. With spasmodic dysphonia I was drowning, sinking, and crying for help. Under such circumstances, self-motivation is virtually nonexistent, or indeed, very limited.

In closing, I must establish that all that which has been written on these pages has been written within the time frame of 7 days following my first botulinum toxin injection, in which the anguished memories of the past 5 years are still so near the surface.

In addition, my interpretation of how I personally perceive, or analyze, the past 5-year period of dysphonia must be accepted as those of a woman who had always felt, prior to that 5-year period, all of life's happenings as strong gusts of maximum extremes. Whenever possible, of optimum extremes.

My inability to maintain my self-dignity in which I had always felt great pride, in retrospect, was the saddest part of my life with spasmodic dysphonia.

Post–Botulinum Toxin Injection

What wonderment!

I am worthwhile again!

The spasms and vocal breaks are no longer heard. It is quite incredible that my entire thinking processes and attitudes have changed so quickly. This is almost, but not nearly, to me the miracle of receiving the botulinum toxin injection.

Not only had my speaking voice cleared, but in the same 24-hour period my brain and my thinking have also cleared.

I am a rocket! I have accelerated to a height that I had forgotten existed. How can this phenomenon occur so swiftly? What new and good plateaus await me?

I had forgotten the sound of my own laughter. I had forgotten the sheer delight of speaking one-syllable words without breaks. I have reverted to the woman I was more than 5 years ago.

I remember me! So soon! So soon! How can this be? I recall now that I was a happy woman, upbeat, joyous.

I expected voice improvement. I anticipated a certain pleasure to replace the sorrow with which I have lived for such a long time. But this? This is unbelievable!

How else to explain the overwhelming exhilaration of being able to do something as basic as ordering a cup of tea in a restaurant. For myself. By myself. For the first time in years to speak in a clear voice. No longer a waitress to tell me she cannot understand me. No longer strangers at nearby tables turning to stare at me.

I have read that with spasmodic dysphonia, not only does a voice change but an entire personality can change. With this fascinating quick rebound that I am experiencing, I wonder about that.

Perhaps the personality is laid dormant, at rest, eager to spring to life anew given the opportunity.

I often cried, "I do not know who I am or even who I was before the dysphonia." I could not recall my persona, so submerged was I in noncommunicative despair.

Yet, within 24 hours I have become the person I had always been, the woman I had completely forgotten.

For this voice, this life, this clarity of thought, I am enveloped in elation.

Conclusion

If I am to benefit from this introspective interpretation of myself as a woman with spasmodic dysphonia, both before and after the botulinum toxin injection, would I, could I, handle it differently the next time around?

Would I, could I, handle it differently the next time around, and there will always be a next time around, if perhaps the botulinum toxin were not available?

Have I learned from these 5 years?

Yes! I'd "do it" better. I'd summon up more courage. I'd find more independence. I'd hold onto my dignity for dear life.

And, I would hope that I would take advantage of all that I have written herein.

M.A.K.

February 21, 1990

The author of this memoir about her spasmodic dysphonia died of multiple myeloma months after providing the above.

References

Aminoff, M.J., Dedo, H.H., Izdebski, K. (1978). Clinical aspects of spasmodic dysphonia. J Neurol Neurosurg Psychiatry 41, 361–365.

Ardran, G., Kinsbourne, M., Rushworth, G. (1966). Dysphonia due to tremor. J Neurol Neurosurg Psychiatry 29, 219–223.

Arnold, G.E. (1959). Spastic dysphonia: I. Changing interpretations of a persistent affliction. Logos 2, 3–14.

Aronson, A E. (1973). *Psychogenic voice disorders: An interdisciplinary approach to detection, diagnosis and therapy.* Philadelphia: W. B. Saunders Company.

Aronson, A.E. (1979). Spastic dysphonia: retrospective study of one hundred patients. Unpublished manuscript.

Aronson, A.E., Brown, J.R., Litin, E.M., Pearson, J.S. (1968a). Spastic dysphonia. I. Voice, neurologic, and psychiatric aspects. J Speech Hear Disord 33, 203–218.

Aronson, A.E., Brown, J.R., Litin, E.M., Pearson, J.S. (1968b). Spastic dysphonia. II. Comparison with essential (voice) tremor and other neurologic and psychogenic dysphonias. J Speech Hear Disord 33, 220–231.

Aronson, A.E., Hartman, D.E. (1981). Adductor spastic dysphonia as a sign of essential (voice) tremor. J Speech Hear Disord 46, 52–58.

Aronson, A.E., Lagerlund, T.D. (1991). Neuroimaging studies do not prove the existence of brain abnormalities in spastic (spasmodic) dysphonia. J Speech Hear Res 34, 801–811.

Aronson, A.E., Peterson, H.W., Litin, E.M. (1964). Voice symptomatology in functional dysphonia and aphonia. J Speech Hear Disord 29, 367–380.

Aronson, A.E., Peterson, H.W., Litin, E.M. (1966). Psychiatric symptomatology in functional dysphonia and aphonia. J Speech Hear Disord 31, 115–127.

Barkmeier, J.M., Case, J.L., Ludlow, C.L. (2001). Identification of symptoms for spasmodic dysphonia and vocal tremor: a comparison of expert and nonexpert judges. J Commun Disord 34, 21–37.

Barton, R.T. (1979). Treatment of spastic dysphonia by recurrent laryngeal nerve section. Laryngoscope 89, 244–249.

Berke, G.S., Blackwell, K.E., Gerratt, B.R., Verneil, A., Jackson K.S., Sercarz, J.A. (1999). Selective laryngeal adductor denervation-reinnervation: a new surgical technique for adductor spasmodic dysphonia. Ann Otol Rhino Laryngol 108, 227–231.

Bielamowicz, S, Ludlow, C.L. (2000). Effects of botulinum toxin on pathophysiology in spasmodic dysphonia. Ann Otol Rhinol Laryngol 109, 194–203.

Bielamowicz, S., Stager, S,V., Badillo, A., Godlewski, A. (2002). Unilateral versus bilateral injections of botulinum toxin in patients with adductor spasmodic dysphonia. J Voice 16(1), 117–23.

Biller, H.F., Som, M.L., Lawson, W. (1983). Laryngeal nerve crush for spastic dysphonia. Ann Otol Rhinol Laryngol 92, 469–476.

Blitzer, A., Brin, M.F., Fahn, S.f et al. (1985). Electromyographic findings in focal laryngeal dystonia (spastic dysphonia). Ann Otol Rhinol Laryngol 94, 591–594.

Blitzer, A., Brin, M.F., Fahn, S., Lovelace, R.E. (1988). Clinical and laboratory characteristics of focal laryngeal dystonia: study of 110 cases. Laryngoscope 98, 636–640.

Blitzer, A, Brin, M.F., Stewart, C.F. (1998). Botulinum toxin management of spasmodic dyphsonia (laryngeal dystonia): a 12-year experience in more than 900 patients. Laryngoscope 108, 1435–1441.

Bloch, P. (1965). Neuro-psychiatric aspects of spastic dysphonia. Folia Phoniatr (Basel) 17, 301–364.

Bocchino, J.V., Tucker, H. (1978). Recurrent laryngeal nerve pathology in spasmodic dysphonia. Laryngoscope 88, 1274–1278.

Borenstein, J.A., Lipton, H.L., Rupick, C. (1978). Spastic dysphonia: an 18-year follow-up. Paper presented at the American Speech and Hearing Association, San Francisco.

Boutsen, F., Cannito, M.P., Taylor, M., Bender, B. (2002). Botox treatment in adductor spasmodic dysphonia: a meta-analyais. J of Speech, Lang and Hear Rsh. 45, 469–481.

Bousten, F., Cannito, M.P., Taylor, M., Bender, B. (2002). Botox treatment in adductor spasmodic dysphonia: a meta-analysis. J Speech Lang Hear Res 45, 469–481.

Bressman, S.B. (2004). Dystonia genotypes, phenotypes, and classification. Adv Neurol 94, 101–107.

Brin, M.F., Blitzer, A., Stewart, C. (1998). Laryngeal dysphonia: observations of 901 patients and treatment with botulinum toxin. Adv Neurol 78, 237–252.

Brin, M.F., Fahn, S., Blitzer, A., Ramig L.O. (1992). *Movement disorders of the larynx. Neurologic disorders of the larynx.* New York: Thieme Medical Publishers.

Brin, M.F., Fahn, S., Blitzer, A., Ramig, L.O., Stewart, C. (1992). Movement disorders of the larynx. In A. Blitzer, M.F. Brin, C.T. Sasaki, S. Fahn, K.S. Harris KS (Eds.), *Neurologic disorders of the larynx,* (248–278). New York, Thieme Medical Pub. Inc.

Brin, M.F., Fahn, S., Moskowitz, C., Friedman, A., Shale, H., Greene, P.E., Blitzer, A., List, T., Lang, D., Lovelace, R.E., McMahon, D. (1987). Localized injections of botulinum toxin for the treatment of focal dystonia and hemifacial spasm. Mov. Disord. 2, 254.

Brodnitz, F.S. (1976). Spastic dysphonia. Ann Otol Rhinol Laryngol 85, 210–214.

Cannito, M.P., Johnson, P. (1981). Spastic dysphonia: a continuum disorder. J Commun Disord 14, 215–223.

Carlsöö, B., Izdebski, K., Dahlqvist, A., Domeij, S., Dedo H.H. (1987). The recurrent laryngeal nerve in spastic dysphonia. A light and electron microscopic study. Acta Otolaryngol 103, 96–104.

Chhetri, D.K., Blumin, J.H., Vinters, H.V., Berke, G.S. (2003). Histology of nerves and muscles in adductor spasmodic dysphonia. Ann Otol Rhinol Laryngol 112, 334–341.

Cohen, S.R., Thompson, J.W. (1987). Use of botulinum toxin to lateralize true vocal cords: A biochemical method to relieve bilateral abductor vocal cord paralysis. Laryngoscope, 96, 534–541.

Cooper, M. (1980). Recovery from spastic dysphonia by direct voice rehabilitation. Proceedings of the 18th Congress of the International Association of Logopedics and Phoniatrics 1, 579–584.

Critchley, M. (1939). Spastic dysphonia (`inspiratory speech'). Brain 62, 96–103.

Critchley, M. (1949). Observations on essential (heredofamilial) tremor. Brain 72, 113–139.

Dedo, H.H. (1976). Recurrent laryngeal nerve section for spastic dysphonia. Ann Otol Rhino Laryngol 85, 451–459.

Dedo, H.H., Izdebski, K. (1983a). Intermediate results of 306 recurrent laryngeal nerve sections for spastic dysphonia. Laryngoscope 93, 9–15.

Dedo, H.H., Izdebski, K. (1983b). Problems with surgical (RLN section) treatment of spastic dysphonia. Laryngoscope 93, 268–271.

Dedo, H.H., Izdebski, K., Townsend, J. (1977). Recurrent laryngeal nerve histopathology in spastic dysphonia. A preliminary study. Ann Otol Rhinol Laryngol 86, 806–812.

Dedo, H.H., Shipp, T. (1980). *Spastic dysphonia: A surgical and voice therapy treatment program.* San Diego: College Hill Press.

Devous, M.D., Pool, K.D., Finitzo, T., et al. (1990). Evidence for cortical dysfunction in spasmodic dysphonia: regional cerebral blood flow and quantitative electrophysiology. Brain Language 39, 331–344.

Dordain, M., Dordain, G. (1971). L'epreuve du "a" tenu au cours des tremblements de lu voix (tremblement idiopathique et dyskinesie volitionnelle, leurs rapports avec la dysphonie spasmodique). Rev Laryngol Otol Rhinol 93, 167–182.

Duffy, J.R., Yorkston, K.M. (2003). Medical interventions for spasmodic dysphonia and some related conditions: A systematic review. Journal of Medical Speech-Language Pathology, 11(4), ix–lviii.

Fritzell, B., Feuer, E., Haglund, S., Knutson E., Scheratzki, H. (1982). Experiences with recurrent laryngeal nerve section for spastic dysphonia. Folia Phoniatr (Basel) 34, 160–167.

Golper, L.A., Nutt, J.G., Rau, M.T., Coleman, R.O. (1983). Focal cranial dystonia. J. Speech Hear Disord 48, 128–134.

Harrison, G.A., Davis, P.J., Troughear, R., Winkworth, A.L. (1992). Inspiratory speech as a management option for SD. Ann Otol Rhinol Laryngol 101, 375–382.

Hartman, D.E., Aronson, A.E. (1981). Clinical investigations of intermittent breathy dysphonia. J Speech Hear Disord 46, 428–432.

Heaver, L. (1959). Spastic dysphonia: II. Psychiatric considerations. Logos 2, 15–24.

Isshiki, N. (1989). *Phonosurgery: theory and practice.* Tokyo: Springer-Verlag.

Isshiki N. (1998). Vocal mechanics as the basis for phonosurgery. Laryngoscope 108, 1761–1766.

Isshiki, N., Haji, R., Yamamoto, Y., Mahieu, H.F. (2001). Thyroplasty for adductor spasmodic dysphonia: further experiences. Laryngoscope 111, 615–621.

Isshiki, N., Tsuji, D.H., Yamanoto, Y., Izuka,Y. (2000). Midline lateralization thyroplasty for adductor spasmodic dysphonia. Ann Otol Rhinol Laryngol 109, 187–193.

Izdebski, K., Dedo, H.H. (1981). Spastic dysphonia. In J. Darby (Ed.) *Speech evaluation in medicine* (105-107). New York: Grune and Straton.

Izdebski, K., Dedo, H.H., Boles, L. (1984). Spastic dysphonia: a patient profile of 200 cases. Am J Otolaryngol 5, 7–14.

Izdebski, K., Dedo, H.H., Ship, T., Flower, R.M. (1981). Postoperative and follow-up studies of spastic dysphonia patients treated by recurrent laryngeal nerve section. Otolaryngol Head Neck Surg 89, 96–101.

Jacome, D.E., Yanez, G.F. (1980). Spastic dysphonia and Meige's disease. Neurology 30, 349.

Jankovic, J., Ford, J. (1983). Blepharospasm and orofacial-cervical dystonia: clinical and pharmacological findings in 100 patients. Ann Neurol 13, 402–411.

Kiml, J. (1963). Le classement des aphonies spastiques. Folia Phoniatr 15, 269–277.

Koufman, J.A., Blalock, D.P. (1988). Vocal fatigue and dysphonia in the professional voice user. Laryngoscope 98, 493–498.

Levine, H.L., Wood, B.G., Batza, E., Rusnov, M., Tucker, H.M. (1979). Recurrent laryngeal nerve section for spasmodic dysphonia. Ann Otol Rhinol Laryngol 88, 527–530.

Ludlow, C.L., Bagley, J., Yin, S.G., Koda, J. (1992). A comparison of injection techniques using botulinum toxin injection for the treatment of the spasmodic dysphonias. J Voice 6, 380–386.

Ludlow, C.L., Schulz GM., Yamashita T., Deleylannis F.W. (1995). Abnormalities in long latency responses to superior laryngeal nerve stimulation in adductor spasmodic dysphonia. Ann Otol Rhinol Laryngol 104, 928–935.

Maloney, A.P., Morrison, M.D. (1994). A comparison of the efficacy of unilateral versus bilateral botulinum toxin injections in the treatment of adductor spasmodic dysphonia. J Otolaryngol 23, 160–164.

Marsden, C.D., Sheehy, M.P. (1980). Spastic dysphonia and Meige disease. Neurology 30, 349.

Marsden, C.D., Sheehy, M.P. (1982). Spastic dysphonia, Meige's disease, and torsion dystonia. Neurology 32, 1202–1203.

McCall, G.N., Skolnick, M.L., Brewer, D.W. (1971). A preliminary report of some atypical movement patterns in the tongue, palate, hypopharynx, and larynx of patients with spasmodic dysphonia. J Speech Hear Disord 37, 466–470.

Merson, R.M., Ginsberg, A.P. (1979). Spasmodic dysphonia: abductor type. A clinical report of acoustic, aerodynamic and perceptual characteristics. Laryngoscope 89, 129–139.

Miller, R.H., Woodson, G.E., Jankovic, J. (1987). Botulinum toxin injection of the vocal fold for spasmodic dysphonia. A preliminary report. Arch Otolaryngol Head Neck Surg 113, 603–605.

Morrison, M.D., Rammage, L.A., Belisle, G.M., Pullan, C.B., Nichol, H. (1983). Muscular tension dysphonia. J Otolaryngol 12, 302–306.

Murry, T., Woodson, G.E. (1995). Combined-modality treatment of adductor spasmodic dysphonia with botulinum toxin and voice therapy. J Voice 9, 460–465.

Nutt, J.G., Muenter, M.D., Aronson A., Kurland L.T., Melton L.J. (1988). Epidemiology of focal and generalized dystonia in Rochester, Minnesota. Mov Disord 3, 188–194.

Parnes, S.M., Lavarato, A.B., Myers, E.N. (1978). Study of spastic dysphonia using videofiberoptic laryngoscopy. Ann Otol Rhinol Laryngol 87, 322–326.

Pearson, E.J., Sapienza, C.M. (2003). Historical approaches to the treatment of adductor-type spastic dysphonia (ADSD): review and tutorial. NeuroRehabilitation 18, 325–338.

Ravits, J.M., Aronson, A.E., Desanto, L.W., Dyck, P.J. (1979). No morphometric abnormality of recurrent laryngeal nerve in spastic dysphonia. Neurology 29, 1376–1382.

Rethi, A. (1952). Role of the stylopharyngeall muscular system in defective phonation due to ventricular bands and in dysphonia spastica. Folia Phoniatr (Basel) 4(4), 2101–16.

Robe, E., Brumlik, J., Moore, P. (1960). A study of spastic dysphonia. Laryngoscope 70, 219–245.

Roy, N., Ford, C.N., Bless, D.M. (1996). Muscle tension dysphonia and spasmodic dysphonia: the role of manual laryngeal tension reduction in diagnosis and management. Ann Otol Rhinol Laryngol 105, 851–856.

Roy, N., Gouse, M., Mauszycki, S.C., Merril, R.M., Smith, M.E. (2005). Task specificity in adductor spasmodic dysphonia versus muscle tension dysphonia. Laryngoscope 115, 311–316.

Sapir, S., Aronson, A., Thomas, J. (1986). Judgment of voice improvement after recurrent laryngeal nerve section for spastic dysphonia: Clinicians versus patients. Annals of Otology Rhinology and Laryngology 95:137–41.

Schaefer, S.D. (1983). Neuropathology of spasmodic dysphonia. Laryngoscope 93, 1183–1202.

Scheer, S., Lee, L. (2001). Acupuncture for the treatment of adductor spasmodic dysphonia. Medical Acupuncture 14, 1–7.

Schweinfureth, J.M., Billante, M., Courey, M.S. (2002). Risk factors and demographics in patients with spasmodic dysphonia. Laryngoscope 1112, 220–223.

Smith, M.E. (2006). Laryngeal reinnervation. In A. Blitzer et al (Eds.), *Neurologic disorders of the larynx.*

Smith, M.E. (In press). Laryngeal reinnervation. In A. Blitzer (Ed,), *Neurologic disorders of the larynx.* New York: Thieme Medical Pub. Inc.

Sulica, L. (2004). Contemporary management of spasmodic dysphonia. Curr Opin Otolaryngol Head Neck Surg 12, 543–548.

Tarrasch, H. (1946). Muscle spasticity in functional aphonia and dysphonia. Medical Woman's Journal 53, 25–33.

Tolosa, E.S., Klawans, H.L. (1979). Meige's disease. Arch Neurol 36, 635–637.

Traube, L. (1871). Spastische form der nervosen heiserkeit. Pathol Physiol 2, 677.

Tucker, H.M. (1989). Laryngeal framework surgery in the management of spasmodic dysphonia. Preliminary report. Ann Otol Rhinol Laryngol 98, 52–54.

Weed, D.T., Jewett, C., Rainey, D.L. Zealer, R.E., Stone, R.E., Ossoff R.H., Nertterville, J.L. (1996). Long term follow-up of recurrent laryngeal nerve avulsion for the treatment of spastic dysphonia. Ann Otol Rhinol Laryngol 105, 592–601.

Zwirner, P., Murry, T., Woodson, G.E. (1993). A comparison of bilateral and unilateral botulinum toxin treatments for spasmodic dysphonia. Eur Arch Otorhinolaryngol 250, 271–276.

Zwitman, D.H. (1979). Bilateral cord dysfunction: abductor type spastic dysphonia. J Speech Hear Disord 44, 373–378.

Additional Reading

Aronson, A.E., Hartman, D.E. (1981). Adductor spastic dysphonia as a sign of essential (voice) tremor. J Speech Hear Disord 46, 52–58.

Aronson, A.E., Brown, J.R., Litin, E.M., Pearson, J.S. (1968a). Spastic dysphonia. I. Voice, neurologic and psychiatric aspects. J Speech Hear Disord 33, 203–218.

Aronson, A.E., Brown, J.R., Litin, E.M., Pearson, J.S. (1968b). Spastic dysphonia, II. Comparison with essential (voice) tremor and other neurologic and psychogenic dysphonias. J Speech Hear Disord 33, 220–231.

Aronson, A.E., Peterson, H.W., Litin, E.M. (1964). Voice symptomatology in functional dysphonia and aphonia. J Speech Hear Disord 29, 367–380.

Aronson, A.E., Peterson, H.W., Litin, E.M. (1966). Psychiatric symptomatology in functional dysphonia and aphonia. J Speech Hear Disord 31, 115–127.

(This series of Aronson et al. articles should be read for a background to both the psychogenic and neurologic forms of adductor spastic dysphonia.)

Blitzer, A., Brin, M.F., Fahn, S., Lovelace, R.E. (1988). Clinical and laboratory characteristics of focal laryngeal dystonia: study of 110 cases. Laryngoscope 98, 636-640.

Brin, M.F., Blitzer, A., Stewart, C. (1998). Laryngeal dysphonia: observations of 901 patients and treatment with botulinum toxin. Adv Neurol 78, 237–252.

(The preceding two articles contain statistical data on the incidence of spastic dysphonia and responsiveness to treatment with botulinum toxin. In a large group of patients who had dystonic movement disorders, the authors illustrate that one type of spastic dysphonia, in all probability, is a manifestation of an extrapyramidal movement disorder of the dystonic variety. The technique of botulinum toxin injection for adductor spastic dysphonia in a large group of patients is reported and voice effects described.)

Bloch, P. (1965). Neuropsychiatric aspects of spastic dysphonia. Folia Phoniatr (Basel) 17, 301–364. (The most voluminous and comprehensive article on spastic dysphonia extant. Has considerable historical significance. Psychoanalytically oriented. Hundreds of references.)

Jurgens, U. (2002). Neural pathways underlying vocal control. Neurosci Biobehav Rev 26, 235–258. (This in-depth review is a must read for any students wanting an understanding of the neural pathways underlying vocal control.)

Ludlow, C.L. (2004). Recent advances in laryngeal sensorimotor control for voice, speech and swallowing. Curr Opin Otolaryngol Head Neck Surg 12, 160–165. (This article reviews research that provides new understanding of laryngeal sensorimotor control. It focuses on the significance of the research and its relevance to the assessment, understanding, and treatment of laryngeal motor control disorders affecting voice, speech, and swallowing.)

Pearson, E.J., Sapienza, C.M. (2003). Historical approaches to the treatment of ADSD: review and tutorial NeuroRehabilitation 18, 325–338. (This review paper presents a tutorial on treatment approaches for ADSD. The tutorial is designed for clinicians interested in treating spasmodic dysphonia and provides background and theory that lay the groundwork for understanding the various treatment approaches.)

Robe, E., Brumlik, J., Moore, P. (1960). A study of spastic dysphonia. Laryngoscope 70, 219–245. (A landmark study, probably the first comprehensive one that advocated that at least one form of spastic dysphonia was neurologic. It served to shift research and clinical thinking about the causes of adductor laryngospasms during speech in new directions.)

AAN. (1990). Assessment: the clinical usefulness of botulinum toxin-A in treating neurologic disorders. Report of the Therapeutics and Technology Assessment Subcommittee of the American Academy of Neurology. Neurology 40, 1332–1336.

American Academy of Otolaryngology-Head and Neck Surgery Policy Statement. (1990) Botox for spasmodic dysphonia. AAO-HNS Bull.

Blitzer, A., Sulica, L. (2001). Botulinum toxin: basic science and clinical uses in otolaryngology. Laryngoscope 111, 218–226.

National Institutes of Health Consensus Development Conference. (1990). Clinical use of botulinum toxin NIH Consensus Statment. 8 (8), 1–20.

(The preceding four papers present the basics on clinical application of botulinum toxin. Three of the articles are position papers on the use of Botox for treatment of spasmodic dysphonia; one is a summary of an NIH consensus conference.)

Chapter 7

Clinical Voice Evaluation

Nathan V. Welham

Voice disorders are inherently complex, and their evaluation should reflect this. The voice can function as a barometer of physical and emotional health; it is closely tied to personal and professional identity; and it is a powerful expressive communication tool. A comprehensive evaluation of vocal function requires a carefully elicited case history, consideration of psychosocial impact, and a complete assessment of laryngeal and vocal fold vibratory function. The clinician should hold a strong knowledge base in laryngeal anatomy and physiology and be able to integrate assessment data within this knowledge framework. The tools available to the contemporary clinician range from his or her auditory and visual perceptual systems, to acoustic, aerodynamic, and endoscopic technologies. In addition, information from the entire voice care team, including a range of medical data from other disciplines (e.g., asthma-allergy, endocrinology, gastroenterology, neurology, oncology, psychiatry, pulmonology, radiology), is often critical in piecing together a complete clinical picture.

◆ Case History Taking

No voice evaluation is complete without a comprehensive case history. The case history assists in determining the path of assessment, points toward potential differential diagnoses, suggests prognosis, and helps to direct treatment. Given this, a successful case history requires a high level of clinical skill. The clinician must be able to efficiently and expertly judge the significance of certain information, remain unbiased by other specialist opinions, know when to pause and listen, and when to probe deeper for clarification or detail. The path of questioning and exploration followed by any given clinician is as varied as the presentation of any given patient. Whereas the clinician brings a depth of clinical knowledge and experience to the situation, the patient brings his or her personal expertise concerning the history

and current status of the presenting voice problem, its implications for daily functioning, and its influences on the patient as a person.

It is important to note that as the voice is influenced by physical, emotional, and personality states, all of these dimensions must be probed in the case history. During the interview and voice evaluation, all plausible etiologies should be entertained. Viewing the presenting problem as an exclusively laryngeal phenomenon can potentially result in misdiagnosis; therefore, the clinician should always consider the possibility of the voice representing a more general disorder of the speech mechanism or entire organism.

The following section details key content areas within a typical voice case history. This section does not address every conceivable history factor relevant to voice but rather covers common issues encountered in the clinic. Of course, it is impossible to master the art of clinical interviewing simply by reading about it, as every clinician's skills are honed with ongoing training and experience. The subsections and order presented here are not inviolable; however, beginning clinicians may benefit from the use of a checklist.

Key Components

Familiarization and Rapport Building

The clinician should strive to facilitate a positive interpersonal environment and relationship with the patient. From early impressions, the clinician perceives the patient's reaction to a new situation and may find signs of tension, anxiety, or depression through facial expression, posture, gestures, and handshake. At the same time, the patient makes important judgments about the clinician: how interested the clinician is in seeing the patient; how secure, at ease, and skillful the clinician is in the interpersonal situation; in short, the kind of person with whom the patient is dealing. If confidence and a sense of trust are established early, the patient will find it easier to discuss his or her personal history.

Nature, Onset, and Course of the Voice Disorder

Nature An often helpful starting point in the clinical interview process is to obtain the patient's description of the presenting problem. The patient's response to an inquiry of this nature may demonstrate insight, motivation, confusion, or misunderstanding. Some patients will simply recast the comments of the referring specialist, whereas others may express dissatisfaction with their current diagnosis. Regardless of the eventual accuracy of the patient's perception, it does have clinical significance. If later intervention is to be effective, misconceptions must be directly addressed and the patient's statement of a primary symptom considered a treatment priority.

Onset Determining the onset of any voice disorder is important in guiding differential diagnosis. Many patients find it difficult to establish the precise onset of voice symptoms because most disorders begin gradually rather than suddenly. Patients who give a vague answer should be pressed to recall the month, day, or even hour when their symptoms first began. Voice disorders associated with musculoskeletal tension, slowly developing vocal fold mass lesions, and progressive neurologic disease tend to develop gradually. Those associated with acute vocal fold lesions (e.g., a hemorrhagic polyp), acute neurologic incidents, and psychogenesis tend to occur abruptly.

It is important to identify significant factors or events associated with the onset of voice symptoms. The patient may associate the onset of symptoms with a significant life event, a period of emotional stress, or an upper respiratory infection. Such reports may be indicative of an underlying psychogenic component (an upper respiratory infection with associated laryngitis can provide a psychogenic trigger for dysphonia); however, it is important to explore these reports carefully, and interpret them within the context of the entire voice evaluation. Many patients with psychogenic voice disorders are notoriously unaware of causative emotional stress or interpersonal conflict. Raising these issues and extracting key information within the context of a clinical interview and later helping patients to understand the link between these issues and their voice disorder requires counseling skills. Because of its indispensability in the evaluation and treatment of voice disorders, a separate chapter on psychologic interviewing and counseling is included later in this book.

Voice symptoms that first appeared alongside speech and swallowing difficulties may be due to a neurologic impairment. The clinician should be alerted to reports of imprecise and effortful speech production, hypernasality, difficulty with chewing and swallowing, and nasal regurgitation. Weight loss should also be noted.

Course It is useful to gauge the degree of variability in symptoms since the onset of the voice disorder, as well as across a typical day. Patients may describe their symptoms as consistent, intermittent and marked by periods of normal voice, gradually worsening or improving over time, or completely unpredictable from moment to moment. Patients with nonorganic voice disorders due to muscu-loskeletal tension or psychogenesis will often report periods lasting from minutes to days when their voices are completely normal, only to worsen again. In contrast, patients with organic voice disorders due to either vocal fold mass lesions or neurologic disease will usually report continuously abnormal voice from time of onset, either consistent in severity or deteriorating gradually or precipitously with time. Myasthenia gravis is characterized by gradual voice deterioration and fatigue during speech and a reversal of these symptoms after rest. Laryngopharyngeal reflux may be indicated by intensified voice symptoms during the first few hours of the day, a result of sleeping in the prone position overnight.

A cautionary note should be made concerning variability in symptoms. All voice disorders, regardless of etiology, generally worsen during physical fatigue and emotional stress. The clinician should not automatically link these variations with a psychogenic etiology. Further, patient descriptions of periods of normal voice production should be questioned carefully. Many patients describe as normal what later proves to only be an episode of improvement.

Associated Factors

It is important to identify factors associated with the presence of voice symptoms, as well as factors that tend to exacerbate or ameliorate symptoms. Reports of fatigue, globus sensation, tightness and pain in the laryngeal region, increased coughing, sensations of irritation and dryness, and heartburn should all be noted. The patient may notice an improvement or worsening of symptoms as a result of various factors. Examples are changes in vocal demand, seasonal allergies, climate, working environment, and eating habits.

Related Health and Medical Issues

Several general health and medical issues emphatically pertain to the voice. The clinician should enquire whether the patient has any diagnosed respiratory disorders (e.g., chronic obstructive pulmonary disease, asthma), gastrointestinal disorders (e.g., gastroesophageal reflux disease), neurologic disorders (e.g., stroke, traumatic brain injury, pseudobulbar palsy, essential tremor, dystonia, Parkinson's disease, multiple sclerosis), allergic rhinitis or chronic sinusitis, autoimmune disorders (e.g., rheumatoid arthritis, systemic lupus), endocrine disorders (e.g., hyperthyroidism, hypothyroidism), psychiatric disorders (e.g., clinical depression, acute or chronic anxiety, schizophrenia), or hearing loss. A description of the current medical and pharmacologic management of these conditions should be obtained. Previous vocal fold, laryngeal framework, head and neck, thoracic, or cardiac surgery should be detailed. It is important to determine whether the patient was intubated during any such procedure and whether radiation therapy was employed in the head and neck region. Other laryngeal trauma, such as from a physical wound or chemical inhalation, should also be noted.

Excessive alcohol, caffeine, tobacco, and illicit drug use is an important area of inquiry and should not be avoided by the clinician. Many substances can have a negative influence on the vocal fold epithelium and lamina propria, and most patients are unaware that the abuse of these substances can exacerbate their voice disorders. When questioning the patient, it is helpful to establish both the quantity and frequency of substance consumption. The discussion of alcohol and illicit drug use may be a particularly sensitive issue with some patients: those who appear reluctant to divulge information should be assured of patient-clinician confidentiality.

Voice Use

Excessive and inappropriate voice use can be a significant factor both in the onset and exacerbation of a voice disorder due to the presumed role of excessive vocal fold impact stress in vocal fold tissue injury (Gray, Hammond, and Hanson, 1995; Gunter, 2004; Titze, 1994b). The clinician should explore the nature and degree of voice use across all domains of the patient's life. Vocational demands can be critical if the patient gives a large number of presentations, spends a significant amount of time on the telephone, in meetings or other group situations, is a performer, or works in a noisy environment. Recreational activities such as amateur or professional singing or acting, attending sports events and concerts, cheerleading, or coaching can all tax the vocal mechanism. When questioning patients about voice use, it is helpful to determine the environment in which the voice is being used (indoor, outdoor, air conditioned, humidified, smoky, noisy, hot, cold), whether aids such as amplification are available and used, and whether the patient has received voice training.

Assessment of Psychosocial Impact

The psychosocial impact of dysphonia on a patient's daily activities and quality of life is a very important area of consideration within overall assessment. It is intuitive that the impact of dysphonia on any individual is the result of personal and professional voice demands, the role of voice in an individual's concept of self, and an individual's ability to manage, cope with, and compensate for disease. In an attempt to accurately measure the psychosocial impact of dysphonia, as well as the functional effectiveness of medical, surgical, and behavioral interventions, several instruments have been developed, most of which are founded on the International Classification of Functioning, Disability and Health (World Health Organization, 2001) or its earlier version, the International Classification of Impairment, Disability and Handicap (World Health Organization, 1980).

The Voice Handicap Index (VHI; Jacobson, Johnson, Grywalski, et al., 1997) is a 30-item instrument designed to examine emotional, physical, and functional responses to dysphonia (**Fig. 7.1**). The emotional domain measures emotional response, the physical domain measures perceived vocal function and laryngeal discomfort, and the functional domain measures the impact of dysphonia on daily activities. The VHI has been validated and data have been published from several patient populations (Jacobson, Johnson, Grywalski, et al., 1997; Rosen and Murry, 2000; Rosen, Murry, Zinn, et al., 2000). An alternative tool, the Voice-Related Quality of Life Measure (V-RQOL; Hogikyan and Sethuraman, 1999), focuses specifically on quality of life changes associated with dysphonia and contains 10 items in two domains (social-emotional and physical functioning) (**Fig. 7.2**). The V-RQOL instrument has been used to measure

---

Voice Handicap Index (VHI), Henry Ford Hospital

Instructions: These are statements that many people have used to describe their voices and the effects of their voices on their lives. Circle the response that indicates how frequently you have the same experience.

F1. My voice makes it difficult for people to hear me.

P2. I run out of air when I talk.

F3. People have difficulty understanding me in a noisy room.

P4. The sound of my voice varies throughout the day.

F5. My family has difficulty hearing me when I call them throughout the house.

F6. I use the phone less often than I would like.

E7. I'm tense when talking with others because of my voice.

F8. I tend to avoid groups of people because of my voice.

E9. People seem irritated with my voice.

P10. People ask, "What's wrong with your voice?"

F11. I speak with friends, neighbors, or relatives less often because of my voice.

F12. People ask me to repeat myself when speaking face-to-face.

P13. My voice sounds creaky and dry.

P14. I feel as though I have to strain to produce voice.

E15. I find other people don't understand my voice problem.

F16. My voice difficulties restrict my personal and social life.

P17. The clarity of my voice is unpredictable.

P18. I try to change my voice to sound different.

F19. I feel left out of conversations because of my voice.

P20. I use a great deal of effort to speak.

P21. My voice is worse in the evening.

F22. My voice problem causes me to lose income.

E23. My voice problem upsets me.

E24. I am less outgoing because of my voice problem.

E25. My voice makes me feel handicapped.

P26. My voice "gives out" on me in the middle of speaking.

E27. I feel annoyed when people ask me to repeat.

E28. I feel embarrassed when people ask me to repeat.

E29. My voice makes me feel incompetent.

E30. I'm ashamed of my voice problem.

Note. The letter preceding each item number corresponds to the subscale (E = emotional subscale, F = functional subscale, P = physical subscale).

Figure 7.1 The Voice Handicap Index (VHI). (From Jacobson, B. H., Johnson, A., Grywalski, C., Silbergleit, A., Jacobson, G., Benninger, M. S., et al., [1997]. The Voice Handicap Index [VHI]: development and validation. Am J Speech Lang Pathol 6, 66–70. ©1997 The American Speech-Language-Hearing Association. Reprinted with permission.)

VOICE-RELATED QUALITY OF LIFE (V-RQOL) MEASURE
UNIVERSITY OF MICHIGAN

NAME:_____DATE:_____

We are trying to learn more about how a voice problem can interfere with your day to day activities. On this paper, you will find a list of possible voice-related problems. Please answer all questions based upon what **your** voice has been like over the past **two weeks**. There is no "right" or "wrong" answers.

Considering both how severe the problem is when you get it, and how frequently it happens, please rate each item below on how "bad" it is (that is, the **amount** of each problem that you have). Use the following scale for rating the **amount** of the problem:

1 = None, not a problem
2 = A small amount
3 = A moderate (medium) amount
4 = A lot
5 = Problem is as "bad as it can be"

Because of my voice,   How much of a problem is this?

1. I have trouble speaking loudly or being heard in noisy situations.	1	2	3	4	5
2. I run out of air and need to take frequent breaths when talking	1	2	3	4	5
3. I sometimes do not know what will come out when I begin speaking.	1	2	3	4	5
4. I am sometimes anxious or frustrated (because of my voice)	1	2	3	4	5
5. I sometimes get depressed (because of my voice)	1	2	3	4	5
6. I have trouble using the telephone (because of my voice)	1	2	3	4	5
7. I have trouble doing my job or practicing my profession (because of my voice)	1	2	3	4	5
8. I avoid going out socially (because of my voice)	1	2	3	4	5
9. I have to repeat myself to be understood.	1	2	3	4	5
10. I have become less outgoing (because of my voice)	1	2	3	4	5

Computational Algorithm

V-RQOL General Scoring Algorithm

$$100 - \left[\frac{(\text{Raw Score} - \text{\# items in domain or total})}{(\text{Highest Possible Raw Score} - \text{\# items})} \right] \times 100$$

Example for Total Score
If a Raw Score is 20

$$100 - \left[\frac{(10)}{(40)} \times 100 \right] = 100 - (0.25 \times 100) = 100 - 25 = 75 \text{ Standard Score}$$

Figure 7.2 The Voice-Related Quality of Life (V-RQOL) measure. (From Murry, T., Medrado, R., Hogikyan, N. D., Aviv, J. E. [2004]. The relationship between ratings of voice quality and quality of life measures. J Voice 18, 183–192. © 2004 The Voice Foundation. Reprinted with permission.)

clinical outcomes in patients with unilateral vocal fold paralysis (Hogikyan, Wodchis, Terrell, et al., 2000) and adductor spasmodic dysphonia (Hogikyan, Wodchis, Spak, et al, 2001; Rubin, Wodchis, Spak, et al, 2004). It also appears to be moderately correlated with clinician ratings of voice quality (Murry, Medrado, Hogikyan, et al, 2004). Ma and Yiu (2001) developed the Voice Activity and Participation Profile (VAPP) in response to evolution in the World Health Organization's classification system for impairment, disability, and handicap. This 28-item instrument assesses activity limitation and reduced willingness to participate in voice-related activities and spans five domains: self-perceived severity job, daily communication, social communication, and emotion. The VAPP has been validated and demonstrates good reliability.

A small number of instruments have been developed for outcomes measurement in specific patient populations. The Voice Outcome Survey (VOS; Gliklich, Glovsky, and Montgomery, 1999) contains five questions designed to measure daily activity and quality of life changes associated with unilateral vocal fold paralysis. The Pediatric Voice Outcome Survey (Hartnick, 2002; Hartnick, Volk, and Cunningham, 2003) is specifically targeted toward the pediatric voice patient and is intended to be completed by caregiver proxy. Both of these devices have undergone initial validation.

◆ Auditory Perceptual Analysis

Auditory perceptual analysis refers to the use of the human auditory perceptual system, often in combination with an external rating system, to make judgments of the nature and appropriateness of an individual's voice pitch, loudness, and quality. Some suggest the ability to relate perceptual judgments to the origin of dysphonias is a kind of art

Equal Appearing Interval

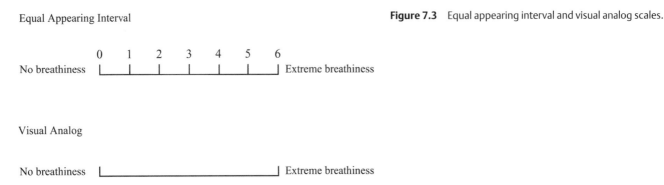

Figure 7.3   Equal appearing interval and visual analog scales.

form not unlike a musician recognizing a chord from a Beethoven symphony or a physician's recognition of a type of pathologic heartbeat or breath sound discerned from auscultation. Although recognized as an important clinical and research tool, perceptual analysis (especially the analysis of quality) has been characterized by questionable validity and poor reliability. It is often unclear which descriptors are the most meaningful in representing both normal and pathologic variations in voice quality. Beyond this, measurement and scaling issues can add further analysis error. Reliability issues have been traditionally associated with such instrument or external task factors; however, it appears that the inherent ability of judges to make reliable judgments must also be questioned (Gerratt, Kreiman, Antonanzas-Barroso, et al, 1993; Kreiman, Gerratt, Kempster, et al., 1993).

Regardless of the critical problems that plague perceptual judgments of voice, this analysis modality holds clear face validity and functional importance. Perceptual voice changes can indicate the presence of vocal pathology and often direct individuals to seek evaluation and treatment. Perceptual judgments are also critical to a patient's evaluation of change after treatment, as well as acceptance by significant others. Further, despite its apparent unreliability, the human auditory perceptual system allows complex and sophisticated judgments of quality, far superior in many ways to the algorithms that underlie acoustic indices. The human auditory perceptual system can process a noisy signal (such as a severely dysphonic voice) with more success than most artificial algorithms (Rabinov, Kreiman, Gerratt, et al, 1995). In some ways, the ability of the auditory perceptual system to make complex and sophisticated judgments is both an advantage and drawback, as judges (particularly experienced judges) appear to assign differing importance to different signal parameters, depending on the nature of the signal (Kreiman, Gerratt, and Precoda, 1990). This may be what manifests as poor reliability among judges.

Contemporary theory (Kreiman, Gerratt, Kempster, et al., 1993), supported by data from a programmatic series of studies (Gerratt and Kreiman, 2001; Gerratt, Kreiman, Antonanzas-Barroso, et al, 1993; Kreiman and Gerratt, 1998; Kreiman and Gerratt, 2000; Kreiman, Gerratt, and Precoda, 1990; Kreiman, Gerratt, Precoda, et al, 1992), suggests that individuals make voice quality judgments with respect to an inherently unstable internal standard, established according to rating experience and exposure to different (normal and pathologic) voices. Voice quality is perceived and processed in a sophisticated multidimensional manner, which is generally problematic for rating systems based on unidimensional scales of specific constructs (e.g., breathiness, roughness). Further, alternative scaling systems may vary in their ability to accurately capture and represent an individual's judgment (**Fig. 7.3**). Equal appearing interval (EAI) scales (which require selecting a value from a series of equally graduated values) allow a discrete response, but if too coarse, may not capture fine perceptual distinctions. Visual analog scales (which require placing a mark on a line with labeled extremes) allow finer perceptual ratings, but if too fine, risk introducing meaningless distinctions. These individual judge and measurement task factors should be carefully considered in the design or selection of any perceptual protocol for clinical application.

Traditional Perceptual Analysis of Voice Protocols

Several perceptual analysis protocols have been developed for the evaluation of voice. Several popular protocols, all developed in different countries, are introduced here. The GRBAS protocol, developed by the Japanese Society of Logopedics and Phoniatrics, contains five 4-point EAI scales: grade (overall severity), roughness, breathiness, asthenia (lack of vocal power), and strain (Hirano, 1981). Each parameter may be rated as 0 (normal), 1 (slightly impaired), 2 (moderately impaired), or 3 (extremely impaired). A training tape is available containing examples of each parameter and various parameter combinations. Developed in the United States, the Buffalo III Voice Profile employs 12 5-point EAI scales spanning both auditory perceptual and other variables: laryngeal tone, pitch, loudness, nasal resonance, oral resonance, breath supply, muscles (hyper- or hypotension), voice abuse, rate, speech anxiety, speech intelligibility, and overall voice rating (Wilson, 1987). Additional subprofiles are provided for specific populations/disorders. The Stockholm Voice Evaluation Approach (SVEA), developed in Sweden, contains 13 parameters: aphonia/intermittent aphonia, breathiness, hyperfunction/tension, hypofunction/laxness, vocal fry/creakiness, roughness, gratings/scrapiness, unstable quality/pitch, voice breaks, diplophonia, modal/falsetto register, pitch, and loudness (Hammarberg, 2000; Hammarberg

Consensus Auditory-Perceptual Evaluation of Voice (CAPE-V)

Name:_____   Date:_____

The following parameters of voice quality will be rated upon completion of the following tasks:
1. Sustained vowels, /a/ and /i/ for 3-5 seconds duration each.
2. Sentence production:
    a. The blue spot is on the key again.   d. We eat eggs every Easter.
    b. How hard did he hit him?   e. My mama makes lemon muffins.
    c. We were away a year ago.   f. Peter will keep at the peak.
3. Spontaneous speech in response to: "Tell me about your voice problem." or "Tell me how your voice is functioning."

> **Legend:** C = Consistent   I = Intermittent
> MI = Mildly Deviant
> MO = Moderately Deviant
> SE = Severely Deviant

<u>SCORE</u>

Overall Severity _____   C   I   ___/100
                MI   MO   SE

Roughness   _____   C   I   ___/100
                MI   MO   SE

Breathiness   _____   C   I   ___/100
                MI   MO   SE

Strain   _____   C   I   ___/100
                MI   MO   SE

Pitch   (Indicate the nature of the abnormality): _____
                 _____   C   I   ___/100
                MI   MO   SE

Loudness   (Indicate the nature of the abnormality): _____
                 _____   C   I   ___/100
                MI   MO   SE

_____   _____   C   I   ___/100
                MI   MO   SE

_____   _____   C   I   ___/100
                MI   MO   SE

COMMENTS ABOUT RESONANCE: NORMAL   OTHER (Provide description):_____

ADDITIONAL FEATURES (for example, diplophonia, fry, falsetto, asthenia, aphonia, pitch instability, tremor, wet/gurgly, or other relevant terms):

Clinician:_____

Figure 7.4 The Consensus Auditory Perceptual Evaluation of Voice (CAPE-V) rating form. Drafted in 2003, this tool for the clinical auditory-perceptual assessment of voice is currently undergoing field testing. [© 2003] The American Speech-Language-Hearing Association, Special Interest Division 3, Voice and Voice Disorders. Reprinted with permission.)

and Gauffin, 1995). Developed in the United Kingdom, the Vocal Profile Analysis (VPA) scheme is an extensive, phonetically based rating protocol containing more than 30 parameters, including vocal tract and prosodic features (Laver, 1980; Laver, 2000).

Regardless of the rating paradigm employed, the clinician should begin attending to the perceptual characteristics of a patient's voice immediately on the initial greeting and continue throughout the case history and various assessment tasks. It is important to gauge both perceptual features as well as the appropriateness of these features for the patient's sex, age, and cultural orientation. In addition, the clinician should note variation associated with particular assessment tasks or trial therapy. Perceptual voice changes under certain conditions may give invaluable insight into the etiology of a condition, as well as prognosis for treatment.

Recent Approaches to Perceptual Analysis of Voice

Several recent approaches to the perceptual analysis of voice demonstrate promise in overcoming (or at least curtailing) the theoretical and practical challenges that are inherent to this area. In 2002, a consensus meeting convened by the American Speech-Language-Hearing Association's (ASHA) Special Interest Division on Voice and Voice Disorders resulted in the development of a pilot assessment instrument, named the Consensus Auditory Perceptual Evaluation of Voice (CAPE-V) (**Fig. 7.4**). The CAPE-V represents the consensus committee's minimum recommended standard for the auditory perceptual analysis of voice disorders and is intended to facilitate increased consistency across individuals in clinical practice. The CAPE-V instrument contains six primary perceptual parameters (overall severity, roughness, breathiness, strain, pitch, loudness), which are rated using 100-mm visual analog scales and judged as either consistently or intermittently present. Ratings are designed to be completed after the production of isolated vowels, sentences, and a connected speech sample. Scales are provided for rating any additional prominent voice parameters, and space is provided for describing resonance and other notable features. At present, the CAPE-V instrument is undergoing field testing, and experimental data on its validity and reliability are forthcoming. Future plans for this instrument include the availability of perceptual referents (anchors) and the development of a training system.

Two recent approaches directly address the presumed variability and instability of the internal standards used by raters in making perceptual judgments. The first approach involves the use of external standards, or anchors, placed at discrete points on a rating scale. By substituting a rater's internal standards with these explicit external standards, rating reliability is significantly improved (Chan and Yiu, 2002; Gerratt, Kreiman, Antonanzas-Barroso, et al., 1993). The second approach, named analysis by synthesis, requires judges to manipulate voice synthesis parameters to obtain an auditory perceptual match with a target sample (Gerratt and Kreiman, 2001). These explicit comparisons bypass the need for internal standard comparisons, also resulting in enhanced reliability across judges.

◆ Acoustic Analysis

Acoustic analysis of vocal function is widely employed in clinical and research settings. By carefully examining sound signals radiated from the mouth, considerable information can be inferred regarding underlying laryngeal physiology. Acoustic studies are typically performed using either live or recorded voice samples and are therefore noninvasive.

Whereas the potential benefits of acoustic analysis are many, it is important that the application and interpretation of these tools is based on a solid conceptualization of relevant theory. Clinicians should hold at least a rudimentary knowledge of source-filter theory and principles of digital signal processing, as well as the algorithmic makeup and potential susceptibility to error of specific analysis tools. By maintaining a balanced and informed perspective across these areas, clinicians will obtain the most benefit from acoustic instrumentation.

Underlying Principles

Source-Filter Theory

First described by Fant (1960), the source-filter theory of speech production forms the foundation of contemporary

understanding in vocal tract acoustics. The central tenet of the theory is that acoustic energy produced by a sound source (the glottal spectrum) is propagated through a filtering system (the vocal tract), resulting in a modified output waveform (**Fig. 7.5**). The glottal spectrum, generated by the vibratory pattern of the vocal folds, is rich in harmonics that decline in energy with increasing frequency. When the harmonically rich glottal waveform is transmitted through the supralaryngeal cavities, individual frequency components are maximized or minimized. Frequency bands allowing maximum acoustic energy transfer are termed *formants*. Formants are analogous to the natural modes of vibration within the vocal tract and can be derived from knowledge of its physical dimensions. Formants may be described in terms of center frequency, bandwidth, and amplitude.

The source-filter theory is based on two primary assumptions: linearity and time invariance (Kent, 1993). Linearity assumes that the model responds equally to several individual inputs as to the sum of those individual inputs. Time invariance states that the model responds indifferently to

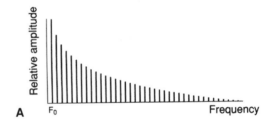

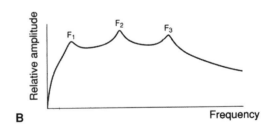

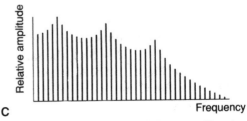

Figure 7.5 Central principles of the source-filter theory. The glottal spectrum (**A**) is propagated through the vocal tract filter (**B**), resulting a modified output spectrum (**C**). (From Titze, I. R. [1994a]. Principles of voice production. Englewood Cliffs, NJ: Prentice-Hall. [© 1994] Ingo R. Titze. Reprinted with permission.)

input that is either time-delayed or time-advanced. These assumptions do not hold under every circumstance; however, they are fairly robust and allow the application and interpretation of several powerful analysis tools. The majority of acoustic analysis procedures described in this chapter will follow source-filter assumptions; however, an introduction to nonlinear approaches will also be provided.

Digital Signal Processing

Contemporary methods in the acoustic analysis of voice are heavily reliant upon computer technology. Initially, however, the acoustic signal must be converted to a digital format that can be readily used by a computer. This process is termed *analog-to-digital conversion* (A/D conversion) and is a form of digital signal processing. A/D conversion comprises translating a continuously varying analog signal to a discretely defined digital signal. Three essential stages are involved: filtering, sampling, and quantization.

The filtering operations employed in A/D conversion consist of equalization of acoustic energy across the entire frequency range (preemphasis filtering), followed by elimination of acoustic energy above the highest frequency of interest (presampling filtering) (Kent and Read, 2002; Owens, 1993). Sampling involves taking discrete measurements of signal energy at regular time intervals (**Fig. 7.6**). Signal information from between these sampling points is discarded; however, assuming an appropriate sampling rate (measured in hertz; Hz) has been selected, the digital waveform can still be considered equivalent to its analog source. Quantization entails translating the amplitude values of the signal into discrete units (**Fig. 7.7**). The greater the number of quantization levels (measured in bit rate), the higher the resolution of the digitized signal.

Each step in the A/D conversion process plays a key role in the preservation of signal integrity for subsequent analysis. Equalization is useful when dealing with speech input to compensate for the characteristic irregularity of energy distribu-

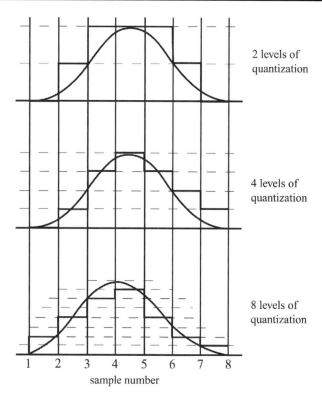

Figure 7.7 Quantization of an analog signal. An increased number of quantization levels results in increased resolution of the digitized signal. (From Kent, R. D., Read, C. [2002]. Acoustic analysis of speech [2nd ed.]. Albany: Delmar Learning. [© 2002.] Reprinted with permission of Delmar Learning, a division of Thomson Learning: www.thomson-rights.com.)

tion across low and high frequencies. Selecting an appropriate presampling filter cutoff and sampling rate is critical to avoid signal misrepresentation in the form of aliasing. Aliasing refers to the presence of a false waveform, reconstructed at a lower frequency than the original signal, and occurs when less than two samples are taken from each waveform cycle (**Fig. 7.8**). Thus, a valid digital representation of a signal requires a minimum sampling rate at least twice the highest frequency of interest, with presampling filtering of all signal energy above the highest frequency of interest. This rule was first stated by Nyquist (1928), and later proved by Shannon (1949).

Guidelines for the acquisition of acoustic voice signals suggest a minimum sampling rate of 20 kHz (20,000 samples per second) and a minimum quantization rate of 16 bits (65,536 discrete levels of signal amplitude) (Titze, 1995). With continual increases in computing power and data storage capacity, these values can be often exceeded with negligible sacrifices in processing speed and storage availability.

Practical Guidelines

Data Collection

The use of appropriate technical and procedural protocols is important in ensuring the integrity of data collected for acoustic analysis (Titze, 1995). Acoustic recording is best performed using a professional-grade condenser microphone, maintained at a distance of 3 to 4 cm and angle of 45

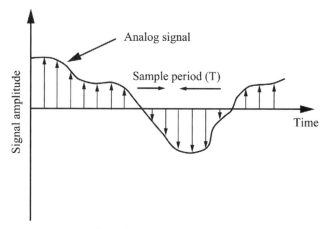

Figure 7.6 Digital sampling of an analog signal. Discrete measurements of signal amplitude are taken at each sampling period. (From Owens, F. J. [1993]. Signal processing of speech. New York: McGraw-Hill. © 1993 McGraw-Hill [U.S., Canada, Mexico] and Palgrave Macmillan [rest of world]. Reprinted with permission.)

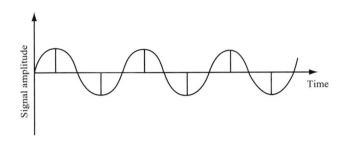

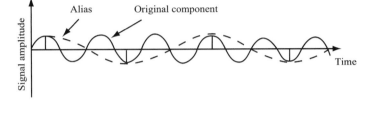

Figure 7.8   Aliasing of a digitized signal due to an inadequate sampling rate (sampling below the Nyquist frequency). (From Owens, F. J. [1993]. Signal processing of speech. New York: McGraw-Hill. [© 1993] McGraw-Hill [U.S., Canada, Mexico] and Palgrave Macmillan [rest of world]. Reprinted with permission.)

to 90 degrees from the mouth. A head-mounted microphone is preferable for ensuring a constant mouth-to-microphone distance. Ambient noise and room reverberation should be minimized and a sound-treated room used when possible. Data should be either directly digitized to computer or stored using digital audio tape (DAT) technology.

For the majority of voice applications, sustained vowels are the most appropriate tokens for acoustic voice analysis. Because of the influence of vowel type, fundamental frequency (F_0), and intensity on vocal perturbation (Gelfer, 1995; Orlikoff and Baken, 1990; Orlikoff and Kahane, 1991), it is important to report these variables when conducting such analyses. Further, accurate and reliable perturbation extraction requires analysis across multiple tokens, each containing several hundred vibratory cycles (Karnell, 1991; Scherer, Vail, and Guo, 1995).

Analysis Tools

The acoustic waveform contains an enormous amount of potentially useful information. A central challenge in the acoustic analysis of voice involves defining and extracting those waveform features that most accurately reflect laryngeal function. As stated, the majority of techniques are dependent upon the source filter theory, exploiting the linear separability of the glottal source and vocal tract function. Though often complex and constantly being refined, many algorithms continue to be vulnerable to error, particularly in the analysis of severely dysphonic voices (Rabinov, Kreiman, Gerratt, et al., 1995). Nevertheless, when appropriately applied and carefully interpreted, acoustic measures hold significant value in describing vocal function.

After a consensus meeting in 1994, The National Center for Voice and Speech (NCVS) issued a summary statement recommending analysis selection based on signal typing (Titze, 1995). Three signals types were differentiated in terms of periodicity and the presence of bifurcations. Signals that are nearly periodic with no bifurcations or strong modulating frequencies (denoted *type 1 signals*) may be appropriately

analyzed using perturbation indices. Signals that contain bifurcations and/or strong modulating frequencies (denoted *type 2 signals*) may be best analyzed using visual displays that permit appreciation of qualitative changes within the analysis segment (e.g., nonlinear phase plots, spectrograms, F_0 contours). Signals that are completely aperiodic (denoted *type 3 signals*) may be best analyzed using perceptual ratings. If adhered to, these consensus guidelines can help protect against inappropriate analyses and maximize the utility of acoustic data. The following section outlines analysis tools commonly employed in the acoustic assessment of voice.

Fundamental Frequency   Fundamental frequency (F_0) corresponds with the rate of oscillation of the vocal folds (expressed in Hz), and is a primary factor in the perception of pitch. The accurate determination of F_0 by computer is extremely challenging and has been identified as a crucial problem in the acoustic analysis of voice (Read, Buder, and Kent, 1992). In an attempt to improve the accuracy of F_0 capture, scientists have approached the acoustic signal using a variety of methods (**Fig. 7.9**). Algorithms such as peak-picking and zero-crossing measure the interval between discrete signal events (such as amplitude peaks or the upward crossing of a horizontal axis) to determine the fundamental period. Strategies such as autocorrelation match the waveform with a time-delayed copy of itself, assuming that the copy with the best match is delayed by the fundamental period. Cepstral analysis involves performing sequential Fourier transformations on the signal and measuring the quefrency (equivalent to the fundamental period) at the point of greatest cepstral energy.

Each of these approaches to F_0 extraction is vulnerable to contamination by signal noise and periodicity, irregularities in waveform morphology, rapid changes in formant structure, and the presence of subharmonics. These difficulties may be partially overcome by low-pass filtering the signal prior to analysis (Titze and Liang, 1993), in addition to appropriate signal type selection (Titze, 1995). Comparison between F_0 extraction methods appears to suggest that strategies based on waveform matching may be the most

Zero-Crossing

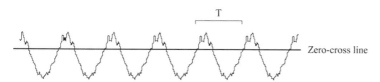

Zero-cross line

Figure 7.9   Illustration of F_0 extraction using zero-crossing and autocorrelation algorithms. In zero-crossing, the fundamental period is determined from adjacent upward crossings of the zero-cross line. In autocorrelation, the waveform is matched with time-delayed copies of itself. The waveform copy with the strongest correlation is delayed by the fundamental period.

Autocorrelation

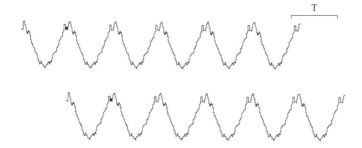

reliable, at least when variations in F_0 are less than 6% (Titze and Winholtz, 1993). Incorporating at least two extraction methods into an analysis and comparing the results across algorithms is another method of guarding against instrument failure (Read, Buder, and Kent, 1992).

F_0 is primarily modulated by changes in vocal fold length, mass, and tension. Variation in one or more of these parameters can occur as the result of normal individual differences or the presence of pathology. Adult vocal folds are longer and have greater mass than those of children, resulting in a lower F_0; likewise, male vocal folds are longer and have greater mass than those of females, resulting in a lower F_0 (Eckel, Koebke, Sittel, et al., 1999; Hirano, Kurita, and Nakashima, 1983). Hormonal changes influencing vocal fold mass and tension may also contribute to changes in F_0 in older adults (Hollien, 1987). Excessively high F_0 may result from restricted vocal fold length and mass (e.g., due to a laryngeal web, or androgen deficiency in pubescent males) or elevated musculoskeletal tension and laryngeal posture. Excessively low F_0 may result from increased vocal fold mass (e.g., due to vocal fold edema or polypoid degeneration or androgen exposure in females) or decreased tension (e.g., due to superior laryngeal nerve neuropathy and impaired cricothyroid function).

F_0 may be measured using a sustained vowel token produced at a comfortable pitch level, a specified target within a patient's F_0 range, or during a speaking or reading task. A sustained vowel production is useful in obtaining an F_0 trace across time, which may reveal the presence of bifurcations or subharmonics, as well as long-term vocal instability such as tremor. Speaking and reading tasks (best performed using nonemotive material) allow an estimation of mean speaking F_0, as well as the standard deviation of speaking F_0 (also called *pitch sigma*). Measurement of F_0 range can highlight difficulties with vocal fold length and tension manipulation, neuromuscular control, or reduced tissue pliability.

Typical speaking, F_0 values vary as a function of age, sex, psychologic state, loudness, and speech task. Normative values have been summarized by Baken and Orlikoff (2000). Prepubescent males and females have comparable F_0 values of around 220 to 240 Hz, which differentiate to ~100 to 120 Hz and 200 to 220 Hz in adult males and females, respectively. This sex difference generally narrows beyond the seventh decade, as speaking F_0 increases in males and decreases slightly in females (**Fig. 7.10**).

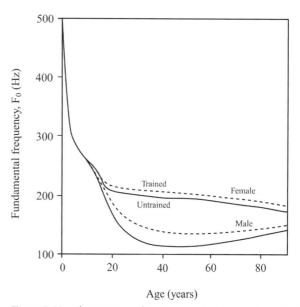

Figure 7.10   Changes in speaking F_0 across the life span, for trained and untrained voices. (From Titze, I. R. [1994a]. Principles of voice production. Englewood Cliffs, NJ: Prentice-Hall. [© 1994] Ingo R. Titze. Based on data reported in Brown, W. S., Morris, R. J., Hollien, H., Howell, E. [1991]. Speaking fundamental frequency characteristics as a function of age and professional singing. J Voice 5, 310–315. Reprinted with permission.)

Intensity   Vocal intensity, the physical correlate of loudness, varies as a function of both subglottal pressure (Ps) and vocal fold vibratory amplitude. Increasing Ps during normal phonation will result in increased vibratory amplitude and mucosal wave excursion. Elevated intensity in a normal conversational situation may reflect difficulty of self-monitoring due to a conductive hearing loss. Reduced intensity may be indicative of poor respiratory support, incomplete glottal closure, or reduced tissue pliability restricting vocal fold vibratory amplitude. In addition, reduced tissue pliability may contribute to difficulty achieving vocal fold oscillation at low Ps, limiting voice production at low intensities.

Intensity is expressed using the decibel (dB) and can be simply measured using a sound-level meter. Alternatively, intensity can be measured using the amplitude of an appropriately calibrated acoustic voice signal. As with F_0, intensity measurements can be made during a production of a sustained vowel token, during a speaking or reading task, or at intensity extremes (for the measurement of dynamic range). Vocal intensity tends to increase alongside increases in F_0, varies as a function of physical and psychologic state, and is typically 2 dB greater in both children compared with adults and in males compared with females (Coleman, Mabis, and Hinson, 1977; Susser and Bless, 1983).

Voice Range Profile   The voice range profile (VRP), or phonetogram, combines F_0 and dynamic range data in a visual representation of the physiologic limits of the vocal system (**Fig. 7.11**). The VRP can be obtained using a keyboard and sound level meter, although automated computer programs are also available to assist with data collection and presentation. Intensity is typically presented in dBs and F_0 using either linear frequency (Hz), logarithmic semitones (ST), or percentage of total range. The VRP for a normal voice has a general form characterized by greater dynamic range in the midfrequency region and tapering near the frequency extremes. The contours for minimum and maximum intensity also tend to increase alongside increasing F_0. The VRP can be described both qualitatively and quantitatively. Variations have been reported as a function of age, sex, history of vocal training, and the presence of vocal pathology (Speyer, Wieneke, van Wijck-Warnaar, et al., 2003; Sulter, Schutte, and Miller, 1995; Teles-Magalhaes, Pegoraro-Krook, and Pegoraro, 2000; Wuyts, Heylen, Mertens, et al., 2003). Methodological considerations have been outlined by Coleman (1993).

Spectrography and Spectral Measures   Spectrography is a powerful analytic technique providing insight into both glottal source and vocal tract filter functions. The spectrogram is obtained by transformation of the acoustic waveform from the time domain to the frequency domain, specifically by the application of Fourier's theorem. The resulting display presents frequency on the vertical axis, time on the horizontal axis, and intensity as the darkness of the plot (**Fig. 7.12**). Spectrograms are extracted using a variable pass-band filter, which at a narrow-band setting (around 50 Hz) captures individual harmonics produced by the glottal source and at a wide-band setting (300 to 500 Hz) captures formants resonating within the vocal tract (**Fig. 7.13**). Precise filter set-

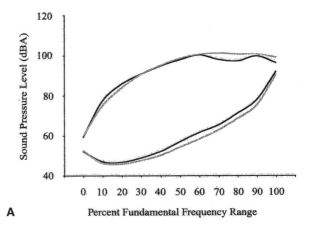

A

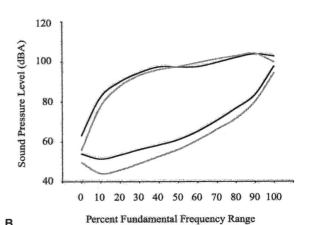

B

Figure 7.11   Mean voice range profiles (VRPs) collected from a series of (**A**) males and (**B**) females. Dark lines represent untrained voices. Light lines represent trained voices. (Constructed based on data from Sulter, A. M., Schutte, H. K., Miller, D. G. [1995]. Differences in phonetogram features between male and female subjects with and without vocal training. J Voice 9, 363–377.)

tings are mandated by the F_0 of the source signal (e.g., a wide-band filter setting for an adult male may result in a narrow-band spectrogram when used with a child's voice).

In addition to providing harmonic and formant information, the spectrogram can provide qualitative insight into abnormal voice quality. Whereas a normal voice signal contains well-defined harmonics/formants, a dysphonic voice signal is often characterized by weak and irregular harmonic/formant patterns and high-frequency noise (Yanagihara, 1967). Bifurcations may also be observed in type 2 signals.

Spectral information can also be extracted using fast Fourier transformation (FFT) or linear predictive coding (LPC) (Owens, 1993). These mathematical procedures allow the derivation of frequency and amplitude data for a short time window. A related measure, the long-term average spectrum (LTAS), provides spectral information across an extended window and can be used with reading and conversational speech samples (**Fig. 7.14**). Differences in peak energy region, as well as spectral shape and tilt, have been reported as a function of sex, age, and the presence of vocal

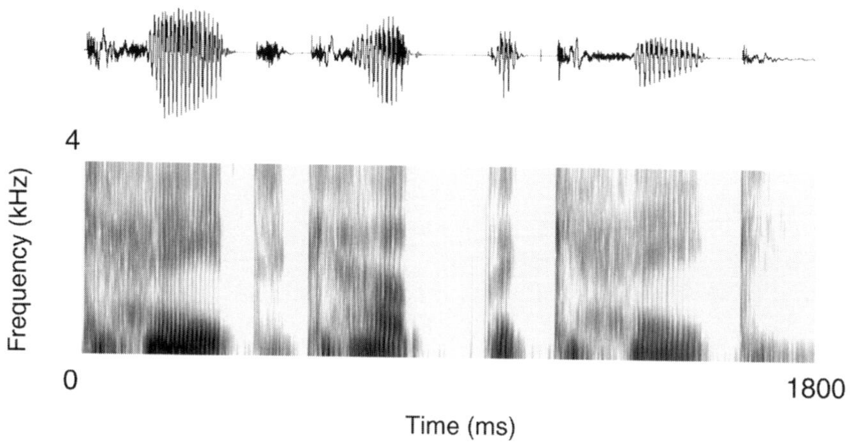

Figure 7.12 Acoustic signal and spectrogram of the phrase "Kate cut the cake."

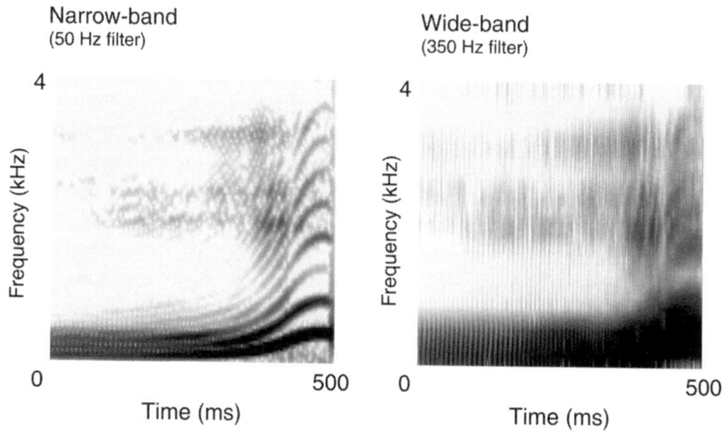

4

Frequency (kHz)

0

1800

Time (ms)

Narrow-band
(50 Hz filter)

4

Frequency (kHz)

0

500

Time (ms)

Wide-band
(350 Hz filter)

4

Frequency (kHz)

0

500

Time (ms)

Figure 7.13 Narrow and wide-band spectrograms of an increasing pitch glide on the vowel /i/. The narrow-band spectrogram shows individual harmonics, whereas the wide-band spectrogram shows formants. The vertical striations seen in the wide-band spectrogram represent vocal fold vibratory pulses.

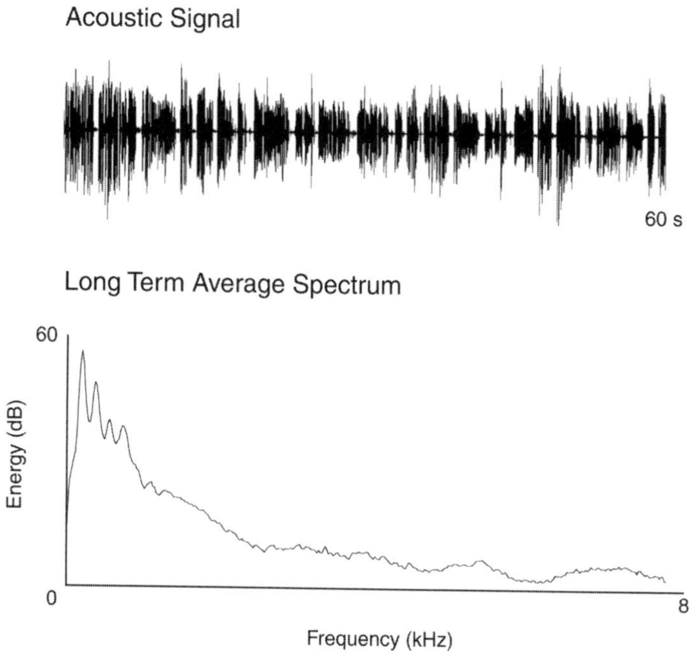

Acoustic Signal

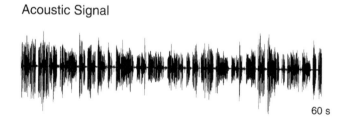

60 s

Figure 7.14 A long-term average spectrum (LTAS) extracted from a 60-second conversational sample.

Long Term Average Spectrum

60

Energy (dB)

0

0

8

Frequency (kHz)

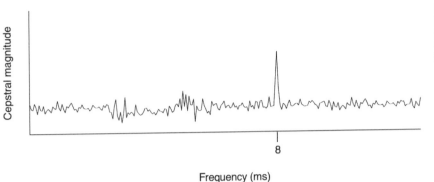

Figure 7.15 The cepstral waveform. The magnitude of the dominant rahmonic, situated at the fundamental period, has been associated with voice quality. Here, a quefrency of 8 milliseconds indicates an F_0 of 125 Hz.

pathology (Kitzing and Akerlund, 1993; Linville, 2002; Mendoza, Valencia, Munoz, et al., 1996; White, 2001).

Cepstral analysis, introduced earlier as a useful tool in the extraction of F_0, also holds application in the acoustic analysis of voice quality. The dominant cepstral rahmonic, situated at the fundamental period, is an indicator of the strength of the rahmonic component of the input signal (**Fig. 7.15**). Several studies have reported an association between dominant harmonic magnitude and perceptual ratings of voice quality (Dejonckere, 1998; Dejonckere and Lebacq, 1996; Hillenbrand, Cleveland, and Erickson, 1994; Hillenbrand and Houde, 1996).

Perturbation Measures   Perturbation refers to the presence of cycle-to-cycle variation in F_0, amplitude, and waveform morphology. Jitter refers to cycle-to-cycle variation in signal frequency (**Fig. 7.16**). Shimmer refers to cycle-to-cycle variation in signal amplitude. Indices such as signal-to-noise ratio (SNR; Klingholz, 1987) and harmonics-to-noise ratio (HNR; Yumoto, Gould, and Baer, 1982) are more general measures of perturbation across F_0, amplitude, and waveform morphology. In normal voices, some degree of cycle-to-cycle perturbation is expected; in contrast, excessive levels of perturbation have been associated with the presence of vocal pathology (Laver, Hiller, and Mackenzie Beck, 1992).

Physiologically, the presence of perturbation in the voice signal is indicative of some degree of irregularity in vocal fold vibration. Several specific contributing mechanisms have been hypothesized. These include momentary fluctuations in neuromuscular activity (Orlikoff, 1989), subtle asymmetries in vocal fold shape and stiffness, aerodynamic

turbulence (Titze, 1994a), and systolic pressure shifts within vocal fold blood vessels (Orlikoff, 1990a,b). Although these factors likely contribute to the small degree of waveform aperiodicity observed in normal voices, more severe perturbations are almost always secondary to pathology.

Whereas the existence of perturbation in the vocal signal is universally agreed upon, no consensus has been reached regarding its precise mathematical definition. As stated by Titze (1994a), there are many ways to approach the quantification of pattern deviation. It is perhaps for this reason that so many perturbation algorithms have emerged. Absolute measures reflect absolute differences in duration or amplitude across sequential vocal cycles and are easily converted into percentage values for the entire analysis window. Relative measures (e.g., relative average perturbation, frequency perturbation quotient, amplitude perturbation quotient) have been developed to account for long-term trends in F_0 or amplitude, often by deriving a second-order perturbation function. SNR and HNR indices calculate the relative presence of harmonic and noise energy within a signal. The NCVS consensus guidelines for perturbation measurement recommend using mean absolute measures by default and second-order measures only when faced with a clear long-term trend (Titze, 1995). Signal typing is always necessary to determine the appropriateness of any perturbation measure.

Nonlinear Measures   Nonlinear approaches to the acoustic analysis of voice are centered on the fact that the complex and often unpredictable nature of vocal fold vibration is not adequately accounted for by linear assumptions (such as which underlie the source filter theory of speech production).

Acoustic signal

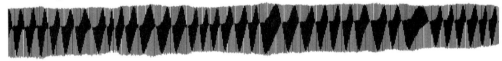

F_0 trace

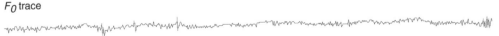

Mean F_0 = 126.3 Hz

Figure 7.16 F_0 trace of a sustained vowel produced by a normal speaker, illustrating subtle irregularities across time. These cycle-to-cycle irregularities reflect frequency perturbation, or jitter.

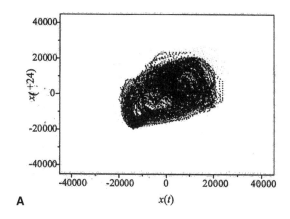

A

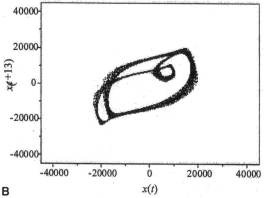

B

Figure 7.17 Phase spaces calculated from acoustic signals collected from a single patient (**A**) before and (**B**) after phonosurgery for the removal of vocal fold polyps. The postsurgical plot reveals greater trajectory stability than the presurgical plot. (From Zhang, Y., McGilligan, C., Zhou, L., Vig, M., Jiang, J. J. [2004]. Nonlinear dynamic analysis of voices before and after surgical excision of vocal polyps. J Acoust Soc Am 115[5 Pt 1], 2270–2277. © 2004 Acoustical Society of America. Reprinted with permission.)

These analysis approaches are rooted in nonlinear dynamic theory, which views the output of certain complex systems as not random but characterized by inherent system nonlinearities. Such systems are termed *chaotic* and by definition must be deterministic (governed by initial conditions and rules), nonlinear, unpredictable, low-dimensional (controlled by relatively few parameters), and highly sensitive to initial conditions (whereby small changes grow exponentially with time) (Baken, 2003).

A popular method for displaying the output of a nonlinear dynamic system is to plot its trajectory in a phase space (**Fig. 7.17**). A phase space represents the independent variables of a system as dimensions in the space. Any variable of interest can be examined (e.g, mass, displacement, velocity, time, and so forth); however, in the case of an acoustic signal represented in the time domain, it is common practice to convert the signal into phase space using a time delay coordinate for each dimension (Herzel, Berry, Titze, et al., 1994). As a signal is represented in phase space over time, it may shift from an

unstable toward a stable or asymptotic trajectory. This stable trajectory is termed an *attractor*. Herzel, Berry, Titze, et al., (1994) described four attractor types: stable stationary states, limit cycles (characterized by a limiting trajectory), tori (representing multiple superimposed oscillators at independent frequencies), and chaotic (nonperiodic).

Several investigators have demonstrated the applicability of nonlinear dynamic analysis to the clinically disordered voice (Giovanni, Ouaknine, and Triglia, 1999; Herzel, Berry, Titze, et al., 1994; Herzel, Berry, Titze, et al., 1995; Zhang, McGilligan, Zhou, et al., 2004). These studies have used phase portraits and other qualitative methods for identifying system attractors, in addition to a range of quantitative measures, such as Lyapunov exponents (which reflect the rate of divergence [or convergence] of initially neighboring trajectories over time), dimension measures, and various entropy measures (which reflect the degree of disorder and rate of dynamic system information loss over time).

◆ Aerodynamic Analysis

Aerodynamic analysis of voice involves measuring changes in air volume, flow, and pressure during phonation. Variation in these parameters allows insight into both respiratory and laryngeal performance. In many cases, a variety of measurement and analysis approaches are available to the clinician or scientist. These approaches vary considerably in terms of the need for specialized equipment, as well as the degree of invasiveness imposed on the patient.

As with acoustic analysis, aerodynamic studies are often dependent upon digital signal processing techniques and, in the case of inverse filtering of the flow waveform, source-filter theory. Contemporary data acquisition systems employ flow and pressure transducers, which produce analog voltage signals for A/D conversion. These signals, as with acoustic signals captured using a microphone transducer, are vulnerable to aliasing in the hands of an inexperienced user. These signals must also be appropriately calibrated using a standard instrument (e.g., a U-tube manometer for pressure, a flowmeter or rotameter for flow).

Volume

Volume refers to the three-dimensional amount of air either present or displaced within a system. Common air-volume measurements include total lung volume, vital capacity (maximum exhaled volume after maximum inhalation), tidal volume (mean volume transported during resting breathing), inspiratory reserve volume (maximum forced inspiratory volume immediately after a resting inspiratory cycle), expiratory reserve volume (maximum forced expiratory volume immediately after a resting inspiratory cycle), and residual volume (volume remaining after forceful exhalation). Whereas these measures provide useful information concerning the integrity of the respiratory system, it is important to note that the air volume required to sustain voice and speech for typical communication is considerably less than that required to sustain life. With the exception of singing, which may be initiated using close to 100% of vital capacity (Watson and Hixon, 1985), most voicing tasks do not tax the volumetric limits of an intact respiratory system.

Pulmonary function values vary systematically with age, sex, and height (Baldwin, Courand, and Richards, 1948), as well as the presence of obstructive or restrictive pulmonary disease. Vital capacity is typically greater in males compared with females, adults compared with children, tall individuals compared with short individuals, and young adults compared with older adults. Racial-ethnic differences have also been reported (Golshan, Nematbakhsh, Amra, et al., 2003; Zheng and Zhong, 2002). Several researchers have offered predictive equations for the estimation of pulmonary function values, traditionally using linear regression but more recently using polynomial regression functions (Glindmeyer, Lefante, McColloster, et al., 1995).

Volume data can be collected using a variety of direct and indirect techniques. Wet spirometry relies on the air-volume displacement of water within a closed system; however, it is not always sensitive to the fast-moving volume displacements associated with speech. Alternatively, volume can be derived from mean flow data collected using a pneumotachograph. Other methods rely on the relationship between volume displacement and movements of the chest wall (typically measured at the ribcage and abdomen), which have been measured using magnetometers (Hixon, Goldman, and Mead, 1973; Hixon, Mead, and Goldman, 1976) and inductance plethysmographs (Russell and Stathopoulos, 1988). Although providing valuable information on the relative contribution of the ribcage and abdomen to volume changes during speech breathing events, these tools are mostly employed in research settings.

Phonation Volume

The maximum volume of air exhaled on a sustained phonatory task (after maximum inhalation) is called phonation volume (PV; Yangihara and von Leden, 1967). PV is the product of maximum phonation time (MPT) and flow (both discussed below) and is directly related to vital capacity. Because of this, PV is influenced by the same factors that influence vital capacity, namely age, sex, and height.

Maximum Phonation Time and the S/Z Ratio

Two traditionally popular indirect clinical measures of respiratory integrity and laryngeal valving efficiency are MPT and the s/z ratio. MPT reflects the maximum duration of a sustained vowel after maximum inhalation and is typically averaged across multiple trials. As inferred above, MPT is a direct function of PV and flow and is also influenced by vital capacity. Thus, any variation in MPT may be a function of altered PV (reflecting respiratory support for phonation) and/or altered flow (reflecting glottal efficiency). In other words, MPT does not allow the differentiation of respiratory versus laryngeal valving issues. MPT is influenced by the same variables that influence PV and vital capacity.

The s/z ratio (Boone, 1977) compares the maximum duration of sustained /s/ and /z/ fricatives after maximum inhalation and across multiple trials. The principle underlying this measure is an assumption that maximum glottal efficiency will result in equal duration for both the /s/ and /z/ fricatives, yielding a theoretical ratio of 1.0. Any reduction in glottal efficiency should result in decreased /z/ duration relative to /s/, resulting in a ratio greater than 1.0. Several studies have reported s/z ratios below 1.0 in the normal population (Sorenson and Parker, 1992; Tait, Michel, and Carpenter, 1980), presumably due to an additional flow impedance source during /z/ production (glottal and lingual) compared with /s/ (lingual only). In an early study of the clinical applicability of this tool, Eckel and Boone (1981) reported ratios in excess of 1.4 for 95% of individuals with documented vocal fold lesions. Subsequent research has failed to replicate this finding (Hufnagle and Hufnagel, 1988; Rastatter and Hyman, 1982; Sorenson and Parker, 1992), lending question to the sensitivity of this measure.

As with any maximum performance task, MPT and the s/z ratio are susceptible to variability both within and across individuals. This variability may be controlled to some degree by detailed instruction, coaching, and repeated trials. Kent, Kent, and Rosenbek (1987), in summarizing the literature on this topic, concluded that it may take as many as 10 trials to obtain a true MPT value. It is important to remember that this may not be clinically practical and may even introduce fatigue. Other (less easily controlled) sources of variability in these indices may include the use of novel glottal valving and lingual articulation strategies in an attempt to sustain constant phonatory/fricative output while compensating for decreasing lung volumes (Christensen, Fletcher, and McCutcheon, 1992; Solomon, Garlitz, and Milbrath, 2000).

Flow

Flow is a measure of volume velocity, or air volume displaced as a function of time. Mean flow (also referred to as DC flow) can be simply derived from volume and time for a given phonatory task. Alternatively, mean flow can be measured using a pneumotachograph (Rothenberg, 1973, 1977) or hot wire anemometer (Kitajima, 1985; Woo, 1986; Woo, Colton, and Shangold, 1987) placed at the mouth, based on the assumption that an open vocal tract (during vowel production) has a negligible influence on flow. Such measurement of mean flow can provide insight into laryngeal valving efficiency. High flow rates may reflect an incomplete closure pattern and/or short closed phase, whereas low flow rates may reflect a pressed phonatory pattern and long closed phase. Normative data for mean flow are highly variable (Hirano, 1981; Wilson and Starr, 1985), possibly reflecting a wide range of laryngeal valving strategies across individuals. Because of this, mean flow is not a sensitive measure in isolation. Several derivative aerodynamic indices, of which mean flow is a component, are discussed below.

Inverse Filtering

Rothenberg (1973) introduced a technique whereby the flow signal captured at the mouth is processed to remove the filtering influence of the vocal tract, yielding an estimate of the actual glottal flow waveform. This process, termed *inverse filtering*, can also be applied to the radiated acoustic signal (Miller and Matthews, 1963). Inverse filtering is inherently appealing, as it allows the noninvasive estimation of a glottal phenomenon; however, it also holds limitations. Most critically, eliminating the influence of the vocal tract requires anticipating its resonating properties. This is often difficult to achieve with complete precision, and so the inverse filters are often fine-tuned to obtain an idealized glottal flow waveform. Although potentially useful with individuals with normal voices, this methodology is susceptible to bias and error when analyzing pathologic voices with deviant glottal waveforms.

The inverse filtered flow waveform, or flow glottogram, can be characterized in several ways (Hillman, Holmberg, Perkell, et al., 1989; Holmberg, Hillman, and Perkell, 1988; Perkell, Hillman, and Holmberg, 1994). Major time-based measures include the fundamental period, open quotient (ratio of total glottal open time to the period), speed quotient (ratio of opening to closing time), and closing quotient (ratio of closing time to the period) (**Fig. 7.18**). Amplitude-based measures include peak flow (maximum flow, presumably at the point of greatest glottal opening during the vibratory cycle), minimum flow (flow during the closed phase of the vibratory cycle, indicative of glottal leakage), and AC flow (the difference between minimum and maximum flow) (**Fig. 7.19**). In making these measurements, it is important to note that the glottal flow waveform is similar but distinct from the glottal area and impedance functions, primarily due to the influence of inertia on the accelerating and decelerating air stream during each vibratory cycle (Rothenberg, 1973). Because of this, measures derived from the glottal flow waveform will not directly correspond with those derived using high-speed imaging or electroglottography (EGG).

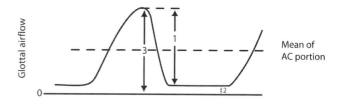

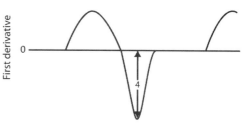

Figure 7.19 The inverse filtered flow waveform and its first derivative. Amplitude-based measures include AC flow (*1*), minimum flow (*2*), and peak flow (*3*). Maximum flow declination rate (MFDR) (*4*) is extracted from the first derivative. (From Hillman, R. E., Holmberg, E. B., Perkell, J. S., Walsh, M., Vaughan, C. [1989]. Objective assessment of vocal hyperfunction: an experimental framework and initial results. J Speech Hear Res 32, 373–392. [© 1989] American Speech-Language-Hearing Association. Reprinted with permission.)

Additional derivative flow measures include the AC/DC ratio (Isshiki, 1981) and maximum flow declination rate (MFDR) (Holmberg, Hillman, and Perkell, 1988). The AC/DC ratio, reflecting the difference between modulated AC flow (the alternating portion of the flow signal induced by vocal fold vibration) and unmodulated DC (mean) flow, is considered a pseudo–efficiency index that does not rely on the measurement of Ps or acoustic output. The AC/DC ratio reflects the efficiency of the vocal folds in converting DC to AC flow energy; thus, any leakage at the glottis during phonation should result in a relative increase in DC flow and corresponding drop in the AC/DC ratio. Isshiki (1981) reported an AC/DC ratio of 0.5 or greater for normal voices; however, other reports have questioned this criterion due to considerable variability across individuals (Holmberg, Hillman, and Perkell, 1988; Wilson and Starr, 1985).

Holmberg, Hillman, and Perkell (1988) introduced the MFDR as an estimate of maximum vocal fold velocity during the closing phase of the vibratory cycle. This index is derived by differentiating the glottal flow waveform and measuring the magnitude of the dominant negative peak (**Fig. 7.19**). Alongside speed and closing quotients measured directly from the glottal flow waveform, MFDR is theoretically associated with the magnitude of vocal fold collision forces, which when elevated may indicate susceptibility to vocal fold trauma. MFDR has been correlated with vocal intensity (Holmberg, Hillman, and Perkell, 1988) and appears to be elevated in the presence of certain hyperfunctional dysphonias (Hillman, Holmberg, Perkell, et al., 1989). It is also greater in men compared with women (Holmberg, Hillman, and Perkell, 1988) and in adults compared with children (Sapienza and Stathopoulos, 1994).

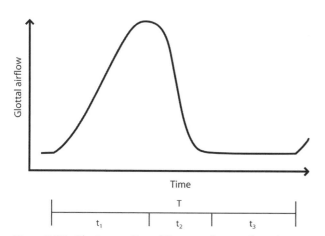

Figure 7.18 The inverse filtered flow waveform, or flow glottogram. The waveform can be delineated into open ($t_1 + t_2$), closed (t_3), opening (t_1), and closing (t_2) phases. Time-based measures include the fundamental period (T), open quotient ($[t_1 + t_2]/T$), speed quotient (t_1/t_2), and closing quotient (t_2/T). (From Hillman, R. E., Holmberg, E. B., Perkell, J. S., Walsh, M., Vaughan, C. [1989]. Objective assessment of vocal hyperfunction: an experimental framework and initial results. J Speech Hear Res 32, 373–392. [© 1989] American Speech-Language-Hearing Association. Reprinted with permission.)

Pressure

Pressure refers to force exerted against the unit area of a given surface. In the establishment and maintenance of vocal fold oscillation, the pressure exerted against the inferior surface of the vocal folds (subglottal pressure, P_s) is of primary interest. P_s can be measured using several approaches, both direct and indirect. Direct measurement approaches are highly invasive and involve either the placement of miniature pressure transducers above and below the glottis (Kitzing and Lofqvist, 1975; Lofqvist, Carlborg, et al., 1982) or tracheal puncture using a hypodermic needle coupled to a pressure transducer (Bard, Slavit, McCaffrey, et al, 1992; Plant and Hillel, 1998). Indirect approaches include placement of an esophageal balloon to measure pressure changes due to displacement of the tracheal-esophageal wall (Lieberman, 1968) or the estimation of P_s from intraoral pressure (P_{io}) during specific speech tasks (Smitheran and Hixon, 1981).

The indirect P_s estimation technique described by Smitheran and Hixon (1981) has gained popularity in both clinical and research applications. This technique requires the patient to produce a train of /pi/ syllables at a constant F_0, intensity and rate, and is based on the assumption that at the moment of bilabial closure and vocal fold abduction for plosive production, the vocal tract is a closed system with equal pressure throughout its length. Measurement is made by averaging adjacent pressure peaks in the syllable train (**Fig. 7.20**). Several reports indicate high correlations between this indirect technique and other direct measurements of Ps (Hertegard, Gauffin, and Lindestad, 1995; Lofqvist, Carlborg, and Kitzing, 1982).

Phonation threshold pressure (P_{th}), the minimum Ps required to initiate vocal fold oscillation, is an index with potentially high clinical relevance. P_{th} is theoretically associated with changes in vocal fold tissue viscosity (Titze, 1988) and should therefore be elevated in disorders characterized by reduced tissue pliability, such as vocal fold scarring and sulcus vocalis. P_{th} appears to vary as a function of hydration status and corresponds with self-perceived ratings of vocal effort (Fisher, Ligon, Sobecks, et al., 2001;

Sivasankar and Fisher, 2003; Verdolini, Titze, and Fennell, 1994; Verdolini-Marston, Titze, and Druker, 1990). A relationship between P_{th} and vocal fatigue has also been reported (Solomon and DiMattia, 2000; Solomon, Glaze, Arnold, et al., 2003).

Several derivative aerodynamic indices rely on the estimation of P_s. Laryngeal airway resistance (R_{law}) is an estimate of glottal resistance to flow and is calculated by dividing Ps by mean flow (Smitheran and Hixon, 1981). High R_{law} may be seen in cases of reduced tissue pliability or hyperfunction; low R_{law} may be seen in cases of glottal incompetence or incomplete vibratory closure. Normative data indicate that R_{law} varies alongside intensity and is typically greater in smaller compared with larger larynges (i.e., in women compared with men, children compared with adults) (Holmes, Leeper, and Nicholson, 1994; Netsell, Lotz, Peters, et al., 1994). Studies addressing age-related changes have reported lower R_{law} values in older males but not in older females (Hoit and Hixon, 1992; Melcon, Hoit, and Hixon, 1989).

Vocal efficiency refers to the efficiency of the laryngeal apparatus in converting aerodynamic to acoustic energy. This index is most often calculated by dividing radiated vocal intensity (acoustic power) by the product of Ps and mean flow (aerodynamic power). Natural power losses may occur during this conversion process due to vocal fold tissue viscosity, turbulent flow at the glottal exit, and the absorption of acoustic energy by vocal tract tissues (Titze, 1994a). The presence of vocal pathology may elevate power loss and reduce efficiency to an even greater extent (Jiang, Stern, Chen, et al., 2004). Vocal efficiency increases alongside increases in F_0 and intensity, requiring careful control of these variables when making comparisons (Titze, 1994a).

◆ Electroglottography

EGG, also called electrolaryngography, is an electrical impedance–based technology for inferring vocal fold contact changes during phonation. The central tenet of this procedure is that electrical impedance across the neck varies systematically with changes in the degree of vocal fold contact. Complete vocal fold contact is associated with low impedance and direct current flow across the glottis. As vocal fold contact decreases, the high impedance of air effects a redirection of current flow around the open glottis, resulting in a reduction in effective voltage across the neck. These voltage changes form the basis of the vocal fold contact (or EGG) signal.

EGG is performed using two electrodes placed on the thyroid laminae. Electrical current passes between the electrodes in both directions, and the neck effectively acts as a variable resistor in a constant current circuit (Orlikoff, 1998). It is important to note that the EGG signal is influenced by a variety of impedance factors besides that of air at the open glottis. Extrinsic laryngeal muscle contraction, laryngeal postural adjustments, and blood vessel dilation and constriction

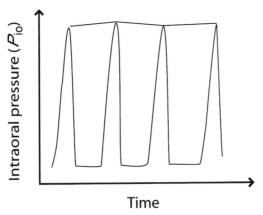

Figure 7.20   Intraoral pressure (P_{io}) waveform for a train of four /pi/ syllables. Adjacent pressure peaks are averaged to obtain pressure values.

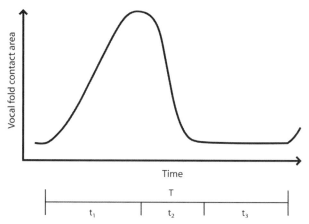

Figure 7.21 The electroglottographic signal. The signal can be delineated into contact ($t_1 + t_2$), minimal contact (t_3), increasing contact (t_1), and decreasing contact (t_2) phases. Time-based measures include the fundamental period (T), contact quotient ($[t_1 + t_2]/T$) and contact index ($[t_2 - t_1]/[t_1 + t_2]$).

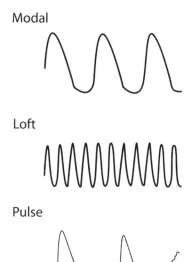

Figure 7.22 Electroglottographic signals collected during voice production in modal, loft (falsetto), and pulse (vocal fry) registers. (From Baken, R. J., Orlikoff, R. F. (2000). Clinical measurement of speech and voice [2nd ed.]. San Diego: Singular Publishing Group. [© 2000]. Reprinted with permission of Delmar Learning, a division of Thomson Learning: www.thomsonrights.com.)

all contribute to gross neck impedance. These factors are typically removed by high-pass filtering of the raw EGG signal. Other potentially challenging impedance factors include excess adipose tissue in the neck, which precludes the use of EGG in some patients, and the presence of mucus strands, which can provide a route for direct current flow across an open glottis, thus mimicking vocal fold contact.

As noted, the EGG signal reflects changes in vocal fold contact area as a function of time (**Fig. 7.21**). It is important to stress that although the EGG signal corresponds with the vibratory cycle, it is clearly distinct from the flow glottogram obtained via inverse filtering and the glottal width and area functions obtained using high-speed imaging techniques. The EGG signal is only meaningful when the vocal folds have some degree of contact; it does not specify the region of vocal fold contact, and it cannot be used to accurately determine the precise moment of initial contact or separation (Colton and Conture, 1990; Orlikoff, 1998). Further, the point of maximum contact in the EGG signal does not necessarily correspond with complete glottal closure. As a consequence of these physiologic realities, the EGG signal has been characterized in terms of a contact phase (marked by clearly increasing or decreasing vocal fold contact) and a minimal contact phase (featuring an apparent lack of vocal fold contact) (Orlikoff, 1998). Based on this delineation, several quantitative parameters have been developed to describe the EGG signal (**Fig. 7.21**). The contact quotient is defined as a ratio of the contact phase duration to the fundamental period (Orlikoff, 1991; Rothenberg and Mahshie, 1988; Scherer, Vail, and Rockwell, 1995). This quotient has a normative range of 0.4 to 0.6 for males and females and is believed to indirectly reflect vocal fold adduction force. Another measure, the contact index, is defined as the difference between increasing and decreasing vocal fold contact durations, divided by total contact phase duration (Orlikoff, 1991). This measure reflects contact symmetry (a value of 0 is associated with perfect symmetry) and is typically between −0.4 and −0.6 for males and females in modal reg-

ister. Pulse register phonation is associated with a contact index around −0.8; falsetto register phonation is associated with a contact index close to 0 (Orlikoff, 2003).

Qualitative changes in EGG signal geometry have been associated with specific alterations in vocal fold dynamics. Characteristic patterns are seen with each of the vocal registers (**Fig. 7.22**). Using modeling data, Titze (1990) described four dimensions of variation in the EGG signal accounted for by specific vocal fold adjustments (**Fig. 7.23**). Widening of the signal peak is associated with increased vocal fold adduction forces alongside an increased contact quotient. Skewing of the signal peak is a reflection of greater increasing contact compared with decreasing contact speed, which is a consequence of the natural convergent nature of the glottis combined with the vibratory phase difference between the upper and lower vocal fold margins. The presence of a bulge in the increasing and decreasing contact portions of the signal (termed *skirt elevation*) is associated with a physical bulge on the vocal fold medial surface. Finally, increased triangularity (termed *skirt ramping*) of the signal is observed with an increased vertical phase difference.

♦ Laryngeal Visualization

Visualization of the larynx during respiratory and phonatory activities is of enormous benefit in the diagnosis and treatment of voice disorders. By observing the laryngeal structures under various phonatory and nonphonatory conditions, critical diagnostic, prognostic, and treatment-shaping data can be obtained. Technological advancements continue to

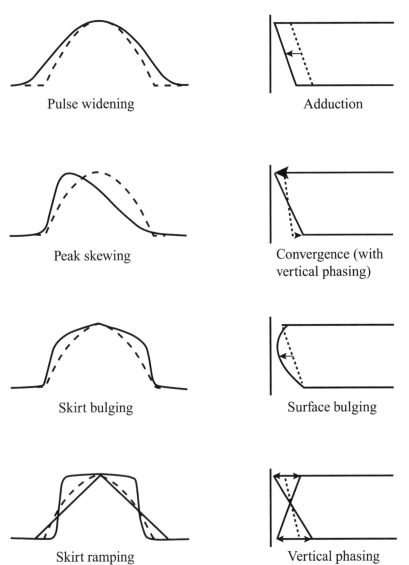

Pulse widening

Adduction

Peak skewing

Convergence (with vertical phasing)

Skirt bulging

Surface bulging

Skirt ramping

Vertical phasing

Figure 7.23 Qualitative variations in the electroglottographic signal and associated vocal fold adjustments. (From Titze, I. R. [1990]. Interpretation of the electroglottographic signal. J Voice 4, 1–9. © 1990 The Voice Foundation. Reprinted with permission.)

improve endoscopic instrument quality as well as image capture, analysis, and storage capabilities. In addition, the appropriate interpretation of complex vibratory patterns is aided by a growing understanding of lamina propria ultrastructure and vocal fold physiology.

Laryngeal visualization is within the scope of practice of both otolaryngologists and speech-language pathologists (American Speech-Language-Hearing Association, 1998). Otolaryngologists use the information gained from interpreting laryngeal images when making a medical diagnosis and planning a medical or surgical intervention strategy. Speech-language pathologists use this information to assess vocal function, evaluate therapy probes, plan behavioral intervention, and administer biofeedback. In many voice-care settings, otolaryngologists and speech-language pathologists work together to interpret all available case history and vocal function data and form a joint intervention strategy drawing on medical, surgical, and behavioral approaches as needed.

Indirect Laryngoscopy

Indirect laryngoscopy refers to a series of clinical procedures designed to allow indirect visualization of the larynx via light reflected against a mirror or prism system or transmitted through a fiberoptic cable (**Fig. 7.24**). These procedures allow evaluation while a patient is awake and in many cases unanesthetized. Although extremely useful in the assessment of laryngeal structure and function, it is important to note that observing the natural physiologic function of the larynx can be challenging in many cases due to individual oral-pharyngeal anatomy, certain hyperfunctional postures, and the gag reflex.

Mirror Laryngoscopy

Mirror laryngoscopy is a traditional technique allowing gross visualization of the larynx. In this procedure, the tongue is drawn forward while a small laryngeal mirror is placed in the oropharynx, positioned to allow visualization of the larynx. A

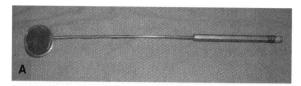

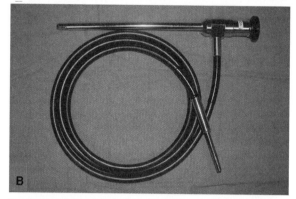

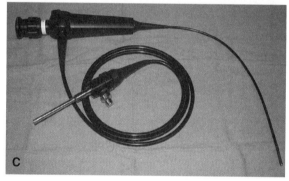

Figure 7.24 Instrumentation used for indirect laryngoscopy. (**A**) A laryngeal mirror, (**B**) 70-degree rigid endoscope, and (**C**) flexible endoscope.

continuous light source is used to reflect light from the mirror. The patient is generally instructed to produce /i/ at a high pitch during this examination. This phonatory posture, combined with holding of the tongue, functions to elevate the larynx and raise the epiglottis, thus allowing maximum visualization of the vocal folds. Although useful for rapid and gross examination, standard mirror laryngoscopy does not facilitate normal physiologic voice production or the evaluation of vocal fold vibratory parameters. A stroboscopic light source can be employed with this procedure; however, permanent image capture is difficult. Finally, the lack of magnification provided by the laryngeal mirror can mask the presence of subtle laryngeal abnormalities with this technique.

Rigid Endoscopy

Rigid endoscopy employs a rigid metal tube device (rigid endoscope) containing a lens and prism system designed to transmit high-intensity light from its proximal to its distal end and a highly magnified image from its distal to its proximal end. A fiberoptic cable provides light from a light source, which is transmitted through a channel of the endoscope's optical array to illuminate the viewing field. A prism providing either a 70-degree or 90-degree viewing angle

facilitates image transmission through an alternate optical channel to the endoscope's eyepiece. A photographic or videographic capture system is usually connected to the eyepiece, allowing permanent image documentation.

For laryngeal visualization, the patient is either seated upright (if employing a 90-degree rigid endoscope) or with the upper body and head extended forward (if employing a 70-degree rigid endoscope). As with mirror laryngoscopy, the tongue is drawn forward while the rigid endoscope is placed in the oral cavity and inserted as far as the oropharynx. Whereas certain patients require the application of topical anesthetic to the oropharynx, most are able to tolerate this procedure well if appropriately positioned and carefully examined. In a small number of cases, however, individual oral-pharyngeal anatomy may preclude the use of this technique altogether. Rigid endoscopy has the advantage of providing a high-quality magnified image (**Fig. 7.25**), adequate for the identification of subtle laryngeal anomalies. Further, the high-intensity light transmission capacity of the rigid endoscope allows the use of stroboscopic and high-speed imaging techniques. The primary disadvantage of this procedure, as with mirror laryngoscopy, is the interference of the endoscope with natural voice and speech production, restricting phonatory samples to isolated vowels.

Flexible Endoscopy

Flexible endoscopy involves the use of a thin fiberoptic cable device (flexible endoscope) containing an array of fibers arranged to transmit light from its proximal to its distal end and an image from its distal to its proximal end. As with the rigid endoscope, an attached fiberoptic cable connects the endoscope to a light source. A control lever allows upward-downward maneuvering of the endoscope tip. An eyepiece is available for direct observation or connection to an image capture system.

Laryngeal visualization using a flexible endoscope is transnasal. This approach holds the benefit of bypassing the gag reflex and allowing evaluation of velopharyngeal structure and function en route to the larynx. Topical anesthetic is generally used for this procedure. The endoscope is gradually advanced through the nasal cavity, nasopharynx, and oropharynx to the laryngopharynx, where it is positioned to provide maximum exposure of the vocal folds or other laryngeal feature of interest.

Flexible endoscopy has the advantage of allowing the evaluation of phonatory function in a natural posture during connected speech and singing. Further, the small diameter of many flexible endoscopes allows for the evaluation of infants and young children. Certain disorders such as functional dysphonia, spasmodic dysphonia, and paradoxical vocal fold motion are best evaluated using this procedure (although often as an adjunct to rigid endoscopy). Stroboscopy can be performed in conjunction with a high-quality flexible endoscope and stroboscopic light source. The primary disadvantages of flexible endoscopy are limited light transmission through the fiberoptic array (particularly with small-diameter endoscopes) and suboptimal image resolution. Optical distortion is an additional consideration (Hibi, Bless, Hirano, et al., 1988). A significant recent development in flexible

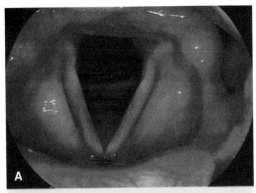

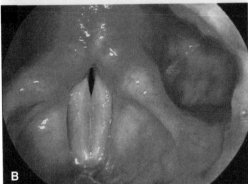

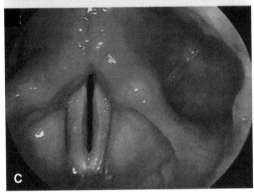

Figure 7.25 Laryngeal still images captured using a 70-degree rigid endoscope. (**A**) The upper image shows the larynx during resting breathing, viewed using a continuous light source. (**B**) The middle image shows a posterior gap closure pattern on phonation, viewed using a stroboscopic light source. (**C**) The lower image illustrates the mucosal wave propagating across the superior surface of both vocal folds during phonation, also viewed using a stroboscopic light source.

endoscopy technology is the availability of endoscopes with a miniature digital camera at the distal tip. This, alongside parallel advancements in fiberoptic technology, holds promise for ongoing improvements in image quality.

Direct Laryngoscopy

Direct laryngoscopy involves direct visualization of the larynx, requiring the patient to be placed in a supine position under general anesthetic. This procedure is performed by the otolaryngologist. A laryngoscope is inserted into the oral cavity and positioned to allow maximum exposure of the vocal folds. The laryngoscope is often suspended to allow the surgeon the use of both hands. Direct laryngoscopy allows close examination of the laryngeal tissues, including palpation of the vocal folds (e.g., to evaluate tissue and lesion pliability) and manipulation of the arytenoid cartilages (e.g., to differentiate ankylosis from paralysis as a cause of arytenoid immobility). A microscope is commonly used for detailed visualization. A contact endoscope combined with methylene blue staining may also be employed to examine cellular, nucleic, and cytoplasmic features of the vocal fold mucosa at high magnification. If indicated, tissue biopsy may be performed.

Direct laryngoscopy is the most invasive of all laryngeal visualization procedures and clearly the most expensive. As the patient is anesthetized, phonatory function cannot be evaluated. Direct laryngoscopy is indicated in cases where tissue changes observed on indirect examination warrant biopsy and in rare cases where indirect laryngoscopy is not possible.

Parameters of Interest

Laryngoscopy performed under continuous light allows the evaluation of structure and gross function. The clinician should examine the laryngeal structures for any signs of acute or chronic irritation or injury and for irregularity or asymmetry. Potentially important structural signs include edema, erythema, pachydermia, leukoplakia, erythroplakia, vascular ectasia and varices, hemorrhage, vocal fold medial edge irregularity and/or roughness, vocal fold length and/or vertical height differences, prolapse, limited airway patency, laryngeal tilt or rotation, asymmetric regions of fullness, sulcus vocalis, and the presence of mass lesions. Gross functional parameters include degree and symmetry of arytenoid excursion during vocal fold adduction and abduction, diadochokinetic ability, cough, stridor, paradoxical vocal fold motion, static or intention tremor, excessive mucus pooling, and supraglottic hyperfunction in the anteroposterior and mediolateral planes.

Studying Vocal Fold Vibratory Patterns

Videostroboscopy

Videostroboscopy refers to the use of a stroboscopic (pulsed) light source for endoscopic visualization of vocal fold vibratory parameters in apparent slow motion. The essential principle of this technique is centered on the visual perceptual phenomenon of apparent motion, whereby successive still images presented at a rate greater than 5 Hz appear to be moving continuously. This concept (also the basis of regular videography) is specifically exploited in videostroboscopy by using a stroboscopic light to illuminate discrete moments of subsequent vocal fold vibratory cycles, which are then perceived as an apparent single vibratory cycle. The stroboscopic light source is synchronized with vocal fold vibratory F_0 captured using a microphone or electroglottographic transducer. The light source may be precisely synchronized with F_0 to provide an apparent motionless image (as each strobe pulse illuminates an identical position in each vibratory cycle), or quasi-synchronized (1 to 2 Hz above F_0) to provide apparent slow motion (as each strobe pulse illuminates successive phases of subsequent vibratory cycles).

Videostroboscopy is a critical tool in any clinical voice setting. It facilitates the evaluation of subtle vocal fold vibratory parameters and provides a basis for making inferences concerning the integrity of the vocal fold body-cover relationship. Several reports have demonstrated the importance of videostroboscopy in reaching an accurate diagnosis, revising a previous diagnosis, and designing treatment (Casiano, Zaveri, and Lundy, 1992; Woo, Colton, Casper, et al., 1991). The primary limitation of this technique is its reliance on the accurate extraction of F_0 for synchronization of the stroboscopic light, rendering the examination of voices characterized by highly aperiodic vibratory patterns impossible. Secondary limitations include an inability to capture vibratory behaviors during phonatory onset and offset, and the fact that the observed vibratory "cycles" are illusionary.

Key vocal fold vibratory parameters observed under stroboscopic light include glottal closure pattern, amplitude, mucosal wave, presence of nonvibrating segments, phase closure, phase symmetry, and regularity (Bless, Hirano, and Feder, 1987; Hirano and Bless, 1993; Poburka, 1999). Glottal closure pattern is observed during the closed phase of the vibratory cycle and generally described using the following labels: complete, incomplete, irregular, hourglass, posterior gap, anterior gap, spindle gap, or variable. An abnormal closure pattern (i.e., not complete at normal pitch and loudness) can result from poor vocal fold adduction due to recurrent laryngeal nerve damage or cricoarytenoid ankylosis, obstruction due to a vocal fold medial edge lesion, laryngeal web, or granuloma, or reduced tissue pliability due to scarring or sulcus vocalis. It is important to note that a posterior gap closure pattern is considered normal in females (Biever and Bless, 1989). Vibratory amplitude refers to the maximum mediolateral excursion of the vocal folds and is typically around 30% of the total vocal fold width in most individuals at normal pitch and loudness. Each vocal fold should be rated independently for this parameter. Decreased amplitude is associated with a decrease in vocal fold length (e.g., in females and children compared with males; or in the case of a laryngeal web), increased vocal fold tension (e.g., associated with increased F_0 or due to hyperfunction), reduced tissue pliability, reduced Ps and loudness, and increased vocal fold mass (e.g., due to chronic edema or a mass lesion). Opposite directional changes in these variables are associated with increased vibratory amplitude.

The *mucosal wave* refers to the phenomenon of a traveling wave moving across the superior surface of the vocal folds in the medial to lateral direction. At normal pitch and loudness, mucosal wave excursion is typically 50% of the total vocal fold width. A reduction in mucosal wave excursion (or complete absence of mucosal wave) is seen in cases of reduced tissue pliability, such as with vocal fold scarring, sulcus vocalis, mass lesions, epithelial hyperplasia, and mucosal dryness. Increased F_0 and falsetto register phonation are also associated with reduced mucosal wave excursion. Increased mucosal wave excursion is often seen in cases of polypoid

degeneration, in children who have an immature vocal fold layer structure, and alongside increases in Ps and loudness. It is important to note that variations in mucosal wave presentation may be regional as a consequence of focal tissue changes. A regional absence of mucosal wave combined with the absence of vibratory amplitude (i.e., complete regional immobility) characterizes what is termed a *nonvibratory segment*. This feature may be constant or isolated to a certain phonatory condition or posture and is typically observed in cases of markedly impaired tissue pliability.

Phase closure reflects the relative durations of the open and closed phases of an observed vibratory cycle. At normal pitch and loudness, the open phase may account for ~40 to 60% of the entire cycle. A vibratory cycle that is predominately open phase is typically associated with a breathy voice quality due to glottal hypofunction. In contrast, a vibratory cycle that is predominately closed phase is often associated with a pressed voice quality due to glottal hyperfunction. Variations in Ps, F_0, vocal effort level, and vocal register all affect phase closure. Measurements can be made by taking a ratio of actual time duration or the number of video frames for both open and closed phases. When measuring this parameter, it is generally helpful to sample multiple vibratory cycles.

Phase symmetry is a measure of the degree to which the two vocal folds mirror each other during vibration. The presence of asymmetry may result from differences in vocal fold mass, length, and/or tension, which in turn may result from a unilateral lesion or edema, unilateral neuropathy, or unilateral differences in tissue pliability or viscosity. In some cases, unilateral vocal fold tension differences may be functional. Any vibratory asymmetry should be described as either constant, intermittent, or specific to a particular phonatory condition or posture.

Regularity, also referred to as *periodicity*, refers to the degree of consistency from one vibratory cycle to the next. Irregularity can result from impaired motor control at the respiratory or phonatory levels, in addition to vocal fold biomechanical asymmetries. A popular method for evaluating this parameter involves the exact synchronization of F_0 and the stroboscopic light source. In this mode, regular vibration appears as an apparent static image, whereas irregular vibration is characterized by cycle-to-cycle movement.

A complete videostroboscopic examination should incorporate a range of tasks, including phonation at normal pitch and loudness levels, at points throughout the pitch and dynamic range, during glissando production, both within and transitioning between different registers, and during inhalation phonation. These tasks are in addition to those used to assess gross laryngeal function under continuous light. If a flexible endoscope is employed, speech and singing samples should also be elicited.

Videokymography

Videokymography is a charge-coupled device-based video technology allowing high-speed single-line scanning of an image of interest. Each line captured by the scan camera is appended to the preceding line to provide a series of stacked images across time. When applied to the larynx, videoky-mography allows the visualization of vocal fold vibratory behavior for a single mediolateral plane. Line scanning is performed at ~8 kHz, which is sufficient to capture actual vibratory behavior in real time. This allows the observation of aperiodic vibratory patterns that cannot be seen using videostroboscopy.

"Commercial videokymography cameras function in two modes. A standard mode is employed for orientation of the endoscope and selection of the plane for videokymography. A videokymographic mode is then employed for high-speed single line scanning and image capture. In first generation systems, standard and videokymographic modes are engaged sequentially and line scanning occurs using the uppermost line of the image observed in the standard mode. As a result, selection of the midmembranous vocal fold as the plane of interest requires appreciable endoscope tilt. This favors the use of a 90° rather than a 70° rigid endoscope. In second generation systems, images from both modes are viewed and recorded simultaneously and the scanning line is not restricted to the uppermost line of the image (Qiu and Schutte, 2006).

As stated, the primary advantage of videokymography over videostroboscopy is its ability to capture actual vibratory cycles and therefore facilitate the study of aperiodic vocal fold vibratory patterns. Its primary limitations are its restriction to a single mediolateral plane (although a series of videokymograms can be captured in different planes), and the potential introduction of artifact by movement of the endoscope or larynx during image capture. To avoid this, the scanning line should be maintained on a steady mediolateral plane, perpendicular to the glottal axis (Švec,

Šram, and Schutte, 2001), and (in first generation systems) the measurement position checked regularly by switching between videokymographic and standard camera modes. Also, when collecting and presenting videokymographic data, it is important to specify the antero-posterior position and any rotational orientation of the scanning line with respect to the glottis; in addition to the pitch, loudness and register features of the phonatory sample of interest."

Videokymography allows the evaluation of many of the same vibratory features as videostroboscopy; however, these features are presented in a different form (**Figs. 7.26 and 7.27**). The glottis is seen as a dark region in the center of the kymogram, varying with respect to changes in vibratory amplitude throughout the cycle. The open, closed, opening and closing phases are easily identified. During the closing phase, the vocal fold medial surface and lower margin can be observed adjacent to the contour of the upper margin. The mucosal wave presents as a thin band that extends beyond the end point of the opening phase, typically maintaining a similar trajectory. Abnormal phase closure, phase asymmetries, and phase irregularities are particularly salient on videokymography.

High-Speed Digital Imaging

High-speed digital imaging is the most powerful technology currently available for the study of vocal fold vibratory behavior. Whereas videokymography is a form of high-speed imaging, complete high-speed systems allow visualization of the entire surface of both vocal folds during phonation

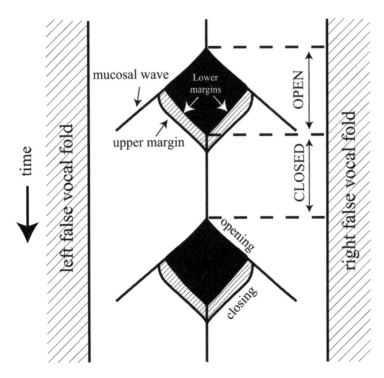

Figure 7.26 Schematic of a videokymogram illustrating key anatomic and vibratory parameters. (From Švec, J. G., Schutte, H. K. [1996]. Videokymography: high-speed line scanning of vocal fold vibration. J Voice 10, 201–205. [© 1996] The Voice Foundation. Reprinted with permission.)

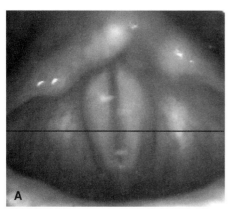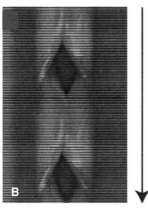

Figure 7.27 A videokymogram obtained during modal register phonation at comfortable pitch and loudness levels. (**A**) The dark horizontal line on the standard camera mode image represents the orientation of the scanning line used to generate (**B**) the videokymogram.

rather than a single line. The primary advantages of this technology are its lack of dependence on vibratory periodicity, its ability to capture subtle vibratory features that may not be evident in apparent motion, and its ability to capture vocal fold dynamics during phonatory onset and offset. Prior to the advent of high-speed digital technology in the 1980s (Hirose, 1988), high-speed laryngeal visualization relied on photographic technology first developed at Bell Laboratories in the late 1930s (Timcke, von Leden, and Moore, 1958, 1959; von Leden, Moore, and Timcke, 1960; Whitehead, Metz, and Whitehead, 1984).

Most commercially available high-speed systems allow visualization of the entire larynx at a frame rate of ~2 kHz. This frame rate can be increased alongside a reduction in resolution or size of the imaging window. Most high-speed digital systems are monochrome; however, color cameras are also available. Adequate visualization of the vocal folds during vibration requires high light intensity and is best performed using a rigid endoscope. A computer with high data transfer rate video memory is also required. Depending on video memory capacity and frame rate, most current systems allow 2 to 8 seconds of data collection at one time.

High-speed digital imaging is a useful research instrument and is beginning to be used in clinical settings. Most of the current challenges associated with this technology (frame rate, resolution, color quality, need for high light intensity, video memory data transfer rate and capacity) are technical and should be resolved with time. The vocal fold vibratory parameters of interest in high-speed digital images are similar to those observed using videostroboscopy, with the addition of preoscillatory and damping behaviors seen during phonatory onset and offset. High-speed images are also well suited to quantitative image analysis.

Analysis of Images

Visual Perceptual Rating

In the majority of instances, laryngeal images are interpreted qualitatively using individual visual perceptual judgments. These judgments feature the same validity and reliability challenges associated with auditory perceptual ratings. Several key factors in maximizing rating validity, interjudge reliability, and intrajudge reliability are quality and duration of training and experience, endoscopic image quality, an appreciation for artifacts associated with image distortion, and the nature of the rating system employed. Poburka and Bless (1998) demonstrated the effectiveness of 4 to 5 hours of computer-aided multimedia training in improving the accuracy of videostroboscopic ratings performed by inexperienced judges. After training, interjudge reliability improved between the inexperienced judges and a group of experienced judges. In a subsequent study, Poburka (1999) developed and evaluated an alternative videostroboscopy rating system based on feedback from the experienced judges (**Fig. 7.28**). Although intuitively easier to use, interjudge reliability with this alternative rating system was similar to that measured using a traditional rating system. Poburka noted that phase closure, phase symmetry, and phase regularity were the most challenging features to rate, regardless of the system employed. In an effort to address artifacts associated with image distortion, Peppard and Bless (1990) demonstrated a transparency tracing procedure to control endoscope-larynx distance and improve image consistency across multiple examinations.

Quantitative Image Analysis

Attempts to quantify the vocal fold vibratory pattern first began with high-speed photography (Timcke, von Leden, and Moore, 1958, 1959; von Leden, Moore, and Timcke, 1960), and have continued with videokymography and high-speed digital imaging (Larsson, Hertegard, Lindestad, et al., 2000; Qiu, Schutte, Gu, et al., 2003). Vibratory pattern data have also been extracted from videostroboscopic images (Lee, Kim, Park, et al., 1998; Lee, Kim, Sung, et al, 2001); however, such data should be interpreted judiciously because of their reliance on apparent motion. The cardinal parameters of interest in these analyses are changes in individual vocal fold position, as well as changes in glottal area over time. From these parameters, glottal width and area functions can be derived and various

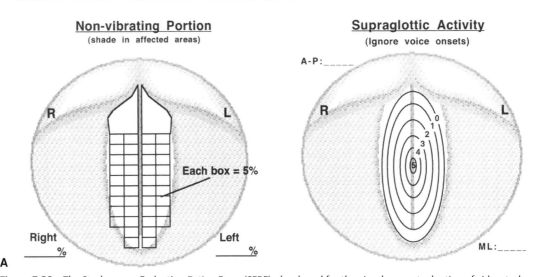

Figure 7.28   The Stroboscopy Evaluation Rating Form (SERF), developed for the visual perceptual rating of videostroboscopic parameters. (From Poburka, B. J. [1999]. A new stroboscopy rating form. J Voice 13, 403–413. [© 1999] The Voice Foundation. Reprinted with permission.) (*Continued on page 158*)

time-based indices calculated. The most commonly used glottal parameters are the open, closed, opening, and closing phases. From these, the open, closing, and speed quotients can be calculated. Recall that these terms are also employed when quantifying key features of the morphologically similar but theoretically distinct flow glottogram. Unfortunately, they (in particular the open quotient) are

often inappropriately applied to the vocal fold contact (EGG) waveform.

Advances in computing power and refinements in imaging analysis technology continue to offer improvement in the speed and accuracy with which key laryngeal and vocal fold vibratory parameters can be measured. Image analysis applications include absolute dimensional calibration based on

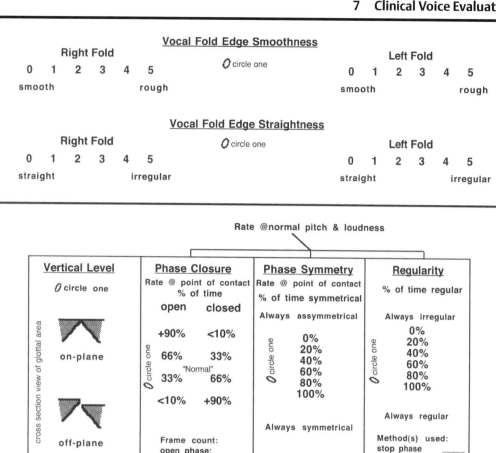

Vocal Fold Edge Smoothness

Right Fold

0   1   2   3   4   5

smooth   rough

O circle one

Left Fold

0   1   2   3   4   5

smooth   rough

Vocal Fold Edge Straightness

Right Fold

0   1   2   3   4   5

straight   irregular

O circle one

Left Fold

0   1   2   3   4   5

straight   irregular

Rate @normal pitch & loudness

Vertical Level	Phase Closure	Phase Symmetry	Regularity
O circle one	Rate @ point of contact % of time	Rate @ point of contact % of time symmetrical	% of time regular
cross section view of glottal area	open closed	Always assymmetrical	Always irregular
on-plane	+90% <10%	0% 20% 40% 60% 80% 100%	0% 20% 40% 60% 80% 100%
	66% 33% "Normal" 33% 66%		
	<10% +90%		
off-plane	Frame count: open phase: _____ Closed phase:_____	Always symmetrical	Always regular Method(s) used: stop phase _____ running phase_____

Glottal Closure

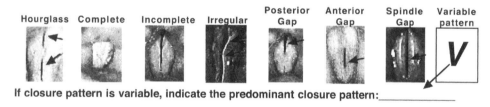

Hourglass   Complete   Incomplete   Irregular   Posterior Gap   Anterior Gap   Spindle Gap   Variable pattern

If closure pattern is variable, indicate the predominant closure pattern:_____

Summary/Additional Comments:

_____

_____

_____

_____

B _____

Figure 7.28   (*Continued*)

laser triangulation (Rosen, Minhaj, Hinds, et al., 2003; Schuberth, Hoppe, Dollinger, et al., 2002), compensation for artifact due to endoscopic image distortion (Deliyski and Petrushev, 2003; Rosen, Minhaj, Hinds, et al., 2003), classification of vocal fold lesion color and texture (Wittenberg, Kothe, Munzenmayer, et al., 2003), extraction of kymograms from high-speed digital images (Tigges, Wittenberg, Mergell, et al., 1999), and detection of the vocal fold edge contour

and/or mucosal wave (Deliyski and Petrushev, 2003; Yan, Ahmad, Kunduk, et al., 2005).

Figures 7.29 and 7.30 illustrate a series of analytic techniques developed by Yan, Ahmad, Kunduk, et al. (2005) to quantify the vocal fold vibratory pattern observed using high-speed digital imaging. An edge detection algorithm is employed to extract the glottal area function. From this, an analytic phase plot (termed *Nyquist plot*) is derived using a

Vocal fold edge detection

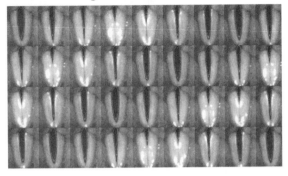

Figure 7.29 Vocal fold edge detection, glottal area waveform extraction, instantaneous frequency measurement, and analytic phase plot construction, based on high-speed digital images. (From Yan, Y., Ahmad, K., Kunduk, M., Bless, D. M. [2005]. Analysis of vocal-fold vibrations from high-speed laryngeal images using a Hilbert transform based methodology. J Voice 19, 161–175. © The Voice Foundation. Reprinted with permission.)

Instantaneous frequency extraction

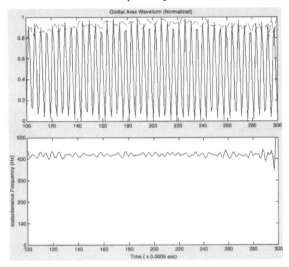

Analytic phase plot construction

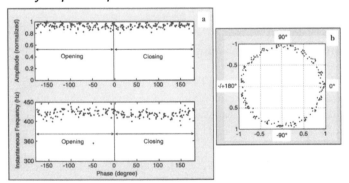

Hilbert transform technique. The Nyquist plot represents a projection of the glottal area function in the complex plane over time and provides a visually salient representation of vibratory behavior. The trace pattern within the plot represents intracycle variation, and the degree of scatter represents intercycle variation. Characteristic pattern deviations have been associated with certain voice quality deviations and vocal pathologies. A second plot, termed the *perturbation plot*, summarizes instantaneous F_0 and amplitude deviations from the mean, as based on analysis of the glottal area function.

◆ Summary

A complete voice evaluation spans a range of domains and yields a clinical data set requiring careful integration and

Analytic phase plot ("Nyquist" plot)

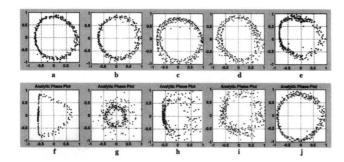

Figure 7.30 Characteristic phase and perturbation plot pattern deviations associated with phonatory and pathologic conditions, extracted from high-speed digital images. Phase plots: (a) normal; (b) normal (high pitch, normal loudness); (c) breathy; (d) stage whisper; (e) hyperfunction; (f) pressed; (g) vocal fold scarring (high pitch, normal loudness); (h) vocal fold stiffness; (i) vocal fold cyst; (j) after surgical removal of vocal fold cyst. Perturbation plots: (a) normal (normal pitch, normal loudness); (b) after surgical removal of vocal fold cyst; (c) vocal fold cyst; (d) vocal fold scarring. (From Yan, Y., Ahmad, K., Kunduk, M., Bless, D. M. [2005]. Analysis of vocal-fold vibrations from high-speed laryngeal images using a Hilbert transform based methodology. J Voice 19, 161–175. © The Voice Foundation. Reprinted with permission.)

Perturbation plot

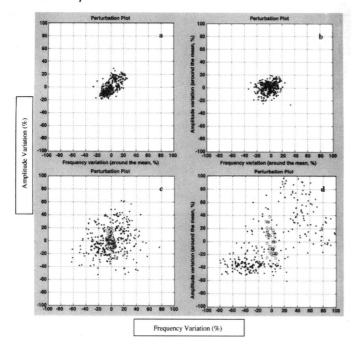

interpretation. It is important to note that not all testing procedures are necessarily required in every case. Test selection should be driven by the case history and symptoms described by the patient. Procedures should be efficient and avoid unnecessary replication. Within each setting, the clinician should be careful to collect data that are comparable from visit to visit and with data reported in the literature. Literature-sourced data should be interpreted critically. The clinician should hold a solid understanding of how a given test or assessment procedure evaluates laryngeal structure and function and its role in making a differential diagnosis or constructing a treatment strategy. It is important to be wary of cases in which the different elements of a patient's assessment data set appear incongruous. Such variation in performance may reflect the nature of the specific disorder, a favorable or unfavorable compensatory strategy, or an assessment error.

Certain elements of voice assessment were not addressed in detail here, either because they are given adequate atten-

tion elsewhere in this book or because they provide supplementary data to those obtained by the speech-language pathologist. Psychologic interviewing is addressed in detail in a separate chapter. Excess musculoskeletal tension assessment is discussed within the context of voice therapy. Radiologic imaging studies are often ordered by the otolaryngologist when evaluating structural defects and when searching for a mass either in the laryngeal region or along the path of the recurrent or superior laryngeal nerves. Additionally, magnetic resonance imaging (MRI) has been used successfully to evaluate soft tissue displacement after vocal fold medialization surgery (Ford, Unger, Zundel, et al., 1995). Laryngeal electromyography (LEMG) holds an important role in the evaluation and characterization of vocal fold movement disorders, including paralysis and paresis, and other neuromuscular disorders such as myasthenia gravis. It is helpful in differentiating paralysis from ankylosis and in making a prognosis for nerve recovery after injury.

References

American Speech-Language-Hearing Association. (1998). The roles of oto-laryngologists and speech-language pathologists in the performance and interpretation of strobovideolaryngoscopy. ASHA 40(Suppl. 18), 32.

Baken, R. J. (2003). Dynamical disorders of voice: a chaotic perspective on vocal irregularities. In J. S. Rubin, R. T. Sataloff, G. S. Korovin (Eds.), *Diagnosis and treatment of voice disorders* (2nd ed.). Clifton Park, NY: Thomson Learning.

Baken, R. J., Orlikoff, R. F. (2000). *Clinical measurement of speech and voice* (2nd ed.). San Diego: Singular Publishing Group.

Baldwin E. de F., Courand, A., Richards, D. W. (1948). Pulmonary insufficiency. Medicine 27, 243–276.

Bard, M. C., Slavit, D. H., McCaffrey, T. V., Lipton, R. J. (1992). Noninvasive technique for estimating subglottic pressure and laryngeal efficiency. Ann Otol Rhinol Laryngol 101, 578–582.

Biever, D. M., Bless, D. M. (1989). Vibratory characteristics of the vocal folds in young adult and geriatric women. J Voice 3, 120–131.

Bless, D. M., Hirano, M., Feder, R. J. (1987). Videostroboscopic evaluation of the larynx. Ear Nose Throat J 66, 289–296.

Boone, D. R. (1977). *The voice and voice therapy.* Englewood Cliffs, NJ: Prentice-Hall.

Brown, W. S., Morris, R. J., Hollien, H., Howell, E. (1991). Speaking fundamental frequency characteristics as a function of age and professional singing. J Voice 5, 310–315.

Casiano, R. R., Zaveri, V., Lundy, D. S. (1992). Efficacy of videostroboscopy in the diagnosis of voice disorders. Otolaryngol Head Neck Surg 107, 95–100.

Chan, K. M., Yiu, E. M. (2002). The effect of anchors and training on the reliability of perceptual voice evaluation. J Speech Lang Hear Res 45, 111–126.

Christensen, J. M., Fletcher, S. G., McCutcheon, M. J. (1992). Esophageal speaker articulation of /s,z/: a dynamic palatometric assessment. J Commun Disord 25, 65–76.

Coleman, R. F. (1993). Sources of variation in phonetograms. J Voice 7, 1–14.

Coleman, R. F., Mabis, J. H., Hinson, J. K. (1977). Fundamental frequency-sound pressure level profiles of adult male and female voices. J Speech Hear Res 20, 197–204.

Colton, R. H., Conture, E. G. (1990). Problems and pitfalls of electroglottography. J Voice 4, 10–24.

Dejonckere, P. H. (1998). Ceptral voice analysis: link with perception and stroboscopy. Rev Laryngol Otol Rhinol (Bord) 119, 245–246.

Dejonckere, P. H., Lebacq, J. (1996). Acoustic, perceptual, aerodynamic and anatomical correlations in voice pathology. ORL J Otorhinolaryngol Relat Spec 58, 326–332.

Deliyski, D., Petrushev, P. (2003). Methods for objective assessment of high-speed videoendoscopy. Proceedings of the 6th International Conference: Advances in Laryngology, Voice and Speech Research, Hamburg, Germany.

Eckel, F. C., Boone, D. R. (1981). The S/Z ratio as an indicator of laryngeal pathology. J Speech Hear Disord 46, 147–149.

Eckel, H. E., Koebke, J., Sittel, C., Sprinzl, G. M., Pototschnig, C., Stennert, E. (1999). Morphology of the human larynx during the first five years of life studied on whole organ serial sections. Ann Otol Rhinol Laryngol 108, 232–238.

Fant, G. (1960). *Acoustic theory of speech production.* The Hague: Mouton.

Fisher, K. V., Ligon, J., Sobecks, J. L., Roxe, D. M. (2001). Phonatory effects of body fluid removal. J Speech Lang Hear Res 44, 354–367.

Ford, C. N., Unger, J. M., Zundel, R. S., Bless, D. M. (1995). Magnetic resonance imaging (MRI) assessment of vocal fold medialization surgery. Laryngoscope 105(5 Pt 1), 498–504.

Gelfer, M. P. (1995). Fundamental frequency, intensity, and vowel selection: effects on measures of phonatory stability. J Speech Hear Res 38, 1189–1198.

Gerratt, B. R., Kreiman, J. (2001). Measuring vocal quality with speech synthesis. J Acoust Soc Am 110(5 Pt 1), 2560–2566.

Gerratt, B. R., Kreiman, J., Antonanzas-Barroso, N., Berke, G. S. (1993). Comparing internal and external standards in voice quality judgments. J Speech Hear Res 36, 14–20.

Giovanni, A., Ouaknine, M., Triglia, J. M. (1999). Determination of largest Lyapunov exponents of vocal signal: application to unilateral laryngeal paralysis. J Voice 13, 341–354.

Gliklich, R. E., Glovsky, R. M., Montgomery, W. W. (1999). Validation of a voice outcome survey for unilateral vocal cord paralysis. Otolaryngol Head Neck Surg 120, 153–158.

Glindmeyer, H. W., Lefante, J. J., McColloster, C., Jones, R. N., Weill, H. (1995). Blue-collar normative spirometric values for Caucasian and African-American men and women aged 18 to 65. Am J Respir Crit Care Med 151(2 Pt 1), 412–422.

Golshan, M., Nematbakhsh, M., Amra, B., Crapo, R. O. (2003). Spirometric reference values in a large Middle Eastern population. Eur Respir J 22, 529–534.

Gray, S. D., Hammond, E., Hanson, D. F. (1995). Benign pathologic responses of the larynx. Ann Otol Rhinol Laryngol 104, 13–18.

Gunter, H. E. (2004). Modeling mechanical stresses as a factor in the etiology of benign vocal fold lesions. J Biomech 37, 1119–1124.

Hammarberg, B. (2000). Voice research and clinical needs. Folia Phoniatr Logop 52, 93–102.

Hammarberg, B., Gauffin, J. (1995). Perceptual and acoustic characteristics of quality differences in pathological voices as related to physiological aspects. In O. Fujimura, M. Hirano (Eds.), *Vocal fold physiology: voice quality control* (pp. 283–303). San Diego: Singular.

Hartnick, C. J. (2002). Validation of a pediatric voice quality-of-life instrument: the pediatric voice outcome survey. Arch Otolaryngol Head Neck Surg 128, 919–922.

Hartnick, C. J., Volk, M., Cunningham, M. (2003). Establishing normative voice-related quality of life scores within the pediatric otolaryngology population. Arch Otolaryngol Head Neck Surg 129, 1090–1093 .

Hertegard, S., Gauffin, J., Lindestad, P. A. (1995). A comparison of subglottal and intraoral pressure measurements during phonation. J Voice 9, 149–155.

Herzel, H., Berry, D., Titze, I. R., Saleh, M. (1994). Analysis of vocal disorders with methods from nonlinear dynamics. J Speech Hear Res 37, 1008–1019.

Herzel, H., Berry, D., Titze, I., Steinecke, I. (1995). Nonlinear dynamics of the voice: signal analysis and biomechanical modeling. Chaos 5, 30–34.

Hibi, S. R., Bless, D. M., Hirano, M., Yoshida, T. (1988). Distortions of videofiberoscopy imaging: reconsideration and correction. J Voice 2, 168–175.

Hillenbrand, J., Cleveland, R. A., Erickson, R. L. (1994). Acoustic correlates of breathy vocal quality. J Speech Hear Res 37, 769–778.

Hillenbrand, J., Houde, R. A. (1996). Acoustic correlates of breathy vocal quality: dysphonic voices and continuous speech . J Speech Hear Res 39, 311–321.

Hillman, R. E., Holmberg, E. B., Perkell, J. S., Walsh, M., Vaughan, C. (1989). Objective assessment of vocal hyperfunction: an experimental framework and initial results. J Speech Hear Res 32, 373–392.

Hirano, M. (1981). *Clinical examination of voice.* New York: Springer-Verlag.

Hirano, M., Bless, D. M. (1993). Videostroboscopic examination of the larynx. San Diego: Singular Publishing Group.

Hirano, M., Kurita, S., Nakashima, T. (1983). Growth, development and aging of human vocal folds. In D. M. Bless, J. H. Abbs (Eds.), *Vocal fold physiology: contemporary research and clinical issues* (pp. 22–43). San Diego: College-Hill Press.

Hirose, H. (1988). High-speed digital imaging of vocal fold vibration. Acta Otolaryngol Suppl 458, 151–153.

Hixon, T. J., Goldman, M. D., Mead, J. (1973). Kinematics of the chest wall during speech production: volume displacements of the rib cage, abdomen, and lung. J Speech Hear Res 16, 78–115.

Hixon, T. J., Mead, J., Goldman, M. D. (1976). Dynamics of the chest wall during speech production: function of the thorax, rib cage, diaphragm, and abdomen. J Speech Hear Res 19, 297–356.

Hogikyan, N. D., Sethuraman, G. (1999). Validation of an instrument to measure voice-related quality of life (V-RQOL). J Voice 13, 557–569.

Hogikyan, N. D., Wodchis, W. P., Spak, C., Kileny, P. R. (2001). Longitudinal effects of botulinum toxin injections on voice-related quality of life (V-RQOL) for patients with adductory spasmodic dysphonia. J Voice 15, 576–586.

Hogikyan, N. D., Wodchis, W. P., Terrell, J. E., Bradford, C. R., Esclamado, R. M. (2000). Voice-related quality of life (V-RQOL) following type I thyroplasty for unilateral vocal fold paralysis. J Voice 14, 378–386.

Hoit, J. D., Hixon, T. J. (1992). Age and laryngeal airway resistance during vowel production in women. J Speech Hear Res 35, 309–313.

Hollien, H. (1987). Old voices: what do we really know about them? J Voice 1, 2–7.

Holmberg, E. B., Hillman, R. E., Perkell, J. S. (1988). Glottal airflow and transglottal air pressure measurements for male and female speakers in soft, normal, and loud voice. J Acoust Soc Am 84, 511–529.

Holmes, L. C., Leeper, H. A., Nicholson, I. R. (1994). Laryngeal airway resistance of older men and women as a function of vocal sound pressure level. J Speech Hear Res 37, 789–799.

Hufnagle, J., Hufnagle, K. K. (1988). S/Z ratio in dysphonic children with and without vocal cord nodules. Lang Speech Hear Serv Sch 19, 418–422.

Isshiki, N. (1981). Vocal efficiency index. In K. N. Stevens, M. Hirano (Eds.), *Vocal fold physiology* (pp. 193–207). Tokyo: University of Tokyo Press.

Jacobson, B. H., Johnson, A., Grywalski, C., Silbergleit, A., Jacobson, G., Benninger, M. S., et al. (1997). The voice handicap index (VHI): development and validation. Am J Speech Lang Pathol 6, 66–70.

Jiang, J., Stern, J., Chen, H. J., Solomon, N. P. (2004). Vocal efficiency measurements in subjects with vocal polyps and nodules: a preliminary report. Ann Otol Rhinol Laryngol 113, 277–282.

Karnell, M. P. (1991). Laryngeal perturbation analysis: minimum length of analysis window. J Speech Hear Res 34, 544–548.

Kent, R. D. (1993). Vocal tract acoustics. J Voice 7, 97–117.

Kent, R. D., Kent, J. F., Rosenbek, J. C. (1987). Maximum performance tests of speech production. J Speech Hear Disord 52, 367–387.

Kent, R. D., Read, C. (2002). *Acoustic analysis of speech* (2nd ed.). Albany, NY: Delmar Learning.

Kitajima, K. (1985). Airflow study of pathologic larynges using a hot wire flowmeter. Ann Otol Rhinol Laryngol 94(2 Pt 1), 195–197.

Kitzing, P., Akerlund, L. (1993). Long-time average spectrograms of dysphonic voices before and after therapy. Folia Phoniatr (Basel) 45, 53–61.

Kitzing, P., Lofqvist, A. (1975). Subglottal and oral air pressures during phonation-preliminary investigation using a miniature transducer system. Med Biol Eng 13, 644–648.

Klingholz, F. (1987). The measurement of the signal-to-noise ratio (SNR) in continuous speech. Speech Commun 6, 15–26.

Kreiman, J., Gerratt, B. R. (1998). Validity of rating scale measures of voice quality. J Acoust Soc Am, 104(3 Pt 1), 1598–1608.

Kreiman, J., Gerratt, B. R. (2000). Sources of listener disagreement in voice quality assessment. J Acoust Soc Am 108, 1867–1876.

Kreiman, J., Gerratt, B. R., Kempster, G. B., Erman, A., Berke, G. S. (1993). Perceptual evaluation of voice quality: review, tutorial, and a framework for future research. J Speech Hear Res 36, 21–40.

Kreiman, J., Gerratt, B. R., Precoda, K. (1990). Listener experience and perception of voice quality. J Speech Hear Res 33, 103–115.

Kreiman, J., Gerratt, B. R., Precoda, K., Berke, G. S. (1992). Individual differences in voice quality perception. J Speech Hear Res 35, 512–520.

Larsson, H., Hertegard, S., Lindestad, P. A., Hammarberg, B. (2000). Vocal fold vibrations: high-speed imaging, kymography, and acoustic analysis: a preliminary report. Laryngoscope 110, 2117–2122.

Laver, J. (1980). *The phonetic description of voice quality*. Cambridge: Cambridge University Press.

Laver, J. (2000). Phonetic evaluation of voice quality. In R. D. Kent, M. J. Ball (Eds.), *Voice quality measurement* (pp. 37–48). San Diego: Singular.

Laver, J., Hiller, S.M., Mackenzie Beck, J. (1992). Acoustic waveform perturbations and voice disorders. J Voice 6, 115–126.

Lee, J. S., Kim, E., Park, K. S., Sung, M. Y., Sung, M. W., Kim, K. H. (1998). Development of videostrobokymography for the quantitative analysis of laryngeal vibratory pattern. Medinfo 9 (Pt 2), 1022–1024.

Lee, J. S., Kim, E., Sung, M. W., Kim, K. H., Sung, M. Y., Park, K. S. (2001). A method for assessing the regional vibratory pattern of vocal folds by analysing the video recording of stroboscopy. Med Biol Eng Comput 39, 273–278.

Lieberman, P. (1968). Direct comparison of subglottal and esophageal pressure during speech. J Acoust Soc Am 43, 1157–1164.

Linville, S. E. (2002). Source characteristics of aged voice assessed from long-term average spectra. J Voice 16, 472–479.

Lofqvist, A., Carlborg, B., Kitzing, P. (1982). Initial validation of an indirect measure of subglottal pressure during vowels. J Acoust Soc Am 72, 633–635.

Ma, E. P., Yiu, E. M. (2001). Voice activity and participation profile: assessing the impact of voice disorders on daily activities. J Speech Lang Hear Res 44, 511–524.

Melcon, M. C., Hoit, J. D., Hixon, T. J. (1989). Age and laryngeal airway resistance during vowel production. J Speech Hear Disord 54, 282–286.

Mendoza, E., Valencia, N., Munoz, J., Trujillo, H. (1996). Differences in voice quality between men and women: use of the long-term average spectrum (LTAS). J Voice 10, 59–66.

Miller, J. E., Matthews, M. V. (1963). Investigation of the glottal waveshape by automatic inverse filtering. J Acoust Soc Am 67, 1876.

Murry, T., Medrado, R., Hogikyan, N. D., Aviv, J. E. (2004). The relationship between ratings of voice quality and quality of life measures. J Voice 18, 183–192.

Netsell, R., Lotz, W. K., Peters, J. E., Schulte, L. (1994). Developmental patterns of laryngeal and respiratory function for speech production. J Voice 8, 123–131.

Nyquist, H. (1928). Certain topics in telegraph transmission theory. Proc IEEE 47, 617–644.

Orlikoff, R. F. (1989). Vocal jitter at different fundamental frequencies: a cardiovascular-neuromuscular explanation. J Voice 3, 104–112.

Orlikoff, R. F. (1990a). Heartbeat related fundamental frequency and amplitude variation in healthy young and elderly male voices. J Voice 4, 322–328.

Orlikoff, R. F. (1990b). The relationship of age and cardiovascular health to certain acoustic characteristics of male voices. J Speech Hear Res 33, 450–457.

Orlikoff, R. F. (1991). Assessment of the dynamics of vocal fold contact from the electroglottogram: data from normal male subjects. J Speech Hear Res 34, 1066–1072.

Orlikoff, R. F. (1998). Scrambled EGG: the uses and abuses of electroglottography. Phonoscope 1, 37–53.

Orlikoff, R. F. (2003). Electroglottographic assessment of voice. In R. D. Kent (Ed.), *The MIT encyclopedia of communication disorders* (pp. 23–27). Cambridge, MA: MIT Press.

Orlikoff, R. F., Baken, R. J. (1990). Consideration of the relationship between the fundamental frequency of phonation and vocal jitter. Folia Phoniatr (Basel) 42, 31–40.

Orlikoff, R. F., Kahane, J. C. (1991). Influence of mean sound pressure level on jitter and shimmer measures. J Voice 5, 113–119.

Owens, F. J. (1993). *Signal processing of speech*. New York: McGraw-Hill.

Peppard, R. C., Bless, D. M. (1990). A method for improving measurement reliability in laryngeal videostroboscopy. J Voice 4, 280–285.

Perkell, J. S., Hillman, R. E., Holmberg, E. B. (1994). Group differences in measures of voice production and revised values of maximum airflow declination rate. J Acoust Soc Am 96(2 Pt 1), 695–698.

Plant, R. L., Hillel, A. D. (1998). Direct measurement of subglottic pressure and laryngeal resistance in normal subjects and in spasmodic dysphonia. J Voice 12, 300–314.

Poburka, B. J. (1999). A new stroboscopy rating form. J Voice 13, 403–413.

Poburka, B. J., Bless, D. M. (1998). A multi-media, computer-based method for stroboscopy rating training. J Voice 12, 513–526.

Qiu, Q., Schutte, H. K., Gu, L., Yu, Q. (2003). An automatic method to quantify the vibration properties of human vocal folds via videokymography. Folia Phoniatr Logop 55, 128–136.

Qui, Q., Schutte, H. K. (2006). A new generation videokymography for routine clinical vocal fold examination. Laryngoscope, 116, 1824–1828.

Rabinov, C. R., Kreiman, J., Gerratt, B. R., Bielamowicz, S. (1995). Comparing reliability of perceptual ratings of roughness and acoustic measure of jitter. J Speech Hear Res 38, 26–32.

Rastatter, M. P., Hyman, M. (1982). Maximum phonation duration of /s/ and /z/ by children with vocal nodules. Lang Speech Hear Serv Sch 13, 197–199.

Read, C., Buder, E. H., Kent, R. D. (1992). Speech analysis systems: an evaluation. J Speech Hear Res 35, 314–332.

Rosen, C. A., Murry, T. (2000). Voice handicap index in singers. J Voice 14, 370–377.

Rosen, C. A., Murry, T., Zinn, A., Zullo, T., Sonbolian, M. (2000). Voice handicap index change following treatment of voice disorders. J Voice 14, 619–623.

Rosen, D., Minhaj, A., Hinds, M., Kobler, J., Hillman, R. (2003). Calibrated sizing system for flexible laryngeal endoscopy. Proceedings of the 6th International Conference: Advances in Laryngology, Voice and Speech Research, Hamburg, Germany.

Rothenberg, M. (1973). A new inverse-filtering technique for deriving the glottal air flow waveform during voicing. J Acoust Soc Am 53, 1632–1645.

Rothenberg, M. (1977). Measurements of airflow in speech. J Speech Hear Res 20, 155–176.

Rothenberg, M., Mahshie, J. J. (1988). Monitoring vocal fold abduction through vocal fold contact area. J Speech Hear Res 31, 338–351.

Rubin, A. D., Wodchis, W. P., Spak, C., Kileny, P. R., Hogikyan, N. D. (2004). Longitudinal effects of Botox injections on voice-related quality of life (V-RQOL) for patients with adductory spasmodic dysphonia: part II. Arch Otolaryngol Head Neck Surg 130, 415–420.

Russell, N. K., Stathopoulos, E. (1988). Lung volume changes in children and adults during speech production. J Speech Hear Res 31, 146–155.

Sapienza, C. M., Stathopoulos, E. T. (1994). Comparison of maximum flow declination rate: children versus adults. J Voice 8, 240–247.

Scherer, R. C., Vail, V. J., Guo, C. G. (1995). Required number of tokens to determine representative voice perturbation values. J Speech Hear Res 38, 1260–1269.

Scherer, R. C., Vail, V. J., Rockwell, B. (1995). Examination of the laryngeal adduction measure EGGW. In F. Bell-Berti, L. J. Raphael (Eds.), *Producing speech: contemporary issues: for Katherine Safford Harris* (pp. 269–289). New York: ATI Press.

Schuberth, S., Hoppe, U., Dollinger, M., Lohscheller, J., Eysholdt, U. (2002). High-precision measurement of the vocal fold length and vibratory amplitudes. Laryngoscope 112, 1043–1049.

Schutte, H. K., Švec, J. G., Šram, F. (1998). First results of clinical application of videokymography. Laryngoscope 108, 1206–1210.

Shannon, C. E. (1949). Communication in the presence of noise. Proc Institute Radio Eng 37, 10–21.

Sivasankar, M., Fisher, K. V. (2003). Oral breathing challenge in participants with vocal attrition. J Speech Lang Hear Res 46, 1416–1427.

Smitheran, J. R., Hixon, T. J. (1981). A clinical method for estimating laryngeal airway resistance during vowel production. J Speech Hear Disord 46, 138–146.

Solomon, N. P., DiMattia, M. S. (2000). Effects of a vocally fatiguing task and systemic hydration on phonation threshold pressure. J Voice 14, 341–362.

Solomon, N. P., Garlitz, S. J., Milbrath, R. L. (2000). Respiratory and laryngeal contributions to maximum phonation duration. J Voice 14, 331–340.

Solomon, N. P., Glaze, L. E., Arnold, R. R., van Mersbergen, M. (2003). Effects of a vocally fatiguing task and systemic hydration on men's voices. J Voice 17, 31–46.

Sorenson, D. N., Parker, P. A. (1992). The voiced/voiceless phonation time in children with and without laryngeal pathology. Lang Speech Hear Serv Sch 23, 163–168.

Speyer, R., Wieneke, G. H., van Wijck-Warnaar, I., Dejonckere, P. H. (2003). Effects of voice therapy on the voice range profiles of dysphonic patients. J Voice 17, 544–556.

Šram, F., Schutte, H. K., Švec, J. G. (1997). Clinical applications of videokymography. In G. McCafferty, W. Coman, R. Carroll (Eds.), Proceedings of the XVI World Congress of Otorhinolaryngology Head and Neck Surgery, Volume 2 (pp. 1681–1684). Bologna: Monduzzi Editore.

Sulter, A. M., Schutte, H. K., Miller, D. G. (1995). Differences in phonetogram features between male and female subjects with and without vocal training. J Voice 9, 363–377.

Susser, R., Bless, D. M. (1983). Vocal intensity measures of normal and voice-disordered children. Folia Phoniatr 35, 176–177.

Švec, J. G. (2000). On vibration properties of human vocal folds: voice registers, bifurcations, resonance characteristics, development and application of videokymography. Ph.D. dissertation. Groningen: University of Groningen. Available at http://www.ub.rug.nl/eldoc/dis/medicine/j.svec.

Švec, J. G., Schutte, H. K. (1996). Videokymography: high-speed line scanning of vocal fold vibration. J Voice 10, 201–205.

Švec, J. G., Schutte, H. K., Šram, F. (1997). *Introduction to videokymography* [videotape]. Prague: Medical Healthcom.

Švec, J. G., Šram, F., Schutte, H. K. (2001). Development and application of videokymography for high-speed examination of vocal-fold vibration. In B. Palek, O. Fujimura (Eds.), Proceedings of LP'2000 (pp. 3–10). Prague: Karolinum Press.

Tait, N. A., Michel, J. F., Carpenter, M. A. (1980). Maximum duration of sustained /s/ and /z/ in children. J Speech Hear Disord 45, 239–246.

Teles-Magalhaes, L. C., Pegoraro-Krook, M. I., Pegoraro, R. (2000). Study of the elderly females' voice by phonetography. J Voice 14, 310–321.

Tigges, M., Wittenberg, T., Mergell, P., Eysholdt, U. (1999). Imaging of vocal fold vibration by digital multi-plane kymography. Comput Med Imaging Graph 23, 323–330.

Timcke, R., von Leden, H., Moore, P. (1958). Laryngeal vibrations: measurements of the glottic wave. Part I: the normal vibratory cycle. Arch Otolaryngol 68, 1–19.

Timcke, R., von Leden, H., Moore, P. (1959). Laryngeal vibrations: measurements of the glottic wave. Part II: physiologic variations. Arch Otolaryngol 69, 438–444.

Titze, I. R. (1988). The physics of small-amplitude oscillation of the vocal folds. J Acoust Soc Am 83, 1536–1552.

Titze, I. R. (1990). Interpretation of the electroglottographic signal. J Voice 4, 1–9.

Titze, I. R. (1994a). *Principles of voice production.* Englewood Cliffs, NJ: Prentice-Hall.

Titze, I. R. (1994b). Mechanical stress in phonation. J Voice 8, 99–105.

Titze, I. R. (1995). *Acoustic voice analysis: summary statement.* Iowa City, IA: National Center for Voice and Speech.

Titze, I. R., Liang, H. (1993). Comparison of F_0 extraction methods for high-precision voice perturbation measurements. J Speech Hear Res 36, 1120–1133.

Titze, I. R., Winholtz, W. S. (1993). Effect of microphone type and placement on voice perturbation measurements. J Speech Hear Res 36, 1177–1190.

Verdolini, K., Titze, I. R., Fennell, A. (1994). Dependence of phonatory effort on hydration level. J Speech Hear Res 37, 1001–1007.

Verdolini-Marston, K., Titze, I. R., Druker, D. G. (1990). Changes in phonation threshold pressure with induced conditions of hydration. J Voice 4, 142–151.

von Leden, H., Moore, P., Timcke, R. (1960). Laryngeal vibrations: measurement of the glottic wave. Part III: the pathologic larynx. Arch Otolaryngol 71, 16–35.

Watson, P. J., Hixon, T. J. (1985). Respiratory kinematics in classical (opera) singers. J Speech Hear Res 28, 104–122.

White, P. (2001). Long-term average spectrum (LTAS) analysis of sex- and gender-related differences in children's voices. Logoped Phoniatr Vocol 26, 97–101.

Whitehead, R. L., Metz, D. E., Whitehead, B. H. (1984). Vibratory patterns of the vocal folds during pulse register phonation. J Acoust Soc Am 75, 1293–1297.

Wilson, D. K. (1987). *Voice problems of children* (3rd ed.). Baltimore: Williams and Wilkins.

Wilson, F. B., Starr, C. D. (1985). Use of the phonation analyzer as a clinical tool. J Speech Hear Disord 50, 351–356.

Wittenberg, T., Kothe, C., Munzenmayer, C., Grobe, M., Volk, H., Hess, M. M. (2003). Automatic classification of leukoplakia on vocal folds using color texture features. Proceedings of the 6th International Conference: Advances in Laryngology, Voice and Speech Research, Hamburg, Germany.

Woo, P. (1986). Phonatory volume velocity recording by use of hot film anemometry and signal analysis. Otolaryngol Head Neck Surg 95(3 Pt 1), 312–318.

Woo, P., Colton, R., Casper, J., Brewer, D. (1991). Diagnostic value of stroboscopic examination in hoarse patients. J Voice 5, 231–238.

Woo, P., Colton, R. H., Shangold, L. (1987). Phonatory airflow analysis in patients with laryngeal disease. Ann Otol Rhinol Laryngol 96, 549–555.

World Health Organization. (1980). International Classification of Impairment, Disability and Handicap. Geneva: WHO.

World Health Organization. (2001). International Classification of Functioning, Disability and Health. Geneva: WHO.

Wuyts, F. L., Heylen, L., Mertens, F., Du Caju, M., Rooman, R., Van de Heyning, P. H., et al. (2003). Effects of age, sex, and disorder on voice range profile characteristics of 230 children. Ann Otol Rhinol Laryngol 112, 540–548.

Yan, Y., Ahmad, K., Kunduk, M., Bless, D. M. (2005). Analysis of vocal-fold vibrations from high-speed laryngeal images using a Hilbert transform based methodology. J Voice 19, 161–175.

Yanagihara, N. (1967). Significance of harmonic changes and noise components in hoarseness. J Speech Hear Res 10, 531–541.

Yangihara, N., von Leden, H. (1967). Respiration and phonation: the functional examination of laryngeal disease. Folia Phoniatr 19, 153–166.

Yumoto, E., Gould, W. J., Baer, T. (1982). Harmonics-to-noise ratio as an index of the degree of hoarseness. J Acoust Soc Am 71, 1544–1550.

Zhang, Y., McGilligan, C., Zhou, L., Vig, M., Jiang, J. J. (2004). Nonlinear dynamic analysis of voices before and after surgical excision of vocal polyps. J Acoust Soc Am 115(5 Pt 1), 2270–2277.

Zheng, J., Zhong, N. (2002). Normative values of pulmonary function testing in Chinese adults. Chin Med J (Engl) 115, 50–54.

Additional Reading

Baken, R. J., Orlikoff, R. F. (2000). *Clinical measurement of speech and voice* (2nd ed.). San Diego: Singular Publishing Group.

Hillman, R. E., Holmberg, E. B., Perkell, J. S., Walsh, M., Vaughan, C. (1989). Objective assessment of vocal hyperfunction: an experimental framework and initial results. J Speech Hear Res 32, 373–392.

Hirano, M., Bless, D. M. (1993). *Videostroboscopic examination of the larynx.* San Diego: Singular Publishing Group.

Kreiman, J., Gerratt, B. R., Kempster, G. B., Erman, A., Berke, G. S. (1993). Perceptual evaluation of voice quality: review, tutorial, and a framework for future research. J Speech Hear Res 36, 21–40.

Orlikoff, R. F. (1998). Scrambled EGG: the uses and abuses of electroglottography. Phonoscope 1, 37–53.

Smitheran, J. R., Hixon, T. J. (1981). A clinical method for estimating laryngeal airway resistance during vowel production. J Speech Hear Disord 46, 138–146.

Titze, I. R. (1995). *Acoustic voice analysis: summary statement.* Iowa City, IA: National Center for Voice and Speech.

Chapter 8

Psychogenic and Other Behavioral Voice Disorders

Voice is more than a mechanical or acoustic phenomenon. It is a mirror of personality, a carrier of moods and emotions, a key to neurotic and psychotic tendencies.

—Brodnitz

When I began my tenure at the Mayo Clinic 45 years ago, I was overwhelmed and uncomprehending of the richness of clinical material. "You can do anything you want here," Dr. Charles Mayo said to me on my intake interview, "so long as you remember that the patient comes first." Then they started coming, the word must have gotten around. They came from every medical and dental specialty conceivable. Referrals came for speech disorders that I had never read or even heard about, undocumented speech, voice, and language signs and symptoms: pharyngeo-laryngeo oculo-linguo myoclonus, foreign dialect syndrome, focal dystonias, borborygmi. I began to specialize in identification of the dysarthrias in neurologic disease and proposed to Dr. Fred Darley that we study the perceptual characteristics of the dysarthrias.

The second disorder that piqued my interest was voice disorders, particularly patients with dysphonias and aphonias referred to me from otolaryngologists—patients who had normal laryngologic examinations and for whom no rational organic etiology was apparent; patients often labeled as having functional or nonorganic etiologies. Being puzzled by the term *functional* caused me to wonder how it was possible for a person to be speaking in a normal voice since early childhood and then, for the first time in adulthood, develop a hoarse, breathy, or loss of voice entirely (as in whispering or muteness). I thought back to my undergraduate and graduate education and realized that the causes of nonorganic voice disorders were never addressed in any logical or convincing fashion. Vocal abuse and vocal hyperfunction were the only categories mentioned.

Then a patient was referred to me who taught me that most nonorganic voice disorders did not occur sponta-

neously or from vocal abuse or faulty habit pattern. A 45-year-old nun, a nurse who worked on the ophthalmology floor of a hospital, had come to the clinic complaining of episodes of whispering. Her laryngologic examination failed to disclose any evidence of laryngeal pathology.

Never having been confronted by someone with an aphonia, I recorded and listened carefully to her voice, searching for words that would describe the complexity of her aphonia. It was a mixture of breathiness and strained hoarseness, interspersed with squeaks and squeals. Then I asked myself, "What was I supposed to do for this patient and her referring physician? Why, if this patient had a normal laryngeal examination, was she whispering and speaking with a squeaky voice?" She was a quiet nun, not yelling at basketball games or arguing loudly with others. I began to search the medical library for articles on aphonia. I discovered that many had been written by otolaryngologists and psychiatrists stating that aphonia is often caused by psychologic conflict, that it could be a hysterical or conversion disorder.

She complained of a pain in the region of her larynx that radiated to her ears and down to her chest. She said that she felt as if she had a lump in her throat, like a ball that was difficult to swallow. At that point, I believed I had two options: to refer her to psychiatry or become the psychiatrist myself and investigate the psychogenic hypothesis. I was in a quandary. Did I have the ethical right to investigate this patient's personal life? Would it be dangerous to her if I did? I had no prior personal training in psychodiagnostic interviewing or psychotherapy. However, in light of the fact that I had been told I could do anything, I wanted to help and was determined to pursue a psychodiagnostic investigation.

At that time, the chairman of the Department of Psychiatry was Dr. Edward M. Litin. He was a tall, rangy man with a deep, resonant voice; he could probably have been cast in the role of God. I had met him at a reception and liked his directness. I phoned him and asked him if he could meet with me, to which he agreed. Where patients were concerned, these were called "curbside consultations." We met over a cup of coffee, and I told him about my patient who was still sitting in my office. I told him about my reservations concerning the ethics and safety of my attempting a probing psychodiagnostic examination. I can see him now; leaning back in his chair, his long legs stretched out in front of him, and with that sepulchral voice of his he told me, "Arnold, I have found that human beings are tougher than that; that each of us possesses a character armor that shields us from divulging painful information. And as for the ethics of investigating emotional causes, I think it is reasonable to say that it would be unethical if you did *not* do so." He continued, "Actually, patients usually feel much better after they have revealed or unburdened themselves of repressed conflicts. Such catharsis provides the patient with a sense of relief for having unburdened themselves. And they are better off for the experience."

I returned to my patient and asked her if any of these aphonic episodes were associated with stresses in her life or personal problems. Tearfully, she told me that her life as a nun had not been what she had expected. At her age, it was overly physically demanding. She was expected to work 80 hours per week, ministering to patients on the ophthalmology floor, and that she no longer had the energy to sustain this kind of workload. But she could not bring herself to tell the mother superior and ask for a reduced workload. It was just against her concept of her responsibilities as a nun and a nurse. As she cried and spoke, her voice gradually returned to normal.

And that was my baptism of fire, a classic conversion disorder—a loss of motor or sensory function of nonorganic etiology as a solution to a conflict. Unconsciously, without a voice she was cast in a sick role, the symbolic function of the voice loss now being that she would be unable to divulge her true feelings to her superior.

Now, I know that many speech pathologists have not been trained as I had, not in this technique, and are reluctant to embark upon such a venture with a patient. But this first lesson has been the mainstay of my practice as a specialist in voice disorders, and ever since I have made it a rule to assume that all nonorganic voice disorders are to be presumed as having a psychogenic etiology and that they all need to be subjected to a psychodiagnostic interview.

◆ Voice as an Indicator of Normal Personality

Personality encompasses those behaviors that distinguish each individual as being different from others (e.g., facial expression, gestures, posture, gait, intelligence, aggressiveness, confidence, attitudes, feelings, sensitivity, and emotional reactivity). Although one might argue that how a person speaks—voice quality, pitch, loudness, stress patterns, rate, pause, articulation, vocabulary, syntax, and ideational content—qualifies as a trait of personality, attempts to demonstrate it have been confounded by several obstacles including individual differences in anatomy, imitation or

learning of parental and sibling voice patterns, and semantic and methodologic impediments:

♦ unsatisfactory definition of personality

♦ questionable validity and reliability of personality tests

♦ difficulty in defining voice variables

♦ variations in research methodology (e.g., selection of subjects as to age, sex, and ethnic background; tests of personality and voice; parameters, methods, and units of measurement)

Nevertheless, there has been no shortage of studies on the relationship between personality and voice. Early investigators attempted to relate auditory perceptual judgments of voice to personality traits such as neurotic tendency, anxiety, introversion, and extraversion. They suggested associations between selected percepts and personality: (1) breathy voice with neurotic tendency, anxiety, low dominance, and high introversion; (2) harsh/metallic voices with high dominance and emotional instability; (3) nasal whine with emotional instability and low dominance; (4) high loudness and low pitch are found with high dominance (Mallory and Miller, 1958; Moore, 1939); (5) hoarseness with reticence and self-consciousness; (6) increased speaking rate with competence and decreased rate with decreased competence and increased benevolence; (7) wide variations in pitch with benevolence and decreased variations in pitch and average level were associated with less competence and benevolence (Brown, Strong, and Rencher, 1974; Williamson, 1945).

At the time these studies were completed, less was known about psychophysical scaling techniques, observer bias, the physiologic processes underlying voice production, and the inherent difficulty in interpreting studies on personality and voice. Accordingly, it is not surprising these interesting observational associations between perceptual qualities and personality have not stood the test of time. This is due, at least in part, to the research methods employed. For example, several of the studies used actors to produce the voice samples. Subsequent studies showed that different actors may attempt to convey the same personality characteristics with widely different voice patterns. In other words, actors are somewhat individualistic in their acoustic preferences in coding personality and speech. Research attempting to relate specific voice features and personality characteristics has conflicting results implying there is not a one-to-one relationship. Differences may relate to personal experiences, interpretation of specific dialogues, bias, and the influence of listeners' personality on judgments. Nevertheless, it is clear that listeners make some judgments about personality characteristics from listening to voice. For example, children with dysphonia were rated negatively on social and personality factors by naïve, young adult judges when compared with those without dysphonia (Ruscello, Lass, and Podbesek, 1988). Specifically, based on voice recordings alone, dysphonic children were judged more negatively on dimensions of "dirty," "cruel," "bad," "worthless," "dishonest," "sick," "sad," "unpleasant," and "ugly" than were their nondysphonic peers ($P < 0.01$). Thus it appears that listeners have psychological percepts relating voice and personality but those characteristics have not yet been clearly defined. Later in this chapter, we will discuss how personality characteristics may relate to specific voice disorders.

◆ Voice as an Indicator of Discrete Emotions

The idea that vocal acoustics are imbued with cues to vocalize emotional state has a long history in human inquiry. For instance, Cicero and Aristotle suggested that each emotion is associated with a distinctive tone of voice—a view espoused by one of the leading contemporary theories of vocal expression. However, it was arguably Darwin who provided the first comprehensive description of the sounds associated with emotion.

Darwin adopted an explicitly comparative perspective, examining emotion-related vocal signals in a variety of species that included nonhuman primates, ruminants, domestic dogs and cats, and humans. In each case, his rich descriptions led him to conclude that both these and other affective expressions are veridical, meaning that there is a direct correspondence between particular signaler states and the communicative display produced. Thus, Darwin treated emotion-related signaling as an inherently honest indicator of internal state.

However, he also made two important observations that suggest a different perspective. The first was that vocal signals can induce emotional responses in listeners; for example, when courting males use calls that "charm or excite the female" during mating season. The second was then going on to say that these vocal signals become associated with the "anticipation of the strongest possible pleasure which animals are capable of feeling." ". . . the critical ideas are that signalers can use species-typical sounds to influence listener affect, and that individually distinctive aspects of these signals come to elicit learned emotional response in recipients that hear them in association with affect-inducing events" (Bachorowski and Owren, 2003).

Affective prosody is defined as the pitch, intonation range, tempo, pausing, emphasis/stress, and rhythm that is automatically and subconsciously injected into speech and signifies emotion of the speaker (Monnot, 2005). When words and affective prosody do not match, as when someone is depressed but professes to be well, healthy listeners attend to the tone of voice rather than the linguistic content and make social judgments based on that subconsciously processed information (Monnot, 2005). Affective prosodic function has been shown to be a dominant and lateralized function of the right hemisphere (Monnot, 2002; Ross, 1997, 1998) that declines with age (Monnot, 2005) and that can be disrupted or destroyed by clinical conditions such as alcoholism, schizophrenia, or by right hemisphere cortical lesions (Monnot, 2002; Ross, 1997; Testa, 2001).

Vocal communication, or affective prosody, includes many elements of emotion such as happiness, joy, confidence, anger, grief, and boredom. Although social emotions are specific to the culture in which they are learned, emotions have been described as short-lived psychologic-physiologic phenomena that represent "honest signals" and are thought to be critical to human communication. In fact, human survival has been hypothesized to be dependent upon vocal communication and language in gregarious species where individuals depend upon the group for safety and protection (Monnot, 2005). A few primary process emotions (anger, sadness, joy/playfulness, fear, disgust, and surprise) are recognized by individuals from diverse cultural backgrounds on the basis of facial expressions and vocal cues. Recent perceptual and acoustic analyses studies indicate that to varying degrees, one emotional state can be distinguished from another using pitch, duration of consonants and vowels, intensity, speech rate, and the means, bandwidth, and spectral shape of the first, second, third, and fourth formants. Reports on perceptual classification of these same emotions ranges from 40 to 60% (Bachorowski and Owren, 2003). These authors suggest that the use of acted rather than natural stimuli may result in emotional portrayals that do not closely correspond with naturally produced vocal expressions of emotion.

Monnot, Orbelo, Riccardo, et al. (2003) have demonstrated that acoustic analyses of fundamental frequency (F_0) are positively associated with subjective judgments of emotion and that detoxified alcoholics who could not vary F_0 were unable to convey emotion accurately to communication partners. This is corroborated by studies of F_0 and emotion demonstrating that speech without F_0, such as whispering, is almost devoid of cues that enable the listener to detect emotion (Monnot, Orbelo, Riccardo, et al., 2003). However, not all recent research on voice and emotions is in agreement. Studies by Kakehi (2005) designed to investigate the perceptual relationship among six basic emotional categories (happiness, fear, anger, disgust, sadness, and neutrality) found that the emotional perception of voice was not categorical.

Similar results were reported by Morosomme and Verduyckt (2005) in a study attempting to compare adolescent with adult listeners' perceived emotions (anger, fear, joy, sadness, neutral, and others) expressed by an actor and patient with progressive muscular atrophy. As in other perceptual studies of emotion, agreement was generally no more than 60%, and differences between adults and adolescents and between males and females were minimal. Perceptual accuracy is reduced when the stimuli presented have been filtered or presented in noise that masks semantic content and are influenced by talker sex and emotional traits and pursuit of social goals and context in which the sample is being produced. Identification of emotions conveyed through voice might be increased by acoustic analyses that does not depend on visual cues and removes listener bias. In a Russian study of actors, recognition rate of a set of emotions (anger, irony, surprise, fear, annoyance, joy, shame, and neutral) was nearly 80% correct using a set of acoustic parameters to describe "prosodic emotions" (pitch, duration of consonants and vowels, intensity, speech rate, means of the first, second, third, and forth formants, bandwidth and spectral shape [Sidorova, 2005]).

Campos, Thein, and Owen (2003) argue that one function of vocal emotional expression is to regulate behavior. In a mother-child dyad, these investigators manipulated exclamations of anger, fear, or joy when an infant was approaching an object and measured how the vocalizations influenced both looking to the mother and behavior toward the toy. Both anger and fear vocalizations produced significant response inhibition with little differences in infant's emotional behavior. On the other hand, the emotional response to joy vocalizations differed from anger and fear in that it produced minimal behavioral disruption of the infant's progress toward the toy and minimal orienting to the mother.

Because emotion links higher brain functions with lower brain functions (Lang, 1994) and the limbic system has strong connections to motor cortex and extrapyramidal tract (Davidson, 2000; Gray, 1991; LeDoux, 2000), it is no surprise that there is some connection between voice and emotions. The challenge is to accurately identify these emotions to facilitate determining etiology of voice problems and appropriate treatment programs.

◆ Voice as an Indicator of Psychopathology

Affective Disorders

If voice reflects both personality and emotional states, one would assume that voice would also serve as an indicator of psychopathology. Indeed, clinicians have often speculated on a link between psychopathology and voice. Affective disorders are psychiatric syndromes characterized by alterations in mood, such as depression, manic or hypomanic states, euphoria, and mood swings. A depressed outlook either may be lifelong or can occur for the first time in a usually cheerful person who unexpectedly becomes chronically sad, tearful, pessimistic, slow of thought, agitated, disinterested, unable to sleep and eat, and who senses a decline in feelings of self-worth. In one such group of 40 patients who demonstrated sadness, retardation of thought processes, anorexia, and insomnia, Newman and Mather (1938) described their voices as dead or listless, with narrow pitch range, infrequent pitch changes, slow rate, frequent pauses and hesitations, and reduced stress or emphasis patterns. In a second group that exhibited chronic gloom, self-pity, and dissatisfaction, speech patterns were different from the first; these had long gliding inflectional pitch changes over a wide pitch range, lively voices, normal rates but frequent pauses, harsh voice quality, and crisp articulation.

Monotonous downward inflectional patterns have been found in depressed patients (Moses, 1954). Whitman and Flicker (1966) found that pitch became higher and loudness lower in proportion to the degree of depression. In agitated depression, they found an increased articulatory rate as patients became more depressed. In a study done by Hargreaves and Starkweather (1964) in which acoustic spectrographic recordings were made during treatment of depression, as patients improved, their overall vocal intensity and their energy in the higher vowel formants increased. In 10 chronically depressed patients, five showed reduced loudness and diminished inflectional changes. Moreover, patients in the manic phase of manic-depressive reactions produce a very different voice and articulation profile: press of speech;

flight of ideas; vigorous articulation; clear, lively, and vital voice; wide pitch range; frequent gliding pitch changes; frequent emphasis and accent; and exaggerated pauses. As these patients become less manic, their pitch range narrows, emphasis patterns are reduced, pauses and hesitations begin to appear, and articulation becomes less vigorous (Newman and Mather, 1938).

Psychiatrists and psychologists have long acknowledged that they can tell much about their patients' emotional state and underlying psychodynamics by listening to their voices. The psychotherapist also uses his or her own voice in ways that will create a more effective relationship with the patient. Reminding us that virtually all methods of psychotherapy involve two or more persons talking together, Bady (1985) wrote:

Since I have been listening to my patients' voices I have also noted that changes in vocal quality accompany their progress. One patient achieved a lighter, less ponderous voice as he became more comfortable with his emotions. Another slowed down his rapid pace. A third achieved a less grating and more fluid tone.

In her own use of voice as a means of making her therapy more effective, the author further states:

In my work I will intentionally use my voice along with my words. Sometimes I attempt through vocal tones to soothe an anxious, agitated patient. Other times I use my voice to stimulate a depressed and hopeless one. On still other occasions I talk to give the patient a human response and my words are less important than the vocal indication of my presence. Sometimes I remain silent to encourage separation from me. Occasionally my voice backfires on me, as when a patient notices my anger or my anxiety through the sound of my voice.

Noticeable differences between "peak" and "poor" therapy hours can be determined by an analysis of psychotherapists' voices. In one study, the therapist's voice during peak therapy sessions was described as more open, lower in pitch, and of softer intensity than during the poor therapy hours, the former giving the impression of warmth, seriousness, relaxation, and closeness (Duncan, Rice, and Butler, 1968).

Considerable controversy surrounds questions concerning if personality factors and psychologic adjustment should be considered causal, concomitant, or consequential to voice disorders. Roy and Bless (1999, 2000a,b) attempted to answer this question by comparing five groups of speakers, a vocally normal group and four groups of disorders, on measures of personality and psychologic adjustment. The majority of functional voice disorders were classified as introverts and the majority of vocal nodules subjects as extroverts. Mirza, Ruiz, Baum, et al. (2001) found similar results in their study of 53 voice-disordered patients. They also noted that patients with vocal fold paralysis may be at risk for subsequent psychiatric problems.

Schizophrenia

The study of voice of schizophrenics has a long history. Although the majority of literature has been based on clinical reports and single-case studies, the similarities between observations suggest there may be distinct developmental vocal characteristics in this population.

In child schizophrenics, Goldfarb, Brownstein, and Lorge (1956) described hypernasality; breathiness; hoarseness; glottalization; flat voice quality; insufficient or inappropriate volume and pitch changes; narrowed total pitch range; tendency toward excessively high pitch; inappropriate rate changes from phrase to phrase; prolongation of phonemes, syllables, and words; chanting quality; insufficient or inappropriate stress; hesitation after and repetitions of sounds or syllables; and flat, monotonous prosody. In another study, Goldfarb, Goldfarb, Brownstein, and Scholl (1972) noted the absence of a single specific clustering of these speech abnormalities in child schizophrenics, with the basic disturbance being loss of control and of regulation of speech.

In adolescent schizophrenia, Ostwald and Skolnikoff (1966) described a 15-year-old male's speech as having a nasal quality, articulatory imprecision or indistinctness, exaggerated intonational patterns, and a high and prolonged rise in pitch toward the ends of questions. As in childhood schizophrenia, there was excessive variability of rate and rhythm. Similarly, Chevrie-Muller, Dodart, Sequier-Dermer, and Salmon (1971) found reduced pitch range, reduced rate, and increased pause time in female adolescent schizophrenics.

In an adult schizophrenic, melody or pitch patterns were found not to glide but to jump at intervals and without relationship to ideational content. Accent (emphasis or stress pattern) was inappropriate, and speech contained rhythmic monotonous repetitions of vocal patterns (Moses, 1954). Moskowitz (1951) described the speech of adult schizophrenics as monotonous, weak, flat, colorless, and gloomy. Saxman and Burk (1968) found significantly slower reading rates in adult schizophrenics than in normal subjects.

◆ Voice as an Indicator of Life Stress

Clinical and instrumental studies prove that otherwise normal voice perceptibly and measurably changes under emotional stress. A smooth, well-modulated voice signifies cortical control over the emotionally primitive, phylogenetically older nervous system. During subcortical emotional release, phonatory and respiratory control disintegrates. Massive automatic fight-or-flight reactions prepare the organism for increased physical work—fixing the upper extremities to the thoracic cage for combat, requiring firm adduction of the vocal folds and wide abduction to facilitate an increased volume and flow of oxygen to meet the body's increased metabolic demands. Such emergency physiologic states are incompatible with fine voice pitch, loudness, and quality control.

Most group studies to determine the effect of stress on voice have induced stress by either exposing subjects to threatening stimuli, asking them to lie, or requiring them to perform difficult tasks. These studies have been criticized, however, because the stresses did not represent real-life situations and therefore their intensity may not have been suf-

ficient to induce measurable emotional responses. Male-female differences were sometimes not taken into account, and subjects have been noted to mask their voice reactions to emotion. Despite these objections, the results of a cross section of studies seem to have established that increased voice fundamental frequency (pitch) is directly related to increased stress. Aviators and astronauts in distress show increased fundamental frequency proportional to the amount of stress experienced. Simonov and Frolov (1973), reporting on the effects of stress and fatigue on the voices of cosmonauts, found that increased heart rate correlated positively with increased intensity of the higher vowel formants. Voice pitch elevation corresponds directly with increased emotional tension in pilots, according to Khachatur' yants and Grimak (1972), Popov, Simonov, Frolov, et al. (1971), and Williams and Stevens (1969).

Voice patterns may also be indicative of personality type of speakers without voice disorders. Males with type A personality were found to be seven times more likely to develop coronary artery disease than type B personalities (Friedman and Rosenman, 1959). The type A personality has such traits as excessive drive, ambition, aggressiveness, impatience, and a habitual sense of time urgency when challenged by the environment. Subsequently, Rosenman, Friedman, Straus, et al (1964) discovered that perceptually type A personalities had similar voice and speech patterns: explosive semiviolent accentuations in prosody that carried a "certain aggressive timbre" but that appeared only when that person was interested in or excited about the subject under discussion. The type B personality spoke in an "unruffled, rather smooth manner without explosive or aggressive accents."

These observations were made at the time by clinical description and were not masked to the observer, introducing a possible observer bias. Subsequently, Friedman, Brown, and Rosenman (1969) completed an acoustic study of voices of a cohort of male subjects with type A or B personalities but free of coronary artery disease. To induce exhibition—the eagerness to win or excel at a challenging activity and to release latent hostility—a two-paragraph diatribe was composed in which an officer exhorts his troops prior to battle. The subject was asked first to look over the paragraph in preparation for reading it into the microphone. The investigators reported that even prior to the experiment itself, the type A subjects ($n = 19$) blurted out the identical question "Do you want me to read this with expression?" whereas no type B subjects ($n = 18$) ever asked that question. Type B subjects had few or no vocal escalations, average noise-free period (45 seconds) nearly identical to the average total time (46 seconds), resulting in an average index of 1.06, the ratio of the total reading time to noise-free time. The majority of type A subjects, 14 of 19, exhibited several vocal escalations, had significantly less average noise-free periods than type B subjects, and a significantly greater average index of 1.50. From this study, the authors concluded that voice analysis successfully segregated the majority of type A from type B personalities.

Psychogenic Voice Disorders

Numerous studies have suggested a link between stress and voice resulting in psychogenic-based voice disorders (Aronson,

Peterson Jr., and Litin, 1966; Bhatia, 2000; Dietrich and Verdolini, 2005; Jain et al, 2000; Lauriello et al, 2003; Mirza et al, 2003; Roy and Bless, 2000; Roy et al, 2000). In the literature and in the clinic, the terms *functional, psychogenic, psychosomatic*, and *nonorganic* are used synonymously in reference to a group of voice disorders that exist in the absence of organic laryngeal pathology. The label *functional* appears most often. However, from a survey of clinicians' usage, Perelló (1962) found no fewer than eight interpretations of "functional voice disorder": (1) no apparent alteration in structure detected by laryngoscopic examination; (2) negative laryngoscopic examination but positive stroboscopic examination; (3) dysphonia disproportionately severe when compared with existing anatomic lesions or inflammations; (4) disorder of nervous origin with variable symptoms and conducive to the formation of organic lesions; (5) disorder reversible (as opposed to organic disorders, which are usually irreversible); (6) function is altered (the disorder disappears when the organ is used correctly); (7) incorrect motor utilization (therefore, it is a dysfunction); and (8) desire to mask ignorance of exact cause.

Objection to the term *functional* mainly has to do with its ambiguity and lack of precision, especially in light of the following realities: (1) There is more than one functional voice disorder. (2) Functional voice disorders not only sound different but also occur for different reasons and, therefore, should be considered as separate subtypes. (3) Most subtypes can be traced to emotional or psychologic causes. More accurate, then, is the term *psychogenic voice disorders*. A psychogenic voice disorder is broadly synonymous with a functional one but has the advantage of stating positively, based on an exploration of its causes, that the voice disorder is a manifestation of one or more types of psychologic disequilibrium, such as anxiety, depression, conversion reaction, or personality disorder, that interfere with normal volitional control over phonation.

Why do only certain persons react to environmental stress and interpersonal conflict by developing an abnormal voice? Why is it that others who have emotional reactions to stress and conflict never have voice problems? Why is it that still others express their personal problems through some organ system other than the larynx? No satisfactory answers to these questions have been found. Perhaps each person is predisposed by personality or physiologic makeup to hyperreact through a particular neuromuscular or visceral system. Those who are prone to develop voice disorders might be called laryngo-responders to designate their predisposition to developing laryngeal and voice disorders as their unique avenue for the expression of emotional distress.

If everyone who was unable to express emotion developed an abnormal voice, not just certain predisposed persons, clinics would be overwhelmed by patients with psychogenic voice disorders. The distinguished director and writer Elia Kazan (1988) gives a casebook description of what it is like not to be able to express one's feelings openly. To anyone's knowledge, he never developed a psychogenic voice disorder, but if he had, the following thoughts would have fit the disorder perfectly.

When someone works in the arts, he works from craft, not emotion. I'd done play after play that I had no true feeling for, and I'd again and again suppressed the feelings I did

have, choked them off, my hands pressing at my throat, stifling the scream that, if it could be heard, would be my true voice.

"Speak now," I said to myself, "release your true feelings before it's too late. Be yourself. Take your place in the world. You are not a cosmic orphan. You have no reason to be timid. Respond as you feel. Awkwardly, crudely, vulgarly—but respond. Leave your throat open. You can have anything the world has to offer, but the thing you need most and perhaps want most is to be yourself. Admit rejection, admit pain, admit frustration, admit pettiness, even that; admit shame, admit outrage, admit anything and everything that happens to you, respond with your true, uncalculated response, your emotions. Work on it. Stir up the lump whenever you can. Raise your voice."

Based in part, on the work of Lazarus and Folkman (1984) Dietrich and Verdolini (2005) offer a psychoneuroimmunologic (PNI) framework to explain the interactions among cognitive, emotional, biological, and behavioral pathways in mediating stress-related voice responses. According to this framework, stress-induced voice changes occur when environmental demands exceed the individual's abilities to cope with threat or challenge (Lazarus and Folkman, 1984). Chronic stressors generate physical disease by causing negative affective states (e.g., anxiety, depression), which in turn affect biological processes that influence disease risk. Of particular concern to voice and the work of Dietrich and Verdolini are stress-induced biological processes involving the autonomic nervous system (ANS). Based on ANS literature on other areas of the body, they speculate that acute or chronic stressors may increase muscle tone, increase or decrease blood flow, and decrease upper airway secretions. Effects on voice would involve muscle tension, capillary abnormalities, and sicca laryngeal conditions, which could influence laryngeal function (e.g., muscle tension dysphonia) and laryngeal structure (e.g., phonotrauma). This intriguing physiologic model provides a practical explanation of musculoskeletal tension disorders.

An alternative nonlinear model of behavior described by Gustafson and Meyer (2003) to explain a case of panic appears to apply equally well to voice. They make several assumptions in their nonlinear model that are different than those models assuming that stress is cumulative; that when environmental demands exceed the individual's abilities to cope with threat or challenge a problem begins. Gustafson and Meyer assume that the dynamics bringing about a pathologic state are nonlinear, that the discontinuity can be expressed in two-dimensional space as a catastrophe where a patient pushes himself or herself from point (a) to (b) in a normal state of affect and suddenly finds himself or herself in high anxiety or panic (c) or collapsed into depression (d). What follow are further catastrophes or complications. Anxiety that is sufficiently threatening to affect functioning leads to drastic compensations to bring it to manageable levels, such as hysterical somatization, or phobic avoidance, or borderline self-destructive acts (Gustafson, 1999). The patient is in a naïve state in which her plan of action is unrealistic (Gustafson, 1997, 2000) even though the strategy may have been successful in the past. For example, a child may have been successful in deflecting harm from abusive parents by being particularly nice only to find out as an adult that the same behavior may lead to being taken advantage of by a spouse or employer and thus she finds herself in a catastrophe of panic or collapse (Gustafson, 1986). It takes little imagination to see how this model applies to voice.

Musculoskeletal Tension Disorders

In the physically healthy individual, states of tension come about in two ways: (1) from exogenous sources, such as overwork, tense working conditions, professional worries, unhappy family life, or unfavorable situations of occupational placement such as poor ergonomic working postures, working in noisy environments, or working around pollutants; and (2) from endogenous sources, such as peculiarities of personality structure that tend to induce tension (e.g., perfectionism, compulsive attitudes, overambitious drives, lack of adaptability through inflexible rigidity, or uncontrolled outbursts of anger). Under such conditions, tensions may build up without appropriate release. States of increased tension eventually lead to augmented nervous irritability. As a result of this continuously increasing state of neural reaction, the musculature is incited to higher tonus, in excess of the actual demands made on it (Luchsinger and Arnold, 1965, p. 15).

One cardinal principle in clinical voice disorders is the following: The extrinsic and intrinsic laryngeal muscles are exquisitely sensitive to emotional stress, and their hypercontraction is the common denominator behind the dysphonia and aphonia in virtually all psychogenic voice disorders. It is unlikely that there is any single factor responsible for the voice problem. Anxiety, anger, irritability, impatience, frustration, personality, response to disease states, stress, and depression may all be contributing factors. On laryngoscopic examination, the vocal folds either are normal, are mildly inflamed, fail to adduct completely, hyperadduct, or are slightly bowed. In general, however, the extent of visible pathology is incongruously minor or absent in comparison with the severity of abnormal voice.

Musculoskeletal tension can be detected manually by the clinician and can be sensed by the patient. The tension produces elevation of the larynx and hyoid bone. The clinician tests for such tension by encircling the larynx with the thumb and middle finger in the region of the thyrohyoid space, feeling to determine whether the space has been narrowed by laryngeal elevation. The larynx and hyoid bone resist being manually moved laterally or vertically. When the larynx and hyoid bone are pressed and kneaded in the areas indicated, the patient will respond with discomfort or pain, sometimes quite severe, depending upon the degree and duration of the muscle tension. The pain will be either unilateral or bilateral, although more often it is unilateral. The normal larynx does not respond in this manner, so that discomfort and pain with normal-appearing vocal folds are most often diagnostic of laryngeal musculoskeletal tension. If the larynx is pulled down after the sensitive areas are kneaded, and if decreased hoarseness and breathiness and increased volume follow, such is proof that musculoskeletal tension was responsible for the dysphonia. This test is also the main component of the therapy for these disorders.

In the Conversion Aphonia section later in this chapter, it is stated that patients who whisper as a sign of a conversion reaction also exhibit extreme musculoskeletal tension, with the larynx suspended high in the neck and the entire hyoid-laryngeal sling remarkably stiff. The aphonic does not whisper because of passivity of the musculature; on the contrary, the musculature is under supercontraction. This fact was demonstrated in the laboratory by Tarrasch (1946), who recorded electromyographic potentials from the sternocleidomastoid and thyrohyoid muscles bilaterally during quiet respiration and attempts to phonate. She found considerable spasticity of the musculature in aphonic patients. Van den Berg (1962) cites Faaborg-Andersen's electromyographic study of the intrinsic muscles of the larynx in normal subjects who whispered voluntarily. Even under such artificial conditions, increased electrical activity was found in the adductor laryngeal muscles. Similarly, in an x-ray tomographic study done by Zaliouk and Izkovitch (1958), a patient with conversion aphonia showed hypercontraction as reflected in increased constriction of the supraglottic larynx.

Not only does laryngeal musculoskeletal tension produce discomfort or pain when the examiner applies pressure in the regions described, but also patients volunteer information about spontaneous pain radiating to the ear, sternum, and midchest. They feel as if a foreign body were stuck in the throat and report difficulty in swallowing, constriction, and swelling or compression in the pharyngolaryngeal area. They have what is referred to as a *globus sensation*. Globus is reportedly related to psychogenic disorders and recently also has been strongly related to laryngeal esophageal reflux as described elsewhere in this book. Takahashi, Hinohara, Ohmori, et al. (1971) reported on 652 cases of a disagreeable sensation in the pharyngolaryngeal region and found a high incidence of neurotic tendencies in this group. Some had carcinophobia after a close friend or relative had died of the disease. They concluded that dysphoric affective states play an important part in producing these sensations. The relationship between dysphonia, musculoskeletal tension, and environmental stress is illuminated in the following case study without any known reflux disease.

Case Study 8.1

A 37-year-old single female, a registered nurse, noted a "cracking" of her voice 5 months prior to coming to the clinic, at first only a few times a week but becoming more frequent, so that by the end of 3 weeks she had become continuously hoarse. She consulted her family doctor, who thought that her dysphonia was due to postnasal drip and prescribed cough syrup, and, later, ampicillin without benefit. She was next examined by an otolaryngologist, who noted irritation of her vocal folds but did not offer a diagnosis or treatment. Two months after onset, her voice returned to normal while she was on vacation in Mexico, but it worsened upon reentry to the United States. She went back to her family doctor, who prescribed Valium (Diazepam) and Decadron (Dexamethasone), which were also ineffective, and attempted to treat her disorder as if it were myasthenia gravis by prescribing Mestinon (Pyridostigmine), which also was of no benefit.

Indirect laryngoscopy showed normal vocal folds, and neurologic examination failed to disclose any evidence of myasthenia gravis or other neurologic disease. Her general medical examination was normal.

Her voice was continuously strained, hoarse, and produced with above-normal physical effort. On vowel prolongation, she produced a clear voice at a higher pitch level. Her cough and glottal coup were normally sharp, indicating good vocal fold adduction. She reacted with discomfort and pain, grimacing in response to pressure over the posterior region of the hyoid bone bilaterally. Her larynx, at rest and on phonation, was positioned high in her neck, close to the hyoid bone. Her voice improved momentarily when the larynx was moved downward by the examiner during vowel prolongation. Asked if her dysphonia could be a reaction to emotional stress, and asked to describe any upsetting events that might have occurred surrounding the onset and development of her dysphonia, she became momentarily silent, frowning, as if taken off-guard by the question. After a few moments' reflection, she smiled and, as if it were occurring to her for the first time, said that in fact, she had been struggling with a distressing situation. Shortly before her dysphonia, a local newspaper editorial had appeared that was critical of the costs of the patient's position as a public health nurse and that argued for the elimination of her job. A bitter conflict broke out between her department and the editor, with accusations flying in both directions. Caught in the middle, the patient grew increasingly angry over the unfairness of the allegations, yet had no means of responding to them.

As she disclosed this information, her frustration and anger became apparent. Her face flushed, and although on the verge of tears, she continued to talk. During the next few minutes, her voice spontaneously returned to normal. She was gratified and surprised at this sudden and unexpected improvement. She said she had suspected that her voice disorder had something to do with the conflict at home but had not appreciated its importance until the question had been put to her directly. She ought to have suspected the connection, she said, when her voice had begun to improve after a resolution of her job problem shortly before coming to the clinic.

This case illustration is not atypical. Consultation with several specialists before arriving at a diagnosis and treatment of the disorder is typical in patients who have musculoskeletal tension dysphonia. Perceptually undramatic and indistinguishable from hoarseness due to other causes, musculoskeletal tension dysphonia is treated erroneously as if it were laryngitis. Diagnostically important in the cited case were the strained voice, tightness, hoarseness, history of voice return while on vacation, and pain in response to pressure in the region of the larynx. The diagnosis was confirmed when the voice returned spontaneously as the patient ventilated her feelings. Loosening of her character armor, physical relaxation, abandoning of defenses, and freeing of affective expression through weeping or laughter are diagnostic and therapeutic in such cases.

Vocal Abuse

Hyperadduction of the vocal folds occurs when there is increased closing force, or adduction time, in the glottal cycle. It can occur as a primary problem resulting in a secondary pathology or as a compensatory movement secondary to an underlying pathology. A problem for clinicians is determining which came first: the chicken or the egg. The vocal consequences of hyperadduction perceptually range from complete aphonia to a mildly hoarse voice. The pathologic consequences of hyperadduction of the vocal folds are typically one of three kinds of secondary laryngeal pathologic states: (1) inflammation and edema, (2) vocal nodules or polyps, or (3) contact ulcers. There is a tendency to think of these as vocal abuse disorders because they are often associated with strenuous speaking, singing, yelling, screaming, coughing, and throat-clearing. But abuse or misuse is too simple an explanation for these complex disorders. These hyperadduction voice disorders may be the consequence of lingering compensatory strategies adopted during bouts of laryngitis secondary to upper respiratory infections (URI), they may be related to personality traits and associated responses to excessive environmental demands or responses to illness, they may be an interaction with tissue irritation from laryngeal-esophageal reflux, or they may be an intermediate link in the chain of causes that begins with an emotionally determined impetus to vocalize aggressively. Regardless of the cause, the effect of such behavior is to produce traumatic lesions, leading many clinicians to categorize vocal nodule or contact ulcer as organic voice disorders. But, from a fundamental etiologic point of view, they are probably better characterized as functional or behavioral, because the lesions were the result of abnormal speaking behavior, lesions are not always present, and they are often motivated, or at least compounded, by personality or emotional factors.

Across the life span, the effects of vocal abuse exist on a severity continuum. School-age children who abuse their voices will have either normal-appearing vocal folds, inflammation without discrete lesions, or discrete lesions. Senturia and Wilson (1968) reported on 32,500 children aged 5 to 18 years and found that 1962 (6%) had abnormal voices. Of that abnormal group, 338 aged 6 to 11 years were given voice, hearing, psychometric, and laryngologic examinations. The males predominated over females by a ratio of 2:1. Of these voice-defective children, 147 were given laryngoscopic examinations, and 47.5% were found to have varying degrees of redness or edema or both in the region of the arytenoid cartilages. Interestingly, redness or edema or both in the region of the arytenoid cartilages is one of the cardinal signs of laryngeal esophageal reflux (Koufman, 1991). On indirect laryngoscopy in these 147 children, only 92 had vocal folds that could be completely visualized. Of those 92 children with abnormal voice, 63 had discrete lesions such as nodules, hyperplasia, and diffuse or localized edema; again, conditions often attributed to laryngeal esophageal reflux with or without accompanying vocally abusive behaviors. The predominance of lesions in males compared with females was almost 3:1 in children having discrete vocal fold lesions and more than 2:1 in those not having discrete lesions. As the vocal folds lengthen during puberty more for males than females, this ratio is reversed because the impact stress of vocal fold contact is distributed over a larger area in males and concentrated in females at the mid-membranous portion of the vocal folds. The voice signs within this group of 92 children consisted of whispering, breathiness, and stridency.

The amount and type of classroom voice use of children diagnosed as having hoarse voices was compared with that of children who had normal voices by Barker and Wilson (1967). The length and loudness of utterances were tabulated for 14 children in the control group (normal voice) and for 14 in an experimental group (hoarse voice). The researchers found that the children with normal voices produced an average of 20.92 vocalizations in a 2-hour period compared with 61.50 vocalizations by the children with hoarse voices within that same time period. The difference between the two groups was significant beyond the 0.01 level. Of interest is the observation that the children with the abnormal voices were more active within the classroom during unstructured periods than were the children with normal voices. These indications of extraversion are consistent with Roy and Bless (1999) data on adults suggesting individuals with vocal nodules are often extraverted and have an inability to inhibit and consequently might be more likely to talk more and louder than their introverted counterparts who developed functional voice disorders with more open glottal postures.

The theme of personality aggressiveness, hyperactivity, emotional reactivity, and family problems in dysphonic children with and without discrete vocal fold lesions is of considerable importance in understanding the factors responsible for vocal abuse. Barker and Wilson, who were social workers, investigated the family structure of both the children with voice problems and those without. Of 153 who were classified as having abnormal voices, 65% came from homes in which there was excessive family conflict, whereas 35% came from homes in which there was considered to be none. Of 97 children whose voices were normal, only 35% came from conflict-ridden homes (i.e., almost twice as many children with abnormal voices came from home environments that were considered pathologic).

One cause of vocal abuse after puberty is cheerleading. Many studies have proved that the result can be chronic dysphonia with or without vocal fold damage. Jensen (1964), for example, found that 12% of 377 cheerleaders were dysphonic. Andrews and Shank (1983) found that 37% of 102 high school cheerleaders had a history of voice problems. Reich, McHenry, and Keaton (1986) surveyed 146 female cheerleaders ranging in age from 15.5 to 18.6 years and found that, at one time or another, 32% had experienced acute aphonia and 86% complained of dysphonia. The average number of times that these students became aphonic during a given season was 4.2 and dysphonic 7.3. Cheerleaders present a particularly interesting group because they are generally believed to be extraverts, and cheerleading engages them in vocally abusive activities.

After high school, occupation scores as one of the major etiologic factors in abuse. Teaching ranks among the highest of those occupations identified as vocally abusive. Teaching is demanding, causes emotional stress, and requires consid-erable talking. The amount of talking is greater in the lower elementary grades where teachers are thought to be at greatest risk for developing voice disorders. Acoustic analysis of teacher talking patterns has demonstrated that teachers in grades K through 3 talk louder, longer, and at higher pitch (Roy, et al, 2004).

Vocal Nodules

Vocal nodules are associated with vocal misuse or abuse. The nodule is a small, white or grayish protuberance on the free margin of the vocal fold at the junction of the anterior and middle third. It is a tissue reaction to frictional trauma between the folds, a growth of hyperkeratotic epithelium with underlying fibrosis. The nodules may begin with a submucous hemorrhage and may develop from the fibrosis of an organizing hematoma. In the very early stages of vocal abuse, there may be nothing more than a localized capillary hemorrhage, swelling of the vocal fold edges, and redness of the folds. Later, fibrosis and the fully developed, roughly semicircular, grayish or white nodule form.

Vocal nodules represent a degeneration of the lamina propria with fibrosis and edema. Both the visual appearance and histologic nature of nodules is controversial though it has been suggested that acute vocal nodules are morphologically different from chronic. In the acute phase, the squamous epithelium is normal but covers an edematous stroma with thin-walled blood vessels, loose fibrous tissue, and lymphocytes. In the chronic phase, the nodules possess a thickened epithelium and demonstrate acanthosis, keratosis, and fibrosis with minimal edema of the underlying connective tissue.

Three stages of vocal nodule formation have been described: (1) a local accumulation of fluid in the subepithelial layer of the vocal folds; (2) an organized inflammatory response with accumulation of protein and increased vascularity; (3) further organization of the lesion with fibrosis and possibly keratosis of the epithelium (Arnold, 1962; Gray, 1991). Nodules vary in size from no larger than a pinhead to as large as a split pea. Early nodules may appear red, gelatinous, and floppy, whereas chronic nodules are typically white and conical or hemispherical and appear hard and fixed to the underlying mass of the mucosa (Vaughn, 1982).

The nodule is located at the midmembranous portion of the vocal fold because it is the point of maximum impact stress, or trauma, to the vocal fold. In cases of loud phonation, the impact stress is greater because of the larger subglottal pressures displacing the tissue to a greater extent, and in cases of singing, or high-pitched productions, the vocal fold collisions occur more frequently. After the nodule has been formed, the resultant dysphonia is perceived as breathy, husky, or foggy in quality, with a tendency toward low pitch. Interestingly when the fundamental frequency of the pitch is determined, the frequency is not lower compared with age-matched controls. The perception of lower pitch comes from the combination of the qualities of breathiness and hoarseness. The dysphonia results from the increased vocal fold mass and change in the vibratory pattern particularly in the hourglass-shaped closing pattern. As the vocal folds project into the glottis, they cause air-stream turbulence and prevent the vocal folds from adducting anterior and posterior to the lesion. The breathy or husky quality is the effect of failure of vocal fold closure in the nonadducted areas around the nodules.

Contributing further to the notion that children who develop vocal nodules may differ in personality and family history from those who do not, Nemec (1961) observed that children with hyperfunctional dysphonia, including vocal nodules, were more aggressive and less mature and had more difficulty in managing stressful situations than children with normal voice. Mosby (1967) studied 25 children, 16 with vocal nodules and 9 with other types of dysphonia, by means of a battery of psychologic tests. He found a high incidence of neurotic personality conflict, overrepressed aggression, feelings of inadequacy, poor relationships with parents, and severe dependency needs. Wilson and Lamb (1973), in a study of 12 children with vocal nodules and 12 with normal voices, concluded that children with vocal nodules had personalities that included marked aggressiveness, lack of control, or passive, overcontrolled adjustment to aggression. By administering the California Test of Personality, Glassel (1972) compared 15 children, aged 7 to 11 years, who had vocal nodules with 15 who had normal voices. He found that the children with nodules scored significantly poorer on all measures of personality adjustment; they had reduced feelings of belonging, a reduced sense of personal worth, withdrawal tendencies, and antisocial feelings. However, not all children with nodules were vociferous according to the popular stereotype, although they manifested the same degree of neurotic tendency as those who were. In a study of 77 children with vocal nodules, Toohill (1975) found that the parents of 62 children with nodules described their children as screamers, incessant talkers, or loud talkers. Sixty-six were described as having one or more of the following personality traits: aggressiveness, hyperactivity, nervousness, tenseness, frustration, or emotional disturbance.

Further suggestion of psychoneurotic tendencies in children who develop vocal nodules comes out of a study by Green (1989). She had the mothers of 30 children with vocal nodules and 30 control mothers rate their children's behavior on a standardized checklist of abnormal behaviors called the Walker Problem Behavior Identification Checklist. The children with vocal nodules, 22 of whom were male and 8 female, ranging in age from 3 to 12 years, received a substantially higher percentage of abnormal ratings than the control group. More than 60% of the children with vocal nodules were rated as positive on the following traits: (1) temper tantrums when the child cannot get his way; (2) argues and wants to have the last word; (3) does not obey until threatened; (4) complains of others' unfairness. Also rated high was the tendency toward overactivity and restlessness and the need for approval for tasks attempted. Not more than 20% of the children with normal voices received ratings for these behaviors. From this study, the author concluded that:

The concept of the development of vocal nodules in children has traditionally conjured a fixed mental picture of vocal abuse in a vociferous child. Current research suggests that such a focus is too simplistic and that the people working with children with vocal nodules may need to consider a multiplicity of etiological and management variables including acid reflux, small vocal folds, laryngeal microwebs, personality, family, and classroom dynamics.

Vocal nodules also have been found in association with velopharyngeal insufficiency independent of any particular personality traits. The need for higher intraoral pressures and for increased loudness causes overdriving of the vocal folds. (See Chapter 4 for a more detailed discussion.)

The etiology and pathophysiology of vocal nodules in adults are basically the same as in children, with minor variations. As previously noted, whereas the incidence of vocal nodules is higher in male children than in females, this trend is reversed in adults. Singing and occupation as primary or contributory causes are strong in adulthood. It is also likely that these females' vocal folds have shorter vibratory lengths so that the impact stress at the midmembranous region where nodules occur is greater. Additionally, adult females with nodules have some of the same personality characteristics and daily habits as children who develop nodules. They are talkative, socially aggressive, and tense and have acute or chronic interpersonal problems that generate tension, anxiety, anger, or depression. Even when the nodules appear to be the sole result of abuse from singing or other strenuous vocal activity, it is often found that these were not the only factors responsible for the vocal overuse; these patients had often also entered a period of their lives in which concomitant emotional stress had surfaced.

A review of a few case histories of individuals with vocal nodules highlights both the similarities and differences often seen between cases.

Case Study 8.2

A 63-year-old married female was referred by the Department of Otolaryngology with a diagnosis of bilateral small vocal nodules. She had begun to complain of hoarseness 8 years previously whenever she had to use her voice strenuously, such as over background noise or during animated conversation. She had been seen by laryngologists and speech clinicians who had made the diagnosis of vocal abuse and given "exercises," which were ineffective. Aside from her voice difficulties, her health had been good, although she complained of general fatigue with prolonged voice use.

On examination, her voice was nearly normal; there was a slight hoarseness consistent with the size of the nodules observed by the otolaryngologist. Complete motor speech examination failed to disclose any evidence of dysarthria, and the remainder of the examination of the speech structures failed to disclose any other defects.

While giving the social-psychologic history, the patient said she believed that her husband was responsible for her voice problems. She described him as a voluble speaker, loud and animated. The patient, during most of her married life, had to raise her voice to compete with him during discussions, not only when they had company but also when they were alone together. "He dominates the conversation, that's his personality, his nature, you're never going to change that . . . he is a shouter and I am a quiet talker." Despite this marriage-long contrast in their personalities, her voice troubles first began when she became interested in activist politics and needed to express her opinions in a more forthright manner. She volunteered that she believed she had gotten into the habit of using her voice excessively and with a great deal of tension as a reaction to her husband's vocal manner. "Now, even when I have to talk to a group, I tense up." When her voice was bad, she complained of shooting pains from her larynx to her ears, and on examination she had pain in response to pressure over the hyoid region and thyroid cartilage.

Joint discussion with the patient and her husband confirmed her testimony; he proudly confessed to being "vociferous, aggressive, dominating," more concerned with his own opinion than hers. He described her as a "sounding board" and not nearly as concerned with her opinions as with his own. "I know it's selfish and cruel. she's a very tranquil individual and I am not. I'm the second last angry man!" She said to him, "You are a monopolizer of conversations, my main complaint is when there are other people in the conversation he interrupts them, and won't let them finish. He'd rather talk than do anything else. Unfortunately, it becomes a monologue."

What emerges from this examination is not only a basic difference in how these two individuals communicate but also an even deeper disagreement as to what ought to be said and what is best left unsaid. Not only is the psychogenic etiology of this woman's vocal nodules substantiated by an in-depth interview as a contributing etiology, but the results of that interview also point to the requirement for more than symptomatic voice therapy.

The balance between vocal abuse and emotional stress is different in each patient with vocal nodules, and it is often difficult to separate the two. Whereas in the previous study, emotional and personality factors were prominent, vocal abuse is more apparent in the following case study of a farm wife, although the patient is not free of stress.

Case Study 8.3

A 39-year-old farm wife and mother of three boys had sung most of her adult life for weddings, funerals, and baptisms. One year before coming to the clinic, she had hoarseness occurring intermittently but did not consult anyone until 7 months after onset. Laryngologic examination showed a thickening of the mucosa of the left vocal fold and a small ectasia on the posterior third of that fold. Laryngologic examination at the time she presented to the clinic, 1 year after onset, showed clear evidence of bilateral vocal nodules at the junction of the anterior and middle third of the vocal folds.

The patient was a pleasant, energetic, healthy housewife and mother of a highly musical family. In addition to her heavy singing schedule, her daily talking habits were prodigious; teaching, singing, talking, using her voice all day long with her children and her neighbors, and speaking on the telephone.

Special cases of vocal nodules in adults occur in the culture of the pop singer, whose voice usage is often one of extreme abuse with or without coexisting fatigue and emotional stress. Greene (1972) had these interesting comments about this subgroup in Britain.

Pop singers claim an immensely important role in entertainment, although professors of singing in the classical style do not recognize their vocalization indeed as singing. The senior coach of the Covent Garden Opera Company has said he would not consider them seriously as candidates for the course. Their members are legion and they give pleasure to millions. They are largely untrained, having musical sense and personality and pleasing voices but some, it must be admitted, have little natural vocal endowment. For many it is a short life but a lucrative one and when the voice is lost through vocal abuse they drop out of "show biz."

The vocal gymnastics and tricks peculiar to each singer, the double notes, acute pitch changes, the scoops and swirls have to be executed against the deafening competition of amplified music. Despite the use of a hand microphone they must still "belt it out" at the top of their voices. The sound-pressure levels created by the bands and rock and roll groups are so great that they exceed the safety levels for avoidance of hearing impairment.

The common run of cabaret and pop-group singers perform for many hours on end starting at midnight and going on into the early hours. When not singing they often are smoking and talking in a dry, hot, and polluted atmosphere. They frequently eat late and have other lifestyle habits that promote laryngeal esophageal reflux. Consequently, it is not surprising that chronic laryngitis and vocal nodes are common in this population.

Case Study 8.4

A 19-year-old nightclub singer complained of intermittent hoarseness for 3 to 6 months. She was a backup vocalist in an eight-piece brass band and sang 6 days a week. Laryngologic examination revealed moderate-sized vocal nodules bilaterally at the junction of the anterior and middle third of her vocal folds.

In addition to the close relationship between singing and dysphonia—the patient complained of less voice trouble when on vacation—she disclosed recent life stresses concerning problems with a boyfriend in the band. At the same time, she began to examine her career goals, summing up her feelings over the past 6 months by saying, "I'm feeling a lot of emotional stress I've never felt before. Just seems like everything is coming down at once." She admitted to being depressed during the time of her voice disturbance and personal problems.

The foregoing case studies are suggestive that multiple factors may contribute to the etiology of vocal nodules, to which personality traits may contribute.

Contact Ulcer

The second vocal abuse–musculoskeletal tension–emotional stress voice disorder having secondary traumatic tissue reaction is contact ulcer, or contact ulcer granuloma. Instead of epithelial tissue developing, as in vocal nodule, a contact ulcer is an erosion of the mucosa. Occurring unilaterally or bilaterally, the ulcers are found at the junction of the middle and posterior third of the vocal folds, the intercartilaginous region, at the tips of the vocal processes of the arytenoid cartilages. The hard cartilaginous undersurfaces of the vocal processes strike the mucosa of the opposite vocal fold, causing hyperemia, the formation of granulation tissue, and, finally, an ulcer crater with its raised, inflamed margins.

Contact ulcer is generally thought to be a consequence of laryngeal esophageal reflux or laryngeal intubation trauma. Since reflux has been identified as a primary etiologic factor, no definitive incidence or prevalence studies have been completed. It is a disorder primarily of adult males in their 40s; adult females are affected less frequently, and children infrequently. Male susceptibility may be due to the male tendency to adopt a low-pitched voice, moving the locus of force of vocal fold contact posteriorly. Ulcerations in the region of the arytenoid cartilage can also result from trauma due to laryngeal intubation.

Clinical and research studies conducted 50 years ago pointed to certain common characteristics among adult males who developed contact ulcer (Peacher, 1947; Peacher and Hollinger, 1947):

♦ hypertonic laryngeal musculature as a component of generalized musculoskeletal tension

♦ habitual use of an excessively low voice-pitch level

♦ explosive speech stress patterns

♦ sharp, abrupt glottal attack (*coup de glotte*)

♦ restricted pitch variability

♦ phonation using excessively high infraglottal pressure with bursts of intensity

Some patients with contact ulcer complain of discomfort or pain coming from deep within the neck radiating to the lateral neck area or ear, a tickle in the throat, an urge to clear the throat, a lump in the throat, and an aching or dryness. At one time, the classic profile of the contact ulcer patient was thought to be a male in his 40s who uses his voice intensively in his daily life and is either a lawyer, teacher, minister, actor, or salesman. In personality, he is tense and hard-driving and is often under chronic stress. Cigarette smoking, alcohol consumption, exposure to air pollutants, and extremes of air temperature and humidity are contributory factors. Smoking and alcohol are both considered causative factors in reflux, and all of the factors contribute to tissue irritation, which when coupled with impact stress may result in ulcerations.

Musculoskeletal tension secondary to emotional stress is also considered to be a predisposing factor responsible for the mechanically damaging hyperadduction of the vocal folds, and some believe that ANS effects are responsible for

vasoconstriction of the laryngeal mucosa, reducing blood supply to that region and thereby increasing its susceptibility to trauma. As previously mentioned, recently this profile of causative factors has been expanded to include laryngeal esophageal reflux.

The dysphonia of the patient with a contact ulcer is characteristically low pitched, hoarse, and grating. Not only does chronic vocal abuse produce contact ulcer, but sudden traumatic yelling or shouting can also precipitate it. It often occurs after laryngitis, particularly when the patient has continued to abuse the voice during a throat infection. The following studies are typical of contact ulcer patients.

Case Study 8.5

A 43-year-old steel plant supervisor had an 11-month history of laryngitis, during which he developed a contact ulcer. His dysphonia had become chronic 4 months after he had begun working in the machine shop of his plant, during which time he used his voice constantly, having to raise it to high loudness levels to be heard over the environmental noise. This environment was also dusty, hot, and dry in the summer and cold and damp in the winter. Moreover, he sang in a male chorus, and he complained of long working hours and general fatigue. On examination, his voice was hoarse and low in pitch with some acoustic evidence of breathy air escape.

A 41-year-old professor of English literature had a 5-year history of episodic hoarseness in association with lecturing, which became worse during resumption of a regular teaching schedule and assumption of new duties as a curriculum supervisor. Indirect laryngoscopy showed a contact ulcer granuloma on the posterior third of the left vocal fold. His voice was hoarse and excessively low in pitch and gave indications of breathy air escape. He described his style of lecturing as "animated" and "forceful," with a tendency to use an unnaturally low pitch. He perfectionistically prepared his lectures and delivered them under conditions of anxiety and tension. He found that his voice would tire toward the end of each lecture, and he would feel muscular tension in his neck and pain in his throat, sometimes expanding into headache.

A 48-year-old automobile plant manager gave a 2-month history of hoarseness with upper respiratory infection. Indirect laryngoscopy showed bilateral contact ulcer granulomas at the bases of both vocal folds. His voice was hoarse with excessively low pitch. Vocal abuse and emotional stress coincided with manufacturing problems, his dysphonia developing shortly after spending 6 hours a day in the shop talking over noise levels approaching 100 dB. Much of his speaking had to do with reprimanding employees for inefficiency, and at the same time, he was regularly involved in public speaking in civic organizations.

A 43-year-old radiologist presented with a 6-month history of hoarseness after an upper respiratory infection. Video endoscopy revealed a unilateral contact ulceration on the left vocal process. His voice was somewhat asthenic and his vocal range significantly reduced. History of vocal abuse was negative. He denied excessive alcohol intake and did not smoke. He had a positive history of esophageal reflux for which he was making lifestyle changes and taking PPIs (Priton Pump Inhibitors) without noticeable change in symptoms.

Ventricular Dysphonia

Closely allied to musculoskeletal voice disorders is ventricular dysphonia, or dysphonia plicae ventricularis, characterized by a continuously strained, harsh, or hoarse low-pitched voice described as rattling, rumbling, cracking, and ticker-like. During ventricular dysphonia, both airflow and frequency are abnormally low and the true vocal folds cannot be visualized. To some, ventricular dysphonia gives the impression of phonating during strangulation, and to others it has a groaning, animal quality suggesting exertion of extreme effort. The voice disorder derives its name from the fact that voice is produced by vibration of the false or ventricular vocal folds rather than the true folds. Its etiology is often unclear. Because it has been noted to occur in muscularly tense people and also because it is extreme hyperfunction, it is probably best classified as a musculoskeletal tension disorder. It is important to note that many patients who have organic disease of their true vocal folds, which are incapable of producing adequate sound, compensate by using their ventricular folds instead.

Conversion Voice Disorders

This group of psychogenic voice disorders originates from the psychoneurosis known as a conversion reaction or conversion disorder. A conversion disorder is any loss of voluntary control over normal striated muscle or over the general or special senses as a consequence of environmental stress or interpersonal conflict. The criteria for conversion reactions are that they:

♦ are specific physical symptoms or syndromes that cannot be traced to any anatomic or physiologic disease

♦ are unconscious simulations of illness, which the patient is convinced is of organic origin

♦ serve the psychologic purpose of enabling the patient to avoid awareness of emotional conflict, stress, or personal failure that would be emotionally intolerable if faced directly

♦ can occur in any sensory or voluntary motor system

Examples of sensory conversions are loss of general sensation in response to touch, pressure, or pain, or impairment of the special senses of vision or hearing. Motor conversions take such forms as weakness, incoordination, complete loss of movement control ("paralysis"), or unusual or bizarre movements anywhere in the body.

The word *conversion* was first used by Freud to explain a mechanism by which an unbearable idea is rendered innocuous by having its energy transmuted into some bodily form of expression (i.e., conversion is a theoretical conception of a clinical finding). Sensory or motor loss in the absence of organic disease is a defense mechanism against a threat from the environment. It is conjectured that somehow the psychic energy generated by that threat is transmuted or converted into a somatic sign, and, as in conversion voice disorders, the somatic sign is symbolically related to certain specifics about the threat or conflict that created it.

The idea that psychic energy can be transformed into physical or "organic" dysfunction is difficult to grasp. Freud's theory of "libidinal" conversion to physical dysfunction has been the subject of much criticism because of its metaphorical quality. It becomes more acceptable, however, if modernized to mean symbolization of the conflict or unbearable idea. In their contemporary interpretation of the meaning of conversion reaction, Ziegler and Imboden (1962) wrote the following clarifying explanation:

We have found it useful to consider the patient with a conversion symptom as someone enacting the role of a person with "organic" illness, symbolically communicating his distress—dysphoric affect and/or unacceptable fantasy—by means of somatic symptoms. In our conceptual model, this somatic mode of communication does not serve to "discharge" pent-up emotion but, rather like any other language, it is useful as an instrument in negotiating interpersonal transactions. Through the conversion reaction, the fact that the patient is in distress is formulated to himself and communicated to others in the egosyntonic terms of "physical illness," and the patient thereby distracts himself (with varying degrees of success) from the more immediate perception of his dysphoric affect. Human beings may communicate their feelings and ideas to themselves and others in a variety of modes such as ordinary consensual language, sign language, dreams, autistic verbal symbols of schizophrenia, or autistic somatic symbols of conversion reaction. Conversion may be viewed as operating, in this way, like other psychological processes. In many conversion reactions seen clinically, the message of emotional distress is communicated primarily in nonverbal ways (to the patient himself as well as the others in his transactional field) in terms of somatic symptoms which are, in effect, an analogic code. The patient unconsciously chooses particular symptoms according to his conception of illness, as derived from his own past experiences with illness or from his observation of others. His particular symptoms will then simulate physical illness in a relatively expert or relatively crude manner, depending upon the degree of congruity between his imagery of illness and that of the observer. Within this context of unconsciously simulated illness, specific symptoms may develop or receive prominence because they are especially suited to the symbolic representation of specific fantasies, affects, and motivational conflicts.

Sometimes *hysteria* is used in place of *conversion reaction* (e.g., *hysterical voice disorder, hysterical aphonia,* or *hysterical dysphonia*), in which case hysteria and conversion are used interchangeably and synonymously. Technically, this failure to differentiate the two terms is incorrect. *Conversion* refers to somatization of an emotional conflict, as elaborated previously, whereas *hysteria* refers to a personality type or behavior pattern. Criteria for hysteria are (1) an immature or egocentric person who has a propensity to develop subjective complaints involving various parts of the body, prompting that person to consult many physicians and to submit to a succession of operations. (2) In the case of a female, one who is seductive or flirtatious, sometimes hostile or manipulative, and who accents or highlights her sexuality by her manner, voice, dress, and gait, thus revealing an insecurity in this sphere. (3) A suggestible, dependent, shallow person, dramatic and theatrical in manner and labile in affect, who takes cues from what seems to be expected according to the environment and who plays a series of superficial roles in relating to other people. Many individuals satisfy one or more of these criteria for hysterical personality but do not have a conversion reaction. Conversely, many patients with conversion reaction bear none of the personality or behavior traits of the hysterical personality.

A conversion voice disorder (1) exists despite normal structure and function of the vocal folds, (2) is created by anxiety, stress, depression, or interpersonal conflict, (3) has symbolic significance for that conflict, and (4) enables the patient to avoid facing the interpersonal conflict directly and extricates the person from the uncomfortable situation. The onset of the voice disorder is almost always associated with emotional conflict. For many years, the misconception abounded that the only voice sign of conversion was whispering or aphonia. However, conversion voice disorders come in many forms: muteness, aphonia, and less dramatic forms of dysphonia, such as breathiness, hoarseness, falsetto pitch breaks, and continuous falsetto. The multiplicity of voice signs of conversion reaction has been substantiated by Aronson, Peterson Jr., and Litin (1966), who found identical criteria for conversion reactions in patients whose problems ranged from muteness to varying degrees and types of dysphonia.

Conversion Muteness

The most extreme and incapacitating conversion voice disorder is muteness or mutism, in which the patient neither whispers nor articulates, or may articulate without exhalation. Entering the room with notebook and pencil, they write their questions and answers, and although unaware of what they are revealing, involuntarily cough, showing their normal vocal fold adduction. The patient will also cough sharply on request without being aware of the incongruity between their normal cough and manifest inability to phonate. Patients who present with one form of conversion voice disorder very likely have experienced other forms.

Common findings in such patients are chronic stress, primary and secondary gain, indifference to their symptom, other manifestations of conversion, poor sex identification, suppressed anger, immaturity and dependency, neurotic life adjustment, and mild to moderate depression. Different as these individuals are from one another, a common denominator runs through their histories: (1) a breakdown in communication with someone important to that person; (2) a conflict between wanting but not allowing oneself to express anger, fear, or remorse verbally; (3) fear or shame standing in the way of expressing feelings via conventional speech and language. A typical case follows:

Case Study 8.6

A 44-year-old female presented with no use of speech structures for communication. All her responses were written. Her history was one of struggle and deprivation from birth. She was the youngest of 10, her family being burdened by five other children from her father's former marriage. By the time she was 20, her father then dead and most of the children gone, she had been saddled with the responsibility of caring for her aging mother and two older sisters. She lived a Cinderella-like existence, doing the household chores and being dominated by her sisters, who rarely allowed her out of the house. Under these circumstances, at age 23, she had her first conversion symptom, a "paralysis" of the right arm lasting 2 weeks. Three years later, she became severely depressed and unable to work for several months. Then, at age 27, her mother, "the only person who ever loved me," died. Shortly thereafter, she developed a "paralysis" of both legs and became an invalid for 1½ years. Physical therapy effected a "dramatic cure." Her doctors, who knew of her hostile and dependent relationship with her sisters, urged her to get out on her own. Six years later, at age 35, she married a 27-year-old man with a son from a previous marriage. She had made an adjustment to life. Financial worries and behavior problems in the son were followed by episodes of dysphonia. During the winter prior to the current interview, she had many episodes of intermittently phonated-whispered voice. Her current episode had begun 9 months before with a period of whispered speech lasting 7 months and finally giving way to muteness and writing notes.

Conversion Aphonia

Conversion aphonia refers to involuntary whispering despite a basically normal larynx. Indirect laryngoscopic examination indicates normal or partial adduction of the vocal folds on vowel production or coughing. Even without laryngoscopic examination, normalcy of the vocal folds can be heard as the patient coughs and makes other glottal sounds unassociated with speech. Similar to dysphonia associated with musculoskeletal tension, the larynx in conversion aphonia is often elevated in the neck along with the hyoid bone, and the entire laryngeal-hyoid sling is rigid and is difficult to move manually in any direction.

Within the category of aphonia falls a considerable variety of whispers: pure or noiseless; harsh, sharp, or piercing; intermittent high-pitched squeaks and squeals; moments of normal voice. The sharpness of the whispering indicates that the intrinsic laryngeal muscles are in a state of hypercontraction, even though the vocal folds are prevented from approximating.

Approximately 80% of patients with conversion aphonia are female. Many have had previous episodes of aphonia or dysphonia that have spontaneously cleared. Onset can be sudden, within seconds or minutes, or over a period of hours, beginning with hoarseness that turns into aphonia. Conversion aphonias and dysphonias are often triggered by colds or flu and associated laryngitis. Upon recovery from the upper respiratory infection, the dysphonia remains, worsening to aphonia. Often, onset is associated with fatigue or exhaustion. Discomfort, pain, and tightness in the larynx and upper and lower neck and chest regions are common in the conversion group, as they are in the musculoskeletal tension group. As in conversion muteness, aphonic patients give histories including either acute or chronic emotional stress, symbolic significance of the voice loss, primary and secondary gain, a tendency toward indifference to the incapacitating effects of the voice, and conversion reactions in other regions of the body at different times in their lives. Additional findings are emotional immaturity, neurotic life adjustment, and mild to moderate depression.

Although the following studies are of patients with conversion aphonia, they could apply equally to patients who are mute or to those who are dysphonic.

Case Study 8.7

A 14-year-old girl's parents were separated and involved in divorce litigation. She had markedly ambivalent feelings toward her father. Her latest episode of aphonia occurred an hour after a violent argument with him on the telephone over her request for Christmas money.

A 58-year-old housewife learned of her brother's death. En route to his funeral, she received word that her sister-in-law had died. She awoke the next morning with aphonia that continued for the next 2 years.

A 31-year-old secretary and mother of three had been carrying on an extramarital affair for 9 years and was fearful that this relationship would be discovered. During the past year, she had been having disagreements with her employer, and her fear of being fired was the only factor that kept her from "telling him off." Her aphonia occurred shortly after her boyfriend lost his job and moved to a new location, preventing her from communicating with him; she had begun to consider breaking off their relationship.

A 26-year-old police officer was not happy in his work but would not tell anyone of his feelings, particularly his parents, for fear of disappointing them, as they had encouraged him to enter police work. He had always been quiet, nonaggressive, and reluctant to lose his temper. He had had previous episodes of aphonia and dysphonia that had cleared spontaneously, but this most recent one failed to improve over a 3- to 4-week period. The main reason for his dislike of being a policeman was an inability to exert authority—a fear that he would say the wrong thing or reap dislike or disapproval from those he tried to reprimand. He would find himself becoming nervous and upset when having to give a motorist a ticket; if the motorist argued with him, he would shake and get mixed up. He had no idea that his voice losses were related to his attitudes toward his work until after symptomatic voice therapy and discussion with a psychiatrist, when he began to realize that his voice loss was an attempt to change jobs. He finally came to realize that he must tell his family

about his feelings and return to his previous job, which was that of a dyer in a textile mill, where he could be alone with his thoughts.

We are reminded of an important personality characteristic of patients with conversion voice disorders: their difficulty in dealing maturely and openly with feelings of anger. The following exchange illustrates the point:

Case Study 8.8

Clinician: You would say, then, that you are not very good at telling people how you feel.
Patient: Certainly not. I look calm to everybody, but I'm not. When something bothers me I get it right here (motions to her throat) and I just tighten up.
C: You're not the type that can talk back and let off steam.
P: (Smiles) With my voice the way it is? Why, that's impossible.

Here is a more detailed case study of a 33-year-old, married woman who went to her otolaryngologist after becoming aphonic. The case illustrates the sheer depth and complexity of human problems that can underlie voice loss, the importance of not approaching aphonias and dysphonias as voice disorders only but rather approaching treatment of the total person, and the importance of delving into the psychosocial history to obtain the underlying etiology of the voice disorder.

Case Study 8.9

Otolaryngology: This 33-year-old woman has a history of recurrent sinusitis. Earlier this year, she noted sore throat and sinus drainage. She has been unable to speak normally for a week, along with difficult and painful swallowing, reduced appetite, tinnitus, and dizziness when she blows her nose. Her vocal folds are inflamed on examination. Impression: Severe upper respiratory infections with bronchitis and laryngitis. Her dysphonia seems out of proportion to the physical findings. She has a good cough. Psychogenic aphonia. See Speech Pathology.

Speech Pathology: History. This 33-year-old, married female with two boys aged 4 and 9 years was referred from the Department of Otolaryngology because of suspected psychogenic aphonia. She says she lost her voice 13 days ago. She awoke with a "scratchy" voice, which disappeared within an hour, and she has been whispering ever since. She had one similar voice loss for 2 days when she was 16 years old.

Examination: The patient was aphonic on examination. However, her cough and *coup de glotte* were normally sharp. She had +2 musculoskeletal tension and discomfort in the thyrohyoid region in the response to palpation.

Diagnostic-therapeutic musculoskeletal tension reduction in the laryngeal-hyoid region produced completely normal voice within 15 minutes.

The psychosocial history portion of the examination disclosed serious and chronic emotional problems, which the patient described with considerable crying.

1. She has been desperately unhappy living in a small town where she feels completely isolated with no one to talk to.

2. She feels overburdened having to care for her two children, the younger of which is exceptionally active and difficult to control.

3. She and her husband fight a great deal over material possessions and about one another's parents. They rarely go out together. He often leaves her alone when he goes hunting and fishing.

4. She complains bitterly about her husband's parents, who dislike her intensely and do not talk to her when they see her in public.

5. She is estranged from her own parents, whom she describes as eccentric and crude. (It is important to note that she lost her voice on the day of an impending visit from her parents.)

6. She cries most intensely while describing her sister's suicide 5 years ago. She has never spoken to anyone about her feelings concerning her sister's death.

7. She is embarrassed and fearful that her husband will continue to criticize her as being like her sister, and she expresses misgivings as to whether or not she might have the capacity to commit the same act.

Impression: Psychogenic aphonia, probably conversion disorder.

Recommendation: (1) Normal voice followed symptomatic voice therapy, as noted. (2) Discussed with patient and husband the importance of psychiatric consultation. They agreed.

Psychiatrist: This 33-year-old, married mother of two sons was referred for psychiatric consultation by Speech Pathology.

She described developing her difficulty with her voice the day she received news that her father had invited himself and her mother to stay with her and her husband for an indefinite time while her husband went on a hunting trip. Throughout the initial part of the interview, the patient repeatedly returned to her father's physical and verbal abuse and his critical and demeaning nature throughout her entire life. On more recent visits, he has become sexually inappropriate toward her. She describes several other recent sources of life stress and perceives herself to be irritable and unhappy during the past 5 years, since her younger sister's death by suicide. Since then, she has been more argumentative and difficult to get along with. Other complaints are social and emotional isolation, finding it difficult to make friends and to get babysitters for her two children. She has a poor relationship with her in-laws, whom she perceives as mean to her and judgmental and

unsupportive of her throughout her marriage, particularly after the birth of her first child, who had a congenital leg deformity. Recently, she impulsively and angrily confronted them. When they responded defensively in anger, she saw this as confirming their lack of caring and their meanness.

She is frustrated within her marriage, perceiving that her husband's work prevents him from spending sufficient time at home, and she feels isolated, unhappy, and unsupported.

Her family history is positive for suicide in her younger sister, who was diagnosed as schizophrenic and who spent considerable time in and out of psychiatric institutions. She has an alcoholic brother and paternal grandfather, and her maternal grandfather committed suicide during the Depression.

She believes that her upbringing was unhappy—that her father was abusive and uncaring and her mother passive and dominated. Her father treated the girls in the family with disrespect, was demeaning and at times physically abusive. He valued only his sons. She is angry with her mother, who did not defend her and her sisters from this behavior. She was particularly close to her younger sister when they were growing up and they served as support and confidant for each other. In her mid teen years her sister became extremely troubled and got involved with a bad crowd at school and with drugs. Her behavior continued to deteriorate, and her sister was disowned by the rest of the family, whereas the patient repeatedly tried to rescue her and help her. This situation continued for several years until this young woman committed suicide. The patient relates having had to deal with funeral home arrangements and visitations and that no one else in the family attended or was supportive. She expresses feelings of guilt and a sense that she should or could have done more despite her repeated attempts to help, although her efforts were undone or rebuffed by her sister.

The mental status examination disclosed the patient to be neatly and stylishly dressed and groomed, appearing younger than her chronologic age. The initial part of the interview consisted of a dramatic litany of many individuals in her life who had or have been "treating me mean." She became tearful while discussing her sister's death and her guilt, remorse, and feelings of isolation. She was able to acknowledge an underlying sense of low self-esteem. At the end of the interview, she was less distraught, more sad, and more comfortable than at the beginning. She acknowledged that she needed to continue to talk with someone. There was no evidence of a thought disorder or gross cognitive impairment. Her voice remained normal throughout the entire interview.

Impression: (1) Adjustment disorder with mixed emotional features. (2) Dysthymic disorder. (3) Histrionic personality traits. (4) Secondary marital discord. (5) Conversation aphonia (by history; voice normal on examination).

Recommendation: This patient needs psychotherapy. I will look into different treatment options that would be available for her.

Conversion Dysphonia

Varying degrees and types of hoarseness—with and without a strained-harsh quality, high-pitched falsetto breaks, breathiness, intermittent whispering with moments of breathy and normal voice, and other variants too numerous, diverse, and indescribable to mention—occur for the same psychodynamic reasons as muteness and aphonia. A study undertaken by Aronson, Peterson Jr., and Litin (1966) comparing mute and aphonic patients with those having varying forms of dysphonia, conducted to determine similarities and differences in the etiology of their voice signs, showed that this dysphonic group was not essentially different in terms of case history, personality, and clinical criteria for conversion reaction from mute or aphonic patients (**Table 8.1**).

An important finding among all these patients, regardless of voice type, is that despite the psychoneurotic explanation for their voice signs, few have incapacitating psychiatric disturbances. In many ways, they have adjusted to their anxiety or depression. Many are willing to continue as they are rather than submit to any therapy. Others are earnest in their desire for a better voice.

Psychogenic Adductor Spasmodic Dysphonia

As described elsewhere in this text, certain patients who have an intermittently strained voice, or complete voice arrests from hyperadduction of the vocal folds during contextual speech, descriptively called *adductor spastic dysphonia*, have excess laryngeal musculoskeletal tension caused by psychologic stress. Some of these patients have conversion reaction, in which the adductor spastic dysphonia is produced by the same mechanisms that produce conversion muteness and conversion aphonia.

In other patients, the adductor spastic dysphonia is a sign of a neurologic disorder, and that is the reason why proper differential diagnosis between the psychogenic and neurologic types of spastic dysphonia is so important. Following is a case study of a young man who developed psychogenic adductor spastic dysphonia, which in all probability was a conversion reaction.

Case Study 8.10

History: A 29-year-old, single, male office worker was referred by Otolaryngology for the evaluation of dysphonia. The patient had complained for several years of an abnormally strained voice. However, laryngologic examination failed to demonstrate any structural lesions or weakness of the vocal folds. He was referred to Speech Pathology for further investigation of the cause of the voice disorder and for therapy.

Examination: This patient has a moderate to severe adductor spastic dysphonia consisting of intermittent waxing and waning of strained hoarseness and moments of complete voice arrests due to adductor laryngospasms. Vowel prolongation is clear some of the time but interrupted by varying degrees of strained hoarseness. The remainder of the oral-physical and speech examinations failed to disclose evidence of motor-speech disorder.

The psychosocial history background to the voice disorder is highly positive. The patient's voice problems began 4 years ago as whispered speech, which lasted 3 years, except for a 10-month interval during which his voice returned to normal. When the abnormal voice reappeared, it had the intermittently strained voice quality identical to his voice on examination. He has no family history of voice disorder or neurologic disease, including tremor.

The patient is a college graduate who majored in business administration. He is unmarried and lives with his parents. He admits to several problems in his emotional and personal life.

♦ He has a history of "fears" that he has difficulty describing. They emerge in the form of nightmares and sudden unpredictable terrors triggered by everyday incidents. For example, he developed a "great fear" a few years ago upon viewing a wax figure in a museum that made him feel as if he were "losing control." For this, and other reasons, the patient has been undergoing psychiatric treatment.

♦ The patient expresses considerable ambivalence about living with his parents. He enjoys the comforts of familiar surroundings, being waited on by his parents. At the same time, he is irritated with himself and with them because of his dependency. He does not wish to hurt his parents' feelings, but he is chronically irritated by his father's continuous, perfectionistic criticism of his habits—how he conducts his life, reminding him to straighten his tie and to get his hair cut, and refusing to allow him to use the family car. His mother, whom he describes as frequently irritable, badgers him to get married, which he would very much like to do, but he has always had difficulty establishing compatible relationships with women. He describes his mother as "nagging" and his father as "intolerant."

The patient moved out of his parents' home for 9 months, during which his spastic dysphonia disappeared. He lived in an apartment, by himself, a few blocks from his parents, but he felt the need to visit them every night. He then moved back into his parents' apartment, whereupon his spastic dysphonia promptly returned.

During a discussion with the patient and his parents, they corroborated their son's description of the family relationships, his father saying, "He is afraid to get out on his own. He is overdependent upon us."

The patient, for his part, and with some irritation, rejected the interpretation that his voice disorder had anything to do with his ambivalence about living at home, although later he reluctantly admitted that there might be some connection. Nevertheless, he continued to ask questions revealing that he was looking for an organic explanation for his spastic voice.

Impression: Psychogenic adductor spastic dysphonia, possibly conversion disorder. His initial voice problem sounds like he had conversion aphonia, and now he has an adductor spastic dysphonia. Both the aphonia and the spastic dysphonia disappeared for long periods, only to return. Organic (neurologic) forms of spastic dysphonia do not remit to this extent.

Table 8.1 Psychiatric Characteristics of 27 Patients with "Functional" Voice Disorders

Psychiatric Factor	Group I Patients (Mute)	Group II Patients (Continually Whispered)											Group III Patients (Intermittently Whispered-Phonated)										Group IV Patients (Continually Phonated)					Total	
	1	2	3	4	5	6	7	8	21	22	23	24	9	10	11	12	13	25	26	14	15	16	17	18	19	20	27	+	–
Acute stress	–	–	+	+	+	–	+	+	+	–	–	–	–	+	–	+	+	–	–	–	–	–	+	–	–	+	–	10	17
Chronic stress	+	+	+	–	–	–	–	–	–	+	–	+	–	+	+	+	+	+	+	–	–	–	–	+	–	–	+	13	14
Conflict symbolism	–	+	+	+	+	+	+	–	–	+	–	–	–	+	–	+	+	–	+	–	–	–	+	+	–	+	+	15	12
Primary gain	–	+	+	+	+	–	+	–	–	+	–	+	–	+	–	+	–	–	+	+	–	–	+	+	–	+	+	13	14
Secondary gain	+	+	+	+	–	+	+	+	–	+	+	–	+	+	+	–	+	–	+	+	+	–	+	–	+	–	+	17	10
Indifference	+	+	+	+	–	+	+	+	+	+	+	–	+	–	+	+	+	–	–	–	+	–	+	–	+	+	+	17	10
Clinical hysteria	+	–	–	–	–	+	+	–	+	+	+	+	+	–	+	+	–	+	–	–	–	–	–	+	+	+	+	12	15
Other conversions	+	–	–	–	–	+	–	–	+	+	–	+	+	–	–	–	–	+	–	–	–	–	–	+	+	–	–	8	19
Somatic complaints	–	–	–	–	–	–	–	–	–	+	+	+	+	–	–	–	+	+	–	–	–	–	+	+	+	–	–	7	20
MMPI conversion	+	–	–	–	–	+	–	–	+	–	+	–	+	–	+	–	–	–	+	–	–	–	–	–	+	–	+	9	18
Marital discord	–	–	–	–	+	–	–	+	–	+	–	–	+	+	+	+	+	–	+	–	–	+	–	+	+	–	+	10	17
Poor sex identification	+	+	+	+	+	+	+	+	+	+	–	–	+	+	+	+	–	–	–	–	–	+	+	+	+	–	+	18	9
Anger	+	+	+	+	+	+	+	+	+	+	+	+	–	+	+	+	+	+	+	–	+	+	+	+	+	+	+	25	2
Immature dependent	+	+	+	+	–	+	+	–	+	–	+	–	–	+	+	+	–	+	+	–	–	+	–	+	+	+	+	18	9
Neurotic life adjustment	+	–	+	–	–	+	–	+	–	–	+	+	–	–	+	–	+	+	+	–	–	+	–	+	+	–	–	16	11
Mild to moderate depression	–	+	+	–	–	–	+	+	–	–	+	–	+	–	–	–	+	+	–	–	–	–	–	–	–	–	–	7	20

Source: Aronson, A.E., Peterson, H.W., Jr., Litin, E.M. (1966). Psychiatric symptomatology in functional dysphonia and aphonia. J Speech Hear Disord 31, 115–127.

MMPI, Minnesota Multiphasic Personality Inventory.

The conflict in which this patient is trapped has to do with his need for his parents' support; however, for this he has had to accept being cast in the role of an adolescent by his parents' continuation of their lifelong overconcern and overcriticism of him. He is unable to separate from his parents and is chronically angry at their overcontrol, but he is unable to vent his anger at them for fear of disturbing them and upsetting the domiciliary arrangements that he enjoys. His spastic dysphonia may be seen as a somatic manifestation of his inability to express his true feelings to his parents.

Recommendations: During an extensive and frank discussion with the patient and his parents, during which the probable underlying dynamics of the voice disorder were discussed, it was reemphasized that the voice disorder was not caused by organic illness and it was strongly suggested that the patient return to his psychiatrist for more intensive psychotherapy with the objective of helping him to become more self-reliant and less dependent on his parents for emotional and physical support. A full report will be sent to the patient's psychiatrist.

Mutational Falsetto (Puberphonia)

The problem of mutational falsetto, or puberphonia, revolves around the subject of the pubertal change of the voice. What we are concerned with here are the physiologic changes of the male and female anatomy associated with pubertal and adolescent voice change, a subject inseparable from the disorder of mutational falsetto, or puberphonia. The mutational period of human development represents a dramatic physical and emotional transformation in the life of the individual. By way of review, we have noted in Chapter 2 that the principal changes that take place during puberty are (1) a considerable increase in vital capacity secondary to an increase in the size and strength of the thoracic musculature, (2) an increase in the length and width of the neck, and (3) a descent of the larynx producing a greater length and width of the pharynx thus enlarging the resonatory system. The length of the male vocal folds increases by approximately 1 cm and the female ~3 to 4 mm.

The basic difference between the pubertal development of the male and the female larynx has to do with the direction of their growth. Until puberty, they are essentially the same in size and form; however, during pubertal development, the male larynx grows especially in the anteroposterior direction leading to the protrusion of the thyroid eminence also known as the pomum Adami, or Adam's apple. In general, the female larynx increases in height greater than in width, the result in both sexes being a deepening of the voice and greater vocal power.

Furthermore during mutational voice change, the mucosa becomes stronger and less transparent; the tonsils and adenoids atrophy; and the epiglottis increases in size, generally flattens out, and assumes a more elevated position.

The timetable for mutation of voice begins with premutational changes consisting of a loss of phonatory power, a slight lowering of pitch, and breaks in the voice. Voice mutation in females starts as early as 9 years of age and in males around

10. The thymus gland diminishes and disappears. The secondary sex characteristics develop, the function and size of the thyroid gland increases, as well as the hypophysis. In males, there is a considerable increase in respiratory capacity; both the length and circumference of the chest increase rapidly providing greater driving force. The above-mentioned lengthening of the neck and relative descent of the larynx are associated with deep voices. As has been noted in an earlier chapter, there are racial, geographic, and climatologic determinants of the advent of mutation occurring earlier in city dwellers, in better educated children, and in warmer climates. Girls' voices tend to change about 1 year earlier than boys' and the change is less dramatic. In temperate climates, the majority of girls begin mutation at 12 to 14 years of age, boys 13 to 15, with greater acceleration nearer the Equator and some retardation of the onset of mutation at the North and South Poles with exceptions to this rule. The average duration of mutation is 3 to 6 months. The so-called break in the voice during pubertal change consisting of a sudden, involuntary change in pitch and quality is not typical of most boys' voices and is more a caricature than anything else. It is probably true that only a minority of young boys experiences the voice "break." In a study by MacKenzie (1871), only 17% of choir boys showed breaks of their voices, and the phenomenon is uncommon in girls. In the literature, the majority of writers suggest that the causes of the break are sudden and alternating contractions of the cricothyroid muscle and the thyroarytenoid muscle. The pubertal voice change begins with a huskiness and unsteadiness of the speaking voice, which may show vacillations of one to two tones, also known as the "forme frust" of the break. The general trend of mutational voice change is a downward direction of pitch. It is generally agreed that boys' speaking voices become one octave lower and girls' one or two tones. Investigations of pubertal change of the singing voice have led to the agreement that the lower limit of girls' voices descends one or two tones and the upper limit may gain the same. The lower limit of boys' voices descends a full octave. The transformation of the boys during mutation seems to take the following direction: a gradual lowering of the lower limit; with steadiness of the higher tones, the low notes slowly become steady (main phase); the stabilization of the low notes marks the end of the mutational period.

Pathologic Mutation of Voice

Abnormal vocal mutation can be subdivided into organic and psychogenic etiologies. Although the symptoms may be similar, the etiologies differ with the organic haring an identifiable physical component. The emphasis in this chapter is on the nonorganic mutations.

Classification of Mutational Disturbances

Organic

1. Endocrinologic

   a. Persistent child's voice

   b. Delayed mutation

   c. Precocious mutation

Psychogenic

1. Mutational falsetto

2. Incomplete mutation

Mutational Falsetto This is the most frequently diagnosed mutational disturbance. The mutational falsetto voice is conspicuously high and casts doubt on the masculinity and maturity of the speaker. Not only caused by problems of sexual identification, mutational falsetto can result in psychologic disturbances because of its effect on others.

The laryngoscopic finding in mutational falsetto is one of an elongated elliptical opening of the glottis typical of normal speaking males.

Incomplete Mutation This disorder consists of incomplete or insufficient lowering of the boy's voice, which may be weak, breathy, and have a definite effeminate quality, especially over the telephone, a curse to its user.

Within the context of voice mutation and mutational voice disorders, it is reasonable and appropriate to bring up the history of the eunuch and the castrato. The word *eunuch* comes from the Greek *eunochos* and the Latin *eunuchus* meaning "keeper of the bedchamber," one of the eunuch's many functions. Men have been castrated from the time of antiquity for several reasons: (1) as a consequence of being taken prisoner during times of war; (2) for the salvation of the soul. In certain Christian sects, men have castrated themselves both testes and penis to suppress temptation; (3) for purposes of revenge. In the Orient, a vengeful husband could demand in court the castration of his wife's lover; (4) to produce male opera sopranos, a subject upon which we will elaborate later. In post-Renaissance Italy, choirboys were castrated so that these youths and adults could sing as full-bodied sopranos in the cathedrals of Europe. Although the Catholic Church discouraged the operation, the Vatican's interest in emasculated men for its choirs maintained the castrati into the 20th century; (5) in Rome, handsome men were castrated to become playthings or "boy toys" of wealthy matrons who could copulate without fear of pregnancy; (6) as guardians of harems. In the East, eunuchs served as the protectors of sultans' harems; (7) as punishment for rape. Through history, castration was employed against rapists; for example, by the ancient Greeks, who used castration to punish rapists. The offender was called a *spados* meaning "to draw out" or "drag," a description of how the testes were removed from the scrotum. These men were despised in Greek society and refused employment. These men who had their testes "dragged" often masqueraded as women, giving rise to the use of the word *drag* for a man dressed in women's attire; (8) as noted above, during the pre-Christian era, the Roman eunuch was fittingly called a *volupatas*, Latin for "pleasure," and the origin of the word *voluptuous* for the soft, rounded, feminine distribution of the eunuch's body fat. Eunuchs became the main attraction in the orgies given by the emperors Octavius, Tiberius, and Caligula, who made no secret of their fondness for castrated men. The satirical poet Juvenal, speaking of Roman women who preferred the flower of marriage and not the fruit, wrote "some women always

delight in soft eunuchs and tender kisses and in the absence of a beard and the fact that the use of abortives is unnecessary."

Eunuchs were even more popular among Roman men. The 2nd century Greek satirist labeled homosexuality with eunuchs as a cause of the corruption of Roman morals by tempting everyone from emperors to generals.

Castration has played a significant role in the history of Christianity. The Christian emperor Constantine reduced the number of eunuchs when he ordered capital punishment for castrators.

The soprano castrato voice is the product of the following anatomic changes that occur as a consequence of castration. To begin with, during puberty in the male, the vocal folds increase in size as a response to the secretion of testosterone from the gonads, and the neck lengthens increasing the size of the pharynx and also increasing the thoracic dimensions. By removing the gonads between the ages of 7 and 10, the boy's soprano never deepens to the baritone or bass, and with increased vital capacity and increases in the size and strength of his respiratory musculature, his thin soprano blossoms into a large expansive soprano that no female could produce. For centuries, the Catholic Church in Rome was the major user of castrated sopranos, employing them in the Vatican Chapel choir until the practice of castration was condemned by Pope Leo. One Italian writer described the castrati soprano as follows:

> *What singing! Imagine a voice that combines the sweetness of the flute and the animated suavity of the human larynx—a voice that leaps and leaps, lightly and spontaneously, like a lark that flies through the air and is intoxicated with its own flight; and when it seems that the voice has reached the loftiest peaks of altitude, it starts off again, leaping and leaping still with equal lightness and equal spontaneity, without the slightest sign of forcing or the faintest indication of artifice or effort; in a word a voice that gives the immediate idea of sentiment transmuted into sound, and of the ascension of a soul into the infinite on the wings of that sentiment. What more can I say?*

This method of castration going back to antiquity was practiced in the Middle East to obtain a eunuch for the harem or to permanently punish a rapist: the male was strapped, arms and legs, to a table, a thin cord was knotted around his genitals, and with a sharp razor, the organs were amputated. The wound was cauterized by the application of a searing hot poker or molten tar. The mutilated youngster or adult was deprived of water for several days to prevent urination, which could infect the healing region. Then, he was forced to drink enormous amounts of water, until the pressure in his bladder literally pushed the urine through layers and layers of scar tissue, providing him with an orifice. The mortality rate was perhaps 80%. If he survived the operation, he began his new job as a docile, sexually unthreatening slave.

Clearly, the castrato voice is not the typical mutational falsetto. Mutational falsetto is not due to any anatomic immaturity of the larynx or vocal folds. The larynx is anatomically and physiologically capable of producing a normal low-pitched voice but fails to do so. In males, the voice may move upward in pitch during puberty, giving the impression of a female voice. This high-pitched falsetto type is weak, thin, breathy, hoarse, and monopitched, giving the overall impression of immaturity, effeminacy, and passiveness. In some males and females, the change in voice pitch may have begun but failed to descend completely, stopping somewhere between the pubescent and the adolescent voice. The pitch is lower than the falsetto type but retains a similar weakness, thinness, hoarseness, and monopitch.

The etiology of mutational falsetto is unclear because it has not been carefully investigated. Some attribute it to faulty learning and others to psychogenic causes. The individual and family background cannot be depicted other than superficially. One opinion is that the pubescent or adolescent, if male, acquired a stronger feminine than masculine attachment and self-identification and a neurotic need to resist the normal transition into adulthood. Variations along these themes include embarrassment about an excessively low-pitched voice developing earlier than the patient's contemporaries, forcing the pubescent male to retain the high-pitched voice, or the unconscious or conscious need to maintain a higher pitched singing voice because of the rewards attendant upon that skill such as that associated with participation in boy choirs.

Psychologic immaturity may not be the only cause of this disorder. Other factors are (1) delayed maturation in endocrine disorders that retards laryngeal development, perpetuating a high-pitched voice that then becomes difficult to abandon because of its longer-than-normal persistence into adolescence, even after the larynx has attained normal size; (2) severe hearing loss preventing the individual from perceiving his or her voice during adolescent voice change; (3) weakness or incoordination of the vocal folds or of respiration because of neurologic disease during puberty; (4) general debilitating illness during puberty, which not only may delay overall growth during puberty but, because of the physical restrictions of being bedridden, may reduce the range of respiratory excursions and, consequently, tidal air volumes, preventing the development of adequate infraglottal air pressure necessary for full vocal fold displacement.

The following laryngeal-respiratory postures and movements are bases for the high-pitched mutational falsetto voice (**Fig. 8.1**).

♦ The larynx is elevated high in the neck.

♦ The body of the larynx is tilted downward.

♦ The vocal folds are stretched thin by contraction of the cricothyroid muscles.

♦ Respiration for speech production is shallow, and on exhalation infraglottal air pressure is held to a minimum, so that only the medial edges of the vocal folds vibrate and do so at an elevated fundamental frequency.

Mutational falsetto is found in patients of all ages, some as young as 14 or 15 years and brought by their parents, and others volunteering themselves for help later in life after a long struggle with this social and psychologic handicap of a voice that does not match gender or sounds infantile. Almost all those seeking help for the first (or 10th) time in their 50s or

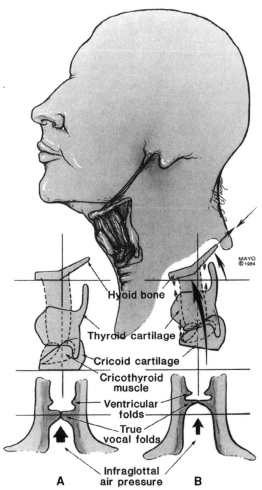

Figure 8.1 Comparison of normal laryngeal position with that of mutational falsetto. (**A**) Normal phonation. Note relatively low position of larynx, ample thyrohyoid space, blunt edges of vocal folds, and high infraglottal pressure. (**B**) Mutational falsetto. Note relatively high position of larynx, narrowed thyrohyoid space, thin edges of vocal folds, and low infraglottal pressure.

60s testify that their voices have broken into deeper or lower pitch levels during shouting or lifting. Characteristically, they fail to recognize the message of normalcy that these downward pitch breaks reveal. The falsetto voice is the only one they know. Producing a sharp glottal attack with or without the examiner exerting downward force on the larynx during phonation elicits the low-pitched voice. The psychologic penalties of mutational falsetto are great, labeling the male bearer as feminine. Use of the telephone is particularly embarrassing, as callers misinterpret the male with falsetto as being female. Teasing of young males in school and rejection for employment are additional problems.

Clinicians often miss the diagnosis of mutational falsetto because of unfamiliarity with the syndrome. Yet it is one of the easiest and most rewarding disorders to treat. Familiarity with the distinctive sound of mutational falsetto and the method of testing for it should be mandatory in the training of all speech pathologists and laryngologists.

Transsexualism Changing one's anatomy to assume the opposite sexual role is called *transsexualism*. The majority of such changes are from male to female. Such individuals need, in addition to an altered physical appearance, speech that conforms to the chosen sexual identity. The effects on the larynx of the administration of female hormones for the enhancement of female characteristics are apparently minimal. The successful elevation of fundamental frequency in transsexuals as a consequence of voice therapy has been reported by Bralley, Bull, Gore, and Edgerton (1978). These researchers were able to elevate fundamental frequency in one patient from 145 to 165 Hz after seven therapy sessions. Kalra (1977) was able to change the fundamental frequency of a male-to-female transsexual from a mean of 168 to 196 Hz after four therapy sessions. These patients reported satisfaction with their increased fundamental frequencies, although as it turned out, voice pitch was not the only method of effecting changes: altered phoneme production, inflectional patterns, and even vocabulary contributed to the total impression of femininity.

Childlike Speech in Adults Adults, adolescents, and children are seen in clinical practice who present with childlike speech patterns. The effect of a mature person speaking like a child is created by a combination of phonatory, resonatory, and articulatory modifications. However, in addition to the speech patterns that simulate those of a child, the impression of immaturity is often augmented by facial expressions, gestures, and postures that convey dependency and passiveness. The aberrant speech patterns usually consist of (1) elevation of habitual pitch; (2) exaggerated and ingratiating inflectional patterns; (3) articulation with reduced mouth opening; (4) open facial expression with raising of eyebrows; (5) cherubic smiling; and (6) demure head movements, bodily postures, and gestures.

Regressive speech serves the purpose of relieving the person from the responsibility of relating to others on an adult plane. It says, in effect, that the person does not wish to be regarded as an adult with the responsibilities for mutual interaction that an adult relationship entails. The following case study illustrates one variation on the theme of childlike speech in adults.

Case Study 8.11

Speech Pathology: This is a 26-year-old, divorced woman with two young children who is a student in a junior college. She was referred by the school counselor, who was concerned about the patient's speech because of its implications for her future ability to succeed academically, socially, and vocationally. She feels self-conscious about her speech and is afraid to start conversations.

On examination, she had a high-pitched voice produced with childlike inflectional patterns. She articulated with small, smiling mouth postures and spoke with her head cocked to one side, using supplicating, ingratiating gestures as she did so.

Prior otolaryngologic examination established that her larynx was of normal size. On phonatory examination, she

was able to lower her pitch considerably when instructed to do so but was unable to sustain a low-pitched voice during conversational speech.

Symptomatic voice therapy was administered during seven voice therapy sessions over a period of 1 month during which the patient was able to lower her pitch and eliminate many of her childlike mannerisms. Having accomplished this change in her external means of communication, she began to express the need for greater independence and complained that she found it difficult to use the more adult speech patterns that she had learned in social relationships because of the persistence of her childlike and dependent self-image.

Psychiatric consultation with the possibility of psychotherapy was recommended, to which the patient acquiesced somewhat reluctantly as she realized that changing her speech alone would not solve all of her interpersonal and self-image problems. A psychiatric consultation was arranged.

Psychiatry: This patient was seen in psychiatric consultation because of her unusual voice and speech mannerisms, which would appear to be associated with her basic personality and self-concept. Her entire demeanor, including her gestures, posture, manner of speech, and tone of voice, come across as a very small, dependent, and naïve child.

Her history suggests that she has always been a very passive and dependent person. As she talks about her current situation and past problems, she does not give any indication that she recognizes that she may have played a part in them. All of the difficulties in her life, as she sees them, are due to unavoidable circumstances or to "not nice" people.

She, herself, does not actually complain about her voice. She indicates that a counselor who is working with her said that it would be better if she had "a more assertive voice." She says that some people act like they think she has a nice voice, whereas others seem surprised by it. In her very childlike way, she indicates that she always has been very shy with people and that she doesn't speak up very often. She says that she can talk to "nice people" but doesn't like to talk to people who are not nice, saying that "some people are rude." These terms *nice* and *not nice* seem to be almost her only adjectives in describing others.

The patient never liked school, didn't see much point to it, and didn't see why she should have to go to school. She said that "a lot of the kids were not nice and some were rude." She had considerable difficulty academically.

Regarding her voice, she comments that before she was 13 years old, her voice was both lower in pitch and louder, but, even then, she said she was shy and would rarely speak up. She rather passively accepted others' opinions that maybe her voice is a problem.

It is my impression that this patient's voice is simply the most obvious component of the overall manner in which she presents herself. Her speech is the external sign of a hysterical personality structure in which she envisions herself in the role of a tiny, passive, dependent child who almost, but not quite, speaks "baby talk" and who is upset by people who are "not nice," people who might challenge her playing of this role. At this time, she does not express any insight or concern about her personality problems or her own pattern of behaving or relating.

Psychotherapy summary: Throughout several months of weekly therapy, this patient continued to speak in a very high-pitched, infantile voice. There were moments when this type of speech would improve throughout the hour, but it was quite unusual for this to happen. During initial therapy sessions, the patient presented herself as someone who is very rigid and moralistic. She would come regularly to therapy; however, she became upset when a session had to be canceled and refused to come or call. She seemed to handle very poorly any absences or fluctuations on the part of the psychiatrist. She seemed relatively uninvested in the therapy and saw to it that the sessions remained superficial. She was quite resistant toward efforts to enable her to gain insight into her interpersonal problems and into the deeper issues causing her childlike demeanor. Any expression of painful affect was usually met by fleeing from the therapy session. She was extremely sensitive to any change in schedule, which was followed by weeks of nonattendance. Finally, she failed to return even after contact with her by telephone. She does not seem capable of handling insight-oriented psychotherapy and does not seem to have the ego strength to tolerate a transference relationship.

◆ Rebound Psychologic Effects of Voice Disorders

To possess a voice disorder, whether psychogenic or organic, is to experience demoralization. Voice is part of the person. Self-alienation occurs when our voices are no longer "us" and identify is lost. Once the patient learns that the voice disorder is not a threat to health, an adverse secondary psychologic reaction sets in triggered by the patient's rejection of his or her own voice and by the reactions of listeners. "What is the matter with your voice? You should do something about your voice!" Change in facial expression of listeners upon hearing the abnormal voice is detected easily by the patient. It is only a brief time from the onset of the disorder until the patient begins to dread meeting others, acquaintances and strangers alike. The individual with a defective voice elects to speak less and less often to avoid such reactions. We observe the depressing effects of voice disorders in well-adjusted patients with organic voice disorders as well as in those whose disorders are psychogenic. In addition to their primary psychologic discomfort, patients with psychogenic voice disorders have amplification of their already unhappy state because of self and listener rejection of the voice.

If the patient's voice disorder is severe enough to interfere with intelligibility, the situation can be even worse. It is difficult to understand these individuals in noisy and even quiet environments, so that their voice disorders seriously interfere with their professional, business, and social lives. Consequently, the effect of the voice disorder on others and on the patient becomes circular and escalating: the patient's frustration and anger elevate musculoskeletal tension, and whatever primary organic or psychogenic voice disorder existed up to that point is worsened to an even greater degree of severity. It is axiomatic that emotional stress exacerbates virtually all voice disorders, whether organic or psychogenic. Those who are privileged to care for individuals who have moderate to severe voice disorders will become convinced that the anger, frustration, anxiety, depression, and discouragement that these patients experience from the social effects of the disorder itself is tantamount to an illness requiring as much attention as the voice per se.

◆ Iatrogenic Voice Rest

In medicine, the term *iatrogenic* means a disorder or illness caused or exacerbated by the treatment or advice administered by the practitioner (e.g., a vocal fold paralysis caused by accidental severance of a recurrent laryngeal nerve during a thyroidectomy). Voice rest can produce or aggravate a dysphonia as in the following narrative of a patient:

They told me not to talk too much. I feel, if I'm all right, why are they asking me to keep quiet? Now that they told me not to talk, I'm worried. Never to scream? Never to sing? They also told me not to cough. I've been holding my voice back. The aggravation is sitting right here (points to neck and chest). I can't let it out.

Any illness induced by the actions of the clinician is called iatrogenic. Voice disorders can be caused or worsened by the actions of the clinician. The patient who undergoes surgery on the vocal folds or on those regions of the neck or chest that may result in edema or paralysis of the vocal folds may experience dysphonia, either temporarily or permanently. What cannot be predicted in such cases is the extent of the patient's suggestibility upon recovery from surgery. Upon hearing the abnormal voice, the patient may become anxious or depressed and may develop a musculoskeletal tension or even a conversion voice disorder superimposed upon the organic one. Some patients upon hearing their normal voices resort to older laryngeal postures to match their preoperative voice, a voice that will be maintained unless there is behavioral intervention to teach ways of using the revised anatomic structure. In others, psychogenic voice disorders after laryngeal surgery have occurred because of unconscious hostility toward the surgeon or for secondary gain.

A second type of psychogenic iatrogenic voice disorder can begin with the sometimes ill-advised prescription of excessive voice rest. Korvin (2005) summarized the legends and realities surrounding recommendations for voice rest. She divides voice rest into three categories: absolute with no vocalization whatsoever, modified with soft vocalizations limited to no more than 5 minutes/hour, and voice conservation. The underlying rationale is based on theories of microtrauma and injury that suggest continued phonation may interfere with restoration of the molecular structure of the vocal fold and healing after some types of surgery. Although opinions vary, studies indicate 1 to 2 weeks is appropriate for majority of remucosalization to occur without any apparent muscle atrophy. Voice rest for longer periods of time may have adverse affects. Korvin suggests the patients at greatest postoperative risk are those who smoke, who have large amounts of tissue resection, and those who use their voice excessively. She also notes that voice rest has psychologic implications and that although the impact of voice rest on the psyche varies by patient, it may induce feelings of insecurity, helplessness, and dissociation from the verbal world. She concludes that although further research is needed, and voice rest should be determined on an individual basis related to type and degree of surgery, voice rest is both possible and necessary for some surgical cases.

An alternative opinion about this controversial issue of voice rest is that with the exception of a few surgical procedures requiring voice rest (and even then only brief rest is required), to advise patients with organic, and particularly psychogenic, voice disorders to whisper or remain mute for days or weeks is the worst advice that can be given a patient with a voice disorder. The larynx and voice are exceptionally suggestible and responsive to anxiety. When a clinician suggests voice rest, a seed of doubt is planted about that patient's basic ability to phonate. The possible result is a secondary psychogenic voice disorder. An added complication of voice rest is that failure to use the vocal folds causes flaccidity of nonuse, possibly creating still another dysphonia in addition to that already present. How the idea of voice rest originated as a "therapy" is not clear. One suspects that it is the choice of clinicians who, knowing little about the care of the patient with a voice disorder, reason by analogy that inasmuch as rest is good for many things, it ought to be good for the voice, too. The following testimony is from a speech clinician who herself was placed on voice rest.

Case Study 8.12

It all seemed so simple, a nodule on the right vocal band would be removed under general anesthesia and 1 or 2 weeks of vocal rest would be advised. The Christmas season appeared the quietest time in terms of diminished teaching responsibilities with the hope that the hoarseness I exhibited for several months would be diminished.

Optimistically, I entered the hospital situation, even having them obligingly do the blood work and allow me to go "out to dinner." Lovely hotel, food lacked style! The surgery was uneventful, occurring early in the morning and I returned home that evening, drowsy but well. Flowers arrived and solicitous calls came constantly. It all seemed a lark! I was perfectly in control of the situation. Clinically, it would be an interesting situation for someone in the field of speech pathology. What followed was a nightmare of psychologic trauma.

As director of a large speech and language center, it seemed only reasonable that I could return to work immediately. My family, who at first seemed delighted with a silent mother and wife, quickly began to realize that this same person would need them to answer her phone calls, make calls, and generally accomplish those things that require voice. This, in itself, would have been no problem. What I didn't plan on was the feeling of isolation. The ungodly sense of being a spectator to the world! We read about this psychologic phenomenon; we talk about it when we teach. Until one experiences the detachment and the profound loneliness, one cannot readily understand what the words *vocal silence* really mean.

Few people enjoy talking to someone who can give only a "yes" or "no" return. Cryptic notes, written on magic slate, soon lose their readability, as well as their interest. My husband as well as my colleagues appeared annoyed at the frequent taps on their shoulders or the snapping of my fingers: two methods I used to focus attention on my slate.

As an individual who has worked long years at creating dialogue in my household, my family showed deep resentment toward the monologue situation. Mother could not talk about her feelings. Her body was fine, why didn't she talk? My disability became almost a personal affront and inconvenience. Even my dearest friends soon tired of calling and waiting for phone taps: one equaled yes, two equaled no, and multiple taps meant goodbye. The burden of conversation on the part of the speaker became more problematic than anticipated. How difficult it must be for the parent who receives little or no response from their child!

Peoples' responses generally ranged from humor to a singing or gestural response that assumed that I could not hear or speak. One bright-eyed stranger asked me if I were a mute.

The frustration of not being in control was devastating. One constantly needs someone else, and locked within you are all the reactions and impressions that for years you have learned to share and enjoy. The very antithesis of one's basic personality was operating.

As I write this I am still silent, eagerly awaiting the end of this journey. My need to write this is based on my need to communicate and to assist those of us who work with aphasia, vocal problems, and other speech and language problems, to attempt to gain some insight into the psychologic and emotional aspects of the problems involved. My entire approach to therapy has altered as a result of this experience. Never again will I read, hear, or advise "vocal rest" with the same lack of understanding or empathy (Fiedler, 1977).

The following study illustrates a repeated finding in the practice of voice disorders: when patients become dysphonic or aphonic, either unconsciously or voluntarily, as in vocal rest, they seem to lose their sense or feel for volitional phonation. It is an experience that teaches the clinician that the patient has undergone some sort of loss of recall, memory, or even praxis for normal voice production. We do not think that the articulatory mechanism is susceptible in a similar way to the effects of nonuse, illustrating again the special nature of the larynx and phonation.

Case Study 8.13

D.S., a 5-year-old boy, was found to have small bilateral vocal nodules. His speech clinician placed him on complete voice rest, which unfortunately was enforced for 5 continuous months. At the end of 5 months, the nodules had disappeared, and the child was instructed by both the physician and speech pathologist to renew normal phonation. Despite all efforts by the child, he could only whisper. He became completely aphonic but conversed easily with all people with much animation and relative comfort. This functional aphonia remained for 2 months after he was instructed, "Go back and talk the normal way, Davey." The child gestured that he wanted to use his voice but that he could not "find it." Therapy efforts to restore the phonation were begun some 7 months after the child's natural phonation had ceased (Boone, 1977).

♦ Summary

♦ Voice may provide clues to underlying personality in normal individuals; however, research to prove this assumption is fraught with problems of defining personality, vocal parameters, and acceptable research methodology.

♦ Specific changes in voice quality, pitch, and loudness have been associated with discrete emotional states, environmental stress, depression, and schizophrenia.

♦ Psychogenic voice disorders are muteness, aphonia, and dysphonia in the absence of organic laryngeal disease, or with disease that is insufficient to explain the voice disorder. These voice disorders can be traced to the anxiety or depression produced by life stress, to psychoneuroses, or to personality disorders.

♦ Musculoskeletal tension due to environmental stress can produce a variety of dysphonias, sometimes even aphonia, that are the effects of hypercontraction of the extrinsic and intrinsic laryngeal musculature.

♦ If hypercontraction of the musculature caused by musculoskeletal tension is combined with vocal abuse, the tissue reactions of inflammation, a vocal nodule, or contact ulcer can develop, causing further dysphonia.

♦ A vocal nodule is a small, white or grayish protuberance on the free margin of the vocal fold at the junction of the anterior and middle third where impact stress is greatest, generally bilateral. Vocal nodules occur in children of both sexes, and most commonly in adult females who use their voices excessively by screaming, yelling, excess talking, or singing. More often than not, children and adults with vocal nodules are extraverts.

♦ A contact ulcer is a superficial ulceration of the mucosa overlying the medial surface of the arytenoid cartilage at the junction of the posterior third of the vocal fold. It develops at the tip of the vocal process of the arytenoid cartilage, unilaterally or bilaterally. The ulcer is caused by forceful and damaging contact between the opposing arytenoid cartilages during forceful phonation under conditions of heightened muscular tension and reduced pitch. Contact ulcer has a predilection for males in their 40s who come from occupational backgrounds involving greater-than-average voice use and who show personality characteristics of aggressiveness and competitiveness. Reflux, smoking, alcohol consumption, and air pollution are often associated findings in the histories of patients who have contact ulcer.

♦ A conversion voice disorder is muteness, aphonia, or dysphonia in which there is an involuntary loss of control over the muscles of phonation as an unconscious attempt to avoid unpleasant confrontations.

♦ Voice disorders can occur in patients who have problems of emotional maturity and sex identification. Mutational falsetto (puberphonia) is the failure of adolescent voice change, most often in males, despite normal laryngeal growth.

♦ Whether organic or psychogenic, all voice disorders produce adverse secondary psychologic effects on the speaker, increasing the severity of the primary voice disorder.

♦ Iatrogenic voice disorders are those caused inadvertently in the course of treatment of other medical or surgical problems and as a result of injudicious advice, the most notable of which is excessive voice rest.

References

Andrews, M., Shank, K. (1983). Some observations concerning the cheerleading behavior of school-girl cheerleaders. Lang Speech Hear Serv Sch 14, 150–156.

Arnold, G.E. (1962). Vocal nodules and polyps; laryngeal tissue reactions to habitual dysphonia. J Speech Hear Disord 27, 205–217.

Aronson, A.E., Peterson, H.W., Jr., Litin, E.M. (1966). Psychiatric symptomatology in functional dysphonia and aphonia. J Speech Hear Disord 31, 115–127.

Bachorowski, J., Owren, M.J. (2003). Production and perception of affect-related vocal acoustics. Ann N Y Acad Sci 1000, 244–265.

Bady, S.L. (1985). The voice as curative factor in psychotherapy. Psychoanal Rev 72, 479–490.

Barker, K.D., Wilson, F.B. (1967). Comparative study of vocal utilization of children with hoarseness and normal voice. Paper presented at the convention of the American Speech and Hearing Association, Chicago, IL.

Bhatia, M.S. (2000). Hysterical aphonia-an analysis of 25 cases. Indian J of Medical Sciences. 54(6), 335–338.

Boone, D.R. (1977). *The voice and voice therapy*. Englewood Cliffs, NJ: Prentice-Hall.

Bralley, R.C., Bull, J.L., Gore, C.H., Edgerton, M.T. (1978). Evaluation of vocal pitch in male transsexuals. J Commun Disord 11, 443–449.

Brown, B.L., Strong, W.J., Rencher, A.C. (1974). Fifty-four voices from two: the effects of simultaneous manipulations of rate, mean fundamental frequency, and variance of fundamental frequency on ratings of personality from speech. J Acoust Soc Am 55, 313–318.

Campos, J.J., Thein, S., Owen, D. (2003). Emotional expressions as behavior regulators. Ann N Y Acad Sci 1000, 244–265.

Chevrie-Muller, C., Dodart, F., Sequier-Dermer, N., Salmon, D. (1971). Etude des parameters acoustiques de la parole au cours de la schizophrenic de l'adolescent. Folia Phoniatr 23, 401–428.

Davidson, R.J. (2000). Affective style, psychopathology, and resilience: Brain mechanisms and plasticity. *American Psychologist*, 55, 1196–1214.

Dietrich M., Verdolini, K. (2005). Acute stress and the effects on voice: potential roles of the autonomic nervous system. VOICE and EMOTIONS XV. Annual Pacific Voice Conference and First International Pacific Voice & Speech Foundation/PIXAR Animation Studios Conference on Voice Quality and Emotions. Emeryville, CA.

Duncan, S., Rice, L., Butler, J.M. (1968). The therapists' paralanguage in peak and poor psychotherapy hours. J Abnorm Psychol 73, 566–570.

Fiedler, I. (1977). Vocal rest. ASHA 19, 307–308.

Friedman, M., Brown, A.E., Rosenman, R.H. (1969). Voice analysis for detection of behavior patterns. JAMA 208, 828–836.

Friedman, M., Rosenman, R.H. (1959). Association of specific overt behavior pattern with blood and cardiovascular findings: blood cholesterol level, blood clotting time, incidence of arcus senilis, and clinical coronary artery disease. JAMA 169, 1286–1296.

Glassel, W.L. (1972). A study of personality problems and vocal nodules in children. Paper presented at the American Speech and Hearing Association Convention, San Francisco, CA.

Goldfarb, W., Brownstein, P., Lorge, I. (1956). A study of speech patterns in a group of schizophrenic children. Am J Orthopsychiatry 26, 544–555.

Goldfarb, W., Goldfarb, N., Brownstein, P., Scholl, H. (1972). Speech and language faults of schizophrenic children. J Autism Child Schizophr 2, 219–233.

Gray, J.A. (1991). Neural systems, emotion, and personality. In J. Madden (Ed.), *Neurobiology of learning, emotion, and affect* (pp. 273–396). New York: Raven Press.

Gray, S.D. (1991). Basement membrane zone injury in vocal nodules. In J. Gauffin, B. Hammarberg (Eds.), *Vocal fold physiology: Acoustic, perceptual and physiological aspects of voice mechanisms* (pp. 21–27). San Diego: Singular Publishing Group, Inc.

Green, G. (1989). Psycho-behavioral characteristics of children with vocal nodules: WPBIC ratings. J Speech Hear Disord 54, 306–312.

Greene, M.C.L. (1972). *The voice and its disorders*. Philadelphia PA: J.B. Lippincott.

Gustafson, J.P. (1977). *The new interpretation of dreams*. Madison, WI: James P. Gustafson.

Gustafson, J. (1986). *The complex secret of brief psychotherapy*. New York: W. W. Norton.

Gustafson, J. (1999). *The common dynamics of psychiatry*. Madison, WS: James P. Gustafson.

Gustafson, J.P. (2000). *The common dynamics of psychiatry*. Madison, WI: James P. Gustafson.

Gustafson, J.P., Meyer, M. (2004). A non-linear model of dynamics. Psychodynamic Practice 10, 479–489.

Hargreaves, W.A., Starkweather, J.A. (1964). Voice quality changes in depression. Lang Speech 7, 84–88.

Jain, S., Bnadi, V., Zimmerman, J., et al. (2000). Incidence of vocal cord dysfunction. Presentation and treatment options. J Voice 14, 99–103.

Jensen, P. (1964). Hoarseness in cheerleaders. ASHA 6, 406.

Kakehi K, Sogabe Y. (2005). Emotional perception in voices: Is it categorical or not? VOICE and EMOTIONS XV. Annual Pacific Voice Conference and First International Pacific Voice & Speech Foundation/PIXAR Animation Studios Conference on Voice Quality and Emotions. Emeryville, California.

Kalra, M.A. (1977). Voice therapy with a transsexual. Paper presented at the American Speech and Hearing Association Convention, Chicago IL.

Kazan, E. (1988). *A life*. New York: Doubleday.

Khachatur' yants, L., Grimak, L. (1972). Cosmonaut's emotional stress in space flight. N.A.S.A. Space TT F-14, 654.

Korvin, G.S. (2005). Voice rest: legend or reality? In J. Abitbol (Ed.), *Phonosurgery and voice care*. Paris: Clinique Sainte-Isbelle/Generale De Sante.

Koufman, J.A. (1991). The otolaryngologic manifestations of gastroesophageal reflux disease (GERD): A clinical investigation of 225 patients using ambulatory 24-hour pH monitoring and an experimental investigation of the role of acid and pepsin in the development of laryngeal injury. Laryngoscope 101(suppl. 53), 1–78.

Lang, P.J. (1994). The motivational organization of emotion: Affect-reflex connections. In Stephanie H.M. van Goozen, N.E. van de Poll, J.A. Sergeant (Eds.), *Emotions: Essays on emotion theory* (pp. 61–93). Hillsdale, NJ: Lawrence Erlbaum.

Lauriello, M., Cozza, K., Rossi, A., Di Rienzo, L., Coen Tirelli, G. (2003). Psychological profiles of dysfunctional dysphonia. Acta Otorhinolaryngol Ital 12(6), 467–473.

Lazarus, R.S., Folkman, S. (1984). *Stress, appraisal and coping*. New York: Springer.

LeDoux, J.E. (1986). The neurobiology of emotion. In J.E. LeDoux, W. Hirst (Eds.), *Mind and brain: diologues in cognitive neuroscience* (pp. 301–327). New York: Cambridge.

Luchsinger, R., Arnold, G.E. (1965). *Voice-speech-language*. Belmont, CA: Wadsworth.

Mackenzie, M. (1871). *Essay on growths in the larynx: with reports, and an analysis of one hundred consecutive cases treated by the author*. Philadelphia: Lindsay & Blakiston.

Mallory, E., Miller, V. (1958). A possible basis for the association of voice characteristics and personality traits. Speech Monogr 25, 255–260.

Mirza, N., Ruiz, C., Baum, E.D., Staab, J.P. (2003). The prevalence of major psychiatric pathologies in patients with voice disorders. Ear, Nose, & Throat Journal 82(10), 808–10, 812, 814.

Monnot, M. (2005). New basic emotions and affective prosody and effective communication. VOICE and EMOTIONS, XV. Annual Pacific Voice Conference and First International Pacific Voice & Speech Foundation/PIXAR Animation Studios Conference on Voice Quality and Emotions. Emeryville, CA.

Monnot, M., Lovallo ,W.R., Nixon, S.J., Ross, E. (2002). Neurological basis of deficits in affective prosody comprehension among alcoholics and fetal alcohol-exposed adults. J Neuropsychiatry Clin Neurosci 14(3), 321–328.

Monnot, M., Orbelo, D., Riccardo, L., Sikka, S., Rossa, E. (2003). Acoustic analysis support subjective judgments of vocal emotion. Ann NY Acad Sci 1000: 288–292.

Monnot, M., Orbelo D., Riccardo L., Sikka S., Rossa E. (2003). Acoustic analyses support subject judgments of vocal emotion. Ann N Y Acad Sci 1000, 110–134.

Moore, W.E. (1939). Personality traits and voice quality deficiencies. J Speech Hear Disord 4, 33–36.

Morosomme D., Verduyckt I. (2005). Recognition of vocal and facial cues of four primary emotions (sadness, happiness, anger, fear) in a patient affected by Steinert Disease and in a professional actor. Matching of vocal and visual signals. VOICE and EMOTIONS XV. Annual Pacific Voice Conference and First International Pacific Voice & Speech Foundation/PIXAR Animation Studios Conference on Voice Quality and Emotions. Emeryville, CA.

Moses, P.J. (1954). *The voice of neurosis*. New York: Grune & Stratton.

Moskowitz, E. (1951). Voice quality in schizophrenic reaction type. Ph.D. thesis. New York: New York University.

Nemec, J. (1961). The motivation background of hyperkinetic dysphonia in children: a contribution to psychologic research in phoniatry. Logos 4, 28–31.

Newman, S.S., Mather, V.G. (1938). Analysis of spoken language of patients with affective disorders. Am J Psychiatry 94, 912–942.

Ostwald, P.F., Skolnikoff, A. (1966). Speech disturbances in a schizophrenic adolescent. Postgrad Med 40, 40–49.

Peacher, G. (1947). Contact ulcer of the larynx: Part IV: A clinical study of vocal re-education. J Speech Disord 12, 179–190.

Peacher, G., Hollinger, O. (1947). Contact ulcer of the larynx: the role of re-education. Arch Otolaryngol 46, 617–621.

Perelló, J. (1962). Dysphonies fonctionnelles: phonoponose et phononevrose, Folia Phoniatr 14, 150–205.

Popov, V.A., Simonov, P.V., Frolov, M.V., Khachatur' yants, L.S. (1971). The articulatory frequency spectrum as an indicator of the degree and nature of emotional stress in man. N.A.S.A. Space TT F-13, 772.

Reich, A., McHenry, M., Keaton, A. (1986). A survey of dysphonic episodes in high school cheerleaders. Lang Speech Hear Serv Sch 17, 63–71.

Rosenman, R.H., Friedman, M., Straus, R., Wurm, M., Kositchek, R., Hahn, W., Werthessen N.J. (1964). A predictive study of coronary heart disease: the Western Collaborative Group Study. JAMA 189, 15–22.

Ross, E.D., Orbelo, D.M., Burgard, M., Hansel, S. (1998). Functional-anatomic correlates of aprosodic deficits in patients with right brain damage. Neurology 50(suppl. 4), A363.

Ross, E.D., Thompson, R.D., Yenkosky, J. (1997). Lateralization of affective prosody in brain and the callosal integration of hemispheric language functions. Brain and Language 56, 27–54.

Roy, N., Bless, D.M. (2000). Personality traits and psychological factors in voice pathology: A foundation for future research. Journal of Speech, Language and Hearing Research 43, 737–748.

Roy, N., Bless, D.M., Heisey, D. (2000a). Personality and voice disorders: A multitrait-multidisorder analysis. *Journal of Voice 14* (4), 521–548.

Roy, N., Bless, D.M., Heisey, D. (2000b). Personality and voice disorders: A superfactor trait analysis. J Speech Lange Hear Res 43, 749–768.

Roy, N., Merrill, R.M., Thibeault, S., Parsa, R.A., Gray, S.D., Smith, E.M. (2004). Prevalence of voice disorders in teachers and the general population. J Speech Lange Hear Res. 47(2), 281–293.

Roy, N, Bless D.M. (1999). Personality traits and psychological factors in voice pathology: a foundation for future research. NCVS Status and Progress Report 191, 201.

Ruscello, D.M., Lass N.J., Podbesek J. (1988). Listeners' perceptions of normal and voice-disordered children. Folia Phoniatr (Basel) 40, 290–296.

Saxman, J.H., Burk, K.W. (1968). Speaking fundamental frequency and rate characteristics of adult female schizophrenics. J Speech Hear Res 11, 194–203.

Senturia, B.H., Wilson, F.B. (1968). Otorhinolaryngolic findings in children with voice deviations. Ann Otol Rhinol Laryngol 77, 1–15.

Sidorova J. (2005). Voice parameters responsible for auditory perception and speech emotion recognition: Error-correcting tree language inference and decision trees. VOICE and EMOTIONS XV. Annual Pacific Voice Conference and First International Pacific Voice & Speech Foundation/PIXAR Animation Studios Conference on Voice Quality and Emotions. Emeryville, CA.

Simonov, P.V., Frolov, M.V. (1973). Utilization of human voice for estimation of man's emotional stress and state of attention. Aerospace Med 44,256–258.

Takahashi, R., Hinohara, T., Ohmori, K., Saruya, S. (1971). Psychosomatic aspects of the complaint of foreign feelings of the pharyngolaryngeal region. In Ear, Nose and Throat Studies (pp. 723–729). Tokyo: Department of Otorhinolaryngology, Jikei University School of Medicine.

Tarrasch, H. (1946). Muscle spasticity in functional aphonia and dysphonia. Med Wom J 53, 25–33.

Testa, J.A., Beatty , W.W., Gleason, A.C., Orbelo, D.M., Ross, E.D. (2001). Impaired affective prosody in AD: Relationship to aphasic deficits and emotional behaviors. Neurology 57, 1474-1481.

Toohill, R.J. (1975). The psychosomatic aspects of children with vocal nodules. Arch Otolaryngol, 101, 591–595.

Van Den Berg, J. (1962). Modem research in experimental phoniatrics. Folia Phoniatr 14, 81–149.

Vaughan, C. W. (1982). Current concepts in otolaryngology: diagnosis and treatment of organic voice disorders. N Engl J Med 307, 333–336.

Williams, C.E., Stevens, K.N. (1969). Emotions and speech: some acoustical correlates. J Acoust Soc Am 52, 1238–1250.

Williamson, A.B. (1945). Diagnosis and treatment of 72 cases of hoarse voice. Q J Speech 31, 189–202.

Whitman, E.N., Flicker, D.J. (1966). A potential new measurement of emotional state: a preliminary report. Newark Beth Israel Hosp 17,167–172.

Wilson, F.B., Lamb, M.M. (1973). Comparison of personality characteristics of children with and without vocal nodules on Rorschach protocol interpretation. Paper presented at the American Speech and Hearing Association Convention, Atlanta, GA.

Zaliouk, A., Izkovitch, I. (1958). Some tomographic aspects in functional voice disorders. Folia Phoniatr 10, 34–39.

Ziegler, F.S., Imboden, J.B. (1962). Contemporary conversion reactions: II. Conceptual model. Arch Gen Psychiatry 6, 279–287.

Additional Reading

Aronson, A.E., Peterson, H.W., Jr., Litin, E.M. (1966). Psychiatric symptomatology in functional dysphonia and aphonia. J Speech Hear Disord 31, 115–127. (This article illustrates the strong influence of interpersonal problems on the development and maintenance of dysphonia and aphonia.)

Bady, S.L. (1985). The voice as curative factor in psychotherapy. Psychoanal Rev 72, 479–490. (This article on the importance and meaning of voice for patient and psychotherapist alike makes extremely interesting reading. The author goes into considerable detail about how the therapist's voice can facilitate therapy and how the patient's voice indicates that person's emotional status. The act of verbalizing one's thoughts is analyzed as a physical as well as psychologic one, having almost tactile effects.)

Elias, A., Raven, R., Butcher, P., Littlejohns, D. W. (1989). Speech therapy for psychogenic voice disorder: a survey of current practice and training. Br J Disord Commun 24, 61–76. (This article is worth reading for information on the attitudes and practices of speech clinicians in the United Kingdom toward patients with psychogenic dysphonia and aphonia. This survey revealed some interesting opinions and practices concerning the inadequacy of their undergraduate education in psychology and psychiatry and the extent to which such education served them later in practice. From the study, the authors were led to conclude that much more background in psychology and psychiatry was necessary in the practical treatment of patients with psychogenic voice disorders. [See Chapter 11 for more details about this study])

Hartman, D.E., Aronson, A.E. (1983). Psychogenic aphonia masking mutational falsetto. Arch. Otolaryngol 109, 415–416. (An interesting case illustrating the coexistence of two psychogenic voice disorders, the second caused by the first.)

Kramer, E. (1963). Judgment of personal characteristics and emotions from nonverbal properties of speech. Psychol Bull 60, 408–420. (Excellent, unbiased critical review of the literature on the relationship between voice, personality, emotions, and psychopathology.)

Peacher, G. (1947). Contact ulcer of the larynx: Part IV. A clinical study of vocal re-education. J Speech Disord 12, 179–190. (One of a series of four landmark studies on the etiology, symptomatology, and therapy of contact ulcer. Check its bibliography for the remaining three. They're well worth reading.)

Ziegler, F.S., Imboden, J.B. (1962). Contemporary conversion reactions: II. Conceptual model. Arch Gen Psychiatry 6, 279–287. (An absolute must for anyone who works with psychogenic voice disorders because it explains so well the modern interpretation of conversion and hysteria.)

Chapter 9

Psychodiagnostic Interviewing and Counseling for Voice Disorders

A quiet hour spent in discussing the problems of the patient will help much to remove anxieties and restore vocal function.

—Brodnitz

A few introductory remarks are in order on the subject of our own voices as clinicians, interviewers, and therapists. Our speech is a medium by which we carry on our work. In the diagnostic and therapeutic situation, all is mediated through speech. Virtually all of what we do involves two or more people talking together where voice is a reflection of the emotional state of the clinician as well as of the patient. It allows both to achieve an empathic understanding.

The quality of the clinician's voice influences the emotional state of the listener. Many psychoanalytic writers have mentioned the voice not only as a means of conveying thought but also as an exquisite representation of emotion. The patient knows the clinician's inner state from various nonverbal cues, including quality of voice. The tone of the voice and the overall prosody of speech reflect conflict in the patient and alert the clinician as to the best times for intervention.

It becomes readily apparent that voice is the primary expression of the individual, revealing general personality as well as transient emotional states. An experienced psychotherapist wrote:

Since I have been listening to my patients' voices I have also noted that changes of vocal quality accompany their progress. One patient achieved a lighter, less ponderous voice as he became more comfortable with his emotions. Another slowed down his rapid pace. A third achieved a less grating and more fluid tone. In my work I will intentionally use my voice along with my words. Sometimes I attempt through vocal tones to soothe an anxious agitated patient. Other times I use my voice to stimulate a depressed and hopeless one. On still other occasions I talk to give the patient a human response and my words are less impor-

tant than the vocal indication of my presence. Sometimes I remain silent in order for me to encourage separation from me. Occasionally my voice backfires on me, as when a patient notices my anger and my anxiety through the sound of my voice.

It may actually feel to the patient as though he is ejecting an angry or sad thought from his body. Perhaps our patients own their spoken thoughts not only with their ears, but with their entire body, which both produce sound and hear it. We all know instances when a patient gives evidence of strong physical distress while verbalizing a disturbing thought and then feels much more relief afterwards. We all have that same experience which addresses itself to the relief and therapeutic value of catharsis; perhaps my patient's comment that talking gives her thoughts air is not only a metaphor for a psychological experience, but also a description of the stream of air that flows through the vocal apparatus in order to produce a sound. Sound is something concrete touching us. Sound is a contact experience. Sound waves are transmitted through the air and create tiny, yet definite impressions on the skin and eardrum. A loud noise is felt as well as heard at lower frequencies. There is a gentle, but definite, vibration distinct from any superimposed on the sound. The voice of the therapist creates both a psychological and physical bridge between herself and her patient. And we stress the importance of the way we touch one another with the sounds of our voices.

If we consider it possible that one person can physically affect another, then vocal intonations of the therapist take on further importance. The therapist's voice is to soothe or stimulate the patient, a voice that reflects the relaxation and the self-confidence of the therapist. A self-assured voice may stimulate hope and courage into the timid voice of the patient. Our voices along with our words help our patients find within themselves the capacity for change (Bady, 1985).

Let us consider the everyday functions of the human voice in our lives so that we can better understand why a voice disorder can have such devastating effects on us. We have already learned that emotional problems cause abnormal voice and that abnormal voice can cause or exacerbate emotional problems.

Following are the values that voice has for us: (1) for the expression of intellect; (2) as a means of emotional expression of anger, grief, and nuances of feeling and thought; (3) as a means of establishing and maintaining our personal identity. We have seen time and again how abnormal voice or loss of voice is tantamount to the loss of the *self:* "my voice is not me anymore" or its equivalent is so often conveyed to the clinician to indicate the patient's loss of personal identity; (4) as a means of self-assertion and of controlling others; (5) to assert our opinions, to project our feelings, to confront the world; (6) as a means of expressing our creativity in the formulation of ideas and as an expression of our artistic selves; (7) to make sound for its own sake as an escape from loneliness and isolation (i.e., as a defense against silence); (8) as an expression of our sexuality during courtship and mating; and (9) as a way of camouflaging our true feelings during interpersonal communication (i.e., to deceive, disguise, and guard our secrets).

You lose all of these human rights and values when you can no longer use your voice (this truth is nowhere better demonstrated than in the DVD, accompanying this text, of Mrs. M.K. who had relied on her voice for most of life's pleasures until she developed adductor spasmodic dysphonia, which nearly destroyed her).

✦ Rationale for the Psychodiagnostic Interview

During the question-and-answer period after the presentation of a paper on voice therapy for transsexualism at a national convention, the speaker had emphasized how, in addition to changing the patient's pitch, inflection, and vocabulary, she found it necessary to provide psychological support for the identity crises that vexed her patient, who was going through a profound life change. A young student's hand tentatively rose, and with a voice and frowning expression that clearly communicated her perplexity and confusion, she hesitantly asked, "But . . . are . . . we . . . psychologists?" In that single question dwelt all the ambiguity, ambivalence, and uncertainty that has characterized our profession's stance on the question of the responsibility for learning, knowing, and practicing psychologic interviewing and counseling with patients who have communicative disorders.

The predominant attitude in our academic training toward this subject has been to avoid it, narrowly defining the clinician's field of practice as retraining vocal habit patterns. We believe it is impossible and unethical to treat people who have voice disorders without weaving into diagnosis and therapy the interviewing skills of the psychiatrist, clinical psychologist, and psychiatric social worker. Any in-depth study of voice disorders forces us to conclude that—so long as clinicians obtain privileged information from patients; so long as people have voice problems because of life stress and interpersonal conflict; so long as voice disorders produce

anxiety, depression, embarrassment, and self-consciousness; so long as patients need a sympathetic person with whom they can talk about their distress—we will need to consider our training incomplete until we have learned the basic skills of psychologic interviewing and counseling. Most psychogenic voice disorders, particularly of the conversion type, are unlikely to improve without a proper balance between direct voice therapy and psychotherapeutic discussion.

As a psychiatrist, Kolb (1971) wrote:

Today the interview is used by members of all the professions directly concerned with sustaining or improving mental health. All are confronted with the abnormal from time to time. All elicit information concerning personality traits and symptoms that are distressing to the patient. All, too, must conduct themselves in such a way as to establish the compassionate understanding of the problem revealed to them by the person being interviewed.

Speech-language pathologists who treat patients with voice disorders require interviewing and counseling skills to aid them in determining the presence of emotional factors and the extent to which they are instrumental in causing or perpetuating voice disorders. They must recognize patients who are in need of professional psychodiagnostic and psychotherapeutic help when their emotional problems overshadow their voice disorders or when the emotional aspect needs to be managed before the voice disorder can be treated. If the speech-language pathologist has neither the skills to bring out the voice patient's troubles nor enough knowledge to recognize serious emotional illness, a disservice is done to the patient. Stated here clearly and unequivocally, we are not advising that speech-language pathologists conduct psychotherapy but rather that they obtain background information to identify etiology and to relieve acute psychologic distress by providing psychologic support. Its purpose is the etiologic differential diagnosis of the voice disorder and the identification and referral of voice patients to psychiatrists, psychologists, and other mental health specialists.

In a study by Butcher, Elias, Raven, et al (1987), an attempt was made to determine the value of the speech-language pathologist functioning as a psychotherapist in collaboration with the clinical psychologist for patients who were unable to respond to direct voice therapy alone. The authors concluded that psychotherapy as a treatment for psychogenic voice disorders was able to achieve a 50% success rate in patients for whom voice therapy alone had been unsuccessful, and that a psychotherapeutic model for patients with psychogenic voice disorders with the speech-language pathologist and the psychologist working as cotherapists was highly workable in treating psychogenic voice disorders that had not responded to traditional approaches. They discovered that speech pathologists using psychotherapeutic techniques with patients who had psychogenic voice disorders achieved in their patients improved voice *and* positive psychologic changes.

After discovering a considerable divergence of training, attitudes, and practice in the treatment of patients with psychogenic voice disorders in the United Kingdom, Elias, Raven, Butcher, et al (1989) surveyed 244 practicing speech clinicians to determine their current opinions and practices in the diagnosis and treatment of psychogenic voice disorders and whether or not they thought they were properly educated to deal effectively with this population. In their survey, they paid particular attention to preparation in psychology and psychiatry and their experiences in relating to these professions within the framework of voice disorders. What they found was that:

♦ About 75% of speech clinicians surveyed said they always treated psychogenic dysphonia or aphonia when patients were referred to them.

♦ Asked how confident they were in their understanding and treatment of these disorders, 4% said they always were, 58% that they usually were, 33% said some of the time, and 5% said never.

♦ About 75% of the clinicians said that their patients usually improved.

♦ A variety of treatment techniques were used by the speech-language pathologist population surveyed, the main ones being relaxation, voice exercises, and counseling. A minority of clinicians used a diversity of psychologic techniques.

♦ The clinicians expressed the opinion that they could expect more improvement from psychogenic dysphonic patients than from aphonic ones.

♦ Although voice exercises, breathing, and relaxation methods were taught at the undergraduate level, psychologic techniques were more likely to have been learned subsequently. The observation that counseling was much more freely advocated than taught corresponded with comments that it was important and not as extensively taught as needed. About 70% would still welcome further training in the treatment of voice disorders from a clinically involved psychologist or psychiatrist, and several respondents believed that more graduate courses ought to be available than there are at present.

♦ More than 75% of the respondents considered their undergraduate course in psychology and psychiatry as "mainly theoretical."

♦ Only 15% rated their psychology lectures as related to their voice disorders lectures; the remainder were equally divided between those who perceived little relationship and none at all.

♦ Referral of patients with psychogenic voice disorders to a psychologist or psychiatrist was practiced by 74% of the respondents, of whom 42% felt uncertain as to when to refer. More than 75% would have liked better access to a psychologist or psychiatrist but indicated that a barrier to cooperation with these professions was the mental health professionals' limited interest in voice disorders; in our experience, lack of knowledge of the field of voice disorders.

Based on their survey, the authors concluded that there is no reason to dispute the textbook advice that patients with psychogenic aphonia and dysphonia should be treated by speech-language pathologists and that improvement usually follows. They expressed their support for the concept that therapy for psychogenic voice disorders should not be addressed solely to the voice itself, quoting Greene (1972):

Recovery of voice, however, is not the sole aim of treatment. Therapy must aim at removing or alleviating the cause and obtaining better adjustment of the patient to his difficulties by gaining some insight into the connection between the voice symptom and the precipitating factors.

In their discussion of the results of this survey, the authors concluded:

It is, therefore, important that any speech therapist[1] treating psychogenic voice disorders, which are not uncommon, should have psychological skills, and a clear idea when cooperation with, or referral to, a different specialist would be the best course. In this context, it is disappointing that education in psychology and psychiatry is perceived as remote from everyday practice. Moreover, many speech therapists have found it necessary to acquire important psychological skills after qualification.

The education of speech therapists should always incorporate counseling and other relevant psychological skills. These are already taught in some centres. This would provide a welcome application of the theory and an appropriate preparation for current practice. Speech therapists should be prepared before qualification for undertaking joint therapy with a psychologist or psychiatrist, since this is not a rare undertaking when there is an interested person available. Post-qualification courses are essential to enable therapists already in practice to acquire the psychological skills they have found they require.

It is difficult to convince most people how deeply voice disorders strike at the heart of the patient's total existence and how special voice is in the average person's emotional and intellectual life. Always impressive is how chronic voice disorders can unhinge even the most stable personality. The following letter was written by a college professor who had undergone recurrent laryngeal nerve resection for adductor spasmodic dysphonia. She was having intermittent difficulties during the postsurgical voice-stabilization period and wrote the following letter to a fellow patient with similar voice-adjustment problems. The letter is illustrative of not only the impact of the voice disorder on the patient but also of the critical nature of the support from her speech-language pathologist.

Case Study 9.1

I was reliving a night ~15 months after my surgery when I read of your recent frustrations. I had been getting along beautifully off and on but then I had about 4 or 5 days in succession when my voice sounded like a scratchy whisper. I just knew that the worst possible was happening—that my remaining vocal cord was giving out and that I would become voiceless. I was actually crying one night at 9:00 PM, filled with fear, and the phone rang. My husband

---

[1]*In the United Kingdom,* speech therapist *is the official term for* speech-language pathologist.

answered. The call was for me. It was the speech pathologist calling to check how I was getting along. Can you imagine getting a call at that hour? Well, I poured out my fears to him and a very noticeable softness and quietness became evident in his voice. He told me that he had never heard of anyone losing the use of the second vocal cord. In that quiet voice that sounded as if he were suffering with me because of my fears, he gave me a great amount of strength by telling me not to worry about it—that he didn't know why I was experiencing what I was going through but that he felt sure that within a short time my voice would be back to what it had been in the weeks before this very frightening period. The assurance, the calming effect, the knowing that he was concerned about me after so long a time was the best medicine that I could have had. And do you know what? The very next morning my voice was back! I can't explain it. Unless the horrible fear of truly losing the ability to speak caused the voice to be worse than it really needed to be.

I think we must both be concerned too much with how we sound to others. Even yet I am very self-conscious of how I sound to others much of the time. I am getting better. Sometimes I actually forget about my voice quality, but most of the time I hear my voice as something less than what I would desire if I had a chance. But I am so thankful for what I have that I don't know why I can't do as you suggest—talk as I do with what I have and forget about what people think about it.

My voice has been strong for the most part during the Christmas holidays. But today it is thick, as though there is a fog within me. I dreaded answering the phone a while ago. Frustrating. I don't know why our voices fluctuate so. Frankly, I do not believe that you should quit your job. You see, since I teach, I have 3 months in the summer when I don't teach. My voice has the same periods of fluctuation then as it has when I teach. I think life itself causes our bodies to change. For a normally healthy person without the voice problem that we have, these changes are not evident as they are in us. And in the summer when I am not working and under no stress and strain, I will have my days of bad voice. On my bad days my voice sounds thick, sort of gravelly, and has very little volume. When I try increasing the volume, some of my sounds come out as air instead of audible sounds. Frustrating? I can't tell you how very much. And of course that just makes it all the worse. But why wouldn't I be frustrated when I am lecturing to college students and my voice comes out in a stupid-sounding way. But the point is that it happens on weekends, in the summer, during Christmas vacation, etc.

Does your voice carry in a large supermarket? Does your voice perform normally in any large area? Mine doesn't. I need walls for the voice to bounce off of, it seems. My voice is always much better in a small room. Nearly all my classes are conducted in rooms that can accommodate 30 people. When I teach in a larger room, I have to work harder. However, I found out just very recently that even when my voice seemingly has very little volume, it has something that causes it to "carry" much better than one would have reason to hope for. But in a noisy large area such as a supermarket, a listener has to come quite close

to me to hear what it is I am saying. And I have a lot of trouble talking to the supermarket clerk when I am being checked out. When they talk to me and ask me something, I answer, but they have problems hearing me. I feel very embarrassed, hurt, and frustrated at such times.

Now, after all that complaining, I must quickly say that I am so thankful for having had the surgery, for having the ability to talk without that horrible strain that I had prior to surgery, for being able to function well enough to be able to keep my teaching job. It still is the best thing that ever happened to me.

The reasons that the speech-language pathologist needs to be trained in psychologic interviewing and counseling are the following:

♦ The high incidence of psychologic causes and effects of voice disorders requires that these etiologic factors be investigated so that they can be understood and dealt with.

♦ Improvement or even disappearance of the voice disorder is common during the patient's disclosure of interpersonal problems causing the disorder.

♦ Parceling out the patient with a voice disorder to psychologic personnel to obtain basic personal examination data and to manage less critical emotional problems is often impractical.

♦ Patients who have psychogenic voice disorders may relate better to a psychologically oriented speech-language pathologist (who is not officially defined as a mental health specialist) during the initial phases of evaluation and therapy than to a psychiatrist or psychologist, because some voice patients tend to reject such referrals. The speech-language pathologist can lead the patient into areas of psychologic sensitivity and gradually educate the patient about the need for professional counseling. Such an approach has salvaged many a patient who otherwise would have become offended and who would have rejected premature referral to mental health personnel.

♦ Many voice disorders are caused by mild, transient interpersonal problems and not by deeply embedded conflicts or life-long psychoneuroses. These patients are not a danger to themselves or to others. They can be safely and conveniently managed by the speech-language pathologist trained in psychologic interviewing and counseling.

♦ In clinics in which speech-language pathologists have easy access to laryngologists, psychiatrists, and psychologists, the risk of encountering trouble dealing with critical emotional problems of voice patients is practically eliminated.

♦ The interviewing and counseling skills learned by speech-language pathologists increase their own self-understanding and their understanding of others. It teaches them how to ask questions and how to deal effectively with people in trouble.

- Mental health professionals often have a full patient load and patients have difficulty being seen immediately, delaying treatment and return of their voices.

Characteristics of a Successful Interviewer

The most important ingredient in successful interviewing and counseling is the speech-language pathologist as a person. Clinicians who communicate best with people who have problems possess the following traits:

- *Their orientation to life and to others is one of equanimity and acceptance.* Voice patients come from all cultural, educational, and economic backgrounds, talk differently, look different, and harbor beliefs and habits of unimaginable varieties, many contrary to the clinician's. If one is by nature hypercritical, judgmental, prejudiced, or threatened by such behaviors, although not verbally disapproving, these attitudes will nevertheless be communicated in other ways. Consequently, clinicians must learn to accept patients' habits, ideas, and lifestyles as belonging to them, separate from their own, and they must deal with patients within a framework of the patient's life orientation.

- *They respond to personal information with understanding and encouragement.* Clinicians must provide an atmosphere in which the patients perceives that the clinician is very much interested and concerned about them.

- *They know how to ask questions.* The speech-language pathologist must learn to ask open-ended questions that will encourage the patient to free-associate. "Tell me about your family, your work, your relationships." The clinician should interrupt only when the patient seriously strays off the track or skirts personal data, reciting names, dates, and places, thereby avoiding disclosure of personal information. The clinician's objective is to elicit how the patient *feels* and not just a recitation of events.

- *They know how to listen.* Clinicians must learn to become attentive listeners and to refrain from giving advice. This rule has exceptions, but in general speech-language pathologists want to help patients solve their own problems by allowing them to rely on their own resources.

- *They are perceived as sympathetic and trustworthy.* As such, patients will find it easier to confide in clinicians. To witness the superficial, defensive, organ-oriented patient give up facades and become more human, reacting on a more personal level, using more personal language, is a satisfying accomplishment. Tears well up in their eyes. They will apologize for losing emotional control; the clinician reassures them that it is proper and desirable for them to express themselves. Full expression of emotion in interviewing and counseling for voice disorders is tension relieving. Such an abreaction has untold clinical impor-

tance. During such release, psychogenic voice disorders, or organic disorders with psychogenic components, often disappear, convincing clinician and patient alike that the voice problem was wholly or in part related to unexpressed conflict and emotions, a point the patient often resists up until such breakthrough. With emotional release, patients suddenly find themselves freed to discuss situations openly that they have been suppressing. The speech-language pathologist is often the *first and only person* to whom they have disclosed this private information, and they feel a tremendous relief for having done so. What often begins as a "voice disorder" ends as a sign/symptom of a larger interpersonal conflict that demands a solution; the voice disorder was only the "tip of the iceberg." Clinicians must recognize and accept that many voice disorders are unconscious substitute solutions for patients who cannot solve larger problems. The speech-language pathologist's job in such cases is to help the patient recognize that the voice is only a surface sign and that they need to face and solve embedded problems before a normal voice can be attainable. Many voice disorders occur because of interpersonal conflicts in which the patient has suffered an injustice for which that person has not had his or her "day in court." To have one's "day in court" is to be able to express one's need for justice, something these patients have been unable to do verbally.

- *They are willing to set aside adequate time for the psychologic aspects of the examination and therapy.* Psychologic interviewing and counseling take time. No matter how knowledgeable or skilled the clinician, if a special block of time is not set aside for leisurely discussion, then rarely will the patient open up. Rushing the examination is antithetical to good interviewing and counseling.

The following scenario is not unusual in the life of the speech-language pathologist specialist in voice disorders:

It is 3:30 in the afternoon on a Friday. One ought not to be distracted by thoughts of the coming weekend's diversions, but one is, nevertheless. This is the last patient of the day, and I wish for something simple. The history is as follows. The patient was referred to me by an otolaryngologist. She had been referred to him by her internist because of dysphonia and throat pain. Her general health was good. Her main reason for coming to the clinic was back pain, neck pain, and hoarseness. She feared cancer. For her low back pain, she had seen a physiatrist, who had prescribed relaxation exercises and who told her to lose weight. No etiology of her pain had been formulated along the way, and she was being treated symptomatically.

The laryngologist found her larynx to be clean—not a shred of evidence of a structural lesion or paralysis, and he reassured her that she did not have laryngeal cancer. She had pain and tenderness, especially on the right side of her neck just beneath the angle of her mandible level with the hyoid bone, and the area was sensitive to pressure. The laryngologist injected lidocaine into the region, which numbed the pain temporarily, but her dysphonia remained. He then sent her for evaluation and treatment of her voice disorder.

She was a neatly dressed, ruddy-faced woman of 56 from Saskatchewan where she and her husband farmed, apparently prosperously. This was her second marriage and had lasted 15 years. There were no children. She described the marriage as happy, and she denied life problems associated with her voice disorder. Gradually, 3 years ago, she became aware of both tightness in her throat and episodes of hoarseness, which became chronic. The throat pain began during her dysphonia.

On examination, her voice was hoarse and strained, resembling adductor spasmodic dysphonia, except that the hoarseness did not fluctuate; it was continuous. It did not have quite the proper spectrum for spasmodic dysphonia. Her entire neck musculature felt rock stiff to the touch, and she winced and withdrew when I touched her neck just below the angle of the mandible.

Did she abuse her voice, I asked? How much, and under what circumstances? Not very much, she shrugged. Once in a while she would shout across a field to her husband, but she was not a talker. I wondered if she felt isolated living on such a large farm with few neighbors. But, she claimed she was content.

The discussion fell off into silence. She gazed at the wall and frowned. "Come to think of it," she said, "I have had to raise my voice in talking to my husband. He seems to be getting hard of hearing. It's irritating. I say something and he asks me to repeat it; it gets tiring. No, he has never had his hearing tested." We talked about the possibility that voice strain and general muscular tension might have been brought on by her having to speak in this way to her hard-of-hearing husband. I encouraged her to get her husband to see an otologist to determine the cause and treatment of his hearing loss.

By now it was 4:30 PM and I was hoping for an ending to this evaluation. But I felt irritated with myself as I lifted half off the chair to extend my hand to say goodbye. The next words came as if from some other jurisdiction in my head. I dropped back into my chair. "There's one more question I'd like to ask, if you'll permit me. How is your sexual relationship with your husband?" For the first time in over an hour, she looked me dead in the eyes. There was an excruciatingly long period of silence. Then she turned her head so that I could not see her face. She turned back, eyes closed, head down. A tear rolled down each cheek and cascaded onto her lap. She was choked up and could not speak but answered with a negative shake of her head. When she regained her composure, she explained that during the past few years her husband's sexual interest had declined to nearly complete inactivity. Until then, their relationship had been good. Then she found that she would have to initiate any relations, and most of the time he would decline, saying that he was too tired or wouldn't be able to perform. "How did you feel about this?" I asked. Tears again welled up in her eyes, and she said that she guessed she'd have to accept the situation, but hadn't quite anticipated such an early sexual demise. She said that she felt guilty for having brought up the subject because she loved her husband and, with that, she cried bitterly. We talked about her husband for a while, that he was only 58, still relatively young. Perhaps, she thought, his growing obesity might have something to do with his declining libido.

By 5:15 PM, at least 50% of her hoarseness had disappeared. We talked about marital counseling, and she was certain that their family doctor could help them find a counselor closer to home. We both sat in wonder at how the larynx and voice react to pent-up emotions and how the throat pain came from the suppression of crying. As she left, she thanked me for bringing her problem into the open: "Nobody else ever had," she said.

♦ *They are patient and persistent.* We have noted the tendency for patients with voice disorders to deny emotional problems. Because patients skirt main issues, which they are either unconscious of or unwilling to divulge, the clinician must be prepared to wait and must not be afraid to press ahead for information when he or she feels that information being obtained is sterile and that he or she detects something beneath the surface that the patient is concealing. With patients who have voice disorders, the completely nondirective approach is not quite the right one. The optimum falls somewhere between the directive and the nondirective.

♦ *They are authentic.* Many professionals have the idea that professionalism is equated with formality, rigidity, and even coldness. They entrench themselves behind their desks. Their posture, the architecture of the room, and harsh lighting restrict verbal and emotional intimacy. The clinician should get out from behind the desk; sit closer to the patient; look the patient in the eyes. It is important to try to feel what the patient is feeling; one should not be afraid to agonize with the patient. If the clinician has had lifelong difficulty expressing emotions, he or she is going to have difficulty doing so with patients. The world is cold and impersonal, and people do not display their feelings easily. It is rare for patients to meet someone who behaves humanly. They are grateful for it.

♦ *They are honest.* Patients respect professionals. Sometimes, clinicians think patients imbue them with more knowledge than they deserve. There is a dangerous temptation for the clinician to erect a facade of superiority and authority. Patients ask many questions about the causes of and therapy for their voice disorders. Could it be caused by this pollution, that postnasal drip, or an unfriendly magnetic field that surrounds them, some incident that happened years ago? At such times, there is a temptation to appear more knowledgeable than reality justifies. If clinicians do not know, they should say so. Patients have to learn to accept the clinician's fallibility as well as their own. Nonetheless, clinicians are being consulted for their knowledge and, therefore, should communicate technical information as clearly and efficiently as possible. For this reason, thorough knowledge of voice disorders *and related fields* is imperative. Speech-language pathologists must be as well read as possible, and if they do not know the answers to certain questions, they should find out for themselves and for their patients.

♦ *They help the patient to form his or her own conclusions.* When it comes to helping patients realize the relationship between a psychogenic voice disorder and events in their lives, clinicians must encourage patients to speculate whether there might be such a connection, and clinicians must not make interpretations for them. People who arrive at their own conclusions believe them more firmly than if they are told. The process is called *insight*. It is a coming together, a gestalt, a realization of the interconnection among things.

◆ Stages of Personality Growth in Patients with Psychogenic Voice Disorders

A patient with voice disorders of primarily psychogenic origin is experiencing a failure to express his or her *self*. Clinicians must help that person learn a greater freedom of verbal self-expression. There is no magic to this kind of therapy. It is nothing more or less than giving the patient encouragement to achieve what he or she has wished for many years: to express the self at any level with a feeling of freedom. The pioneering originator of client-centered psychotherapy, Carl Rogers (1961), has analyzed the process of change from lesser to greater communication with the self and the outside world as a result of psychotherapy.

The process is one of change from *fixedness* to *flowingness:*

Stage I

- ◆ unwillingness to communicate with the self
- ◆ feelings and personal meanings neither recognized nor owned
- ◆ rigid personal constructs. Communicative relationships construed as dangerous
- ◆ no problems recognized by the patient
- ◆ no desire for change
- ◆ considerable blockage of internal communication

Stage II

- ◆ Expression begins to flow on the subject of non-self topics.
- ◆ The patient perceives problems as being external to the self.
- ◆ There is no sense of personal responsibility for those problems.
- ◆ Language indicates that patient does not "own" ideas expressed, and he does so in the past.
- ◆ Feelings expressed are unrecognized and unowned.
- ◆ Experience is bound by the structure of the past.
- ◆ Contradictions are expressed with little recognition by the patient that they are contradictions.

Stage III

- ◆ freer flow of expression about the self as an object

Stage IV

- ◆ expresses more intensive feelings
- ◆ greater expression of feelings in the present tense
- ◆ loosening of the matter with which experience is intertwined
- ◆ greater feeling of self-responsibility for problems

◆ Common Psychopathology in Patients with Voice Disorders

Patients who have voice disorders are often in need of help because of psychopathology either related or unrelated to their voice disorders. Recognition and referral for psychiatric consultation may or may not be productive. The following material has been abstracted from *The Psychiatric Interview in Clinical Practice* by MacKinnon and Michels (1971), which is strongly recommended reading.

Psychopathology is concerned with emotional disorders—neuroses and psychoses. Behavior and character disorders are included; they interfere with the patient's ability to function properly at home, at play, at work, and in affectional relationships.

The distinction between neurotic and character traits is that neuroses consist of compromises between repressed wishes and unconscious fears in which the individual is trying to deal not only with the real world but also with inner anxieties. The neurotic is aware of something foreign in his or her makeup and wishes to be free of it, whether depression, anxiety, phobias, obsessions, compulsions, or conversion reactions. Character traits, on the other hand, are more basic to the individual's personality, and the individual feels relatively comfortable with them. Nevertheless, such people may be irresponsible, impulsive, aggressive, and mistrustful. The following are common clinical syndromes found in patients with voice disorders.

The Obsessive Patient

The main character traits of the obsessive personality are punctuality, conscientiousness, tidiness, orderliness, and reliability, stemming from a fear of violating the rules of social conduct. Parsimony with time and money is characteristic, as is exaggerated concern about proper social codes and competitiveness. Intellect is used to avoid confrontation with the emotions; the obsessive is a cerebral individual. Vocabulary and theoretical constructs are highly developed, and the language used in communicating with others is often confusing rather than clarifying. An overreliance on detail often masks the major point of the commentary.

The interview is characterized by a tendency for the obsessive to control the interviewer and the interviewing situation to avoid the expression of deeper feelings. Definitions, terminology, and other intellectual aspects of behavior are chosen by the patient for discussion rather than underlying feelings and emotions. Sometimes the obsessive overcontrols the interview to such an extent that the roles of interviewer and interviewee appear reversed. To avoid disclosure of underlying feelings, the patient may show characteristic speech patterns, particularly in the voice. Loudness may be low or speech articulated so poorly that the interviewer will not be able to hear what the patient is saying. Silence often occurs; it is another technique used to avoid emotional contact.

The Hysterical Patient

The hysterical personality is warm, imaginative, charming, and exuberant. Such patients are often attractive physically, as well as in personality. Verbal communication is characterized by the expression of inner feelings of emotion in relating experiences. Exaggeration is a common quality of their language. Overdramatization is at the core of their communications.

The reason that these traits are considered pathologic is that they are superficial, and the patient is often devoid of any real feeling of affection, love, or intimacy. Although in outward appearance the patient may seem at ease and confident, beneath may lie anxiety and insecurity. Female hysterics are often seductive and are possibly a trap for the male clinician, but the purpose of this behavior is to obtain approval and admiration rather than sexual intimacy. Helplessness and dependency may pervade the clinical relationship, with the patient attempting to maintain a childlike relationship with the clinician.

In contrast with the obsessive patient, the hysteric lacks orderliness and punctuality. Ordinary daily tasks are boring and avoided. Thinking is impulsive and intuitive. Commonly, there are marital or sexual problems because of the fear of emotional expression. Apropos to voice disorders, patients with hysterical personalities frequently develop conversion voice disorders as well as other somatic complaints.

Although interviewing hysterical patients is often personally and socially pleasant, such patients can produce sterile interview results because of their inability to discuss deeper feelings. Overdramatization and role-playing become irritating to the clinician attempting to get beneath the surface. The language of the hysteric impedes communication of the true self, as does the obsessive's overintellectualization. In the hysteric, the language is different, however; it is one of overdramatization, exaggeration, and distortion. The clinician gets the uneasy feeling of a lack of congruence between the patient's language and what the patient is actually feeling or the facts the patient is disclosing about his or her background and experience.

The Depressive Patient

Sadness, helplessness, and reduced self-esteem are mild signs of depression with which all humans must contend. Clinically depressed patients lose interest in life, however, and have diminished appetite and little enthusiasm for the general pleasures of life. Such people are preoccupied with themselves, ruminating about the past. Anxiety can be part of the syndrome, and so can anger. Overall, the depressed patient is slow of thought and movement, is preoccupied with bodily complaints and health, has difficulty in sleeping, awakens early, is fatigued, and often has changes in appetite.

Although many depressions stem from lifelong family pathologic conditions, others are considered constitutional or biologic. Many individuals become depressed over the loss of friends or relatives through death or separation. Paradoxically, certain people become depressed after promotion or other forms of recognition that threaten to expose incompetence, either real or imagined, or because success is equated with hostile aggression.

Patients with voice disorders are usually depressed. It is either a cause of the voice disorder or a result of the voice disorder's interfering with their enjoyment of life. If the depression is the effect of the voice disorder, voice improvement often resolves the depression. Otherwise, psychiatric consultation and therapy are necessary. Often, patients with voice disorders are depressed because they are under the misconception that they have "caused" the disorder. Their depression is often alleviated when they are reassured that such is not the case; clinicians have an important educational function in this regard. In addition, the hope that can be generated from voice therapy, as well as the encouragement of the speech pathologist, can contribute considerably to the alleviation of depression. Information and reassurance go a long way in helping the patient with a voice disorder to attain a happier frame of mind.

Which of the above mentioned personality types do you recognize in the following histories?

Case Study 9.2

A 30-year-old mother of three children has been under stress from several sources: She works at a supermarket full-time to supplement the family income while having to maintain her household. She is dominated by her mother, who is hypercritical of how the patient manages her life. The patient and her husband disagree on many matters, and communication between the two is very poor because both have emotional problems. She has had several previous episodes of aphonia and dysphonia, but on interview her voice is nearly normal. Laryngologic examination was normal.

Clinician (C): Your voice sounds fairly normal to me. Is this the problem that you came to the clinic for?

Patient (P): Well, I've had trouble off and on for about the last 2 years.

C: Do you actually lose your voice completely so that you have to whisper?

P: Back on the 18th of September, I could hardly get it up at all. I felt as if I was dragging everything right on out. But usually it is mostly a whisper.

C: What is the longest period of time that you have lost it?

P: Well, I wouldn't say that I've completely lost it, except for this last time on the 18th of September. But it's always been hoarse, almost gone.

C: How long a period of time had you lost it starting with the 18th of September?

P: Well, it sounded like I had laryngitis for about a week before. And then it just left.

C: Did you go around whispering then?

P: Well (laughs), I could hardly do even that. I mean, I felt like I was pulling everything right on out. My husband called the doctor and he gave me some medicine. It took ~24 hours before it took hold.

C: And did you lose it again?

P: It got hoarse, but I never lost it again.

C: Then why did you come here?

P: My doctor sent me here to see this guy (laryngologist) that looked down my throat, and he referred me to you.

C: Did anything happen on or about September 18th that might have upset you?

P: I wouldn't say it's any one thing. I can go back several years. I work, and I was hired to work 3 days a week. Well it so happens that I think the first time it happened was when I got left alone—we usually have three girls working—and I handled the whole burden plus three children at home, housework. Ever since then I have been carrying more of a load. They've been quitting, coming and going, and now we've been one gal short since the last of March, and this hoarseness has been pretty steady since then. So I think it's an emotional thing.

C: Why do you say it's emotional?

P: Well, I think it's my nerves because I'm trying to do too much. You know, putting in 5 days a week, 8 and a half hours a day, plus taking care of a home, children.

C: As you tell this to me, you seem to be on the verge of crying. (Mention of this brings tears to the patient's eyes.)

P: Nerves. (Smiling, holding back tears.)

C: How about people who are close to you at home and at work? Are you having any problems with any one individual?

P: Hmmm. Not now, not since this one gal quit. She wanted a job. She had to have a job to get out of the house because she was tending to be an alcoholic, but she didn't really want to work and I was more-or-less carrying her load and my load both. Well, she was getting on my nerves. Other than that, I don't know. My kids get on my nerves.

C: How about your husband? (Note at this point her unawareness or her unwillingness to divulge the problem of her husband as a major source of her unhappiness and how it comes to the surface later in the interview.)

P: Very seldom.

C: How about your relatives?

P: (Laughs) My mother.

C: What about your mother?

P: (Patient gives a long sigh.) Well, oh, she keeps trying to run our lives, I guess telling me what to do and what I shouldn't do, sometimes running me down.

C: How does she try to run your lives?

P: Well, I don't know. Since we've been first married, well, I don't know, she says my husband hasn't got a good enough job, or I don't call her often enough. She has never approved of the doctor we go to, and (long sigh) she's started in on the dentist I go to, and I don't know, I never keep my house clean enough. She seems to think I am not strict enough with the kids, training them, you know, to say "thank you" or "please." I don't know, it's a lot of

things in general (close to tears again). I guess I let too many people bother me, I think.

C: What else?

P: Gee, I don't know. I don't know if there is anything else. My husband and I are perfectly happy, we don't have very many arguments. I know we don't see eye-to-eye on a lot of things.

C: Like what?

P: But I try not to contradict him, I let him have his own way.

C: What kinds of things don't you see eye-to-eye on?

P: Politics, a few things at church (laughs, long pause). We-l-l-l (word prolonged), we've been rivals through high school (becoming mildly indignant). Now, this is a silly thing. Every year at this time (becomes more tearful, voice beginning to quaver), he runs down my school, talks up his, every time sports start—especially basketball (laughs).

C: Does he do it good-naturedly, or does he do it maliciously?

P: Well, I'm always wrong. No matter what I say, he runs it down.

C: Everything you say?

P: Other things, too.

C: So, there is some problem between you and your husband.

P: Hmmmmm. I suppose you could say that. Let him have his way. Don't argue with him. What's there to do? Instead of causing an argument, I keep my mouth shut.

C: Has this been going on since you were married? Or has it been more recently?

P: Well, I don't know. When he used to listen to his ball games, I used to walk out of the house. He used to get on my nerves.

C: Why?

P: I don't know. He sits there telling me all of the faults of what they are doing or what they should have done, and it doesn't interest me. And if I tell him I don't want to hear about it, well, then he gets mad. I mean, if there are times when I want to talk to him, if the sports news is on or a political thing or something (closer to tears) he wants to watch, I've got to keep my mouth shut, but if there is something I want on and he wants to talk, I've got to sit there and listen or he gets mad.

C: Is he a short-tempered person?

P: I am. I don't know, he is calmer (crying now). But it seems like he's got to have more of his way. Not really his way, I don't know just how to put it. If he wants help with something, you just have to jump to it right away or else he gets mad. When I do things, I just go ahead and do it. I don't stop and ask whether I should do it this way or do it that way or do it all. But, with him he's got to discuss every little detail. If he should do it or how it should be done. So often he's got to have help with everything.

C: Is he a perfectionistic person? It sounds as if he wants things to be done just so.

P: I'm more that way. I don't know, maybe it comes down to money problems. We don't really have money problems. But to him it's a mighty big thing. At times I just like to go out and have a good time, go to a dance. But he doesn't dance. If I want to take the girls to a show, I do it myself. He'd rather sit home and watch those damn ball games. (Cries bitterly.) It seems that I can't say anything. I can't express my point of view. Because I'm never right. I mean, when it comes down to politics, well, he'll say, "Vote this way. There is no sense in voting against me. That will only cancel both our votes." I just don't know what it is. Like, coming here today, he says the only thing my doctor sent me over for was to see whether there was something wrong with my throat. He says, "How many times are you going to come back here, run up a big bill?" He says, "This is it, this is the last time. You can't be chasing back and forth." There he's telling me again (extremely angry) and, as far as I'm concerned, I want to get down to the bottom of it, to find out why I'm losing my voice. (Breaks down again.) And I don't care how much money it costs! (Long pause while patient composes herself.)

C: How long have you been married?

P: Oh, a little over 11 years.

C: How do you basically feel about your husband?

P: Oh, I love him. He is a good man. I don't know, maybe the thing that bothers me the most is he's too much of a perfectionist on how the house should be run. I know his own mother told me she was glad to get rid of him, because she could sweep the floor and he'd go right after her and sweep it again. This thing about having the house being just so, so often he'll refer to back to being in the Army. I have to hang the shirts on the hangers all one way, all facing one way. The roll of toilet paper even has to be on one way. Even with the girls, if they don't make their beds just right, he threatens them. He says that he'll come up there and rip them all apart and start'em all over. He says, "That's what they do to you in the Army." So, I don't know if it's got to do with that or what. (Long pause.) But, I didn't think it was any of this that was causing my trouble, I figured I was just working too many hours trying to be a good guy, trying to fill in until they got somebody hired but I just keep getting further and further behind in my housework, and this bothers me, too.

Patients with psychogenic voice disorders are referred to speech-language pathologists who practice in hospitals as well as in clinics.

Case Study 9.3

The following experience concerns a young woman from a South American country who came to the United States for surgery unrelated to the larynx. She had had endotracheal anesthesia and awoke with a severely breathy dysphonia. The laryngologist wrote:

> "She gets a good glottic closure and has a normal voice at times. Should be a functional [sic] dysphonia. Get speech pathology to see her."

The door to the hospital examination room opened, and a nurse escorted the patient into the room and then disappeared.

The patient collapsed into the chair opposite mine and then jackknifed forward, her head falling into my lap. She burst into great sobs, through which she managed to blurt out, "Oh, doctor, doctor, my family, they are driving me crazy!" Her sobbing subsided, replaced by great sniffling noises. Then she was quiet and finally sat up in her chair. I withdrew a clean handkerchief into which she noisily blew her nose, then smiled. Her eyes, although wet and red, were large and dark, and her skin had a reddish hue. Her lips were full, red, and etched in a cupid's bow. When she smiled, her teeth shone in white contrast against her dark skin. She spoke again, "I'm sorry, doctor, for having troubled you like this." Her English was excellent, delicately graced with a Portuguese accent. Her voice was severely breathy bordering on aphonia, but it retained the faint outlines of pitch and inflectional changes, which gave her voice expression. Her cough was sharp, giving evidence of her fundamentally sound larynx. What did she mean, I asked, that her family was driving her crazy. Angrily, she told of how, just before I had arrived, she had a telephone call from her mother, who had reprimanded her for not telling her she was going to leave the country for surgery.

Born in Brazil, the daughter of a coffee plantation owner, the patient had been educated in a Catholic girls' school in the United States where she had met her husband, aged 38 years, 6 years older, who was also a student in the United States studying chemistry. She withdrew from her wallet a color photograph of her husband perched high upon a chestnut brown horse. He wore a red beret and an ascot and was, she said, an excellent polo player. She also showed me photographs of her two sons, 10 and 12 years old, both blond and handsome.

Then she lowered her head, and when she looked up again, tears were in her eyes. Her jaw was clenched, and her eyes were wide, and, in what seemed like mock anger, she rasped, "But, he is like so many Latin men. He makes me so angry." Then she stopped and smiled at me through her tears, her head cocked to one side, waiting for me to respond. "What do you mean?" "He treats me like a child, and he doesn't pay enough attention to me. When he comes home at night, he sits and reads the newspaper or a book and doesn't speak a word." Her lower lip bulged and set. "What else?" I asked. She paused. Her eyelids fluttered three times. She smiled sheepishly. "You'll think I'm silly." "No I won't," I insisted. A long pause. "Well, I don't like him to look at other women. You are surprised?" She smiled, and proudly flicked her head obliquely upward. "You don't understand Latin men. They all think they are great lovers and spend every minute trying to prove it. We were at this big banquet and he was sitting next to me and across from us was a girlfriend of mine, and he kept staring at her decolletage all evening!" We both laughed.

Then we talked more seriously, and she told me she had, a year ago, lost a child at birth. Then 2 weeks before her surgery, she received a phone call from her cousin that she too had lost her baby during childbirth. I tried symptomatic voice therapy but was unsuccessful. I saw her the day before she left the hospital, and except for her voice, she looked and felt well. I apologized for being unable to help her toward a more normal voice, but she reassured me that my visits, she called them "moral support," were more helpful than I could realize.

Three months later she wrote:

The first time I had a real voice was in New York, 3 days before coming home. I had a dream that night. I dreamed that I was sitting down in a drawing room with my cousin and his wife, the ones I told you had lost their second baby. I was doing all the talking, and I could listen to my own voice. I was cheerful and happy, telling them all about my visit to the United States. Suddenly I told them: "How funny. Do you know what happened to me when I heard of your baby's death? I lost my voice." As soon as I said this I woke up and knew I could speak again. I screamed, and my own voice came out! You cannot imagine how happy and delighted I was. I could not believe it. It was 7 o'clock in the morning. Since then, my voice began to come back for moments: 15 minutes, 10 minutes, half an hour. The day after the trip, which I made all by myself, I had no voice whatsoever. I felt depressed, sad, and very ill. I arrived at my home after a long flight and was excited to see my husband, children, parents; happy to be back home and to think that all I had gone through was over. After my arrival, my voice improved gradually, over a period of days. It has been 3 months since I had my operation,

and sometimes when I get upset I notice a slight sore throat and I feel that my voice begins to change. But that is all. Luckily I feel very well; strong, happy, and so mentally different from what I felt last year.

♦ Summary

- ♦ Knowledge of the principles and possession of the skills of psychologic interviewing and counseling are indispensable in the diagnosis of and therapy for voice disorders.

- ♦ Virtually all patients with voice disorders, whether organic or psychogenic, have some degree of emotional disequilibrium, either as a cause or as an effect of the voice disorder.

- ♦ Many nonorganic voice disorders diminish or disappear during discussion of life stresses responsible for those disorders.

- ♦ Sensitivity to more serious emotional illness in patients who have voice disorders can facilitate referral to proper mental health specialists.

- ♦ The speech pathologist who is most likely to succeed in providing psychologic support of the patient with a voice disorder is one who has a high degree of acceptance of self and others, is understanding, is skillful in asking questions, knows how to listen, is sympathetic and trustworthy, and is persistent.

References

Bady, S.L. (1985). The voice as a curative factor in psychotherapy. Psychoanal Rev 72, 479–490.

Butcher, P., Elias, A., Raven, R., Yeatman, J. (1987). Psychogenic voice disorders unresponsive to speech therapy. Br J Disord Commun 22, 81–92.

Elias, A., Raven, R., Butcher, P., Littlejohns, D.W. (1989). Speech therapy for psychogenic voice disorder: a survey of current practice and training. Br J Disord Commun 24, 61–76.

Green, M.C.L. (1972). *The voice and its disorders*. 3rd ed. London: Pitman Medical.

Kolb, L.C. (1971). Section one: major clinical syndromes. In R.A. MacKinnon and R. Michels (Eds.), *The psychiatric interview in clinical practice. philadelphia*, PA: W.B. Saunders, 89–360.

MacKinnon, R.A., and Michels, R. (Eds.), (1971). *The psychiatric interview in clinical practice*. Philadelphia, PA: W.B. Saunders.

Rogers, C.R. (1961). *On becoming a person*. Boston, MA: Houghton Mifflin.

Additional Reading

Butcher, P., Elias, A., Raven, R., Yeatman, J. (1987). Psychogenic voice disorders unresponsive to speech therapy. Br J Disord Commun 22:81–92. (This interesting article on the feasibility of speech clinicians administering counseling and psychotherapy to patients with psychogenic voice disorders conjointly with psychologists is an innovative and forward-looking approach to the treatment of psychogenic voice disorders.)

Hejna, R.F. (1960). *Speech disorders and nondirective therapy*. New York. Ronald Press. (Deals exclusively with the issue of counseling and psychotherapy for all communicative disorders. See especially pp. 22–25 on voice problems.)

MacKinnon, R.A., Michels, R. (1971). *The psychiatric interview in clinical practice*. Philadelphia, PA: W.B. Saunders. (A practical, basic, and eminently readable textbook on the technique of the interview. Introduces the student to psychologic interviewing and lucidly distinguishes among different psychoneurotic and personality disorders.)

Rogers, C.R. (1961). *On becoming a person*. Boston, MA: Houghton Mifflin. (This collection of the best articles and lectures by the well-known clinical psychologist provides a deeper understanding of the objectives of clinician and client in interviewing and psychotherapy.)

Chapter 10

Studies in Clinical Diagnosis

The first principle is that you must not fool yourself—and you are the easiest person to fool.

—Richard Feynman, physicist

The purpose of this chapter is to help the student develop a comprehensive grasp of the clinician-patient relationship in voice diagnosis and treatment. The clinician needs to know much more than "techniques" to successfully treat patients who have voice disorders. An understanding of the overall picture is indispensable because, although the range of voice disorder types in the human population is limited, no two individuals present their voice disorders in the same manner owing to the following variables: age and gender; duration, etiology, and severity of the voice disorder; concurrent physical illnesses; personality; premorbid and concurrent psychiatric predisposition; nationality and cultural background; education; socioeconomic level; occupation and social situation; motivation; verbal ability; genetic heritage; and insight.

Inherent, and necessary, in the traditional textbook format is that material be presented in a logical, orderly manner. Textbook knowledge is one thing; clinical thinking and action are another. In practice, the clinician becomes a detective and is required to work backward from fragments of data: in this case, the victim is the abnormal voice, and the clinician-detective must use surface auditory-perceptual and visual-perceptual signs as means of reasoning toward probable abnormal laryngeal physiology and, even further remotely, to the underlying etiology behind that physiology.

◆ Voice Clusters

Recognizing this practical necessity, the voice cluster concept was devised to help us organize our thinking about abnormal voice unknowns. The concept is based on the fact that abnormal voices have a tendency to group themselves into perceptually distinctive colonies. A voice cluster is an abstraction, or prototype—it is no single patient's voice. For example, one cluster is the husky breathy whispered–continuous group under which all breathy voices are gathered. The common anatomic denominator is that the vocal folds do not meet firmly to form a tight seal. The specific anatomic, physiologic, and etiologic reasons can be very different from patient to patient, however, and finding out the reasons will require further investigation. The point to be made is that we have to begin somewhere to categorize the sound of the voice in order to further our logical thinking about its cause. Following are eight distinctive voice clusters. After listing them, each will be discussed in detail. The clusters are:

- ◆ the husky breathy whispered–continuous group
- ◆ the strained hoarse–continuous group
- ◆ the strained hoarse voice arrest–intermittent arrhythmic group
- ◆ the strained hoarse voice arrest–intermittent rhythmic group
- ◆ the voice tremor group
- ◆ the breathy whispered–intermittent group
- ◆ the low-pitched hoarse group
- ◆ the high-pitched group

Clinical case studies for the purpose of enabling the student to apply the cluster concept will be presented. These studies have been selected as much for their unusual as for their ordinary occurrence in clinical practice. A prevalent misconception abounds that the atypical case is not worthy of attention for the very reason of its rarity; specifically, that time should be spent on the more commonly occurring voice disorders. Experienced clinicians, particularly those who have medical differential diagnostic experience, will testify as to the danger of that idea. The reason is that the least frequently seen voice problem almost always provides the clinician with the greatest chance of making a mistake. It is important to emphasize that the case studies selected here are not intended to be all-inclusive or systematic accounts of every kind of voice sign or disorder that could occur in clinical practice. Rather, the objective is to give the student a sense of the often convoluted nature of the diagnostic and decision-making process. While reading these studies, the student should keep in mind that matters are not always as they appear to be and clinicians should look for alternative, and sometimes surprising, explanations to what might have begun as a simple, straightforward diagnostic unknown. These studies can be somewhat confusing and frustrating, and this is intentional, to reflect actual practice. At selected points during each presentation, questions are asked that will encourage the student to consider alternatives in problem solving. After each case study is a discussion that contains the answers to most of the questions raised during the narrative. They can be used as bases for class discussion. Case studies and answers also can be found in other chapters of the book.

Husky Breathy Whispered Continuous Group (HBW-C)

When we hear a voice that deviates from normal, the first question asked should be "What might be happening at the vocal fold level to produce this kind of voice?" When we hear a voice that is continuously or steadily husky, breathy, or whispered, the answer is "incomplete glottic closure" (**Fig. 10.1**).

"What are the possible reasons for such incomplete approximation of the vocal folds?" One major and potentially lethal cause is a mass lesion that produces a rough or irregular surface on one or both vocal folds preventing them on closure from forming a smooth seal along the vibrating glottal margin and causing turbulent airflow that we perceive as breathiness (**Fig. 10.2**).

"What specific kinds of lesions are capable of producing such interference?" The most common are polyps, nodules, webs, and carcinomas. Glottic insufficiency from postsurgical loss of tissue, such as after cordectomy, can produce similar results, and so can loss of mass from senile bowing of the vocal folds or a sulcus vocalis.

The clinician must ask, "How do these various conditions affect the glottal margin and ability of the vocal folds to vibrate?" The more irregular the surface or the greater the opening between the vocal folds, the greater will be the breathy component. The larger the mass of the lesion, the lower the pitch, unless the lesion is sufficiently stiff that it inhibits and limits vibration to a smaller area of the vocal folds. The more heterogeneous the vibrating surface of the two vocal folds, the more irregular the vibration and hence the harsher the vocal quality. Thus, in the case of vocal nodules, cysts, or polyps, most of the surface is smooth and the vocal changes less dramatic than in the case of a voice emitted from unilateral irregular-surfaced glottic carcinoma. Similarly, a large glottic gap with total absence of closure is going to be significantly more breathy and weak, often nearly atonal, compared with a glottal gap but near closure. Thus, there are a myriad of possibilities, and clinicians are not trying to make a diagnosis from their perceptual judgments but merely to begin making hypotheses to help them ultimately discover the etiology of the problem and need for additional diagnostic tests (**Fig. 10.3**).

Whether any of these laryngeal pathologies is responsible for the breathy type of voice found within this cluster will be determined by endoscopic examination.

Assume that such examination has taken place and has failed to identify any of the lesions just described. The next question should be, "What other causes could produce a voice that falls within this cluster?" The answer is neurologic disease, which is the next major cause within the husky breathy whispered (HBW)-cluster group (**Fig. 10.4**).

"What is the reason that a neurologic lesion could produce a voice of this cluster description? Where could such lesions in the nervous system take place to produce such a voice? With which neurologic syndromes could such voice be associated?"

Neurologic lesions can prevent adduction of the vocal folds. Any interference with functioning of the tenth cranial nerve will produce unilateral or bilateral vocal fold paralysis or paresis preventing their approximation (**Fig. 10.5**).

Careful laryngologic examination will probably establish whether or not such adductor weakness has taken place.

Assume that such examination has failed to disclose paralysis. We must then entertain another possibility, that of myoneural junction disease, or myasthenia gravis, having a prominent laryngeal representation (**Fig. 10.6**).

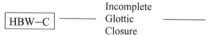

Figure 10.1 Flow chart of Husky breathy whispered continuous voice group (HBW-C) showing answer to first question of "What might be happening at the vocal fold level?"

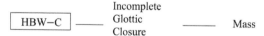

Figure 10.2 Flow chart of Husky breathy whispered continuous voice group (HBW-C) depicting second step in detecting possible causes of incomplete approximation of the vocal folds.

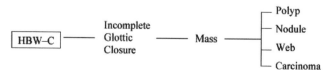

Figure 10.3 Flow chart of Husky breathy whispered continuous voice group (HBW-C) illustrating some of the myriad of possibilities of masses that could cause incomplete glottal closure.

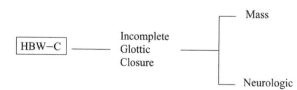

Figure 10.4 Illustration of an additional cause of Husky breathy whispered continuous voice group (HBW-C) that should be considered when by endoscopic exam the vocal folds appear normal.

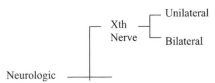

Figure 10.5 Diagram of flow chart showing one probably cause of neurologic Husky breathy whispered continuous voice group (HBW-C) is either unilateral or bilateral paralysis of the X cranial nerve.

Further neurologic examination, including motor speech examination, would be necessary to confirm or rule out this disease.

A third possibility is early parkinsonism, because breathy voice is one of its first indications. The location of the lesion is within the basal ganglia (**Fig. 10.7**).

Further possibilities are apraxia of phonation producing loss of recall for phonatory movements and frontal lobe disease producing defects of personality, motivation, and insight (**Fig. 10.8**).

The importance of a complete neurologic examination to clarify the differential diagnosis among these various possibilities is obvious. It should also be apparent that these dysphonias are classifiable under such larger categories as dysarthria, apraxia, and dementia.

The sequence of clinical diagnostic screening from organic to psychogenic causes follows a practical rationale based on three important premises: (1) It is mentally difficult to think about organic and nonorganic causes together without becoming disorganized and even confused. Thus, taking these two major categories one at a time will keep us from becoming entangled in a morass of conflicting clinical signs and symptoms. (2) The reason that organic causes are examined first is because they are potentially life-threatening. (3) It is easier to communicate with patients and inform them of nonorganic causes once we are convinced no such organic causes are present, because all patients who have discomfort and/or sensory or motor changes believe their dysfunction is organic.

At this point in our schema, let us say we have satisfied ourselves that the patient who presents with a voice of this cluster does not have any of the mass lesions or neurologic diseases suspected. "Where do we go from here in our thoughts and procedures to help explain this type of abnormal voice?" We must seriously consider that the abnormal voice is not caused by organic disease and begin to look for psychogenic, behavioral, or other medical causes such as reflux (**Fig. 10.9**).

In order to find out if psychogenic causes exist, it is mandatory that a serious, probing psychosocial history be administered. In the broadest general terms, we are looking for evidence of acute situational conflicts or chronic life stress, time-related to onset and development of the abnormal voice. Depression, anxiety, and conversion reaction are the most common effects of such stresses. They produce laryngeal musculoskeletal tension, laryngeal elevation and muscle tension pain, and *globus* (**Fig. 10.10**).

To summarize, the majority of voices that fall within the cluster under discussion can be analyzed according to the composite schema that follow in **Fig. 10.5–Fig. 10.14** and **Fig. 10.17–Fig. 10.20**.

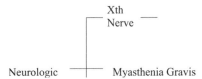

Figure 10.6 Illustration that Myasthenia Gravis is an additional possible etiology of neurologic based Husky Breathy Whispered Continuous Voice Group (HBW-C).

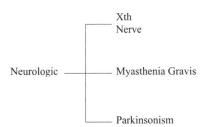

Figure 10.7 Flow chart depicting the additional neurologic causal possibility of Parkinsonism in the Husky Breathy Whispered Continuous Voice Group (HBW-C).

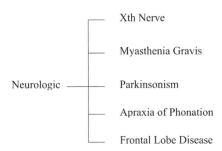

Figure 10.8 Flow chart showing common etiologies of neurologic Husky breathy whispered continuous voice group (HBW-C) that clinicians need to consider in completing voice assessment.

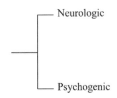

Figure 10.9 Flow chart adding psychogenic as a possible reason for incomplete approximation of the vocal folds reminding clinicians there are numerous possible causes of Husky Breathy Whispered Continuous Voice Group (HBW-C).

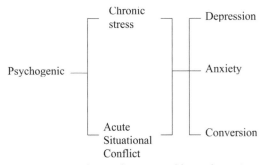

Figure 10.10 Schema of some possible psychogenic causes of Husky Breathy Whispered Continuous Voice Group (HBW-C).

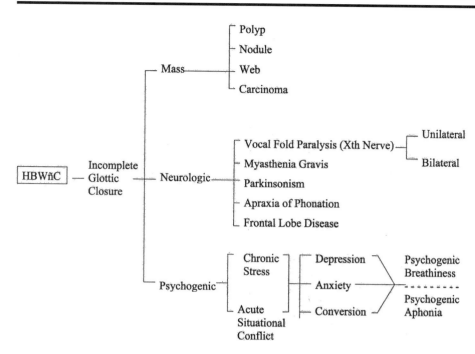

Figure 10.11 Composite schema illustrating decision making branching in determining possible causes of Husky Breathy Whispered Continuous Voice Group (HBW-C).

It is important to note that while dividing the problems into organic and nonorganic provides a functional schema that aids clinicians in systematic decision making, most patients do not fall into a purely organic or nonorganic category. Clinicians need to be mindful that chronic stress may result in esophageal reflux, muscle tension, and associated lesions. Neurologic disorders and associated dysphonias may result in secondary depression and anxiety. Part of the clinical detective work is differentiating the primary and secondary relationships in the complex problem of vocal dysphonias (**Fig. 10.11**).

The following specific case studies illustrate in detail the evolution of voice disorders requiring the kinds of procedures and reasoning heretofore discussed. After this first series of case presentations, schematic flow diagrams will be presented for the remainder of the cluster groups, although without detailed commentary as in this one, allowing the student to work out the meaning of the charts independently.

Case Study 10.1

A 40-year-old, female, unemployed high school science teacher married with three children had a normal voice until 2 years prior to examination when she underwent thyroid surgery. Upon recovering from the anesthesia, she was alarmed to discover that her voice was almost a whisper, and she would choke on liquids unless she swallowed small amounts at a time.

Q1: *What do you suspect is the etiology of her dysphonia?*

Her nurse had written that her cough sounded "mushy and weak." On laryngoscopic examination, the surgeon found a right unilateral vocal fold paralysis. He told her that it would be wise if she used her voice very carefully, whereupon he prescribed voice rest for 1 week. When she resumed talking, she found that her breathiness was as bad as or worse than before. She received no information

concerning the prognosis of her voice. The surgeon referred her for voice therapy. She was treated twice a week for 2 months and showed "considerable improvement," but she retained a degree of breathiness that left her dissatisfied. She returned to her otolaryngologist, who recommended Teflon injection, but the patient, wary of further surgery, declined.

Q2: *What is the rationale for recommending Teflon (Teflon® Dupont Company, Wilmington, DE), fat, Gelfoam (Gelfoam® Pfizer Inc., New York, NY), or collagen injections?*

The psychosocial history is normal. She describes her relationships with her husband and children as happy, and she expresses much optimism about her life, but she does become upset by her voice, particularly under noisy conditions. She wants to return to classroom teaching and knows she will not be able to do so as long as her voice is abnormal. She is dismayed that her poor voice deprives her of pleasurable social conversation. She cries frequently during the examination.

Her voice quality is moderately breathy, loudness level is reduced, and mild friction noise is heard during inhalation. She sustains the vowel /a/ with a remarkably low volume. You are startled by her ability to triple her volume on demand, during which she produces nearly normal voice. Her cough and glottal coup are normal, and she no longer has difficulty swallowing. A repeat laryngoscopic examination shows that the right vocal fold is still paralyzed.

Q3: *Explain, anatomically, why thyroid surgery should have produced a unilateral vocal fold paralysis in this patient.*

Q4: *Draw a superior view of the patient's vocal folds during phonation immediately after surgery.*

Q5: *How does your drawing explain the patient's voice signs and symptoms immediately after surgery?*

Q6: *Why was she having trouble swallowing liquids?*

Q7: *What is the explanation for the nurse's note that, immediately after surgery, her cough sounded "mushy and weak"?*

Q8: *How might you explain the fact that, on your examination, even though the right vocal fold was still paralyzed, her cough and glottal coup were normally sharp?*

Q9: *How might you explain the fact that when the patient was asked to sustain vowels loudly, her volume tripled and her voice quality became nearly normal despite the persistence of her vocal fold paralysis?*

Q10: *What information in the history gives a clue to the etiology of her persistent dysphonia?*

Q11: *Is there an alternative hypothesis as to the etiology of her persistent dysphonia?*

Q12: *From the data given, how would you proceed with therapy?*

Discussion

This patient's voice disorder teaches an important lesson about the psychologic repercussions of organic voice disorders. Here is a woman who obviously had a unilateral vocal fold paralysis after thyroidectomy, a not uncommon occurrence owing to the proximity of the thyroid gland and the recurrent laryngeal nerve. She was frightened when she awoke from the anesthesia to discover that, in effect, she could not talk normally and had problems swallowing. The emotional trauma of sudden voice deprivation in a basically healthy woman who has the responsibilities of a family and a career, both of which place a high demand on the ability to speak, may not be as well appreciated as it ought to be. Such anxiety is further heightened by the fact that no one could give her a satisfactory answer to her question as to when, or even whether, her voice would return to normal. The surgeon then places her on voice rest, which communicates to her that not using her voice is good, which must mean then that to use it is bad. The speech clinician who subsequently sees her for therapy and brings about voice improvement fails to reverse the patient's concept of guarded voice use, and she reaches a plateau in therapy that she never surmounts.

The clue to her potential for better voice should have been the discovery that the patient's cough was disproportionately sharp in contrast with her breathiness and reduced loudness. This suggests, despite the persistence of her unilateral vocal fold paralysis, there is good compensatory approximation of the normal vocal fold against the paralyzed one. This was subsequently confirmed by laryngoscopic examination. The final proof of her untapped capacity for a nearly normal voice was when she produced a loud, clear voice on demand. Her discovery that she could do this provoked in her genuine surprise; she had not been aware of her potential. What she had done, quite unconsciously, was to partially shut down her depth of respiration and force of vocal fold adduction in a misguided attempt to avoid damaging her vocal folds. Audible sound during inhalation also suggests that the

paralyzed fold was in the median or paramedian position making compensatory adduction easier.

Therapy consisted of using behavioral modification techniques to increase loudness and helping the patient divest herself of the notion that vigorous use of her voice was bad. On the contrary, the more she used it, the better her voice would become. She was given supervised practice using a much louder, clearer voice. She wrote 1 month later saying that her voice was nearly normal under most speaking conditions. She still had a unilateral vocal fold paralysis but was able to compensate with her unaffected vocal fold and better respiratory support.

Case Study 10.2

The 47-year-old wife of an American industrialist living in London, England, came to the clinic because she has been unable to find a satisfactory explanation or help for the following complaint: During the past 6 months, her voice had been getting softer. It had reached the point where people had to ask her to repeat what she was saying. She was examined by two laryngologists before coming to the clinic. One said her vocal folds were normal; the other said that the posterior region of the folds were not closing completely but could make nothing of this finding. He described her voice complaint as "functional."

She had just been reexamined by a laryngologist and, for the first time, a neurologist. Neither was able to diagnose her problem. The laryngologist wrote, "Her voice sounds pretty normal to me." The neurologist, having just completed her residency, was perplexed by the case because the complaint was confined to the patient's voice and she "didn't have much else to go on." She eventually decided that the voice complaint was "nonorganic." The referral note said, "Evaluation and therapy for functional voice disorder."

The patient was a tall, exceptionally well-groomed woman whose manner and language revealed a keen intelligence and capacity for detailed recall. She reported that she was at a cocktail party for her husband's executive friends when she first noticed she could not speak loudly enough to make herself heard over the noise. Since that occasion, more than 6 months ago, she has had several similar episodes, and within the past 3 months she's noticed it even when there was little or no extraneous noise. She stated that the problem was no longer just occasional but was "present more and more of the time."

The psychosocial history was completely unremarkable; the patient and her husband were well suited to one another. Their children were grown and successfully on their own; their daughter was an attorney for a utilities company, and their son was finishing a surgical residency. The patient admitted that when she was under the stresses of everyday life, her voice was noticeably worse.

Voice evaluation revealed that her conversational loudness level was, in fact, reduced, and her voice was mildly breathy or husky. Her cough was so near normal that you are unable to consider it anything other than that or, at most, a mild variant of normal. One thing you note is that she does not use much pitch or loudness variation. When you point this out to her she quickly agrees, because a close friend had told her just the other day that, on the phone, she sounded "flat and depressed" and had expressed concern about the patient.

Q1: *What might be the diagnostic possibilities of the voice findings obtained up to this point?*

Q2: *What is the diagnostic significance of the finding that the patient's voice is worse when she is under stress?*

You ask her to sustain the vowel /a/ as long and steadily as she can. The first time she does this, you note that her voice definitely is breathy, but you think you hear something else, a faint irregularity of some kind. On the second and third trials, you are certain that buried within the breathy quality is a rapid tremor, so subtle as to escape any but the most discriminating ear.

Q3: *What conclusions might you draw about the breathy voice quality?*

Q4: *What are the possible interpretations of the rapid tremor?*

Q5: *Why was the tremor heard only on vowel prolongation?*

On routine motor speech examination, you find that her alternate motion rate and regularity on /pʌ/, /tʌ/, /kʌ/ repetitions are normal, but here, again, you find yourself further perplexed that she does not open her lips very widely as she repeats the syllables.

Q6: *Comment on the possible significance of the lip movements just described.*

Q7: *How might this finding relate to those accumulated thus far?*

Finally, because you have been taking special note of the patient's facial expression during the latter part of the examination, you remark to yourself that it is not expressive, except when she speaks with emotional emphasis or smiles. Toward the end of the examination she volunteers, "for whatever help it might be," that her golf game has deteriorated during the same period as her voice complaint.

Q8: *What do you think are the possible causes of the patient's voice disorder?*

Q9: *What steps would you take at this point in the examination?*

Discussion

This study illustrates the importance of being sensitive to the fact that signs of neurologic syndromes in the very early stages of their evolution often appear to others as "functional," and that we are not often blessed with their full, classic clinical characteristics. Here is a diagnosis that was missed by four physicians, primarily because the patient's signs and symptoms were limited to her speech. This is common in early voice signs of neurologic disease; after all, breathiness and reduced loudness are also signs of psychogenicity. That is why as clinical detectives, we

must leave no stone unturned. We must investigate the physical, social, neurologic, psychologic, environmental, and genetic possibilities. We must look for any additional signs, which, when assembled, may form a pattern that might explain the patient's dysphonia or other chief speech complaint. The first clue we get about this patient is that her demeanor does not fit with the typical patient with psychogenic or "functional" dysphonia. Her psychosocial history was unremarkable, she was happily married and financially secure. We then learn that, in addition to her breathiness, one laryngoscopic examination showed that the interarytenoid portions of the vocal folds were not approximating completely. In addition to the breathiness, we have evidence of a loss of pitch and loudness variations. During the speech examination, she had a barely detectable, rapid voice tremor on vowel prolongation that could never have been detected during running speech owing to its mildness. The failure of her lips to make normally wide excursions on alternate motion rate for /pʌ/ now became an important finding. The information that her voice was worse under stress proved nothing either way; patients with both organic and psychogenic voice disorders report this complaint as often do speakers without voice complaints. Thus, only after putting these findings together did her lack of facial mobility take on importance.

By now it should be apparent that the suspicion of early parkinsonism has been raised. You telephone the neurologist who had last examined her and ask if you might speak with her about your findings. You tell her that the patient's voice and associated speech findings may be suggestive of early hypokinetic or parkinsonian dysarthria, which might be revealing itself primarily via her larynx. After expressing ill-disguised surprise, she thanks you and suggests that another neurologist who specializes in Parkinson's disease examine the patient. He does. His note reads: "This patient has mild masking of facies, mild rigidity of her upper extremities to passive movement, and mild reduction in arm swing and distance between her steps as she walks. This, in all probability, is early Parkinson's disease. The mildness of her signs does not warrant any treatment at this time. The patient should be scheduled for reexamination in 6 months."

Case Study 10.3

A 24-year-old airline stewardess comes to you for advice concerning vocal nodules. The referring laryngologist describes "bilateral well-developed, probably encapsulated, nodules in the middle of the membranous section of the vocal folds." The patient went to the laryngologist after a friend had advised her that she ought to have an examination because someone else she knew had a similar voice quality and she was found to have serious organic disease.

The patient says that her voice has been "kind of husky" for as long as she can remember. She was a cheerleader in high school and describes herself as one who talks incessantly; even when she is alone, she talks to her dog. She does not smoke and drinks only socially with moderation. On examination, her voice has a noticeably breathy-husky quality.

Q1: *What is the physical explanation for the patient's "breathy-husky" voice quality?*

Q2: *What is the most likely etiology of her vocal nodules?*

Q3: *Do you feel comfortable making a therapy decision at this point? If so, what do you think ought to be done? If not, what further information do you think you need?*

The psychosocial history is as follows. After high school graduation and 2 years of college, she was accepted for flight attendant training. One year later, she married an accountant and continued to work at her airline job. She says her marriage is "quite satisfactory," although recently she has been unhappy about her husband having to work long hours because of increased responsibilities. She wishes she could see more of him. She conveys the impression that there are no deeper problems.

As far as she is concerned, her voice has never been a problem. Other than being unable to sing high notes, she has no voice limitations. Many people even tell her they like the quality of her voice. Actually, her main reason for coming to the clinic was that she feared a disease of her larynx, not because she wanted help for her voice.

Q4: *Do you think this patient is a candidate for voice therapy? Why?*

Q5: *Should this patient's vocal nodules be removed surgically? Why?*

Q6: *What would you have done if the laryngologist had recommended surgical removal?*

Discussion

The "breathy-husky" voice quality in this patient is typical of those who have vocal nodules. The voice quality is the effect of the nodules projecting medially into the glottis from the vocal folds so that when they approximate during phonation, the vocal edges do not form a complete seal; instead, spaces are left in the region of the nodules allowing air to escape during phonation, hence the breathy quality. At high pitch, when only the edge of the vocal fold cover participates in vibration, the lesions may approximate momentarily stopping vibration, much like would happen if you touched a vibrating guitar string. The nodules may also cause a slight increase in mass that contributes to the perception of a husky voice. From the history provided, and the laryngologist's description of probable encapsulation, it would appear that these nodules have been present for a long time. Quite likely, they were formed when the patient was a cheerleader or before. Her greater-than-average voice use and working as a flight attendant in a dry, noisy environment have probably caused them to persist.

There is serious doubt that voice therapy is necessary or even desirable. The patient is satisfied with her voice even though most clinicians would agree it was defective. In many vocal abusers, excessive voice use is inseparable from their basically extroverted personalities, making voice modification difficult to achieve. If she were motivated to change, teaching methods of projection without abuse coupled with vocal hygiene might diminish the abuse but would not modify the excessive amount of talking. However, even if she were motivated, reducing vocal abuse probably would not significantly diminish the size of the nodules owing to their encapsulation. In view of the poor prognosis for reducing encapsulated vocal nodules by means of voice reeducation, there is a strong tendency to advocate surgical removal. Although in some instances this might be advisable, there are risks associated with surgery; there may be scarring or other tissue defects, and the dysphonia may remain or even become worse. Moreover, if the surgical treatment brought about a normal voice, the patient might be unhappy with the outcome because she currently gets positive feedback from friends stating they like her voice.

Case Study 10.4

A patient is sent to you with the following history. She is a 52-year-old woman who complains of general fatigue and episodes of voice loss for about 2 years. Twenty years ago, she had an episode of anxiety, hyperventilation, and a sense of impending doom. She was helped with psychologic counseling and has had only rare occurrences of these complaints ever since. Three years ago, she choked on a carrot; said it stuck in her windpipe and that she nearly died. Two years ago, she began to have what she describes as "severe fatigue, no stamina, generalized weakness, a need to walk slowly—like I'm 90 years old." She says her symptoms are getting progressively worse.

When she talks on the telephone for long periods, her "voice loses volume and becomes a whisper" accompanied by chest discomfort and a pulling sensation in her epigastrium. She feels more fatigued and weak during these spells, and three or four times she felt light-headed when she had them. At first these episodes occurred only once or twice a week, but now they occur daily "anytime I talk." All of her symptoms are now worse.

The neurologist who wrote these findings also noted that when he asked her to count to 100, her "voice deteriorated to a whisper."

Q1: *At this point, what causes of her voice disorder might you consider?*

During your examination, you discover that her voice is intermittently breathy during contextual speech. Her cough is normally sharp. She complains of pain in the region of her larynx. She gives no evidence of hypernasality or nasal emission, and her articulation is normal. You ask her to count vigorously from 1 to 150. She becomes nearly aphonic by the time she reaches 60 but with no signs of hypernasality or articulatory disturbance accompanying the voice change. Her cough during her aphonia retains its sharpness.

Q2: *Does this patient show the classic signs of the dysarthria of myasthenia gravis?*

Q3: *What is the neuroanatomic type of dysarthria that can accompany myasthenia gravis and what are its classic signs?*

Q4: *Is it possible for someone to have myasthenia gravis localized to the larynx only?*

Q5: *If the voice had deteriorated to aphonia for reasons of muscular weakness after the stress test of counting, what do you think the quality of her cough ought to have been?*

You discuss your findings with the neurologist, who suggests that Tensilon (ICN Pharmaceuticals, Inc., Costa Mesa, CA) be administered after voice deterioration but, in this case, he suggests injecting sterile water prior to the Tensilon test.

Q6: *Why do you think the neurologist wanted to inject sterile water before Tensilon?*

The neurologist inserts the needle of a syringe filled with sterile water into the patient's arm, but she has not been informed that water is the substance being injected. Her voice, which begins as a whisper after having been first fatigued, becomes steadily louder and clearer as she counts, even before the neurologist has injected the water. The patient complains of "feeling funny." The water is then injected with no further effect.

Q7: *What do you conclude from the events just described?*

Q8: *How do you think you (the speech-language pathologist) and the neurologist should proceed with the patient from this point?*

Further discussion with the patient reveals, for the first time, that ever since she had been placed in a cardiac intensive care unit 2 years ago for cardiac arrhythmia, she has been chronically anxious about her heart. Even though the cardiac findings were diagnosed as benign, she still becomes extremely anxious whenever her heartbeat is irregular.

Q9: *Discuss the relevance of this latest information to the patient's total neurologic and speech signs and symptoms.*

Q10: *What further action do you think should be taken?*

Discussion

On the face of it, any speech deterioration during prolonged or effortful speaking ought to bring to mind myasthenia gravis. The question that often confronts us is whether a given patient with myasthenia gravis needs to demonstrate all of the classic signs of flaccid dysarthria; that is, whether all speech systems—respiratory, phonatory, resonatory, and articulatory—need to be implicated before we can reasonably suspect this type of dysarthria. The answer is "no." Although rare, bulbar myasthenia gravis can become manifested at the laryngeal level only, so it is reasonable that this patient was reasonably suspected of having the disease, especially when her voice had deteriorated during stressful counting. But, all findings did not fit with the idea of progressive muscular

weakness as the underlying cause of her bouts of dysphonia. Rarely, if ever, does the myasthenic patient's voice deteriorate into a complete whisper, as this patient's had. However, most telling was the preservation of her sharp cough during the time she was aphonic. This exhibits an inconsistency and is a clinical red flag telling you something in the picture does not fit. The typical patient with flaccid dysphonia from true muscular weakness of the laryngeal adductors will produce a weak or "mushy" cough proportionate to the degree of dysphonia present. The neurologist suspected that something about his entire examination did not fit with organic disease and when presented with evidence of the sharp cough decided to do a placebo test—sterile water instead of Tensilon—first to see if the patient would respond as if she had been given the drug. Our suspicions were confirmed when the needle had been inserted into the vein and her voice began to improve as if she had been given Tensilon, *even before the water had been injected.* The test was discontinued with confirmation of psychogenic dysphonia.

It is curious that a small percentage of patients will develop nonorganic musculoskeletal reactions (which in some cases are conversion reactions) that simulate neurologic syndromes relatively well-known to the general public, such as myasthenia gravis or multiple sclerosis. Often, the idea is inadvertently suggested by prior medical consultations or by the patient's experience with a relative or friend who had the disease.

In this patient, the reason was never found as to why she happened to acquire a nonorganic dysphonia that resembled myasthenia gravis, but the neurologist strongly suspected that it had something to do with her anxiety about her heart. His course of action from that point was to schedule a complete examination by a cardiologist for a new opinion, with the intent of educating the patient as to her true cardiac status. Held in reserve was a psychiatric consultation should the cardiologist's counseling prove ineffective.

Strained Hoarse Continuous Group (SH-C)

Case Study 10.5

A 47-year-old, male, community college economics instructor comes to you with the complaint of hoarseness that began developing at the onset of the fall semester. Now Christmastime, his voice is worse than it has ever been. He thinks he has been under stress because of a change in his teaching duties, having been given increasing responsibilities owing to the loss of a faculty member. He finds that about halfway through a lecture, his hoarseness increases and he feels pain in his throat. He recently visited an otolaryngologist who said that his vocal folds looked nearly normal except for some slight reddening. Until his voice disorder began 4 months previously, he had been in excellent health and had had no previous trouble with his voice in spite of an active teaching career spanning 20 years. On voice evaluation, you hear a continuously strained hoarse voice quality. On vowel prolongation, there is a "wet" sounding noise superimposed on the hoarseness, and, at times, it sounds as if there is a very subtle, rapid tremor or "flutter" in the patient's voice. The psychosocial history reveals that he is happily married with two teenage children, both of whom are doing well in school. His wife is a social worker employed part-time. The patient admits that he has always been high-strung, that lecturing has always been extremely important to him, and that he derives most of his work satisfaction from teaching, finding students stimulating and challenging. This past semester has been more upsetting than previous years owing to having to teach two additional courses, which interferes with preparation for his lectures and reduces the amount of time he has to spend with individual students. Being compulsive and meticulous, he becomes anxious if he has not prepared adequately for every lecture.

Q1: *What possible etiologies of this patient's dysphonia do you entertain?*

Q2: *What evidence can you muster to support your position?*

Q3: *What is the significance of the specialist's observation of erythema of the vocal folds?*

Q4: *What significance do you give to the observation that his voice sounded "wet" on vowel prolongation?*

Q5: *What interpretation do you give to the observation of a rapid tremor or "flutter" during vowel prolongation?*

Q6: *How would you progress with the examination and the management of this patient from this point? What is your rationale?*

The patient's cough sounded reasonably normal. However, his glottal attack on a vowel seemed to be produced with less than normal percussion.

Q7: *If valid, what interpretation would ordinarily be given to a less than normal glottal attack on a vowel?*

Q8: *Why would the cough be sharper than the glottal attack on a vowel?*

You decide to perform an oral-physical examination. With a tongue depressor, you stroke the patient's lips from the angles of the mouth toward the center and think you see a slight pursing of his lips. Upon opening his mouth, you find that his mouth glistens with a coating of saliva, and you ask if he has noticed any wetness of his pillow upon arising in the morning. Upon protruding his tongue approximately one-half inch beyond his incisor teeth and resting it there, you think you see an irregular surface of his tongue along both sides. Every now and then you see dimpling movements in different areas of the surface of the tongue along the sides.

Q9: *What interpretation do you give to the wetness on the surface of the mouth and tongue?*

Q10: *What is the significance of the question about the wet pillow in the morning?*

Q11: *What is the meaning of the irregular tongue surface along the sides?*

Q12: *Of what relevance are the dimpling movements scattered over the edges of the tongue?*

During the interview, you note further that two or three times when you touched on personal issues, the patient seemed to be on the verge of crying. When asked about it he said, almost puzzled by his own loss of control, that he had been doing that quite often during the past 2 months, sometimes with only the slightest provocation. You note also as he speaks that in addition to the hoarseness, his prosody is somewhat lacking in pitch variations.

Q13: *What thoughts come to mind about the patient's tendency to cry easily?*

Q14: *Does the observation of a tendency toward monopitch contribute anything to your differential diagnostic thinking?*

Continuing with a routine motor-speech examination, you are further alerted to the possibility that on testing alternate motion rate for /pʌ/, /tʌ/, and /kʌ/, his ability to repeat these syllables may not be quite within the normal speed range, something that did not appear abnormal during contextual speech. You decide to measure his rate and discover that for the /pʌ/, his maximum rate is 5 Hz; for /tʌ/, 4 Hz; and for /kʌ/, his rate fluctuates between 3 and 4 Hz.

Q15: *What significance do you give to the alternate motion rates obtained?*

Further background information reveals that the patient has been having difficulty lately swallowing liquids, tending to choke occasionally unless he drinks slowly. His gag reflex, on your continued motor-speech examination, is quite hyperreflexive, and, yet, even though you do not hear any hypernasality, he has mild nasal emission producing moisture on a mirrored surface, confirmed with nasal airflow studies.

Q16: *What is the potential significance of the patient's occasional tendency to choke on fluids?*

Q17: *In view of the hyperactive gag reflex, of what significance, if any, is the mild degree of nasal emission observed?*

Q18: *What diagnostic possibilities are you entertaining concerning this patient's voice disorder?*

Q19: *What decisions would you make concerning further procedures to be taken with this patient?*

Discussion

The case depicted here is not unusual. A patient comes with a focal voice disorder in which most or all attention by various clinicians has been directed toward the larynx, obscuring other deviations of speech, which admittedly can be borderline and appear normal until scrutinized carefully. Such was the situation with this patient who, because of no mass lesions and because of symmetric movements of the vocal folds, was considered to be free of organic disease. The inflammation noted by the otolaryngologist is common in patients, and especially in those who have a tendency toward vocal misuse or who may have esophageal reflux; in this case, it is considered to be insignificant. It would have been reasonable for the average clinician to attribute the strained hoarse dysphonia to vocal misuse in a teacher under stress in his job, but concurrent events are not necessarily causally related, once again, highlighting the necessity of looking carefully at the whole picture so as not to identify a correlational or contributing factor as the causal factor.

Piecing together, the evolving historical and examination findings the clinician should have become increasingly suspicious that there was more going on with this patient's speech mechanism than a phonatory disorder. In retrospect, we see a picture forming of a man developing emotional lability, dysphagia, reduced ability to swallow accumulating saliva, possible tongue atrophy and fasciculations, velopharyngeal insufficiency (which can occur even in the presence of an active gag reflex), a positive sucking reflex, and borderline slow reciprocating muscle movements as demonstrated on alternate motion rates.

The differential diagnostic choices in this patient are multiple **(Fig. 10.12)**. He may be misusing his voice, he may be compensating for an underlying laryngeal disorder, he may be exhibiting a psychogenic voice disorder, or the signs and symptoms may reflect very early spastic (pseudobulbar) dysarthria-dysphonia having a major laryngeal-phonatory expression.

The decision at the termination of the speech pathologist's examination ought to have been, and was, to refer the patient for a neurologic examination, whereupon signs of spasticity were found elsewhere in the body, as was evidence of muscle denervation on electromyographic examination, implicating the lower motor neuron system in addition to the upper motor neuron pyramidal system. The neurologist's diagnosis was motor neuron disease, probably amyotrophic lateral sclerosis.

Strained Hoarse Voice Arrest–Intermittent Arrhythmic Group (SHVA–IA)

Case Study 10.6

A 32-year-old woman enters your office. Three chairs line the wall, each extending further from your desk. She sits on the one farthest from you, piling her coat, purse, and paperback book on her lap. She smiles, sits erectly, and leans away from you (**Fig. 10.13**).

Q1:   *What early inferences might be made about this person based on the information given?*

Q2:   *Which statement to the patient do you think would be the most appropriate to make at this juncture in the examination?:*

A.   *"I see you've been reading the latest bestseller. I've been wanting to get it myself. What do you think of it?"*

B.   *"Your doctor sent me a report about your voice disorder. From his letter, it looks as if you've been abusing your voice quite a bit lately."*

C.   *"You might be more comfortable if you put your belongings on that chair and sat next to my desk. I think we'll be able to converse more easily that way."*

Clinician (C): What brings you to the clinic?

Patient (P): My voice. It's been like this for 3 months, and it's like about to drive me up the wall.

C: Could you describe it? What's different about it now compared with the way it used to be?

P: Gee, that's going to be hard . . . Well, I guess it's kind of hoarse. Well, not exactly hoarse; it's different from the hoarseness I usually get from laryngitis. It's, uh, kind of strained or raspy; like I'm pushing or pulling everything from way down here. (She lays the flat of her hand on her abdomen.) It's very tiring. Sometimes it gets so bad I just don't talk.

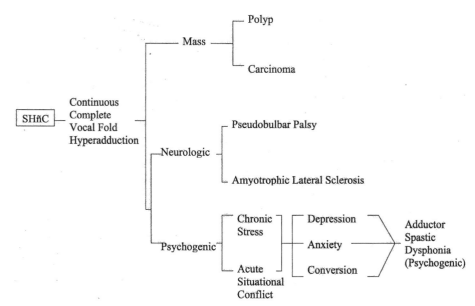

Figure 10.12   Flow chart of the multiple differential diagnostic choices of Strained hoarse continuous group (SH-C).

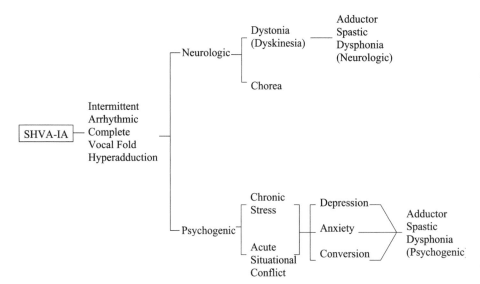

Figure 10.13 Differential diagnosis schema for Strained hoarse voice arrest - intermittent arrhythmic group (SHVA-IA) illustrating steps in detecting cause of intermittent arrhythmic complete vocal fold hyperaddution.

C: How did this voice trouble start?

P: It actually began with a cold and sore throat. (Laughs wryly.) Then, the cold went away, but the hoarseness didn't. My neck feels sore, too. (She runs her hand from her chest to under her chin.) And, I get this pain in my ears. The doctor looked but he couldn't find anything wrong with my ears or my lymph nodes.

Q3: *Why didn't the clinician launch directly into a voice evaluation instead of conducting a preliminary discussion?*

Q4: *Even though you have not performed a formal voice evaluation, what might you deduce about your patient's vocal fold activity from her description of her voice?*

Q5: *What do you think is the physical basis for her complaints about increased efforts to talk?*

Q6: *What do you make of her statement that her voice trouble persisted?*

Q7: *What might be the significance of her complaints of neck and ear pain?*

C: So, if I have this correctly, your voice trouble began about 3 months ago with a cold and persisted after the cold cleared. I want to go into the history of the voice disorder in greater detail, but before we do, I want to examine thoroughly your speech mechanism and voice.

C: First, read this paragraph aloud while I tape record your speech.

P: (She reads the "Grandfather Passage" aloud.)

C: Now I want you to sustain the vowel /a/ as long and steadily as you can. Do that 3 times.

P: (As she reads the passage you hear irregular, fluctuating moments of strained hoarseness and slight voice stoppages. On vowel prolongation, her voice is also strained but not as much as during oral reading. You hear moments of clearer voice, which is even more apparent at higher pitch levels.)

C: All right, now will you cough as sharply as you can?

P: (She does so with a sharp, well-defined glottal attack.)

C: What we want to do now is to examine your speech mechanism. I'd like you to sit up straight and rest your hands in your lap. Look straight ahead.

P: (The clinician observes her during complete rest for several seconds.)

C: Now, open your mouth, but keep your tongue at rest on the floor of the mouth.

P: (The tongue is of normal size and shape and is symmetric.)

C: Now, gently rest the tip of your tongue over your lower teeth.

P: (The tongue surface remains quiescent.)

C: Stick your tongue straight out of your mouth.

P: (She does so symmetrically.)

C: Wiggle it from side to side as fast as you can.

P: (These movements are performed rapidly with good range of motion.)

C: Put your tongue in your left cheek and don't let my finger press it in.

P: (This is done in the right cheek as well. Her tongue resists pressure well.)

C: Press your tongue forward against the tongue depressor as I push in.

P: (She does this with good strength.)

C: Lift the tip of your tongue and touch your upper lip.

P: (This is performed normally.)

C: Hold your mouth open quietly again while I look at your soft palate.

P: (It hangs quietly and symmetrically.)

C: I'm going to take this tongue depressor and stroke the sides of your soft palate and pharynx.

P: (She gags easily and both sides of the soft palate rise symmetrically and with good medial pharyngeal wall movement.)

C: Open and close your mouth.

P: (She does so without any deviation of the mandible.)

Q8: *What words might you use to describe the patient's voice signs?*

Q9: *What kinds of information did you expect to obtain from asking her to read a standard paragraph aloud?*

Q10: *What kinds of information did you expect to obtain from asking her to sustain a vowel sound as long as she could?*

Q11: *What is the significance of her clearer voice at a higher pitch level?*

Q12: *What is the purpose of asking her to cough as sharply as possible?*

Q13: *In light of the fact that she has been referred to you with a voice disorder, for what specific reasons did you perform a complete oral-physical examination?*

Q14: *What was the purpose of asking her to sit as quietly as possible while you observed her head, neck, and other bodily structures?*

C: If you will look straight ahead, now, I'm going to feel your neck.

P: (Her larynx is rigid; it is difficult to move from side to side. Her thyroid cartilage is pulled up high in her neck, and her thyrohyoid space is narrow. You encircle the hyoid bone with the thumb of your left hand over the tip of the left major horn of her hyoid bone and the middle finger over the right, and pressing inward, rotate your fingers over this area.) "Ow. Do you have to do that?" (Then, with the thumb and middle finger over the superior borders of the alae of the thyroid cartilage and your index finger in the thyroid notch, you try to maneuver the larynx downward, away from the hyoid bone. As you are doing this, you ask the following.)

C: How does that feel?

P: Oh, it hurts. It really does. (As she says this, you hear a sudden clearing of her voice. She looks at you with surprise.) Say, that sounded different (her voice returning to its strained hoarseness).

Q15: *What is your interpretation of the elevated larynx, laryngeal rigidity, and diminished thyrohyoid space?*

Q16: *Name the muscles most likely to be involved in these physical findings.*

Q17: *Why did she respond with pain when you pressed your fingers and rotated them in the hyoid region?*

Q18: *How does this information contribute to your understanding of the etiologic diagnosis of her voice disorder?*

Q19: *What is the significance of the momentary clearing of her voice as you pulled downward on her larynx?*

C: Let's continue with the history of your voice trouble. Tell me, from the time it began, is it getting better, worse, or staying the same?

P: It fluctuates. Sometimes it's better, sometimes worse.

C: How about time of day; does that affect it?

P: Yes. It's usually better in the morning. In fact, there are times when I first get up in the morning it's normal, and that may last for 15 to 20 minutes.

C: Have there been other times that the voice has returned to normal?

P: Yes. About a month ago it was normal almost the whole time I was on a trip alone to San Francisco, but it got worse again after I came home.

C: So, your voice disorder is not a steady thing; it fluctuates with time of day and where you are. Your doctor wrote in his referral letter that you are in TV production. Tell me about that.

P: I'm an assistant manager.

C: How long have you been in that kind of work?

P: About 10 years. I joined the station right out of college.

C: Do you use your voice much in your work?

P: (She smiles and angles her head toward you for emphasis.) You bet I do. I'm on the phone all day talking to salesmen, technicians, personnel. Some days by late afternoon I can barely talk.

C: And, have you always had to use your voice a lot in your work?

P: Yes. It's been that way from the beginning when I took the job.

Q20: *What is your reaction to the information that the patient's voice fluctuates depending upon situations and time of day?*

Q21: *What is your reaction to the information that at times the voice has returned to normal for several minutes to several days?*

Q22: *What conclusions do you draw about the possible etiology of her voice disorder from the information that she uses her voice far more than the average person in her daily work?*

Q23: *With the information you have at this point, are you satisfied that you understand the etiology of her voice disorder and are ready to begin therapy? If so, what procedures would you next initiate?*

Q24: *If you are not satisfied that you have the entire picture of her voice problem, what further information would you wish to obtain?*

C: Let's stop at this point and review what we have so far. Did your doctor explain the results of his laryngologic examination?

P: Yes. He said my vocal folds were normal except for some slight reddening that couldn't account for my abnormal voice. He said the redness could have come from a cold or it could be due to irritation from abusing my voice.

C: Good. Because I want you to understand that basically there is nothing physically wrong with your vocal folds. There are no growths, infections, or paralyses that might account for your voice trouble.

P: Well, I'm certainly glad to hear that. You hear so much about cancer and things like that. I was really worried . . . But, then why does my voice sound this way? Are you going to tell me this is all in my head?

C: That's a good question, because, here you have this very abnormal-sounding voice and we're telling you there's nothing physically wrong with the voice mechanism.

P: Yes. And, that feeling of stiffness and pain—if that's not physical, what could it be?

C: I appreciate how confusing this must be, so, I want to introduce an idea to you that, for the time being, might help to explain your complaints. A person can have considerable changes in voice along with real feelings of stiffness and pain because of excess contraction of the throat muscles. Most people have had similar tension and pain in other parts of the body. When such tensions occur in the throat muscles, they can cause changes in the voice along with these abnormal feelings.

P: All right. So, what causes the tensions? I think I'm pretty well adjusted. (Slight note of irritation in her manner at this point.)

C: Let's talk about that, if we may. Specifically, was there anything unusual in the way of personal problems when you started having trouble with your voice?

P: Not that I can think of. I was working as usual. Everything is going real well at the job. In fact, I just got a promotion and a raise. No, there's nothing. (As the patient tells you this, she averts her gaze and frowns, looking down at her lap. There is a long pause.)

Q25: *Which of the following steps would you take at this point?*

> **A.** *Accept her denial of problems and continue on to another subject.*
>
> **B.** *Point out to her that she seems upset by something.*
>
> **C.** *Discontinue the examination and make another appointment.*
>
> **D.** *Wait and say nothing.*

(She looks up at you, smiles and shrugs her shoulders as if to say: "That's it; nothing else comes to mind.")

C: This is a difficult question for most people. Sometimes we are unaware that certain things are bothering us.

P: Well, like what kinds of problems are you referring to? I mean, uh, I guess maybe there has been something bothering me, but I didn't think it would have anything to do with my voice. (Pauses) Now that you mention it, I have been unhappy in a situation that I haven't done anything about. Normally, when I'm unhappy in a situation, I change it. (Pause) The marriage.

C: Would you mind telling me more about that?

P: Well, he is very . . . he doesn't want to accept the fact that we don't have a marriage, and it's very difficult for him. He doesn't understand a lot of things about it which I understand. I've never been a nervous person or shaky, you know, about anything, and just since we've been married, I've been fighting divorce or separation. For my husband's sake, I want to stay married.

C: What, in your opinion, is wrong with the marriage?

P: I guess the fact that I don't like closeness. I loved being single. My favorite things are to ride my horse out in the woods for days or read books. Of course, I love being with people also. I am an executive, so I have to be with people. But, marriage isn't anything like I thought it would be.

C: What did you think it was going to be like?

P: Well, I thought it would be a great deal of sharing emotionally and materialistically—all the things that you share—but I didn't think it would be sharing everything, meaning the husband; he doesn't want to do anything unless I do it with him. To me, it has been very draining, because I never in my life, even when I lived with a big family, had all that closeness. I've never had that much closeness in that way; to me, it's like 24 hours of . . . (pauses, searches for the right word).

C: Being stifled?

P: Yes. And I've told him that and explained it to him and he doesn't do it purposely. I think it's the first time he's ever been in love, and he's gotten carried away with it. And the difference being he's a person that needs me and I don't need him. I don't need him in the way, I mean, to fulfill my life, and that is a big difference in our relationship.

C: Did you have trouble confronting your husband with your feelings about the marriage?

P: Not at all, In fact, before we got married, I was really fighting getting married.

C: Why did you?

P: I wish I knew, because it just happened real suddenly, and my husband is very persuasive, and I've always really cared for him, too. (Long pause)

C: How and when did you meet him?

P: We were attending the same advertising convention. That was about 9 months ago. He's older, 52, and has made a lot of money and had been recently divorced. It was a sort of a whirlwind courtship, at least for me. He sort of pursued me during the whole convention. We started going out together. After that, he was very insistent; said he needed me desperately. We were married after 3 months.

C: So, that was about 6 months ago, and your voice trouble started 3 months ago. But, in spite of your feelings about wanting to remain single, you went ahead with the marriage anyway. Did you express your misgivings to your husband before you were married?

P: Very much. I told him I was not a touchy-feely person. I mean, I'm loving, and I have a lot of love to give, and I can accept love, but he is starved for love in the way that he really needs constant patting on the head and a lot of attention, and a lot of what I can't, I guess, give. And, I don't know if there is any reason for him to lack that just because of me.

C: Do you and your husband have much in common?

P: Oh gosh! We have everything in common. We are both very adventuresome; we love to travel, camp, ski.

C: Do you think your voice is better right now than when we started?

P: Much better.

C: I'm glad you recognize that. It's 50 to 75% improved since we began discussing this marital situation. Do you feel better about having talked about that?

P: Yes. Much better. Up until now, I kept rejecting talking to anybody professional about it. I kept thinking, well, whatever it is it will go away tomorrow, because tomorrow would be fine. I got to the point where it was so frustrating not being able to converse and express or even go to a counter and order a bottle of perfume without somebody asking, "What are you saying?" This confirms my feeling that my voice has something to do with keeping things in. In other words, I've always been a happy person, and I'm always jovial and never depressed, and just lately I've been in a state of depression.

C: Can you estimate for how long?

P: Well, I'd say about 3 or 4 months.

C: That's about the time you've had your voice problem.

P: I feel like it has. Because I feel like it, in other words, as I said earlier, I've never been a nervous person. Well, lately I've been very, very tense. I lay down to go to sleep and try to sleep and then just start thinking.

C: Do you think our discussion has been helpful?

P: I'm sure it has. Before, I thought this voice thing was physical, but I realize now I don't have something physical. I feel more comfortable about that. I also feel more comfortable because until now, I hadn't talked to anybody at length about this.

Q26: *What would you say next to the patient? Why?*

C: How do you think we should proceed from here?

P: (She becomes silent for almost a minute, thinking deeply.) Obviously, my voice is better. Sounds almost normal, now. I came to have my voice helped, but here I am with an entirely different problem. That I didn't expect.

C: That's something you're going to have to deal with, isn't it? What do you want to do?

P: I think a separation is worth a try; be away from each other for 6 months or so and for me to seek whatever therapy I need during that 6 months.

C: Therapy? What did you have in mind?

P: Counseling, marital counseling I suppose.

C: Do you know of anyone locally who could help? Or, would you prefer that we arrange for you to see someone?

P: No, I know someone who's really good, has a good reputation. May I ask that you send a report of your examination to her?

C: Of course. And, I'll send a full report to your laryngologist within the next few days.

P: But, do you really think all this has caused my voice trouble?

C: What do you think?

P: (She smiles.) I think it has.

C: I'll say goodbye, then. Please keep in touch and let me know how things turn out?

P: I will. I promise.

Q27: *Is there a relationship between her marital problem and her voice disorder? Or, are they just coincidental? What precipitating factors might have contributed to the problem?*

Q28: *How do you think the clinician in this case handled the situation?*

Q29: *Do you think the patient was in need of psychiatric help? Explain.*

Q30: *What formal diagnosis would you give to her voice disorder? Why?*

Q31: *What do you think is the prognosis for her voice disorder and her relationship with her husband? Why?*

Q32: *Should the patient have been given conventional voice therapy?*

The patient wrote the following letter to the speech-language pathologist:

It has been 2 months since I came to see you about my voice disorder, and I hope you will recall the circumstances surrounding the disorder. As we had decided then, I went to see a psychiatrist in my home town who specializes in marital problems. Both my husband and myself had several sessions with her, and after getting our differences into the open, which took several consultations, we decided, with the approval of the psychiatrist, to separate, This happened 3 weeks ago, and while my voice had remained improved after having seen you, it continued to do so after our separation and as I write my voice is completely normal.

I would like to thank you for all your help and for enabling me to see what was bothering me.

Instructions

1. Write a clinical report of your examination of this patient.

2. Write a letter to the referring otolaryngologist.

Sample Report of Clinical Voice Examination Mrs.____ is a 32-year-old television station assistant manager who was referred by Dr.____ , laryngologist, with a diagnosis of a "voice disorder secondary to vocal abuse." Based on his laryngoscopic examination, except for some evidence of vocal fold irritation, the vocal folds were essentially normal in structure and movement.

The patient began noticing signs of strained voice quality approximately 3 months after her marriage. It has persisted since then, although it fluctuates, depending upon time of day, fatigue, and whether or not she happens to be experiencing an optimistic or pessimistic outlook. On one occasion, the voice was completely normal while she was alone on vacation.

Oral-physical examination failed to disclose any evidence of facial, lingual, velar, or mandibular weakness or asymmetry. She gave no evidence of unusual movements about her face or other parts of her head, neck, or extremities. Articulation, both during contextual speech and on alternate motion rate, failed to disclose any evidence of a motor speech disorder.

The physical history indicates that although Mrs._____ has been under considerable pressure at work using her voice a great deal, this situation has existed for many more years than the short duration of her current voice disorder. After initial reluctance, she disclosed that she was dissatisfied with her marriage owing to its confining nature. As the patient disclosed this information her voice gradually improved. She recognized the improvement and understood the relationship between her voice disorder and her martial dissatisfaction.

We discussed the advisability of her obtaining counseling in order to help her resolve her marital problem. Symptomatic therapy of the voice disorder would be ill-timed in view of her emotional conflict and its priority over her abnormal voice.

We decided that the patient would seek professional help for her marital problem. She will keep us informed as to her progress.

Sample Letter to the Otolaryngologist   Thank you for your kind referral of Mrs._____. I have enclosed the report of my clinical speech evaluation. While I think that vocal abuse might have exacerbated her voice disorder, it was my impression, as noted in the enclosed report of clinical examination, that the fundamental cause of her dysphonia has been psychologic and related to an unresolved marital problem. I think you would be gratified to learn that her dysphonia improved significantly during her disclosure of her dissatisfactions, and that she recognized the relationship between her voice disorder and these tensions. My impression was that symptomatic voice therapy would have been premature at this point inasmuch as her entire attitude shifted from attention to her voice to that of her martial dissatisfaction.

I offered the patient the names of psychiatrists and clinical psychologists in her local area, but she elected to see someone of her acquaintance with an excellent reputation. I will keep you informed as to her progress. I suggested that she contact you at some date in the future to let you know how she is doing.

If there is any further information that you would like to have, please do not hesitate to call or write.

Discussion

It is usually a good idea to begin with general conversation rather than going directly into the mechanics of the voice examination. To do so is not only a sign of personal interest in the patient but also gives the clinician an impression of the patient's total communication in addition to the voice (i.e., resonation, articulation, language, ideation, and affect).

From the transcript, we read the description "strained or effortful." Although it is difficult to know what the voice was like without hearing it, the term *strained* ought to have conjured up hyperaduction of either the true vocal folds, false vocal folds, or both. Complaints about increased effort to talk along with strained hoarseness is also evidence of vocal fold hyperadduction. The increased physical effort indicates that the patient had to exert abnormally intense thoracic and abdominal muscle contraction in order to force air through the hyperadducted vocal folds. The patient's complaint of neck and ear pain is often a sign of chronic excess intrinsic and extrinsic laryngeal muscle contraction.

The statement that the voice disorder began with an upper respiratory infection that disappeared whereas the voice disorder persisted is not an uncommon finding associated with the onset of voice disorders. It is often considered to be indicative of psychogenic dysphonia, as a high percentage of psychogenic voice disorders begin in this way. At the onset of the upper respiratory infection (URI), there may have been some laryngeal edema for which the patient needed to compensate. Whether there are secondary gains of extra attention or reduced workload from having laryngitis or simply that the extraneous muscle effort was maintained to the detriment of voice or some combination of the two is part of what the clinician attempts to determine.

Laryngeal elevation, rigidity, and diminished thyrohyoid space are usually signs of chronic hypercontraction of the extrinsic, and probably the intrinsic, laryngeal muscles and are associated with musculoskeletal tension disorders. The muscle groups most likely involved in such laryngeal malpositioning are the suprahyoids and infrahyoids. Pain when the tissues around the hyoid bone and thyroid cartilage are kneaded supports the inference of excess musculoskeletal tension. (Many clinicians are reluctant to touch the patient, let alone cause pain. Yet, it is essential to determine if, in fact, pain and tension exist if a proper etiologic diagnosis is to be made.)

Momentary clearing of the voice as the larynx was pulled downward reinforces the suspicion of a musculoskeletal tension voice disorder. That the patient's voice fluctuated depending upon situation and time of day further supports psychogenicity; however, it must be strongly emphasized that organic voice disorders also vary in this manner, although they rarely return to normal. That her voice returned to normal, not just improved, from several minutes to several days, almost certainly indicates that the entire voice disorder is psychogenic.

From the written descriptions of the voice, such words as *spastic*, *spasmodic*, *hyperfunctional*, or *strained hoarseness* come to mind. Asking the patient to read a standard paragraph aloud not only provides information about how the dysphonia fluctuates with the production of phonemes in different contexts, but it also reveals other aspects of motor speech. Asking the patient to sustain a vowel provides information about the quality, pitch level, and steadiness of the voice. During such steady-state activity, the clinician can listen carefully for subtle voice aberrations and for fluctuations in laryngeal-respiratory control. Also, in certain voice disorders, vowel prolongation can produce a very different voice than during contextual speech, which may have important differential diagnostic significance.

The fact that the patient's voice was clearer at higher pitch levels should have led the clinician in the direction of considering the voice disorder to be one type of adductor spasmodic dysphonia, in which there is strained voice at conversational pitch levels but clear voice at higher ones.

Asking the patient to cough or produce a sharp glottal attack provides important information about her ability to adduct her vocal folds adequately. In patients who have organic weakness, the cough and glottal coup lack sharpness. A complete oral-physical examination is always important, even when the clinician suspects that the disorder is confined to the larynx, because motor-speech disorders can begin with a dysphonia, predominately, while very careful examination of remaining motor-speech structures may disclose the beginnings of a dysarthria in other regions of the speech musculature.

Asking the patient to keep her mouth, tongue, and jaw at rest while the clinician observes her head and neck structures is important to determine the presence of subtle neurologic movement disorders that have a tendency to show themselves only when the patient is quiescent.

Three factors suggested there was a definite link between the patient's marital problem and her voice disorder. Only during her marriage did she develop the voice disorder for the first time in her life. Her voice became normal while she was away from her husband. Her dysphonia improved during the interviews as she described the conflicts created by her marriage. There was little question that the patient needed counseling. She was in a serious conflictual situation that was already having somatic repercussions, and it was apparent that she was unable to manage this situation on her own.

Based on the intermittent strained voice quality and associated laryngospasm, the history, and the changes in voice, it would be appropriate to conclude that this patient had adductor spasmodic dysphonia, psychogenic, probably of the conversion-reaction type.

Case Study 10.7

A 43-year-old married woman with grown children who worked for a real estate firm came to the clinic for help with a voice problem of 1-year duration. She describes her voice as "tense, strained, and high in pitch, and some words won't come out at all." Her disorder began gradually with a nondescript hoarseness that continued to deteriorate to its current strained quality. It had improved on occasion; she had been receiving voice therapy "to produce a more relaxed and clearer voice." Whereas she found that she could, in fact, produce a clearer voice with concentration, these techniques did not hold up in most speaking situations outside of the clinic. She volunteers that her voice disorder has interfered with her supervisory responsibilities at work and has been equally damaging to her social life. This most important ability had gone out of her life, she said, and at fleeting moments during the past few months, she has had suicidal thoughts.

Lately, she has been complaining of "a tight neck and shoulder," and that especially when driving, she has noticed a tremor of her head. At about the same time, she began to notice a tremor in her voice, but this was prior to its worsening.

Voice examination revealed a pronounced strained-strangled voice, but vowel prolongation was clear and steady, except at a higher pitch level where mild tremor was detected. During the oral-physical examination, she had intermittent head tremor and a tendency for her head to turn to her right side.

The psychosocial history was nonproductive. She was not under any particular stress or anxiety at work, and her marital and other domestic relationships, including those with her children, were pleasant and free of all but the usual day-to-day variations in stress.

The ear, nose, and throat examination report came back with the notation, "normal laryngoscopic examination; functional dysphonia."

Q1: *From this description of the patient's voice, what terminology would you use to describe the voice signs and symptoms?*

Q2: *What muscular actions within the larynx and surrounding structures could be producing this kind of voice?*

Q3: *What significance, if any, would you give to the patient's complaint of turning of her head and head tremor?*

Q4: *What are your thoughts, your reactions to the examination report of a normal larynx and that the disorder was "functional"?*

Q5: *With the information that you have in hand, what next steps would you take in the management of this patient?*

Because of her complaint of mild turning of her head and head tremor, a neurologic examination was scheduled. After a complete examination, the neurologist summarized his findings as follows: "For the past 2 years, the patient has been aware of a sense of aching in the back of her neck in the region of the left trapezius muscle. A few months after the onset she began to be aware of a tendency for her face to turn to the left and the vertex of her head to the right, which she can voluntarily straighten with her left hand. No one else observed these movements owing to their mildness. She is most aware of this movement while driving a car and watching television or a movie. Also a few months after the onset of aching in her neck, she became aware of a horizontal head tremor, intermittently, most noticeable when she was in a motor vehicle. A few months after that she began to detect a tremor in her voice. Laughing or yawning transiently corrected the aberrant head posturing. Because of her voice disorder, her future career is at stake, and if something is not done about her voice she may lose her position in her firm. She admits to a reactive depression to her voice that has also caused her to become withdrawn. In addition to the voice and head and neck findings, it is also important to note that she holds a writing instrument tightly and comments that, within the past year, her penmanship has declined. The remainder of the examination is normal. Impression: The neurologic examination gives evidence of extremely mild, but observable, spasmodic torticollis and associated head tremor."

Q6: *What is spasmodic torticollis?*

Q7: *What is the significance of the head tremor in association with spasmodic torticollis?*

Q8: *What is the connection, if any, between the spasmodic torticollis, head tremor, and the patient's voice disorder?*

Q9: *What is the significance of the change in her writing?*

Conference with both the laryngologist and the neurologist discloses that there is no therapy that could be suggested from the standpoint of their specialties; that there were some drugs that have been used to treat a variety of movement disorders but that none had shown definite promise.

Q10: *What steps would you now initiate with this patient in order to help her with her voice disorder?*

Q11: *The patient is now back in your office and it is your responsibility to summarize the results of everyone's examinations and to counsel the patient further pertaining to future therapy, if any. What would you tell the patient as to the nature of her voice disorder, its cause, and the options for treatment?*

The patient was told that she had a disorder that has gone by the name of *adductor spasmodic dysphonia*, and that in some cases the disorder is psychologic and in some cases it is neurologic. In her case—in addition to the fact that previous psychiatric and psychologic studies had failed to show any significant psychopathology, and that the neurologic examination had disclosed mild but positive signs of a movement disorder—in all probability (although no one can say with complete certainty), this was an adductor spastic dysphonia of the dystonic type involving both torticollis and tremor. Because previous therapy performed by a competent speech pathologist had failed to produce an enduring improvement in her voice, the patient was told the only remaining therapy option available at that time was the recurrent laryngeal nerve resection procedure.

The patient, it turned out, had studied this disorder and its causes and she knew about the surgery for it. She expressed skepticism owing to the conflicting reports about its effectiveness, especially in the long-term, and was concerned about the kind of voice quality that would result from the surgery. On the other hand, she said that she was thoroughly "fed up" with the voice, that she had to do something, and that she was willing to risk failure if there was any chance the surgery might prove to be of benefit for her.

After evaluating videotapes of previous patients who had undergone the surgery, the patient decided to proceed with the lidocaine injection procedure.

Q12: *What is the purpose of the lidocaine injection? Explain, physiologically, its effects on the patient's vocal folds, the kind of voice that will result from the injection, what it can predict about the effects of surgery, and indications and contraindications to surgery based on the injection procedure.*

Sitting upright in the laryngologist's examining chair, a needle filled with 1% lidocaine was injected in the region of the cricothyroid space on the right side of the neck.

Q13: *Why was the injection made at this particular anatomic site?*

Q14: *How soon after the injection should the voice change?*

Q15: *How long should the effects of the injection last?*

Q16: *How can you tell if the injection has paralyzed the vocal folds?*

Q17: *What kinds of voice testing material should be used to enable patients and clinicians to evaluate the effects of the injection?*

It required four injections before the laryngologist was able to hit the nerve and the voice became smooth, slightly breathy, and completely free of spasm. The patient expressed immediate gratification at these voice and physical changes and said that she wished to proceed with surgery without further need for contemplation. The patient underwent a preanesthesia medical examination during the afternoon of that day, entered the hospital at suppertime, and went into surgery at 7:30 the next morning. The patient was anesthetized, a primary, collar incision was made at the base of her neck, and the right recurrent laryngeal nerve was identified. After certainty of

identification by mechanical stimulation of the presumed nerve and looking for momentary vocal fold movement via direct laryngoscopy, a section of the nerve was taken and the neck was closed. The pathologist's report identified the specimen as nerve tissue.

During the next few hours, the patient became increasingly alert, remained in her hospital room that night, and was wheeled to the speech pathologist's office the next morning for a 24-hour postsurgery evaluation.

Q18: *What would you expect the patient's voice to sound like at this postsurgical period?*

Q19: *What would you tell the patient when she asks whether this is the way the voice is going to be or whether it will change?*

Q20: *What advice should be given to the patient at this point as to how to use the voice?*

The 24-hour postsurgical voice was breathy, and each time the patient increased the intensity of her voice, it became raspy and contained falsetto pitch breaks. She expressed satisfaction, at this point, mostly with the increased ease of voice production. She looked calm, her facial expression having changed from one of strain to one of relaxation. Her voice was recorded.

The next morning, 48 hours after surgery, her voice had lost some of the breathiness and was louder. She looked less groggy and continued to express approval of the sound and feel of the voice. Her voice was recorded again and she returned to her hospital room.

On the third morning, 72 hours after surgery, her voice had continued to improve in clarity and loudness. She had just been discharged from the hospital and was going home. She was advised to use her voice fully and not to be afraid of using it, although loud abusive talking would obviously be ill-advised. One week later the patient wrote:

> It is still difficult for me to believe this "miracle" has really happened. Each day is a gift from God. The most wonderful change is that I can again enjoy being with people I love rather than wishing they would go away and let me have some peace.
>
> I am still a little hesitant to talk too much; I don't want to "wear it out."
>
> I can barely remember the constant fatigue and depression I felt only a week ago. The future looks bright and sunny. I believe faith and a realistic expectation of success will keep this "miracle" working.
>
> There are no words adequate to express our gratitude. You have touched our lives in a very special way.

One year after surgery, her voice could be described as nearly normal. It is smooth, melodious, free of any hint of spasm, and, most importantly, has remained consistently so without any sign of deterioration.[1]

---

[1]In the ensuing years, much has changed in the medical world. Hospitalizations are shorter and additional treatment options such as botulinum toxin injections and thyroplasties are available. Recurrent laryngeal nerve procedures remain a viable option, often combined with laser thinning of one of the vocal folds, and as in this case is successful with some patients.

Q21: *What accounts for the voice improvement as time passes after surgery?*

Q22: *Can all patients who have recurrent laryngeal nerve surgery expect the degree of improvement experienced by this patient? What would you say to a patient who asked about the probabilities of improvement as a result of surgery?*

Discussion

This patient had the neurologic adductor spastic dysphonia of the dystonic variety with associated tremor. The strained-hoarse arrests of the voice arose from intermittent hyperadduction of the true and false vocal folds. The first clue to the neurologic nature of her spastic dysphonia was the tremor in her voice and head and the complaint of turning of the head. Tremor and spasmodic torticollis commonly occur in association with each other, and adductor laryngeal spasms can often be a sign of either disorder. The patient's complaint of difficulty grasping a writing instrument may have indicated some dystonic involvement of her hand. After ruling out primary psychogenic factors and obtaining a neurologic examination, and knowing that previous efforts toward voice therapy were unsuccessful and that the patient was approaching the desperate stage of her experience with the disorder, it was obvious that something more drastic needed to be done. Informing the patient as much as possible was necessary. The advantages and disadvantages of surgery needed to be presented, preferably with actual case demonstrations to show the patient what might be expected from the surgery.

The purpose of the lidocaine injection is temporarily to paralyze one vocal fold, simulating the surgery. The kind of voice that results from the injection is not exactly like that from the surgery owing to the frequent involvement of the superior laryngeal nerve affecting the cricothyroid muscle. The patient has to be informed of this fact, and the rule of thumb is that if the patient can accept the lidocaine voice, acceptance of the postsurgical voice will certainly be as good or better. The injection is made in the cricothyroid space because that is the entrance site of the nerve into the larynx. The injection lasts anywhere from 10 to 45 minutes, depending upon how much of the anesthetic infiltrates the nerve. The laryngologist can tell if the injection has paralyzed the vocal fold by performing a laryngoscopic examination after injecting the anesthetic. The speech pathologist can hear the loss of sharpness of the cough, and the voice changes—sometimes rather suddenly—to a husky smoothness, and strained voice arrests suddenly disappear. The voice should be recorded during this period for a further evaluation using the same test materials as those used prior to evaluation, usually a standard paragraph, vowel prolongation, and production of coughing and the glottal coup.

The immediately postsurgical voice is usually breathier and weaker than after the passage of several days owing to the fact that the glottis is widest at this time and that the intact vocal fold has not yet learned to compensate. The patient needs to be reassured that this immediately post-surgical voice will not be permanent and that improvement can be expected within a matter of days. Because there is some evidence to indicate that maintenance of a higher, smoother voice may help to avert spasm in the future, the patient is advised to phonate in a slightly higher pitch than usual and that this be felt in the "mask" region of the face. Feeling in the mask region indicates good resonance balance. Finally, it is always wise to maintain contact with the patient and request follow-up recordings or return visits to monitor the progress of the voice, to provide counsel and voice therapy, as necessary.

Strained Hoarse Voice Arrest–Intermittent Rhythmic Group (SHVA-IR)

Case Study 10.8

A 47-year-old married woman, referred by her family practitioner, complains of a voice disorder that she has had since age 25 years. Until 5 years ago, it was intermittent, but since then it has been persistent. She describes her voice as tremulous. One doctor years ago said she probably had parkinsonism.

The internist's note states that her voice symptoms occurred at first only when she was excited or under stress, but over the years they have become persistent. Tension or stress aggravate her voice disorder. Although not disabling, it is embarrassing.

The patient has had hypertension for 4 years, which is controlled by medication. Her dentition is in poor repair with numerous caries, and she has gingivitis. There is no history of diabetes, hypothyroidism, or any other metabolic disease. Her cardiovascular status is normal. She complains of heartburn once or twice a week. She had a hysterectomy 10 years ago when she was 5 months pregnant. She has had hot flashes for 2 to 3 years, which are not troublesome. She does not take estrogens. She has a mild suprapatellar aching arthralgia when she sits for long periods of time.

The patient divorced her first husband 15 years ago because of physical abuse. Her present marriage is satisfactory. She is employed full-time as an office administrator. She and her husband have four children.

Laryngologic examination fails to disclose laryngeal disease, and the laryngologist thinks her tremulous voice may be "functional" (**Fig. 10.14**). During speech examination, you find a pleasant, mildly obese woman who says her voice disorder was intermittent when it started, but she has become concerned about her voice recently because it has grown worse over the past 3 years. It is now a definite communication problem and interferes with her work as an administrator.

During conversational speech, she has staccato voice arrests. When she sustains the vowel /a/, you hear rhythmic voice arrests of the type heard during contextual speech. You record the vowel prolongation on audiotape and obtain an oscillographic tracing (**Fig. 10.15**). Speech intelligibility is poor owing to the voice arrests. You also

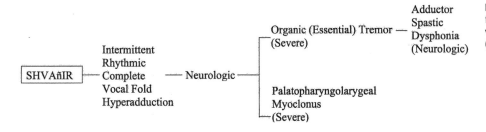

Figure 10.14 Decision making schema for possible causes of Strained hoarse voice arrest-intermittent rhythmic group (SHVA-IR).

notice an almost imperceptible head tremor and possibly tremors around her lips and chin as she speaks, but which are absent when she is silent. Except for her dysphonia, motor speech examination is normal. The patient straightforwardly denies any personal problems during the onset or development of her voice disorder.

Q1: *From the oscillographic tracing, what is the approximate frequency of the patient's voice arrests?*

Q2: *What is the significance of the observation that the patient's voice, head, lips, and chin are tremorous during speech but not during silence?*

Q3: *What could be the connection between the voice arrests and tremor in other parts of her body?*

You schedule a neurologic examination for the patient. This examination confirms the history of the voice disorder and adds other important information: that the patient's legs are beginning to shake and she feels as if her body is getting quivery also. Once or twice a week she chokes while eating, and she thinks she has some quivering of her breathing as well. She has previously been told that her symptoms are "all in her head." The neurologic examination discloses a rapid, forward-backward head tremor, voice tremor, and respiratory tremor. Her hands and feet are quite steady. She has a small-fiber peripheral neuropathy in her legs and mildly decreased reflexes. Her blood pressure is elevated.

The neurologist is the first person to ask the patient about any family history of voice or associated tremors; previous examiners had failed to do so. From this single question emerges the most important information of the entire series of examinations—that tremors in different parts of the body are rampant in the patient's family. The department of genetics produces the pedigree in **Fig. 10.16**. They reported the following data:

♦ The patient's maternal grandmother had tremor of her body and voice.

♦ Her maternal-maternal great grandfather had tremors of his voice, arms, legs, and head.

♦ Her maternal-maternal great aunt had no outward tremor but is said to have "shook inside."

♦ The mother has tremor of her voice and hands, cannot use her hands, and has to be dressed and fed.

♦ One maternal aunt has tremor of her voice and arms and cannot use her hands.

♦ One maternal aunt has tremor of her body, voice, and hands but is able to use her hands.

♦ Two maternal first cousins are said to have voice and general tremor.

♦ Her sister has tremor of her head.

♦ Her brother has tremor of his hands.

♦ One son has a "halting" speech pattern.

Q4: *What is the etiologic diagnosis of this patient's voice disorder?*

Q5: *With what other voice disorders is this one often confused?*

Q6: *How does the physiology of the voice disorder explain the patient's voice tremor and voice arrests?*

Q7: *What relevance is the history that the voice worsens under stress?*

Q8: *What therapy would you suggest for the voice disorder?*

Q9: *How would you counsel a person with this type of voice disorder as to its prognosis?*

Discussion

This patient's voice arrests are momentary laryngospasms produced by intermittent hyperadduction of

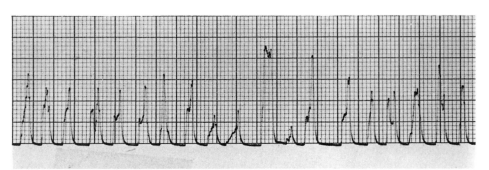

Figure 10.15 Oscillographic tracing of audio recording showing voice arrests produced during vowel /a/ prolongation. Each time the tracing returns to baseline represents no voice, or voice break. 1 second equals 25 mm revealing that arrests occur approximately 4 times/second.

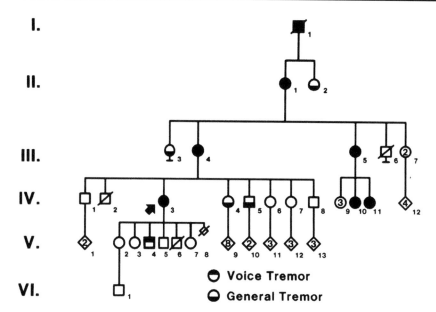

Figure 10.16 Family tree of patient in Case Study 10.8 Strained hoarse voice arrest-itermittent rhythmic group (SHVA-IR) determined to be adductor spasmodic dysphonia of essential (heredofamilial) tremor. The arrow indicates the patient described in the text.

the vocal folds. Their regularity or rhythmicity is more apparent during vowel prolongation than during contextual speech. **Figure 10.15** shows that these arrests occur at a rate of approximately 4 Hz. Rhythmic voice arrests and tremor elsewhere in her body (but only on initiation of movement, not at rest) mean that she has an intention tremor involving her larynx, head, and other body parts. In this particular patient, tremor is present in other members of the patient's family. She qualifies for the diagnosis of essential (heredofamilial) tremor.

Her voice disorder, which some clinicians might have labeled adductor spasmodic dysphonia without qualifications, needs to be further specified as the adductor spasmodic dysphonia of essential tremor, which is to be distinguished from other forms of the disorder. The voice disorder is clearly neurologic and highly resistant to voice or drug therapy though many pharmaceutical agents have been tried with varying degrees of success. At present, the best that can be done for the patient is to educate her as to the etiology of the disorder—many patients are confused about this and are at least relieved to know that it is a recognized neurologic entity and that, although its prognosis is one of continued dysphonia, the disorder is not life-threatening. Education also helps the patient become a better consumer and able to be watchful for development of new and effective treatments. When the adductor spasmodic dysphonia of essential tremor becomes severe enough to threaten speech intelligibility, and not all do, consideration of recurrent laryngeal nerve resection should be given with the understanding that its effects may be temporary. However, experience and clinical studies establish that Botox injection can be highly therapeutic for this disorder, but some patients opt for the nerve resection rather than undergoing Botox injections every 3 or 4 months. Use of amplifiers and/or speaking softly may prolong the effects of botulinum toxin injections.

Voice Tremor Group (VT)

Case Study 10.9

This is a 68-year-old, retired female telephone operator referred by a laryngologist who writes that the patient has a tremor of her voice, that it is "functional," and that voice therapy is recommended. The patient is a heavy smoker and has bilateral polypoid changes on both vocal folds (**Fig. 10.17**).

The patient enters your office, and you notice her right hand shakes as she extends her hand in greeting. For a moment, as you look at her sitting in silence, her head seems to be nodding rhythmically, but her hands rest quietly in her lap. Upon responding to your question as to when her voice trouble began, you hear a coarse, low-pitched, quavering voice. The patient says she has been to several doctors about her voice, which is embarrassing to her. She is apologetic about not heeding her local physician's advice to stop smoking. Recently she was told that her voice was a sign of mild Parkinson's disease. Her voice tremor had begun 8 years ago, so gradually she was hardly aware of it. However, her head tremor began 30 years ago. Her brother, who is 3 years younger, has had head and hand tremor for 4 or 5 years, but his voice is normal.

The voice tremor came on after the extraction of three teeth for pyorrhea. She was given thiopental sodium anesthesia. All went uneventfully. Two weeks after surgery, her teeth were fitted and she had some trouble with her articulation. Six weeks later, a quaver in her voice first appeared. Since then, both the voice and head tremor have gradually worsened. Her tremor is worse when she is tired or upset.

Q1: *What is meant by voice tremor?*

Q2: *What would you expect to see on laryngoscopic examination during vowel prolongation in a patient with voice tremor?*

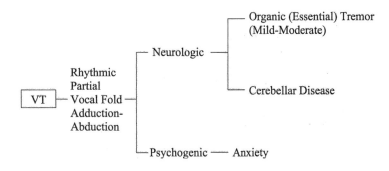

Rhythmic Partial Vocal Fold Adduction-Abduction

VT —

- Neurologic —
  - Organic (Essential) Tremor (Mild-Moderate)
  - Cerebellar Disease
- Psychogenic — Anxiety

Figure 10.17   Flow schema of diagnostic decision making for cases of Vocal tremor group (VT) as illustrated by Case Study 10.9.

Q3: *From the data given, what arguments can you muster in support of the diagnosis of parkinsonism as a cause of the voice tremor?*

Q4: *From the data given, what arguments can be made against parkinsonism as a cause of her dysphonia?*

Q5: *What evidence do we have that the voice tremor is "functional" or psychogenic?*

Q6: *Why does the patient have a low-pitched hoarseness in addition to the tremor?*

An oral-physical and motor speech examination revealed the following information:

♦ The patient's voice tremor on vowel prolongation averaged 5 Hz. The tremor smoothly varied, but occasionally she would produce a complete voice arrest.

♦ Synchronous with the voice tremor were pharyngeal and tongue tremor. Almost unnoticeable were also lip and mandibular tremors.

♦ Although no tremor was noticed when the upper extremities were at rest, the patient had fine hand tremor when she extended her arms with fingers spread.

♦ The patient casually mentioned during this examination that she has used an alcoholic beverage to reduce the severity of her tremors.

Q7: *What formal etiologic diagnosis would you postulate for this voice disorder?*

Q8: *How would you proceed from this point on?*

Suspecting a neurologic etiology, you arrange for the patient to have a neurologic examination, which showed the following:

♦ terminal tremor of both upper extremities

♦ tremor of her head and mandible

♦ mild reduction in sensitivity to touch over the dorsum of both feet

♦ mild incoordination on finger-to-nose testing, bilaterally

♦ mild incoordination on heel-to-knee testing

The neurologist's conclusion from the history and physical examination: "This seems to be a nonspecific tremor—probably of basal nuclear origin and possibly familial. It falls within the scope of organic (essential) tremor or heredofamilial tremor. I doubt that anything is likely to be helpful."

Discussion

Outside of neurologic circles, tremor of the voice is often misdiagnosed as either "functional" or psychogenic or as associated with parkinsonism. On laryngoscopic examination, during vowel prolongation the vocal folds are easily visualized rhythmically adducting and abducting, the pitch rising during adduction and falling during abduction. When severe, the vocal folds will tightly adduct stopping vocal fold self-oscillation, producing voice arrests. If these are pervasive, the voice disorder takes on the characteristics of adductor spasmodic dysphonia.

Parkinsonism does not usually produce voice tremor. In some parkinsonian patients, one can hear a highly subtle tremor like "flutter" on vowel prolongation, but it does not possess the coarser type of tremor as in this patient who has organic (essential) tremor, probably familial. Patients with parkinsonism have tremor, but it is a rest tremor. Essential tremor is an *action* or *intention* tremor.

The patient under discussion was quiescent at rest and exhibited her tremor only during the volitional acts of phonation and extension of her extremities. The student might ask why, then, did she have head tremor at "rest"? The answer is that holding up the head is not actually a resting activity; doing so requires active muscle contraction to overcome the effects of gravity.

Support for psychogenic etiology was unsubstantiated, although stressful events can aggravate and even precipitate tremor, as they do in most neurologic diseases.

The low-pitched hoarseness was consistent with the polypoid changes of the vocal folds secondary to the long history of tobacco abuse and had no relation to the voice tremor.

Alcohol consumption frequently (not always) reduces the amplitude of organic voice tremor and is useful information in diagnostic history-taking.

Management of organic voice tremor is not easy. Symptomatic voice therapy may reduce some of the counterproductive compensatory muscle patterns but is ineffective in eliminating the tremor. No convincing evidence of the effectiveness of essential tremor medications for voice tremor has been reported, even though such medications are often beneficial for tremors elsewhere in the body. Although many patients spontaneously employ alcohol as a palliative for voice tremor, it is hazardous because of its potential for producing dependency.

Educating the patient about the etiology of the voice tremor is more valuable than clinicians may realize. As with many other disorders about which patients have been given an incorrect diagnosis, or none at all, to learn that essential tremor is organic rather than psychogenic, that it is benign, that it does not necessarily have to worsen, and may even improve, and that the dysphonia is common and is acceptable to many listeners can be a genuine relief to patients seeking help for this disorder.

Breathy Whispered Intermittent Group (BW-I)

Case Study 10.10

A 39-year-old clergyman is referred to you by a speech-language pathologist colleague. The patient has had a complete laryngologic examination that failed to disclose any organic laryngeal disease. The referring speech clinician was not experienced in voice disorders and had administered therapy without success. He requests another opinion on diagnosis and treatment of the dysphonia because he is unsure of the diagnosis of abductor or adductor spasmodic dysphonia (**Fig. 10.18**).

The patient, a tall, blond man of striking appearance, has penetrating eye contact and exudes an air of solidity and authority. He is pleasant and straightforward. His language is explicit. He gives the impression of someone who genuinely wants help and will cooperate in any way he can to get it. After completing the preliminaries, he interrupts the examination by asking if his wife could join in the examination, explaining that she has been worried about his voice.

During conversational speech and oral reading of a standard paragraph, you note the following:

♦ Every few seconds, his normal voice cuts out and becomes breathy or whispered. Then, just as suddenly it returns to normal.

♦ These moments of breathiness most often follow unvoiced consonants.

♦ They are more often triggered by plosives than by fricatives.

♦ These plosives are almost invariably unvoiced.

♦ The unvoiced plosives trigger breathiness nearly always when they are in the initial rather than the medial or final positions of words.

♦ The patient can produce several sentences without any segments of breathiness.

♦ During vowel prolongation, his voice is continuously normal (i.e., free of breathy segments).

♦ Each time he produces a moment of breathiness, you notice an abrupt inward movement of his abdomen.

A complete oral-physical and motor-speech examination fails to disclose any evidence of structural or motor disturbances in the remainder of his speech mechanism. The ear, nose, and throat examination is normal. His cough is normally sharp.

You take a careful history. "When and how did your voice disorder begin?" He tells you that it came on 5 years ago very gradually, increasing to its present level of severity within 6 months. It has remained this way ever since. He notices that sometimes his voice is better when he is relaxed and worse when he is under stress, such as while delivering a sermon. He tells you that his voice has never returned to normal for more than a few minutes during the entire history of his voice disorder.

One year after his dysphonia had begun, he sought the help of a speech pathologist who, although not a specialist in voice disorders, agreed to a trial of therapy, because there was no one else available in the patient's locality. For 3 months, twice a week, the patient was given therapies consisting of grunting, chewing, and relaxation exercises associated with biofeedback sessions during which electrodes were placed over his forehead and jaw muscles. These ministrations were mildly and temporarily helpful, but they benefited his voice least when he needed it most, namely, during the counseling and public-speaking

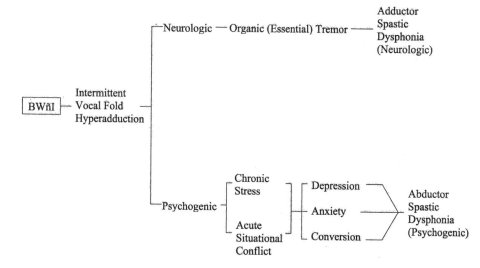

Figure 10.18 Decision making schema for Breathy whispered intermittent Group (BW-I) illustrated by Case Study 10.10 demonstrating abductor spasmodic dysphonia.

demands of his profession. After what he felt was a fair trial of therapy without acceptable results, he broke off further appointments and did nothing about his voice for 3 years.

"Did the speech clinician ever take a history of any psychologic or emotional problems that you might have had at the time your voice disorder started?" The patient answers that he had been asked by the speech-language pathologist some general questions but did not go into any depth; he seemed to emphasize voice retraining over other considerations.

You begin to probe the subject of emotional stress. The patient readily accedes to this line of questioning. You ask him about his relationship with his wife and his professional associates and are comfortable with his responses that indicate (1) he has a stable, amicable relationship with his wife; (2) he is effective and well-respected as a pastor of a small, upper-middle-class suburban community.

"Did anything upsetting happen at the time the voice disorder started 5 years ago?" The following information emerges.

The voice trouble began during a period when their oldest daughter had been arrested for shoplifting. Father and daughter began to have angry "blowups" during which the father was frequently driven to the verge of striking her. The parents tried desperately to help but they had never sought professional assistance.

Commenting on his voice during the height of his conflicts with his daughter, he says: "The more I would yell, the worse my voice would become." During the patient's narrative of this difficult period, his moments of breathy voice are more frequent and of longer duration. Toward the end of his narrative, as he brings the history up to the present, he has fewer and briefer moments of breathiness than at the beginning of the interview.

During trial-and-error therapy, you discover that if the patient makes an effort to sustain voicing during unvoiced consonants, he has fewer and shorter breathy and aphonic breaks.

Q1: *Describe the movements of the vocal folds responsible for the voice aberrations during the patient's contextual speech.*

Q2: *What is the most likely (physiologic phonetic) explanation for the fact that the breathy and aphonic periods are more severe after unvoiced plosive consonants?*

Q3: *Why are the breathy moments less severe or absent in association with unvoiced consonants in medial and final rather than in initial positions of words?*

Q4: *How do you account for the patient's ability to sustain vowel sounds without breathy or aphonic breaks?*

Q5: *What is the most plausible explanation for the abrupt inward abdominal movements simultaneous with moments of breathy voice?*

Q6: *What symptomatic diagnosis would best describe this voice disorder?*

Q7: *What do you think is the etiology of this patient's voice disorder? Support your interpretation.*

Q8: *How would you proceed in the treatment of this patient's voice disorder?*

Discussion

Patients who have alternately normal voice and breathy or aphonic segments during contextual speech may be described as having abductor spasmodic dysphonia. This is a descriptive term only; it tells us nothing about its cause, which requires further investigation. A fiberscopic examination of the vocal folds during contextual speech discloses that each time we hear an aphonic break, we see the vocal folds abduct, and each time we hear a voiced segment, we see them adduct. The sudden inward movement of the patient's abdomen with each aphonic segment occurs because of the sudden drop in vocal fold resistance to the air stream being forced from the lungs by abdominal contractions.

In abductor spasmodic dysphonia, the loss of muscle tension seems to be worsened by unvoiced, as opposed to voiced, consonants, especially voiceless plosives. Apparently, there is some pressure-timing factor that with these phonemes inhibit timely contraction and closure after vowels, and as a result they overshoot, releasing more than the usual amount of air. Their propensity to do so is greatest when the plosives are in the initial positions of words rather than in medial positions, where they are bounded by voiced phonemes, or the final position of words where they are preceded by voiced phonemes. Presumably, that is why vowel prolongations usually contain few or no aphonic breaks; the larynx works less as an articulator and does not require as much in fine motor control adjustments required for connected speech, and vocal folds are adducted and held in a steady state during the entire period of phonation and are not required to shift from voicing to unvoicing and back again.

The psychosocial history strongly points to the probability that this patient's dysphonia is psychogenic, having begun during a period of intense anger and public humiliation brought on by the daughter's antisocial behavior. What is curious is that the dysphonia persists despite resolution of the daughter's difficulties, although the parents still harbor some concern about her. As of this writing, symptomatic voice therapy has not been successful. Although this suggests deeper psychiatric investigation is probably warranted, in cases like this voice therapy should always be tried, and if it fails Botox would be another option. Teaching the patient to voice all consonants may help the patient override the breathy or voiceless segments. The etiology of this patient's voice disorder has not been firmly established and, for the present, must be considered idiopathic.

As a final note, we should be aware that, like adductor spasmodic dysphonia, the abductor type can be of neurologic as well as psychogenic etiology. Two signs of the neurologic type are an absence of a positive psychiatric history and, on vowel prolongation, instead of steady voice, there are rhythmic unvoiced interruptions that may indicate abductor spasmodic dysphonia of essential voice tremor.

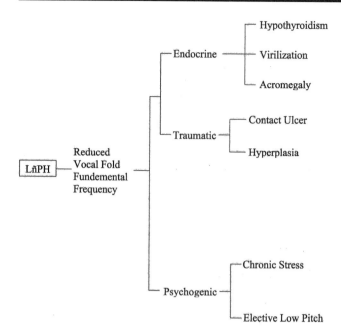

Figure 10.19 Flow chart demonstrating schema of decision making in cases of Low-pitched hoarse group (L-PH) as described for Case Study 10.11.

Low-Pitched Hoarse Group (L-PH)

Case Study 10.11

The following case is that of a 41-year-old professor of English literature with a 5-year history of episodic hoarseness related to lecturing.[2] The hoarseness that brought him to the clinic began 7 months prior to evaluation and coincided with the beginning of a regular teaching schedule and new duties as a curriculum supervisor. Indirect laryngoscopy showed a contact ulcer granuloma on the posterior third of the left vocal cord (**Fig. 10.19**).

Patient (P): Why, I suspect I've had this kind of voice irritation for several years. The last time I had an examination of the larynx was, I think, about 5 years ago, and there was some irritation there but no growth. It has just been this fall that I, as I said, had the laryngitis, at least that's what I call it. I was concerned about it and sinus headaches and so forth. But it was the hoarseness and the irritation and the voice loss that concerned me most, and I work hard at teaching. I move around a lot, I push myself. My style is a kind of Socratic, excited, let's-move-ideas-around kind of style, and I work hard at it, and I force, I know I push my voice. I'm pushing it. I don't sit quietly and let my voice assert itself. When I lecture, particularly in a larger group, and I've had classes of 35 and 40 and 50, I tend to really move out, and I do know that I push my voice beyond its, certainly its normal speech level.

Clinician (C): In terms of loudness?

P: In terms, I think, of volume.

C: Volume. That's what I meant. How about pitch? Do you think you strive for a low-pitched voice, consciously or unconsciously?

P: I don't know. I may do that. I don't know. I may push toward a lower voice range or frequency. I don't know why I might do that. Generally, I'm not conscious of it. I may be doing it and not be conscious of it.

C: Can you think of any ideas as to why you might be pushing for a lower frequency or a lower pitch?

P: Oh, I don't know. I suspect it might be more comfortable in a higher range.

C: Any other thoughts come to mind?

P: I don't know whether I feel this is more impressive, if I'm doing this because I think it's more impressive.

C: There's a possibility that that may be true?

P: I can't isolate that.

C: It's a possibility, but not necessarily true.

P: I know that when I can start speaking in Norwegian I can allow a kind of higher range that's easier.

C: It's easier to speak at a higher pitch?

P: Well, it is when I go into a different language.

C: How about in English; think you should go into a higher pitch?

P: I don't know, but it seems to be a little easier and I seem to be pushing it. I seem to be speaking farther forward or getting the vibration farther forward in my head or something. It does hurt more, like when I drop down now, as opposed to speaking maybe up like this.

C: Do you lecture in a large room?

P: Yes, I have.

C: Are the acoustics good or bad?

P: They vary tremendously; generally speaking, they're not very good.

C: Why is that? What is the nature of the acoustics?

P: Just flat. There is a sense that you have to really get up and project. Most of my colleagues have mentioned this, too. I don't think students could really hear you in the back, you know, if I sat and talked as I'm talking now, for example. Even if it were very quiet, some of the students in the back row simply couldn't hear me in those rooms. I have to push more than I'm pushing right now with my voice. I move toward them. I've done everything I can spatially to get close to them, at least in physical proximity. I do think that right now I can feel a little irritation and hoarseness.

C: How about noise levels, background noise levels, as you're trying to lecture?

P: It's very quiet. I've never had a problem with that. I suspect it might be in secondary education, but certainly there's none. I think I am nervous. I'm always overprepared. I'm always very anxious about doing well. I always have, so that I feel very satisfied, and I've always had good responses, but I've had to work hard at it, and I sweat a lot. I know I'm working hard. I'm in there, I get ready for the class, I prepare very carefully, I plan courses very carefully. I work with them very carefully, so I suspect that I am nervous about class.

C: Now, how will your voice fare during the course of, say a 50-minute lecture, when you are in this particular

---

[2]An actual audio recording of the transcription of the following interview can be heard in Aronson, A.E. (1973). *Audio seminars in speech pathology, psychogenic voice disorders*. Philadelphia, PA: W.B. Saunders. Cassette no. 1, side 1.

mood and you have this degree of tension or anxiety? Will it last or not?

P: It will last, but I feel the strain will last 10 minutes or so. In fact, there will be a more pronounced hoarseness. I can feel the tightening. On the other hand, well I suspect that no matter whether I'm using the Socratic method or not, or just moving into a kind of casual, easy going kind of dialogue of some kind, that the differences are a difference of degree, and in those instances I feel the strain and tightening.

C: Will that tightening also be accompanied by, say, a dull aching in your larynx?

P: You're asking me to become conscious of things I haven't really paid much attention to, and I'm always a little suspicious of my own recall and my own awareness of my physiologic processes, but I think that's true. And I think there is even a tendency to bring about some sort of headache, a little bit of a headache from it. That is, I can feel irritation here starting to bring about a headache reaction . . . But it's never been easy for me to talk. I was always very quiet when I was younger, and through my whole career as a teacher I've worked hard to project, to get away from this. I was fairly introverted and quiet, and I've always had the feeling that other people have had stronger voices, that I have not had a particularly strong voice. But, as I said, I can always remember this kind of, this tendency toward this, this hoarseness, and when I talked for a long time or lectured, I taught high school for 4 years, and I had 5 hours of class a day, I would be darn sore at the end of the day. I would tend to become very quiet and my wife would say that I would, for the rest of the day, speak very, very quietly if I could.

C: Would you feel sort of worn out in general from talking, sort of fatigued?

P: From that more than anything else. Just the physical business of talking. Not the classroom dynamics or anything like that. It was just talking. It has never been particularly easy for me. And I'm in a profession where that's the medium, you see, that's the demand.

Q1: *What is the physical explanation behind the excessively low pitch of this patient's voice?*

Q2: *What is the reason for the contact ulcer being located at the posterior third of the vocal fold?*

Q3: *What is the contribution of the patient's artificially lowering his pitch to his voice disorder, and what would you predict the stroboscopic image would look like?*

Q4: *What might be the causes of the patient's complaint of tightness and dull aching in his throat?*

Q5: *Comment on the relative contributions of vocal abuse, personality, and emotional stress to the development of this patient's voice disorder.*

Discussion

This patient has a poor acoustic working environment coupled with poor vocal technique of long-standing dura-

tion. It is likely that he uses excessive muscle tension to artificially lower and to project his voice resulting in some discomfort. The tightness and dull aching in the throat may emanate from a combination of muscle tension, contact ulcers, and tissue irritation from reflux. Some clinicians would choose to directly observe the patient teaching or ask him to bring in a videotape of his teaching in a large classroom to determine how his teaching voice differs from his conversational speech. As in most other disorders, it is also likely that emotional stress increases his vocal difficulties and lowering his pitch may increase his adduction quotient, the amount of time in which glottal cycle vocal folds are closed relative to the time opened, increasing the probability of tissue damage. You would predict his videostroboscopic examination would show anterior-posterior and medial-lateral constrictions of the supraglottis and a long closed phase similar to that seen during glottal fry. Both amplitude and mucosal wave would be severely reduced but the tissue of the membranous portion would appear during inspiratory phonation to be pliable. Contact ulcers generally occur on the posterior third of the glottal margin at the vocal process where the vocal fold tissue is its thinnest.[3] Approximately 80% of males close this portion of the glottis whereas most females have a posterior glottic chink. This suggests one of the reasons contact ulcers are seen in males but rarely occur in females who have not experienced intubation trauma. Contact ulcers are difficult to treat but generally benefit from voice therapy combined with a strong antireflux regimen. Surgical removal without concomitant behavioral and medical management often results in recurrence. Behavioral modification is generally directed at improving vocal fold vibratory patterns by finding appropriate pitch, reducing posterior glottic closure and hard glottal attacks, improving vocal projection, and, when necessary, using amplification.

High-Pitched Group (HP)

Case Study 10.12

A 23-year-old college student comes to the clinic complaining of general fatigue. She has a history of mononucleosis. Six months ago, she noticed a drooping of her left eyelid that was diagnosed elsewhere as a sign of myasthenia gravis. However, a Tensilon test was negative. During the neurologic history, she does not complain of difficulty chewing or swallowing, double vision, or limb weakness; in fact, she says she runs 3 miles a day. Her neurologic examination is normal; however, her history of left ptosis leads the neurologist to conclude that she does have ocular myasthenia that is currently asymptomatic. After discussing the pros and cons of continuing her medication, she is referred for evaluation of an accompanying speech disorder.

---

[3]Contact ulcers havc been attributed to esophageal reflux, intubation, and vocal trauma.

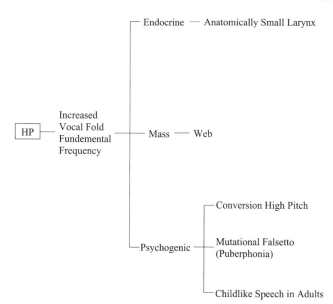

Figure 10.20   The High-pitched group [HP] schema demonstrates the possible causes of increased vocal fold fundamental frequency exhibited by the patient described in Case Study 10.12.

The patient enters your office casually dressed and looking younger than her 23 years. From the moment she speaks, you are startled by her high-pitched, though not falsetto, voice and the way in which she articulates with a slight pursing of her lips and a subtle interdental lisp. Her prosody is that of exaggerated pitch changes. Her speech gives you the uncomfortable feeling that you are talking with a child rather than an adult college student.

She says her speech began to change about 4 years ago. Two years ago, an otolaryngologist said she had a high voice because her larynx was too small. Laryngologic examination here mentions nothing about an abnormally small larynx (**Fig. 10.20**).

Q1: *How do these speech signs relate to myasthenia gravis?*

Q2: *What further tests would you recommend to determine if her speech had anything to do with that disease?*

Q3: *What are the cardinal speech signs of myasthenia gravis?*

Testing her speech musculature fails to disclose any evidence of lip, tongue, mandibular, laryngeal, or respiratory weakness. The all-important stress test of counting fails to produce deterioration of her speech. Her cough is normally sharp. You can find no signs of motor-speech disorder. She can lower her pitch level on demand, but she does not maintain it during conversation speech.

Q4: *What would be the next step in your investigation?*

The psychosocial history discloses that between the ages of 10 and 17, the patient and both of her parents were alcoholic. She gives a history of physical abuse and psychotherapy on and off since age 13. She says she is just beginning to get hold of her problems with the help of a school counselor. Asked if she would like to have help with her speech, she replies that, for the time being, she would prefer not to

because "My voice is me. I don't have a problem; my problem is that other people have a problem with my voice."

Q5: *What do you think is the diagnosis of this person's speech disorder?*

Q6: *How would you proceed in handling this case?*

Discussion

This is an instance of the relatively rare psychogenic disorder known as childlike speech in adults. Technically, it is not solely a voice disorder, as articulation is integral to the total syndrome. It bears many of the features of conversion disorder in that the patient's abnormal use of the speech musculature is unconsciously determined, that the childlike speech "selected" serves to communicate something very important about the self, and that the disorder probably affords the patient primary or secondary gain in her daily life. The prior diagnosis of an abnormally small larynx was presumptive; the speech examination proved she was capable of producing a lower pitch appropriate to her age and sex. Nothing in her speech remotely resembled the flaccid dysarthria of myasthenia gravis with its breathy, weak voice, hypernasality, and consonant imprecision that worsen during effortful speaking. Her myasthenia gravis, limited to her ptosis, was completely independent of her speech disorder.

This patient was adamant in her rejection of our offer of speech therapy; in fact, her insight was so poor that she did not even think her speech was abnormal; recall her conclusion was that the problem was other peoples', not hers. Her denial that her speech was abnormal, also common in conversion reaction, and her rejection of help for the "symptom" require respect, for this patient is telling us that she is not ready to relinquish the protection afforded by her childlike speech. Her frankness in disclosing seriously damaging childhood experiences and her acknowledgment that she needs, and is getting, counseling probably indicate that she may one day be well enough to be able to give up her inappropriate speech and return to a normal speech pattern that she once had. We wished her well and sent her on her way.

♦ Summary

♦ In actual clinical practice, differential diagnosis of a voice disorder begins with categorizing the abnormal voice and then working backward to its etiology by means of logical correlation with laryngologic, psychologic, physical, and neurologic evidence.

♦ Abnormal voices tend to cluster into perceptual groups, but diagnosis cannot be made by voice alone.

♦ Although the voices within these "clusters" may sound similar, they can arise from mass lesions, neurologic diseases, medical conditions, vocal misuse, or psychologic disorders, which can only be determined by further clinical studies.

- Interaction between organic and psychogenic factors must be borne in mind in the assessment of all voice disorders.

- Patients may have two, or more, coexisting problems that are independent.

- Regardless of the primary etiology, patients may have comorbid factors that contribute, if not to the etiology, to the maintenance of the voice problem.`

Chapter 11

Treatment of Voice Disorders

Voice therapy may be defined as an effort to return the voice to a level of adequacy that can be realistically achieved and that will satisfy the patient's occupational, emotional, and social needs. Not everyone, especially not those who have irreversible neurologic or vocal fold lesions, can achieve a normal voice. In such cases, the objective is the best possible voice within the patient's anatomic and physiologic capabilities. It is to the credit of most patients that they understand and accept their voice limitations.

Some voice disorders are so mild that one has difficulty deciding if an abnormal voice actually exists—though it makes it no less significant to the patient as in cases of professional voice users where a mild voice disturbance can cause maximum distress and loss of income. In some instances, the voice disturbance may only exist in the singing voice, or after a strenuous day of talking, or during periods of emotional stress, or may be related less to the voice than to increased vocal effort. In other cases, the voice problem may be severe but the patient may be unaware of or unconcerned about the voice but very concerned about vocal fatigue. Who, finally, is to decide if voice therapy is necessary? Ultimately, it is a team decision, and the patient is a critical member of the team. If a reasonable effort has been made to increase awareness of voice potential, but therapy is declined, such is the patient's right. Where children are concerned, the clinician will usually try more aggressively to obtain the child's cooperation, with the consent of the parents. With experience, clinicians learn that not everyone needs to be helped, can be helped, or wishes to be helped. However, for those who can be helped and are motivated to change, the therapeutic process can result in an improved voice and quality of life.

◆ General Principles

General principles and methods of behavioral voice therapy are continuously evolving. The literature advocates different techniques for the same disorder, and useful therapies have yet to be developed for many disorders. Capable clinicians sometimes are at a loss to say exactly what they do to bring about voice improvement. Reading the literature on voice therapy produces uncertainty as to who is right and which alternatives work because there are limited evidence-based references available. Underneath all of the apparent alternatives, however, lie some common principles.

Remove Obstacles

Progression from abnormal to normal voice takes place as a product of the patient's conscious, volitional response to the clinician's instruction and encouragement. Yet, at the same time the larynx has a natural propensity toward normal function in nonorganic disorders. There is a sense one has about therapy for nonorganic voice disorders that, rather than the need to teach the patient how to use voice again, the clinician's task is to remove obstacles to normal laryngeal function and, by so doing, allow the natural inclination for normal voice to break through. Humans do not have to be taught how to phonate in the first place. There is no reason to believe that our capacity for normal voice does not exist throughout life, though clinicians need be mindful that "normal voice" differs across the age span.

Provide Feedback

Feedback occupies a pivotal position in voice therapy, cutting across all voice disorders. Individual learners respond in different ways to tactile, proprioceptive, visual, and auditory feedback.

Look for Emotional Distress

Voice disorders resulting from emotional stress ought not be treated as only mechanical problems. Consideration of the patient's self-concept, daily life problems, and dysphoric affect ideally is incorporated into therapy. On the other hand, although treating the cause of a voice disorder may be as important as voice production training, the cause may either never be found, may be unalterable, or may be beyond the scope of practice of the treating speech-language pathologist.

Offer Individual Therapy

Voice therapy has to be tailored to the individual. Although the fundamental principle of therapy for a given disorder does not vary, differences in age, gender, hearing, acquisition to feedback, vocal awareness, motivation, intelligence, education, culture, occupation, vocal needs, and general health require that techniques be modified to suit these variables. Thus, voice therapy is individually tailored to each individual.

◆ Specific Principles

For many years, the notion has been fostered that voice disorders follow the same laws of learning as do, for example, articulatory or language disorders, and, as such, are treated in the same way by applying those laws to the larynx and voice. Whereas traditional learning does have application in voice therapy (e.g., practice, targeting, trial-and-error, and the like), special facts about the larynx and voice that do not apply to articulation and language need to be recognized.

Phonation

Phonation is built into the organism as an innate neurophysiologic function. It is not "learned" in the same sense as is articulation or language. The source of sound is the larynx, which also serves sometimes competing functions of airway control, swallowing, laughter, and crying.

Organic Disorders

In organic disorders caused by vibratory disturbances resulting from vocal fold mass lesions or neurologic disorders of paralysis or movement, the main principles of therapy are either muscle strengthening, or reducing force of closure, or improving resonance balance and vocal tract coordination, or adaptation to the mechanical problems by means of positive compensatory phonatory and respiratory maneuvers.

Behavioral Voice Disorders

Behavioral voice disorders, disorders of misuse, abuse, or compensation, exist for one or more of the following reasons and often exist in combination with organic problems. They can occur at the level of the vocal folds or occur at the supraglottic level resulting in resonance imbalance. They may or may not have the presence of a lesion. They may or may not be related to vocal use, vocal environment, or occupation.

Hyperfunctional Voice Disorders

The vocal folds are adducted with excessive force for a variety of reasons including general laryngeal muscle tension as a reaction to the stress of life (e.g., acute or chronic depression or anxiety or excess vocal loading related to occupational or recreational needs) or because of personality traits or to compensate for underlying pathology. These are called hyperfunctional or musculoskeletal tension voice disorders. They are treated primarily according to the principle that when the muscular tension is reduced, the larynx's capacity for normal phonation will normally return *if* the tension is not compensatory. Koufman and Belafsky (2002) state that, "As many as 90% of patients with abnormal laryngeal biomechanics have an underlying organic disorder and are not simply vocal misuse, poor technique or abuse." Based on a prospective analysis of 2000 consecutive patients seen at the Center for Voice Disorders of Wake Forest University School of Medicine, they developed a multifactorial model of voice disorders (the B.I.N.N. [behavioral, inflammatory, neuromuscular, neoplastic] model) and, based on their data, suggest that the average patient with a voice disorder has two or more diagnoses. Typically these are behavioral (90%), inflammatory (70%), neuromuscular (30%), and neoplastic (20%). This is interpreted to mean that most voice disorders have a behavioral component, but it is often not the entire source of the problem. Thus, modifying vocal tension may optimize laryngeal biomechanics or reveal the underlying problem. Voice therapy, then, aims at releasing the inherently normal voice suppressed by excess muscular tension, an objective that can be accomplished in three complementary ways:

◆ by mechanically (manually) relaxing the musculature

◆ by psychologically releasing the anxiety causing the tension

◆ by creating improved aerodynamic muscular balance within the vocal tract

The vocal folds may fail to adduct (hypoadduct) because they are muscularly flaccid or flabby due to nonuse or incomplete use or change in feedback. These are called hypofunctional voice disorders and when behavioral in origin are usually secondary to prolonged use of a weak breathy voice, prolonged illness, prolonged voice rest, faulty learning, or age. Behaviorally, these disorders are treated primarily according to the principle of increasing the tonicity of the vocal folds by means of their full employment during phonation.

Conversion Voice Disorders

The vocal folds fail to adduct because, unconsciously, the patient has a need to be partially or completely without voice. These are the conversion voice disorders. The original loss or diminution of the voice produces three secondary effects:

Patient Can't Produce Normal Voice   Soon after the aphonia or dysphonia sets in, the patient loses the feel for how to produce normal voice, a dissociative-type reaction that persists even after the interpersonal or situational conflict causing the voice disorder has been resolved.

Elevated Musculoskeletal Tension Conversion voice disorders are not as passive as their whispering and breathiness suggest but are actually produced with elevated musculoskeletal tension. In other words, they contain within them a hyperfunctional component involving a variety of combinations of muscles of the larynx.

The conversion voice disorders are primarily treated with behavioral therapies directed at exposing and, if possible, resolving the interpersonal or situational conflicts causing them, educating and physically guiding the patient into increasing degrees of phonation, and balancing musculoskeletal tension.

Voice Abuse Disorders

Cultural, personality, and emotional factors can lead to phonation with excessively sharp glottal attack or long closed phase, which traumatizes the vocal fold mucosa, producing general inflammation or discrete lesions. These are the vocal abuse disorders. Excess musculoskeletal tension is often a component of vocal abuse disorders. They are treated according to the principle of reducing habits of hard glottal attack, excessive loudness, environmental stress, and personality problems.

Precipitating Factors

Internal and external environmental factors can lead to tissue irritation that combined with excessive vocal loading leads to vocal fold trauma. These are called precipitating factors and include laryngeal esophageal reflux disease, poor hydration, exposure to pollutants, and upper respiratory infections. They are treated according to the principle that changing lifestyle, modifying environment, or receiving medical treatment will reduce or eliminate the offending factors.

Occupational and social factors can lead to excess talk time, loudness, or pitch that can lead to vocal abuse. These are called aggravating factors and are treated according to the principle that increased awareness will reduce or eliminate the aggravators and improve voice.

Lesion

The vocal folds may fail to completely adduct because of the presence of a lesion. Some of these lesions resolve with voice therapy aimed at reducing precipitating and aggravating factors along with direct symptom management. Others require surgical management or a combination of surgical and voice therapy.

◆ General Voice Therapy

Voice therapy is performed on two planes: (1) a specific one in which techniques are tailored to the requirements of a

specific voice disorder type, and (2) a general one, composed of generally applicable methods. Both planes are interwoven in voice therapy, their proportions determined by the patient's requirements and the clinician's knowledge of treatment.

Evidence-Based Medicine

No introduction to voice therapy approaches would be complete without a concomitant discussion of evidence-based medicine. As in other areas of medicine, many treatments in common use have never been evaluated (Frattali, 1998). Increasingly, insurance companies, referral sources, and patients want "evidence-based" treatment. Although most realize there is never a treatment guarantee, they want to know what outcome can be expected for a given treatment and how long it will take to achieve it. Frattali lists five primary outcomes and example factors that relate to voice therapy: (1) clinically derived outcomes (e.g., ability to sustain phonation or produce a lower pitch); (2) functional outcomes (e.g., ability to use the telephone or be heard in a noisy environment); (3) financial outcomes (e.g., cost-effective care, average number of sessions); (4) social outcomes (e.g., employability, ability to interact with others); and (5) patient-defined outcomes (e.g., satisfaction with services and quality of life). Treatment outcome research has a hierarchy ranging from the highest level of experimental, or class I, classification to the lowest level of nonexperimental, or class III, classification. Class I includes randomized controlled clinical trials and time series research, whereas class III has no clear comparison groups and includes case studies or reports, registries and databases, and group judgments or expert opinion. According to Fratalli, "Traditional thinking in the medical field reserves randomized controlled clinical trials as the only accepted method of experimental research—a position refuted by clinical researchers who employ small-group or single-subject designs." Verdolini, Ramig, and Jacobson (1998) organized by decade more than 100 voice therapy articles. Few of the articles were class I, but they derived six conclusions about the benefits and success of treatment:

♦ Functional aphonias may benefit from facilatory, vegetative voicing maneuvers.

♦ Some types of intensive therapies benefit voice problems related to Parkinson's disease.

♦ Conventional voice therapy may provide a protective effect against recurrence.

♦ Conventional voice therapy and resonant voice therapy may produce benefits in treatment of nodules.

♦ Intensive hydration treatments may be beneficial in treatment of nodules.

♦ Hyperfunctional voice disorders may benefit from systematic electromyography (EMG) or laryngeal relaxation training.

The conclusions reached from Verdolini and colleagues' scholarly literature review does not mean treatments not listed are not effective. Rather, it suggests that at the time of their review, we did not have evidence of the efficacy of the other techniques. In this chapter, we do not limit techniques to those that are evidence-based because too many of the techniques commonly used do not have class I or II outcomes and would have to be omitted. Rather, we provide an overview of the major techniques and methods described by experienced clinicians providing their expert opinion (class III). Some of these methods also have case reports but few have randomized controlled clinical trials.

Auditory Training

Voice lacks finite acoustic boundaries. A mildly defective voice can become incorporated into the self without much notice, especially in children, whose concerns over its social acceptability are minimal. Even in severe voice disorders, the person may be upset over the voice but has long forgotten the sound of the normal voice and, therefore, any notion of how it ought to sound again.

For these reasons, direct or indirect auditory training, defined as teaching the identification of and discrimination among different voices, is part of most voice therapy. Auditory training may simply be heightening a patient's awareness of differences between normal and defective voices without directly discussing the differences. It can be indirect auditory feedback indicating when a patient hits or falls short of the target voice. In direct auditory training, the underlying assumption is that before a better voice can be achieved, the person has to know how his or her voice sounds. This assumes that patients of all ages need to hear the differences between normal and defective voices before they can produce a normal voice. After comparing other voices with their own, they discuss those differences with the clinician. In the not too distant past, *ear training* was the initial prescribed phase of voice therapy. Ear training included listening to *special sounds* such as clock ticking and car horns, tapping or clapping in imitation of a sound pattern, differentiating between sound pairs of /m-n-n-n-m/ versus /n-n-n-m-n-n-n/, comparing doorbells with car horns or telephone rings, and listening to "good" and "bad" voice. This still may be useful in helping direct children's attention to sound production but generally is not necessary in working with adults.

Whether auditory training is direct or indirect, of major importance is instantaneous auditory feedback. What is singular about voice therapy is that in the early, critical stages, improved voice will break through suddenly and momentarily, milliseconds in duration; although the clinician may hear and identify these gains, the patient usually does not. Consequently, the clinician needs to listen carefully and, when the voice changes, for the better or worse, communicate that change instantaneously to the patient. Initially, this instant feedback ("That's it," "Too high," "Too low") may come with each change or attempt to hit a target voice. Once the patient understands the target and can detect the change, the clinician's feedback is quickly faded.

Respiratory Control

If expiratory air volume is patently insufficient because of neurologic weakness or incoordination, vocal loudness and steadiness will suffer. In such cases, improving a patient's ability to produce a constant pressure by increasing lung volumes available for voice and control of smoother exhalation may be desirable ends. However, often for voice patients, respiration is anatomically and physiologically normal. Abnormal breathing patterns may be due to poor habits or posture, anxiety and tension, paradoxical vocal fold dysfunction, or poor coordination or lack of respiratory support that is often related to neurologic disease. These abnormal breathing patterns frequently result in failing to provide sufficient breath support for optimum voice. Abdominal breathing, often misrepresented as diaphragmatic breathing, affords the greatest lung volumes. Cooper and Cooper (1977) enhance abdominal awareness and breathing coordination to encourage maximum support giving the following advice.

Lying supine, the patient is asked to:

♦ Place one hand on the chest and the other on the abdomen.

♦ Inhale easily through the nose and exhale through the mouth, concentrating on inflating and deflating the abdomen but not the chest.

♦ Inhale quickly through the mouth only and exhale gradually, using the same abdominal breathing method just described.

Sitting, and then standing, the patient is asked to repeat numbers (1) to (3), incorporating the abdominal breathing into phonation at proper pitch and loudness levels.

Gravitational forces and consequent work of the abdominal muscles are different for the supine posture compared with sitting and standing (Hoit, 1995). Thus, the supine position because of the work against the weight of the abdominal contents enhances awareness, and the upright postures help transfer the breathing patterns to phonation. Some clinicians take the supine step a bit further by placing a book on the abdomen and/or by using a mirror or online video recording to aid the patient in observing his or her abdominal movements.

For development of abdominal-intercostal breathing coordinated with phonation, Greene (1972) advocates the following method:

♦ Breathe in slowly and then out, counting in a quiet voice up to 4 and then gradually increasing the count at a rate of one per second. No breath should escape between each count.

♦ Inhale deeply, and, keeping the ribs elevated, count to 15, gradually letting the ribs descend between the count of 15 and 20.

♦ Inhale and, on exhalation, sustain /s/ or /f/ steadily, trying not to let it fluctuate or fade toward the end. Feel the gradual contraction of the abdominal wall as breath is exhaled.

♦ Repeat this, except with a crescendo and diminuendo or in different rhythmic patterns.

For reinforcing the proper respiratory rhythm for speech, she instructs the patient to:

- Breathe in and out slowly several times and then imitate the clinician's rapid intake and slow exhalation. The abdomen should jump forward on inhalation and subside gradually on exhalation.

- Inhale quickly and exhale slowly, counting to 6. Gradually increase the count on exhalation to 20.

Accent Method

The Accent Method, developed by Svend Smith of Denmark more than 50 years ago (Dalhoff and Kitzing, 1989; Smith and Thyme, 1976; Thyme-Frokjaer and Frokjaer, 1987, Thyme-Frokjaer, 1998) is a holistic method that relies heavily on changing abdominal support for voice and incorporates paced rhythmic movements into new motor speech breathing patterns. Based on aerodynamic principles of phonation, Smith incorporated abdominal accents and open airway into speech breathing to facilitate easy clear phonation with appropriate resonance balance. This programmatic method refocuses voice production from the larynx to the abdomen and promotes free open flow of air through the vocal tract. Several studies have documented the changes that take place as a result of this treatment program. Thyme-Frokjaer and Frokjaer have documented that breathy untrained voices achieve a longer glottal closure and creaky untrained voices achieve a shorter glottal closure suggesting that phonatory function has been normalized. They have also demonstrated acoustic changes: energy is increased in the F2 and F3 regions; irregular pitch disturbances are reduced; and variations in voice timbre are increased. Similarly, Kotby, Shiromoto, and Hirano (1993) have documented increased airflow, reduction in lesions, and improved voice in individuals with functional voice disorders and in individuals with mass lesions. Bassiouny (1998) demonstrated significantly better results for voice-disordered patients who had Accent therapy combined with vocal hygiene than for those who had vocal hygiene alone. She attributes the better intervention results to the holistic approach of the Accent Method. Verdolini (1998) suggests its effectiveness may be related to training new motor patterns. She reasons that because timing is fundamental to the development of skilled behavior, the Accent Method's emphasis on timing and rhythmic movements of the body may facilitate new motor programs.

There are four major stages in the Accent technique, which is also coupled with individually tailored vocal hygiene programs. The training stages are supine; sitting; standing; and carry-over. The training stages include accentuated phonatory pulsations on both voiced and voiceless sounds and reading of special texts that help facilitate patient awareness of differences between accentuated and unaccentuated contexts. As originally conceived, the program took 30 or more sessions, which is generally impractical for functional voice disorders being treated in today's clinics located in the United States and has been modified accordingly. The respiratory training is designed to produce a dominant abdominal respiration pattern. Exercises of accentuated phonatory pulsations, often done in response to drumbeats, are used to help the patient become aware of accent patterns. Like the respiratory training of Cooper and Cooper (1977), the Accent treatment program begins in the supine position with hands placed on the abdomen. The patient is asked to take in a deep breath and breathe out slowly against slightly pursed lips in imitation of the clinician producing distinct rhythmic accented breath pulses. The clinician initially uses hand motions to direct the patient when air should be flowing into or out of the body simulating the pattern modeled by the clinician. Both length and speed of exhalations are varied between 2 and 6 seconds. Once the patient has accomplished this slow inhalation/exhalation breathing pattern, slow accented beats are added. With each beat, the patient gives a punch, or stress, to the exhaled air using the abdominal muscles. No sound is added until the patient can stress to the beat on voiceless exhalation. This rhythmic movement is repeated using /s/ /S/ /f/. The beats may be changed from the slow and broad largo to fairly slow andante and then the more rapid allegro. The next step returns back to the slower beat and adds voiced continuants /z/ /dz/ /v/ produced in a light rhythmic manner. This sequence is then repeated in a sitting position. One of the patient's hands is placed on the chest and the other on the abdomen to continue making him or her aware of the role of the abdominal muscles and chest-wall movement patterns. Nonsense syllables and inflection patterns are gradually added. The training sequence is repeated with the clinician and patient standing and adding body movements swaying to and fro and slighting swinging relaxed arms. If at any point the patient fails, the clinician goes back to earlier successful steps before proceeding. Up until the point the new breath support pattern is to be incorporated into conversation, the patient's task is always to imitate the clinician to the beat presented. Clinicians who favor this technique generally use bongo drums to provide the target beats. To learn this technique, clinicians generally need to practice with an experienced clinician or audio or video samples (Khidr, 2005; Khidr, Lantz, and Senatore, 2005; Kotby, 1991; Kotby, Shiromoto, and Hirano, 1993; Thyme-Frokjaer and Frokjaer, 2001, Kotby, 1995).

Davenport and Sapienza (2004) suggest that the term *breathing exercises* encompasses a broad spectrum of treatments, ranging from relaxation exercises to music therapy, which may be taught in a mystic manner with few physiologic guidelines. They state that although the validity of these exercises has not been verified, the successful techniques "may work by facilitating production of the voice at higher lung volumes or by taking advantage of the appropriate gravitational effects that direct breathing in an expiratory direction."

After many years of experience administering voice therapy and attempting to deal with problems of respiration that often accompany voice disorders, Boone (1988) has taken a more conservative stand on its relative importance in voice therapy, although he continues to believe in the importance of modifying respiration in voice disorders. For the patient who demonstrates faulty respiratory patterns, he believes that some modification of respiration for speech is important, using feedback and patient education about optimum respiratory actions. However, over the years, he has observed that many patients develop overconcern about how they are breathing, and their attention to the breathing process has actually interfered with a smooth and easy respiratory style, often increasing their laryngeal tension.

Our thesis might well be that we best alter respiratory patterns by working to extend expiratory control, matching target models, and learning how effortlessly to renew breath. The best technique for altering respiratory patterns, or the degree to which this is necessary to bring about best voice, has not been determined.

Relaxation

Relaxation as an adjunct to voice therapy is commonly advocated to combat excessive musculoskeletal tension. A plethora of descriptions of voice therapy techniques suggest that a more relaxed means of phonation is a primary goal. Relaxation as a primary or augmentative technique is exemplified by the progressive relaxation techniques of Jacobson (1938, 1964, 1976) and McClosky (1977). These techniques try to teach recognition of the difference between feelings associated with muscular tension and those associated with relaxation by having the patient alternately contract and relax head, neck, thoracic, and abdominal muscles. Biofeedback methods have also achieved relaxation, with the patient auditorily and visually monitoring the degree of muscle tension of the face and neck.

Another technique designed specifically to facilitate relaxation of the laryngeal, pharyngeal, and oral structures is chewing. The chewing method of speech muscle relaxation (Froeschels, 1952) is based on the theory that chewing, being a primitive, reflex-like, semiautomatic function, relaxes the lingual, mandibular, hyoid, and laryngeal musculature. The method advocates phonation while performing chewing or munching movements with the tongue and jaw. The progression of steps includes heightening awareness of chewing movements while chewing on a bland cookie or cracker, chewing silently like a savage with exaggerated mouth and tongue movements, adding vowels while chewing, speaking nonsense words while chewing, speaking short meaningful phrases while chewing, and finally carrying the relaxed, improved movements into conversation. This chewing progression often involves mirror work to help emphasize the importance of increased orality. Its value may be limited in patients who are embarrassed by the unusual nature of this therapy.

Yawn-Sigh

Boone and McFarlane (1993) advocate using yawning to open the inlet to the larynx and promote relaxation of the pharynx. The technique is simple to execute. Clinicians simply instruct the patient to yawn and then exhale with a long, breathy sigh. This technique helps patients contrast a hyperfunctional constricted airway with one that is more open. Xu, Ikeda, and Komiyama (1991) used respiratory kinematic sensors to provide biofeedback of a yawning breath pattern (YBP) to 91 voice-disordered patients. They reported significantly better results on voice tests and subjective evaluations for those patients who had the ability to master the YBP. Recent research has demonstrated that yawning has a physiologic basis that promotes relaxation. Yawning is induced by dopamine receptor agonists.

Tone Focus

Deeply ingrained in the history of therapy for voice disorders is the concept of optimum pitch (i.e., that there is a pitch level best suited to the supraglottic resonators that produces the most resonant voice with the least physical effort), located approximately one-fourth of the total pitch range from the bottom (Fairbanks, 1960). Whereas there is little doubt that balance of resonance and range are disturbed in virtually all voice disorders, it is not necessary to make a point of finding a correct pitch level and purposefully teaching it to the individual. In fact, one might argue that clinicians would be misguided to search for a single optimal pitch and rather should work to produce a *tone focus* that is a balance of resonance across the patient's pitch range. Hence, the speaking level best suited to the supraglottic resonators that produces the most resonant voice with the least physical effort will relate to the size and shape of the vocal instrument and the power provided by the respiratory driving force. Each person who has a nonorganic voice disorder has the inherent capacity to phonate with a proper tone focus, but the muscular tensions underlying the disorder have pulled the larynx out of optimum position. When the musculature has returned to its normal state, the correct pitch usually follows often, though not always, accompanied by a natural balance of resonance. When the voice disorder is one of incorrect pitch and resonance, the clinician can roughly demonstrate both how far off the patient is and the extra effort required to produce voice, by helping the patient find the best pitch level that is physically easiest to produce. The "um-hum" method proposed by Cooper (1973) is ideal for this purpose.

The patient is asked to say "um-hum" using rising inflection with the lips closed, as though he or she were spontaneously and sincerely agreeing with what was just said. It is vital to underscore the fact that this "um-hum" be spontaneous and sincere. A natural "um-hum," which is easy and gentle, will be felt around the sides and lower portion of the nose and around the lips. To help identify the placement of tone focus, the fingers of one hand should be placed lightly on the bridge and sides of the nose while the other hand is placed lightly on the throat. As one says the "um-hum," there should be a slight vibration or tingle in the mask area.

Resonant Voice Therapy

In their classic review of voice therapy techniques, Verdolini, Devore, and Ostrem (1998) state ". . . that there are probably many different ways to produce 'good voice.'" They include "forward focus" or "resonant voice" as one of the successful approaches. Based on work described by Arthur Lessac, Verdolini developed a programmatic approach to resonant voice. The program is based on the knowledge that when resonant voice is produced, the vocal folds barely touch while producing a strong, clear voice requiring the least amount of lung pressure resulting in low-impact stress on the vocal fold tissues (Verdolini, Druker, Palmer, et al, 1998). Verdolini's systematic 8-week program teaches the resonant voice gesture by placing emphasis on sensory information and exploration. This is based on mind-brain models of skill acquisition that suggest feeling, hearing, and seeing are more important in learning new skills than are explanations of the physiology of production. Rammage (1997) developed patient practice handouts on resonant voice therapy to supplement treatment. The 10-step instruction summary helps illustrate the systematic approach to this technique.

1. "Sit as tall as you can with your head resting comfortably on top of your spine. You should be able to move your head easily from side to side. Take care not to slouch or raise your chin in the air. Once seated comfortably with your arms resting at your sides and your shoulders relaxed, take a few deep breaths. When exhaling, maintain a continuous breathstream. If you feel any resistance in your chest or neck when exhaling, take a few more breaths until you are exhaling freely. You are now ready to begin to explore your resonant voice."

2. "On a light tone that feels comfortable to you, hum at a comfortable pitch to begin feeling 'buzzing' or vibratory sensations in your head bones and facial tissue. Your lips should be closed lightly and your neck, throat, shoulders, and jaw should continue to feel free. Repeat the hum several times, noticing where you feel 'buzzing.' The buzzing sensation that you feel is resonance."

3. Patient sustains a hum. "Hmmmmmmmmmmmmmmmmmmmmmmmm . . ."

4. "Where do you feel the buzz? In the lips, nose, sinuses, forehead, top of your head, hard palate, teeth, elsewhere?"

5. "After noticing where you feel the buzzing, or resonance, vary the pitch on which you are humming. Hum on a sigh and slide down several pitches, keeping your neck, shoulders, and jaw free and relaxed."

6. "Hum while doing a siren, varying the pitch up and then down."

7. "Do you notice that some pitches feel more buzzy than others? Repeat the siren several times and pay attention to the most resonant, or loudest, pitch. If you find a pitch or tone that feels particularly effortless and powerful, hold that pitch for a moment and then say the word 'man.' Feel the resonant buzz throughout the word."

8. "Hum." Hmmmmmmmmmmmmmmmmmmm . . . .

9. "Let your pitch vary naturally. Focus on the feeling of resonance as you say the entire word or phrase and allow the pitch to vary naturally. The intensity of the resonance or buzzing will vary with pitch. The following words, phrases, and sentences were chosen because they contain the most resonant consonants that we produce, 'm' and 'n.'" Here patients are provided a list of 50 to 60 words such as *mime, moan, running*.

10. "Feel the resonance through the final consonant. Your throat, jaw, shoulders, and neck should feel free and relaxed while you are using resonant voice." Patients are then given short phrases, such as "more money" and "home team," to practice. This is followed by lists of longer sentences such as "Many men were mining" and "Come with me and have some of mom's marvelous homemade jam" and "Mark and Mary may be married in the end of May." Additionally, Lessac's "Ybuzz" sounds are practiced in syllables, words, and sentences. These are sounds that incorporate frontal lip and tongue placements for production of /b/ /f/ /l/ /p/ /s/.

It is interesting to note that humming may have additional health benefits particularly to the extent that sinus infections are thought to be a contributory factor to voice problems. Weitzberg and Lundberg (2002) reported that production of nitric oxide (NO) increased 15-fold during humming compared with quiet exhalation. These researchers suggested that NO helps blood vessels dilate, thereby allowing oxygen-carrying blood to flow more freely. Humming appeared to facilitate exchange of air from the sinuses to the nasal passages, which may, in turn, help ventilate the sinuses, protecting them from developing infections.

Lip Trills

An alternate method to achieve resonance balance is the use of trills. Lip and tongue trills are used to provide the patient a feeling of proper tone focus. Patients are asked to glide up and down their pitch range while doing either lip or tongue trills. During the trill, the aerodynamic balance within the vocal tract is optimal and there can be no strain on the laryngeal apparatus. Patients who initially have difficulty producing trills often find placing their hands gently against their cheeks facilitates the production of lip trills or lip bubbles.

Trial and Error

It may seem paradoxical, but despite established principles and techniques of voice therapy, trial and error is an essential methodology. Far from being a science, voice therapy is pragmatic and demands that the clinician take advantage of accidental, unplanned voice improvements during therapy. Boone (1977) states this principle clearly when he says that the clinician must continually "search for the patient's best and most appropriate voice production. This searching is necessary because so much of our vocal behaviors are highly automatic. The patient cannot volitionally break vocalization down into various components and then hope to combine them into some ideal phonation. Our therapy techniques are primarily vehicles of facilitation; that is, we try a particular therapy approach to probe and see if it facilitates the production of a better voice. If it does, then we utilize it as therapy practice material. If it does not, we quickly abandon it. As part of every clinical session, we must probe and search for the patient's best voice. We use it as the target model in therapy."

The question then is not whether we should use probe therapy but how we use trial and error to elicit the target voice. How long do we try a facilitating technique before abandoning it and moving on to another? How much of each therapy session should we probe to search for the patient's best voice?

There is no single answer to these questions. With experience, clinicians learn to listen to the voice presented by the patient during the first few minutes of an encounter to make judgments about the origin of the disordered voice. During the initial diagnostic session, probe therapy is used to see if a "better" voice can be produced by increasing or decreasing closure, loudness, pitch, resonance, or breath support. It may, or may not, involve use of visual feedback of the acoustic, aerodynamic, or visual image of some part of the vocal tract. Time is usually limited to no more than 15 minutes. Facilitating techniques used are generally those that require little explanation and have the highest probability of making change. For example, with a patient presenting with a weak breathy voice, techniques directed at increasing closure or breath support are the most likely to facilitate change. Using vegetative initiators like a cough or laugh, tried three to four times, is often enough to provide the clinician with a target model of a better voice or with knowledge that an alternative treatment may be indicated. Similarly, with a patient presenting with a loud strained voice, three to four imitations of the clinician sighing, or using a breathy voice, might be sufficient to determine the initial target. In subsequent session(s), as the patient's voice improves, the target of "best voice possible" often changes and is determined by perceived vocal differences, or lack thereof, in therapy. As in most behavioral changes, movement toward achieving the target is rarely a straight line. The patient gets better, regresses, and gets better again. When the patient becomes stuck or discouraged with progress using a particular technique, the clinician often uses trial and error with other techniques to help select a different technique to move the patient forward. A few basic principles may help the beginning clinician in using trial and error searching for a target voice:

♦ Trial and error should not be used as an excuse for a shotgun approach. Clinicians should be systematic in their approach and selective in techniques used taking care to match treatment and problem.

♦ Trial-and-error therapy should not be the major focus of every treatment session. Once a treatment plan is developed, trial and error are used to readjust targets and determine if a new technique could return the voice to greater heights.

♦ Trial-and-error failure at one point in therapy does not mean the technique would not work in the future. Trial-and-error success does not mean that it is the only technique that would work for an individual patient. Voice is dynamic: as the patient gains voice, techniques that did not work well in the beginning may later become excellent facilitators.

♦ Efficient application of trial-and-error therapy requires clinicians to understand the physiology of voice production. Clinicians select techniques to try based on their understanding of the physiology being used to produce the aberrant voice.

♦ To help improve efficiency of practice, clinicians should model trial-and-error tasks before requiring the patient to produce them.

♦ Although both use the same facilitating techniques to determine vocal status, trial-and-error therapy should not be confused with the use of prognostic probes. In therapy, the technique is used until it is no longer functional. When the same technique is used as a prognostic probe, the technique is used briefly to predict if and how the voice might improve further.

This suggests that all direct voice therapy could be considered a facilitating technique. In their book on voice therapy, Boone, McFarlane, and VonBerg (2005) table facilitating approaches alphabetically and the parameters (pitch, loudness, and quality) of voice they affect. Because these are the perceptual parameters clinicians use to judge the effectiveness of a technique, it makes good sense to list them this way though the parameters are not independent, and often changing one parameter will affect one or several other factors. Another way to look at these techniques would be by the physiologic parameters of vocal fold vibration they change. Rattenbury, Carding, and Finn (2004) use a different schema for listing voice therapy techniques. They divide them into indirect voice therapy techniques, direct techniques, and techniques used as prognostic probes. They base their list of prognostic probes on the Morrison and Rammage (1993) classification of voice disorders and muscle misuse. This physiologic schema classifies techniques based on whether they affect isometric closure pattern, glottic contraction, supraglottic (lateral) contraction, anterior-posterior contraction, or total incomplete adduction. This, too, makes sense, particularly when clinicians have means to visualize the larynx, because not all voice problems are resolved even when effort level or vibratory patterns are improved. For example, if vocal fold closure were judged to be excessive, techniques of confidential voice, digital manipulation or laryngeal massage, relaxation, visual feedback, and yawn-sigh might be tried. Conversely, probes for inadequate approximation might include increased or effortful loudness, respiration training, pushing, pitch glides, and visual feedback. The advantage of the latter approach is that clinicians can be more precise in their selection of a facilitating technique and hence more efficient. For example, not all problems of vocal loudness emanate from the same etiology. Probes for loudness problems caused by inadequate closure would be different than probes selected for loudness problems caused by poor breath support, by laryngeal scarring, or by poor motor control. Thus, the clinician needs to know the underlying physiologic effects of each technique to select and apply them in a meaningful manner to determine target models, plateaus, and time to select additional techniques or terminate therapy.

Voice Rest

Voice rest is an indirect voice therapy technique calling for reduction or abstinence of vocal use. It is based on the assumption that the absence of vocal fold impact stress promotes tissue healing, reduces scar formation, enhances healing in the injured larynx, and reduces vocal fatigue. Based on these assumptions, physicians may prescribe voice rest as part of postoperative care, as a preventative measure to reduce vocal fatigue, in the case of vocal fold hemorrhage to prevent further bleeding, and in benign lesions to reduce the size of the lesion. Like most other voice therapy techniques, there is little evidence either to support or refute these assumptions nor is there much consensus on either its necessity or efficacy. Nevertheless, any treatise on vocal treatment would be incomplete without a thorough discussion of the theory and role of vocal rest in treatment of dysphonias and the controversies surrounding its use.

In the past decade, research on changes in the microstructure of the larynx in canines after tissue trauma has led to theories about what happens to the healing structure with microtrauma, which in turn has led to recommendations for voice rest after phonosurgery. In theory, any interruption of microcirculation in the vocal folds leads to temporary ischemia, disruption, and increased permeability of capillaries and ultimately to reorganization of the affected structure and fibrous mass or edema. Gray Pignatori, and Harding (1994) demonstrated some of these organizational changes in the basement membrane zone (BMZ) and the superficial layer of the lamina propria. The histoarchitecture of the BMZ became disrupted, and the structural glycoproteins and fibrous proteins normally seen in the speech language pathologist (SLP) were nearly absent. Durkin, Duncavage, Toohill, et al (l986) injured the vocal folds of eight canines and examined the folds at 1, 2, 3, 5, 7, 10, and 32 days postoperatively to follow the healing process. They observed edema and tissue necrosis at all time points. These findings were augmented by a Korean study adding an additional twist on the influence of phonation on basement membrane zone recovery after phonomicrosurgery (Cho, Kim, Lee, et al, 2000). These investigators used 20 dogs placing 10 in a situation to simulate iatrogenic voice rest and 10 allowed to phonate normally. Healing process was observed histologically at 1, 2, 4, 8, and 12 weeks after surgery. In the voice rest group, the basement membrane was completely re-formed in 2 weeks, and the "cover" appeared completely rearranged by 8 weeks. In contrast, the phonation group had delayed healing and basement membrane changes. Based on these canine results, the authors suggested that voice rest of at least 2 weeks after surgery may be beneficial and that vocal hygiene should be maintained for as long as 8 weeks. However, it has been long known that the canine larynx is not identical to that of humans (Jako, 1972). Jako was one of the first to note that compared with humans, the canine has only a rudimentary vocal ligament and a thicker lamina propria, though it does have a similar basement membrane. Thus, clinicians must be cautious in making direct extrapolations from canines to humans.

Whereas systematic histologic studies of the daily change in the ultrastructure of the vocal fold cannot be observed in humans, the quality of the voice and endoscopic image can be sequentially observed after phonosurgical treatment. In one such study, Wang and Huang (1994) studied 25 patients placed in a sequence of three postoperative programs (voice rest, vocal hygiene, voice treatment) and concluded that voice rest appeared to promote healing and should be used as part of a holistic voice treatment plan after phonosurgery. Ye, Yang, Zhao, et al (2002) were also interested in the role of voice rest in tissue healing postoperatively. They approached the problem by following the voice recovery of 20 patients who had polypectomies. Daily voice assessments revealed the worst voice occurred in day 1, recovered significantly by day 10, and reached normal by day 14. They concluded from these observations that after polyp removal, patients should be placed on 14 days of vocal rest.

In combination, these experimental time-series studies appear to provide some evidence of the effectiveness of voice rest, yet it is unclear the frequency with which clinicians employ voice rest in treatment. In a prospective study attempting to determine if voice rest was the standard of care after excision of benign mucosal vocal fold lesions, Behrman and Sulica (2003) mailed a 16-item survey to all active members of the American Academy of Otolaryngology ($n = 7321$). The majority of the 1208 respondents favored some form of postsurgical vocal rest for 7 days, but only 18% of them recommended complete vocal rest, and 15% did not recommend any type of voice rest.

A recent vocal advocate of voice rest, Gwen Korovin argues a strong case for including voice rest as part of phonosurgical care but does not limit it to postoperative care and recognizes voice rest is not the only contributing factor to vocal fold healing. In her comprehensive discussion of issues related to voice rest, Korovin's recommendations for nonoperative vocal rest include acute edema, prenodules, hemorrhage, mucosal tears, and ulcerations. Similarly, Sataloff and Hawkshaw (2006) state that,

Voice rest (absolute or relative) is an important therapeutic consideration in any case of laryngitis. When no professional commitments are pending, a short course of absolute voice rest may be considered, as it is the safest and most conservative therapeutic intervention. This means absolute silence and communication with a writing pad. The patient must be instructed not to whisper, as this may be an even more traumatic vocal activity than speaking softly. Whistling through the lips also involves vocal fold activity and should not be permitted. So does the playing of many musical wind instruments. Absolute voice rest is necessary only for serious vocal fold injury such as hemorrhage or mucosal disruption. Even then, it is virtually never indicated for more than 7 to 10 days. Three days are often sufficient.

Korovin's advice for voice rest associated with phonosurgery depends on the site and extent of the vocal fold lesion, the type of corrective surgery, and is often combined with behavioral management. This combination of treatment is also advocated by Murry (2001) and Behlau (2005) particularly in cases at greater postoperative risk for healing problems such as patients who are smokers with polypoid corditis or patients who have had significant tissue resections.

The vocal rest program elucidated by Korovin is a four-stage postoperative treatment (preoperative, initial postoperative, first postoperative exam, and subsequent postoperative).

During the preoperative period, the patient is provided education about the medical condition and voice production and provided medical management for problems contributing to tissue irritation. Voice therapy is focused on minimizing the associated edema. The initial postoperative period, which immediately follows surgery, includes voice rest, education about subsequent stages, support systems, and preparation for easy voicing. The first postoperative exam is completed at 1 week. The larynx is visualized to determine the patient's ability to transition from voice rest to voice conservation and the subsequent postoperative treatment. The patient needs to understand the importance of voice conservation for the initial critical healing period. The extent of voice conservation varies by a patient's voice needs, ability to comply with recommendations (i.e., specific time limits recommended for vocal usage vs. good judgment), and the degree and type of surgery. Subsequent postoperative treatment includes practice of vocal hygiene: hydration and humidity, mucolytics, antitussives, and tuning in to listen to body and voice. Postoperative vocal hygiene also includes avoiding smoke, throat clearing, coughing, reflux, and allergens. Korovin (2005) suggests clinicians consider perioperative medications that may affect healing (steroids, antireflux medications, antibiotics, antifungals, oral inhalers, hormone therapy, and blood thinners). Other factors influencing postoperative voice rest recommendations include the availability of an experienced voice care team, extent of preoperative voice therapy, compliance with vocal hygiene, primary or secondary surgery, and appearance and speed of healing. During periods of absolute vocal rest, patients are instructed to use pen and paper, children's write/erase boards, unvoiced noises such as hand clapping, finger snapping, hissing, and e-mail and cell phone text messaging. For the period of voice rest, any unnecessary behavior that has the potential to approximate the vocal folds is to be avoided. Patients are instructed that they should not whisper, mouth words (because they might subvocalize), play wind instruments, whistle, or lift heavy objects. An equally important part of the vocal rest is to avoid crying because it causes increased subglottal pressure and upper thoracic tension, rapid vocal fold closure, and prolonged closed phase. During voice conservation behavioral therapy instruction on use of confidential and resonant voice, vocal function exercises and/or the Accent technique are often employed. Korovin argues against concerns about voice rest resulting in muscle atrophy. Though cognizant that opinions on this topic vary, she makes a case that wound-healing studies indicate 1 to 2 weeks is appropriate for the majority of remucosalization to occur, and that there are no studies demonstrating atrophy after 2 weeks of voice rest. She also addresses the notion that voice rest has negative psychologic ramifications. Again, with little data it is difficult to discern the psychologic implications because there is so much variance between patients. She argues that in select patients, voice rest may induce feelings of insecurity, helplessness, and dissociation from the verbal world, but with proper preoperative counseling/education, the feelings should be temporary.

A perennial problem underlying voice rest recommendations is different notions as to what constitutes "voice rest."

Behlau is very clear in her set of voice recommendations for patients after benign lesion surgery. When voice rest is recommended, she tells patients, ". . . do not use your voice in any circumstance, don't whisper or murmur, don't cough with effort and sound, don't clear your throat and don't speak while doing activities such as defecation or sexual intercourse." Although she does not describe specific stages, she suggests patients return to voice activities gradually, initially being restricted only to necessary situations. She further recommends that during the first 2 postoperative weeks, patients be instructed when returning to voice to avoid speaking on the phone, especially on cells; avoid noisy places; and to refrain from speaking loudly or for long periods.

The need to incorporate vocal rest into treatment programs is also supported by Hoover, Sataloff, Lyons, et al (2001). They suggest that although there are no scientific studies to confirm its efficacy, a brief period of complete voice rest is the standard of care and appears to be helpful in avoiding adverse sequelae and advancing the healing process in the case of mucosal tears.

Murry and Rosen (2000) also support the use of voice rest. They successfully treated three cases of vocal fold hemorrhage, secondary to crying, with voice rest and subsequent phonomicrosurgery for lesions.

Summary of Voice Rest

Thus, voice rest seems logical based on what we know about healing characteristics but remains controversial. Voice rest recommendations generally fall under one of three classifications: complete/absolute voice rest, relative/modified voice rest, or voice conservation. Commonly complete voice rest advice given to patients with voice disorders is to refrain from using the voice; this means not talking at all including no whispering, humming, or throat clearing. Relative voice rest limits vocalizations in time, intensity, and frequency, often suggesting talking at a reduced volume, as if you were no more than an arm's length away from the listener, and for no more than 5 minutes/hour. Advocates of voice conservation advise patients to limit vocalizations to times when they must speak and otherwise conserve the voice using voice rest coupled with hydration.

The duration of voice rest, modified or complete, recommended to patients can range from 24 hours to several weeks, and there is no accepted standard of care probably because of the lack of data and controversial issues associated with extended periods of silence.

♦ Although some data suggest that 2 weeks of silence has therapeutic value, the advice is commonly ignored because of its impracticality. Moreover, there are conflicting studies in the literature suggesting vocal rest is of little value. Based on a study of 127 patients who had surgery for vocal nodules, polypoid degeneration, granuloma, cysts, polyps, leukoplakia, and carcinoma, Koufman and Blalock (1989) concluded that voice rest provided no greater protection against postoperative dysphonia than did an alternate program of voice conservation, that is, soft glottal attack, loudness monitoring, and avoidance of abusive vocal patterns.

♦ Some clinicians believe that absolute voice rest can do harm. It implants the idea in the patient's psyche, especially in those who have susceptibility to psychogenic voice disorders, that the larynx and voice are foci of weakness and that normally energetic voice use is damaging. This idea may persist beyond the duration of the prescribed voice rest and, unless reversed, can lead to anxiety and to a secondary voice disorder or respiratory inhibition. To say it another way, when the recommendation of voice rest creates, perpetuates, or exacerbates a voice disorder, as it often does, voice rest can be considered an iatrogenic[1] cause of a voice disorder. Overcautious voice use is often elected by patients even when not advised to rest their voices. In actuality, the opposite kind of voice use is desired in some patients with voice disorders, that is, rather than voice rest, they need to adopt firm, normally loud voices produced with equally firm exhalatory force.

For some patients, an alternative to voice rest is use of *confidential voice*. Like voice rest, the technique is designed to protect the vocal folds by reducing impact stress. According to Colton and Casper (1990, 1995, 2005), confidential voice is using a quiet breathy voice as if you were speaking confidentially to a person no more than an arm's length away. Clinician modeling a confidential voice and contrasting it with undesirable stage whispers is critical to success of this treatment. Clinicians using confidential voice therapy should make sure that the patient knows and can produce the differences and should limit the time the patient is placed on confidential voice to no longer than is necessary for the vocal injury to heal. Studies of the microstructure of the vocal fold suggest that 1 to 2 weeks should be adequate.

Vocal Hygiene

One of the most commonly used treatment regimens is vocal hygiene. Vocal hygiene focuses on reducing or eliminating behaviors that contribute to the cause or maintenance of voice problems and, by so doing, is thought to improve tissue characteristics and vocal fold vibration. It may include some form of voice rest and antireflux directives (discussed elsewhere in this chapter) and specific lifestyle changes such as diet changes, not eating immediately before retiring, avoiding speaking over noise, alternating talk time with quiet time, speaking within the middle of one's pitch and loudness range so as to avoid phonatory extremes, and increasing hydration. Vocal hygiene programs are individually tailored to the habits and needs of the patient. Clinicians need to be cautious that they are not overly ambitious in program development. Too many demands for lifestyle change can be overwhelming and result in none of the directions being adhered to.

---

[1]Iatrogenesis is defined as illness induced by unavoidable or improper diagnosis or therapy.

♦ Feedback Devices in Voice Therapy

It cannot be overstressed how important a role feedback plays in voice therapy. Because there is minimal tactile and proprioceptive sensation arising from the larynx during phonation, most patients rely primarily on audition. Audition appears to be the primary channel through which voice is monitored, as proved by the congenitally deaf who are known for their severely aberrant voices, which are typically monopitched, poorly modulated in loudness, and abnormal in nasal resonance. When voice becomes defective, intensification of its parameters during therapy is needed. Audio recordings are probably the most common feedback device used by clinicians to enable the patient to examine voice after it has been produced. However, delayed presentation of the voice may have limited benefit as it is often difficult for the patient to relate what he or she produced to what he of she hears moments later, and instantaneous feedback is also necessary. Amplification of the voice, feedback through earphones, is one means. Even simpler is cupping the hand around the ear or phonating while facing the corner of a room, where the voice rebounds off the walls. Feedback devices should be considered as adjuncts to therapy but should not be substituted for the interpersonal and environmental techniques integral with the mechanical aspects of therapy.

Many devices have been developed to enhance sensory feedback of voice production. One of the first specially devised instruments for vocal abuse disorders is the Voice Intensity Controller, which instantly warns the speaker when vocal intensity becomes excessive. Worn like a hearing aid, with the microphone attached to the base of the neck anteriorly and an earphone in the ear, the device can be set so that when the speaker's voice exceeds a certain intensity level, a warning tone is triggered. Holbrook, Rolnick, and Bailey (1974) reported on the complete resolution of vocal nodules, polyps, and contact ulcers in 32 patients who used this device, the mean treatment time being 5.3 weeks. Sound spectrography provides visual feedback display of voice spectra, intensity, and duration, which can be effectively used as feedback in therapy and home training. Both clinicians and patients have easy access to this type of feedback through either commercially available units or freeware obtained over the Internet. We have already been introduced to these devices as clinical evaluation and research instruments, but they clearly serve dual purposes when they provide an instantaneous visual display on a computer screen. Because of their sensitivity to noise in the voice spectrum, these devices are especially useful for the treatment of voice-quality disorders.

The ability to visually monitor voice pitch or loudness is afforded now by a myriad of instruments. Typically, either a head- or neck-mounted microphone transduces the acoustic voice produced by the patient into a visual signal enabling the speaker to read the frequency or intensity. Often, this is in the form of needle deflection, vibration, digitized numbers, or bars reflecting voltage change. Selected instruments provide storage of data useful to the clinicians monitoring treatment as well as direct feedback to the patient.

For example, Cheyne, Hanson, Genereux, et al (2003) in concert with Kay-Pentax has developed a vocal accumulator that monitors vocal load and provides individual patients with feedback about their frequency, intensity, and duration of phonation throughout the day. This portable device holds considerable promise in heightening patient awareness of excess vocal loads and voice-production problems, informing patients about harmful vocal behaviors and assisting clinicians in helping patients get increased practice.

Vocal Function Exercises

Vocal function exercises comprise a treatment program designed by Stemple to build strength and endurance in the laryngeal muscles and in so doing improve range and control of voice production (Sabol, Lee, and Stemple, 1995; Stemple, Lee, D'Amico, et al, 1994). The exercise program is based on the notion that laryngeal muscles are skeletal and thus should respond to exercises similar to those used to improve limb control. Thus, exercises are organized into warm-up and cool-down, stretching and contraction, and power modules. The exercises were first described by Briess (1959) and were based on his extensive work with laryngeal EMG. The program specifies that patients complete a prescribed series of nasalized vowel prolongations and pitch glides twice a day for several weeks. The patient is given a recording diary to keep track of the length of time he or she is able to sustain phonations, the number of trials practiced, and the number of tones produced. Patients going through this prescribed program seem to gain better control over airway valving and in so doing reduce hyperfunctional behaviors.

Lee Silverman Voice Therapy

The Lee Silverman Voice Therapy (LSVT) was initially developed by Ramig and colleagues to improve the voice and speech of individuals with Parkinson's disease (Ramig, Sapir, Fox, and Countryman, 2001; Sapir, Pawlas, Ramig, Countryman, O'Brien, Hoehn, and Thompson, 1999; Sapir, Pawlas, Ramig, Seele, Fox, and Corboy, 1999; Ramig and Dromey, 1996; Ramig, Countryman, Thompson, and Horii, 1995; Dromey, Ramig, and Johnson, 1995; Ramig, Countryman, Thompson, Horii, 1995; Smith, Ramig, Dromey, Perez, abd Samandri, 1995; Countryman, Ramig, Pawlas, 1994; Mamig, Countryman, Thompson, and Horii, 1994; Ramig, 1993). Since the initial development, LSVT has also been successfully applied to individuals with other neurologic disorders, to geriatrics with presbyphonia and to individuals with Down syndrome. LSVT is an intensive treatment program that focuses on increasing loudness. Therapy sessions are held daily, 4 times per week, for 4 weeks, generally with certified LSVT trainers. In both the daily treatment and home practice sessions, patients attempt to recalibrate themselves to speak louder without feeling they are yelling. Tasks focus on loud vowel prolongations at different pitch levels and production of increased loudness in short phrases building up to conversational speech. Patients are taught to "think loud." Outcome measures of LSVT training have demonstrated that not only do patients get louder, but they also have improvement in pronunciation, inflection, and facial animation. Follow-up studies have also shown that as long as 12 months after completion of treatment, patients continue to speak with louder voices. This is impressive as many of the individuals

have progressive neurologic disease. It has been postulated that one of the reasons this technique is effective is that it is simple and by focusing on a single parameter, the patient is able to improve control and coordination of the respiratory-phonatory apparatus. The developers of LSVT underscore the importance of clinician training, reinforcing target behaviors, and recalibrating patients as to what constitutes "normal" production levels.

◆ Reactive Anxiety

In planning treatment, clinicians need to recognize the potential for a serious dilemma in the diagnosis and treatment of voice disorders that can get in the way of helping patients and their ability to help themselves: the strong tendency for patients to become anxious and overprotective of their larynges as a reaction to the diagnosis of organic or psychogenic voice disorder. The larynx is particularly vulnerable to emotional disequilibrium, mild or severe, transient or chronic. One reason for the oversensitivity of the larynx is its vital importance in everyday life for intellectual and emotional expression. We cannot appreciate the importance of a normal voice until the larynx undergoes structural or physiologic changes producing dysphonia or aphonia. The most stalwart person sooner or later will become frustrated, embarrassed, and hypersensitive to the obstacle that abnormal voice presents.

A second reason for the patient's vulnerability to overconcern and emotional reactivity to dysphonia is that the larynx is well known in the public mind as a site of malignancy, and the most common concern that patients express when they develop abnormal voice is that they may have cancer of the larynx.

Thus, our problem, diagnostically and therapeutically, is that, despite our best efforts to prevent it, patients will generate overanxiety about their larynges and voices. Any advice given to them about the need to avoid certain kinds of abusive vocal activities, or even simply the administration of voice therapy, reinforces the patient's belief that the larynx has to be protected at all costs. This attitude easily translates into anxiety and its associated muscle tensions. The patient elects to phonate with less than normal expiratory effort, breathing shallowly and phonating weakly. That is why the laryngologist and the speech-language pathologist, who on the one hand need to give advice and therapy for voice improvement, on the other hand must neutralize the tendency toward the patient's overconcern by not advising it too strenuously and by reassuring the patient that full voice use is desirable as soon as possible. Particularly, we need to emphasize that the patient need not protect the larynx by using reduced loudness and respiratory volumes. In some cases, the clinician does more for the patient by giving simple advice on proper voice instead of a long series of voice therapy sessions, which risk reinforcement of the patient's apprehensions.

Telemedicine

A question raised by students and insurance companies concerns whether the voice-treatment objectives can be obtained by anything other than individual treatment sessions, which are expensive and an inefficient use of clinician time. Efficacy studies comparing group versus individual voice therapy outcomes have not been completed. Mashima, Birkmire-Peters, Holtel, et al (1999) initiated a novel project to investigate the potential of remediating voice disorders remotely using telemedicine. With computer technology and Web cams, this type of treatment becomes an increasing reality and may be particularly beneficial for patients living in rural areas or patients who have difficulty taking time off work to come to a voice center for treatment. Telemedicine makes it possible to receive voice treatment in the privacy of one's computer wherever it might be located.

♦ Phonosurgery

Phonosurgery is laryngeal surgery done solely, or primarily, to improve phonation. This requires some glottic adjustment, and when closure is improved, often gains are achieved not only in voice but also in breathing, vocal effort level, and swallowing. One way of understanding the myriad of phonosurgery techniques is to classify them in one of five categories: removal of pathologic tissue; correction of the position, shape, or tension of the vocal fold; restoration of neuromuscular function; reconstruction for partial loss of the larynx; and reconstruction for entire loss of the larynx. Reconstruction for partial or total loss of the larynx is outside the scope of this text. A brief overview of the other three categories follows.

Various procedures designed to remove pathologic tissue are commonly used in cases of polyps, cysts, nodules, and papillomas. This extirpation surgery can either be done with a laser or a cold knife. Special microsurgical instruments have been developed for this delicate surgery. Laser surgery is controlled destruction by thermal evaporation. The advantage of this technique is the precision and healing. The disadvantage is possibility of error and unwanted destruction of tissue.

As with all surgery, there is a possibility of encountering problems. Although poor outcomes are rare when surgery is done by a "phonosurgeon," voice clinicians should have knowledge of the potential adverse affects. The patient may develop excessive edema and have airway problems that in the worst case cause death or require a tracheotomy. It is also possible that the patient will have an allergic reaction to the anesthesia or to a material being used for an implant. Any time there is tissue damage, there is also possibility of laryngeal scarring. There is no consistently successful treatment for scarring. Thus, this iatrogenic problem is considered to be the most difficult of laryngeal problems to treat and one of the worst adverse consequences of laryngeal surgery. When scarring develops, the voice is often worse than before treatment. On occasion, the scarring may be so extensive as to render the patient aphonic.

The literature is replete with phonosurgical procedures that come under the category of correction of position, shape, or tension. Most of the procedures are either considered to be vocal fold augmentation, or cordal injection, or cartilaginous framework surgery.

Laryngeal framework surgery was first described by Isshiki (1989a,b). Isshiki proposed remodeling the laryngeal framework to achieve better glottal closure and/or to improve pitch. He divided these "thyroplasty" procedures into groups based on whether the removal resulted in a change in position, shape, or tension: type I, lateral compression to achieve median shift of the vocal folds; type II, lateral shift to expand distance; type III, shortening or relocation; and type IV, lengthening to increase tension and elevate pitch by cricothyroid cartilage approximation.

The most common thyroplasty procedure is type I. This procedure is used to correct glottic incompetence when the vocal folds fail to come together. This procedure has been successfully used in patients with vocal fold paralysis, vocal fold bowing, sulcus vocalis, Parkinson's disease, and in abductor spastic dysphonia. A small window is cut in the thyroid cartilage. A muscle, Gore-Tex (PTFE, poly-tetraj-fluoro ethylene; Gore Medical Products Division), fat, or some other alloplastic or biological material is placed in the window to push the vocal fold medially. The procedure is done under local anesthesia so that the surgeon can not only see how well the vocal folds are approximating but also can elicit vocalizations from the patient to see how well he or she is functioning. Windows are drilled in only one side for a unilateral procedure or both sides for a bilateral procedure. One of the beauties of this procedure is that the delicate layer structure of the vocal fold lamina propria does not get disrupted. Moreover, if in follow-up evaluation the procedure is deemed less than ideal, the thyroplasty can be revised.

Cordal injections have a long history (Ford, 2004). Brunning (1911) described correcting vocal fold paralysis by injecting paraffin, bone paste, and a variety of other materials. Arnold (1963) proposed Teflon injection. Initially, Teflon appeared to be an ideal substance. Results were immediate and appeared to be effective. However, as with many such procedures, the immediate glow of success was overshadowed by subsequent reports of long-term consequences of migrating Teflon particles, lack of control as to placement of bolus of Teflon, foreign-body reactions, and Teflon granulomas. Today, most clinics use Teflon only with terminally ill patients or patients in their eighth decade of life.

The last category of phonosurgery to be discussed is laryngeal reinnervation. The concept of replacing a paralyzed or injured nerve is not new. Nearly 100 years ago, Horsley reported repair of an injured recurrent laryngeal nerve (RLN). Subsequently, numerous surgeons have reported success with reinnervation of the RLN with a branch of the ansa cervicalis (Crumley, 1982, 1991; Crumley, Izdebski, and McMicken, 1988; Frazier, 1924; Goding, 2005; Paniello, 2001, 2001; Smith, 2006). The objective of laryngeal reinnervation is to restore physiologic movement and sensation to a paralyzed larynx. The most useful donor nerve in laryngeal paralysis treatment is the ansa cervicalis nerve (Smith, 2006). According to Smith, it matches favorably with RLN, has little to no dysfunction from transection of the branch to the sternohyoid or omohyoid muscles, can be obtained from either ipsilateral or contralateral sides, and can be connected to the larynx by direct neurorrhaphy, nerve-muscle-pedicle, or direct muscle implant. Of these three techniques, the direct neurorrhaphy appears to be most effective and is thought to have "theoretical advantages with restoring viscoelastic symmetry and not just geometric symmetry" (Smith, 2006), as in the case of medialization procedures using implants or injectables. However, clinicians need to recognize that the voice after the neurorrhaphy may be unchanged or worse for the first 3 or 4 months until reinnervation begins. The voice can then be expected to continue improving over a 12-month period. In instances when the patient requires immediate resolution of the voice disturbance, the procedure may be combined with a temporary injectable such as Gelfoam (Surgicel; Pfizer, Inc., New York, NY) or collagen. The neurorrhaphy generally improves adduction but does little for abduction. Zealear and associates (2002) have suggested using electrical stimulation of the denervated muscle to promote selective reinnervation by native over foreign motoneurons. In repeated studies in canines and preliminary human clinical trials, they have demonstrated that paced muscle stimulation using an implantable commercial stimulator results in preferential repressed reconnection by foreign motoneurons, thereby promoting selective reinnervation.

◆ Management of Specific Voice Disorders

The remainder of this chapter is devoted to therapy that has evolved for specific voice disorders based on the special requirements of each disorder.

Musculoskeletal Tension (Vocal Hyperfunction)

The majority of cases we shall find suffer from some excess of muscular function (hyperfunction) in various degrees. However, this refers not to the vocal folds themselves but rather to the whole tensor mechanism of the vocal organ, which comprises all the muscles surrounding the cartilages of the larynx. We have generally not found it necessary—and often not possible—to decide which specific muscle or muscles were at fault (Weiss, 1971).

Life stress elevates general muscle tension, including that of the laryngeal muscles, and can produce an array of voice defects: aphonia, breathiness, hoarseness, or excessively high pitch. No single voice type is associated with musculoskeletal tension. Vocal hyperfunction is the most important concept in the etiology and treatment of nonorganic, and many organic, voice disorders. Intrinsic and extrinsic laryngeal muscle tension expresses anxiety, depression, or anger. In organic voice disorders, it may occur as a result of efforts to compensate for the organic deficit. All patients with voice disorders, regardless of etiology, should be tested for excess musculoskeletal tension, either as a primary or as a secondary cause of dysphonia. The degree of voice improvement after therapy for musculoskeletal tension is proportional to the reduction of musculoskeletal tension.

Following are the principles basic to therapy for musculoskeletal tension associated with vocal hyperfunction.

◆ Extrinsic and intrinsic laryngeal muscle cramping is responsible for the abnormal voice. Reducing musculoskeletal tension releases the inherent capability of the larynx to produce normal voice.

◆ When gently rubbed or kneaded, muscles relax and become less painful.

◆ Lowering laryngeal position in the neck permits more normal phonation.

Testing for Muscular Tension

The first procedure for implementation of these principles is to assay signs of musculoskeletal tension. Its presence is suspected when patients complain of spontaneous pain in the region of the larynx shooting up to the ears and down to the chest and a feeling of a lump, a ball, or tension in the larynx or pharynx. Testing for muscle tension is subdivided into determining three things: (1) extent of laryngeal elevation, (2) pain in response to pressure in the region of the larynx, and (3) extent of voice improvement after tension reduction (**Fig. 11.1**):

1. Encircle the hyoid bone with the thumb and middle finger, working them posteriorly until the tips of the major horns are felt.

2. Exert light pressure with the fingers in a circular motion over the tips of the hyoid bone and ask if the patient feels pain, not just pressure. It is important to watch facial expression for signs of discomfort or pain.

3. Repeat this procedure with the fingers in the thyrohyoid space, beginning from the thyroid notch and working posteriorly.

4. Find the posterior borders of the thyroid cartilage just medial to the sternocleidomastoid muscles and repeat the procedure.

5. With the fingers over the superior borders of the thyroid cartilage, begin to work the larynx gently downward, also moving it laterally at times. One should check for a lower laryngeal position by estimating the increased size of the thyrohyoid space.

6. Ask the patient to prolong vowels during these procedures, noting changes in quality or pitch. Clearer voice quality and lower pitch indicate relief of tension. Because these procedures are fatiguing, rest periods should be provided.

7. Once a voice change has taken place, the patient should be allowed to experiment with the voice, repeating vowels, words, and sentences.

Rate of improvement varies. If the dysphonia has been due to musculoskeletal tension alone and has been present only a short time, the voice may become normal within minutes. Those who have been dysphonic longer may require several hours of therapy administered in separate sessions. The voice rarely changes from aphonia or dysphonia to normal without first passing through several dysphonic stages. The clinician should not hesitate to attempt normal voice within

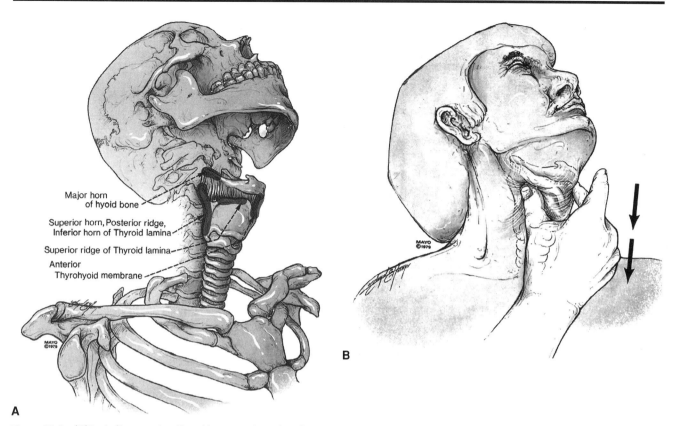

Figure 11.1 **(A)** Loci of laryngeal and hyoid bone pain from digital pressure (shaded areas). **(B)** Maneuvering the larynx to a lower position in the neck.

one session, for the majority of patients can be helped considerably, if not completely, within that time. Patients whose voices fail to improve despite the above ministrations may not be ready to relinquish the abnormal voice because of musculoskeletal tension secondary to conversion reaction. One should watch for the first signs of improvement. Recovery takes on its own momentum. A switch then should be made from repetitions of speech sounds and simple nasal sentences to spontaneous speech beginning with more automatic responses such as the patient's name, address, and occupation.

Once the normal voice has returned, most patients ask why it did and why they were not able to accomplish this by themselves. The clinician explains the effects of muscle tension on voice in terms the patient can understand. Often, after voice improvement, the patient recalls unpleasant life situations giving rise to the voice disorder. A frank and open discussion of such situations and the extent of their seriousness is necessary to determine the need for more intensive psychologic investigation and therapy. Commonly, musculoskeletal tension is not due to a specific problem but is the patient's lifelong way of reacting to stress. Such patients overdrive themselves, and changing daily habits may serve to preclude future abnormal voice episodes. Realistically, the normal voice may be short-lived, and the dysphonia may return when the tension returns. Not much is known about the long-term fate of such therapy or ways to prevent further occurrences.

The literature on voice therapy is replete with advocacy of chewing therapy, progressive relaxation, and biofeedback for

vocal hyperfunction as described earlier in this chapter. These therapies have the same objective as the method just described. However, musculoskeletal tension is a powerfully resistive force, and less aggressive methods often fail. Here, as elsewhere, the best approach is trial and error.

Maneuvering the patient's laryngeal and hyoid anatomy as just described is safe as long as it is performed with good judgment. This technique is not offered as an alternate therapy but as a primary one. It is hard work for both clinician and patient and would not be advocated were it not useful in achieving its aims. Patients will complain of soreness in the region of the larynx after such therapy, but they can be assured that it will disappear within a day or two.

Finally, in addition to elevation of the larynx and hyoid bone, the tongue may be elevated, integral with the total pattern of extrinsic laryngeal muscle contraction. The tongue is carried high in the mouth, and the submental musculature is tense and painful. The tongue should be pressed down along with the hyoid bone and larynx, either with the finger or with a tongue depressor, while simultaneously listening for voice improvement.

Voice Abuse

Vocal Fatigue

Fatigue is defined as an inability to maintain a power output or force during repeated muscle contractions (Powers and Howley, 1990). In limbs, fatigue is often remedied by rest and by exercise building up strength, endurance, and flexibility. A one-to-one relationship cannot be made between limb and laryngeal fatigue because laryngeal fatigue involves both muscle (body) and tissue (cover including epithelium and lamina propria). Consequently, to understand its treatment, it is necessary to look at the assumptions underlying vocal fatigue, and the physiologic limitations of the vocal apparatus. According to contemporary researchers, it is assumed that vocal fatigue relates to the ability of the laryngeal apparatus to withstand various vocal loads. In other words, there is a limit to the mechanical stress that can be placed on the vocal system. But like all systems, there is a range of strength, and some instruments are inherently stronger than others. The ability to sustain a vocal load is, in part, related to the strength of the apparatus but also to the age, the use, and the conditions under which it is used and the material it is made from. Apparatus strength or lack thereof may be offset by training that improves duration of withstanding a given load. For any given individual, the strength of the apparatus may vary and be more vulnerable, or at risk, during times of stress, specific medical conditions, after ingestion of various pharmacological agents and recreational drugs that either dilate blood vessels (vasodilators) or dry out tissue (diuretics), or after periods of excessive use of the vocal instrument particularly when the external environment is poor (dusty, noisy, or dry). This being the case, there are several occupational hazards because of vocal load requirements. Foremost among these hazards is teaching where teachers are required to talk with a loud voice for long periods of time often in less than ideal speaking environments: the rooms often have poor acoustics, are dusty, and contain noisy children. Thus, much of the recent research on workload and vocal fatigue has been accomplished on teachers.

In voice, prolonged phonation is one way to view the laryngeal apparatus's ability to maintain a power output or force. Titze (1999) suggests there are five possible physiologic limitations to prolonged phonation resulting in vocal fatigue: (1) fatigue of laryngeal muscles that provide tension and stability; (2) fatigue of respiratory muscles that provide subglottic pressure; (3) relaxation of passive tension (ligaments, joints, and membranes); (4) increase in tissue viscosity resulting from increased friction from dehydration or chemical changes in fluid compensation; and (5) change in blood circulation where there may be either constricted blood vessels impeding regenerative processes and reduced capacity to transfer heat away from the vocal folds or vasodilation resulting in increased mass.

The symptoms of vocal fatigue are innumerable. Among the most common symptoms reported by patients are voice gives out at the end of the day; increased vocal effort; change in vocal quality (increase in breathiness or glottal fry); decrease in vocal range, flexibility, or endurance; abnormal throat sensations such as hurting, burning, drying, or scratchiness; a tight chest or increased difficulty breathing; or increased throat clearing or coughing. Generally, these symptoms are reported as being worse at the end of the day or after vocalizing (singing, teaching, talking) for some period of time. Most notable is that the patient notices a change in vocal ability and effort.

How then does one treat vocal fatigue, a condition that often changes during the course of the day and does not necessarily result from the presence of pathology but rather from too heavy a vocal load for the apparatus? Research completed in the past 5 years suggests that any treatment that reduces the load will in turn reduce vocal fatigue. This may include increased hydration, periods of vocal rest, exercises building endurance, and use of amplification. The effectiveness of these treatments has been documented in a series of studies by Roy and colleagues (2000, 2001a,b, 2002, 2004), Smith and colleagues (1996, 1998a,b), Jonsdottir and colleagues (2001, 2002, 2003), Sapienza, Crandell, and Curtis (1999), Yiu and Chan (2003), and McCabe and Titze (2002).

Yiu and Chan (2003) investigated the effect of hydration and vocal rest on vocal fatigue in 20 young amateur karaoke singers. Half of the singers were given water to drink and short duration of vocal rests at regular intervals during singing, and the other half sang continuously without taking any water or rest. The subjects who were given hydration and vocal rests sang significantly longer, and the subjects who sang continuously without drinking water and taking rests showed significant changes in jitter measure and the highest pitch they could produce during singing. The authors interpreted these results to suggest that hydration and vocal rests are useful strategies to preserve voice function and quality during karaoke singing. Whether similar results would be found in other singers suffering from vocal fatigue or found with vocal rest without hydration could not be determined from the study. Like amateur karaoke singers, preschool teachers have vocal heavy loading factors and little voice training. Sodersten, Granqvist, Hammarberg, et al (2002) suggest that one way to reduce the vocal loading for this occupation is to "include pauses so that preschool teachers can rest their voices." Chan (1994) took a different approach with kindergarten teachers. He found that teachers who followed a vocal hygiene program for 2 months improved their vocal health by reducing vocal abuses and practicing healthy voice strategies. However, conflicting results were reported by Roy (2002). Roy and colleagues studied the effects of using vocal hygiene versus vocal exercises in 58 teachers with voice problems who were randomly placed in three groups (no treatment controls, vocal hygiene, and vocal function exercises). Only the teachers who were persistent with vocal function exercises showed improvement. However, although teachers in the vocal hygiene group did not improve, they did not get worse as did the no-treatment group. In another study conducted by Roy and colleagues (2005), 64 teachers were randomly assigned to one of three treatment groups: resonant voice therapy, amplification use, or respiratory muscle training. Teachers in the amplification and resonant voice therapy showed improvement with those in the amplification group exhibiting the greatest change. Similar results about the benefit of amplification in reducing the vocal fold and reducing vocal fatigue have also been reported by Sapienza, Crandell, and Curtis (1999) and Jonsdottir (2001, 2002, 2003). Chant therapy also appears to be effective in remedying vocal fatigue (McCabe and Titze, 2002) by decreasing the vocal load through improving resonance balance and reducing adductory forces

Table 11.1   Clinical Clues to Distinguish LPR from Other Causes of Hoarseness

	LPR	Infection	Rhinosinusitis (Postnasal Drip)	Allergy	Benign Vocal Fold Lesion	Malignant Vocal Fold Lesion
Hoarseness characteristic	Fluctuates	Acute, resolves	Acute/chronic or recurrent	Fluctuates	Constant	Progressive
Throat pain	Common (with cough, throat clearing)	Yes	Uncommon	No	From secondary muscle tension	Late (local and referred)
Laryngeal findings	Edema, granuloma, erythema, pseudosulcus	Erythema, edema	Secretions (thick, discolored), edema	Edema, clear secretions, bluish mucosa	Nodules, polyps, cysts, scars	Ulcerative or exophytic (red-white mass), stiff
Aggravating factors	Smoking, obesity, diet/lifestyle	Systemic infection, immunosuppression	LPR, allergy, smoking	Environment, seasonal	Smoking, vocal trauma, LPR	Smoking (common), LPR, ethanolism

LPR, Laryngopharyngeal reflux.

of the vocal fold. It is not surprising to learn that reportedly chant therapy, Accent technique, and resonant therapy all have positive results in reducing vocal fatigue. These treatment techniques promote relaxation, easy phonation, and resonant balance and in so doing reduce the vocal load. Amplification reduces the load by reducing the vocal intensity of the speaker.

Based on existing assumptions and research completed primarily on teacher populations, it appears that a treatment program successful in reducing vocal fatigue and improving vocal quality focuses on reducing vocal load by providing the patient with (1) education as to good vocal hygiene, (2) amplification for speaking in noisy environments, (3) interspersed periods of vocal rest, and (4) treatment techniques that improve vocal resonance, relaxation, vocal flexibility, and endurance (vocal function exercises).

Reflux

Esophageal reflux is included under vocal abuse because it irritates, or abuses, the laryngeal tissues and creates a condition ripe for development of laryngeal pathology. The Committee on Speech, Voice and Swallowing Disorders of the American Academy of Otolaryngology–Head and Neck Surgery's position statement of laryngopharyngeal reflux (LPR) states that LPR refers to the backflow of stomach contents into the throat and differs in mechanism and manifestations from classic gastroesophageal reflux disease (GERD) (Koufman, Aviv, Casiano, et al, 2002). The primary problem in LPR is upper-esophageal sphincter dysfunction, which can occur at any age. Koufman and her colleagues (1985, 1991) have demonstrated the detrimental effects of reflux and they have also demonstrated experimentally that as little as three LPR episodes a week can result in severe laryngeal damage because the larynx lacks the epithelial defenses present in the esophagus. The most common symptoms of LPR are hoarseness, globus pharyngeus, dysphagia, cough, chronic throat clearing, vocal fatigue, and sore throat (Ford, 2006; Koufman, Amin, and Panetti, 2002). It has been estimated by Koufman, Amin, and Panetti (2002) that up to half of patients

with laryngeal and voice disorders have reflux of varying degrees. The severity of the disease determines the treatment. Treatment often includes recommendations for dietary and lifestyle changes to reduce the factors thought to precipitate reflux (e.g., smoking, drinking alcohol, ingesting coffee, eating spicy foods, eating just before bed, sucking on mints, wearing tight belts, bending at waist level, and sleeping without elevation of the head of the bed). In treating LPR, behavioral modification alone often is insufficient, and medical management of acid suppression and esophageal motility is also indicated. Ford (2005) developed a schema to provide clinicians with the clinical clues necessary to distinguish LPR from other causes of hoarseness (**Table 11.1**). He underscores the importance of case history taking and suggests that when the history is suggestive of diagnosis, patients be put on a 3-month trial of behavioral change and gastric acid suppression by adequate doses of proton pump inhibitor (PPI) medication. Patients failing this trial should be referred for multichannel intraluminal impedance and pH-monitoring studies to confirm LPR and assess the magnitude of the problem. Koufman, Amin, and Panetti (2002) state, "For most patients with LPR, twice-daily dosing with a PPI is recommended for an initial treatment for a period of no less than 6 months, and lifetime treatment may be required" (**Fig. 11.2**).

Vocal Nodules in Children

In children and adults, vocal abuse produces general inflammation or focal lesions that result in breathiness, huskiness, or hoarseness. It may occur secondary to LPR, coincidently

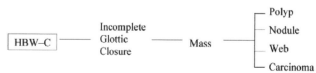

Figure 11.2   Algorithm for assessment and management of LPR from Ford.

with LPR, or alone. Musculoskeletal tension is often the physiologic basis of the abuse, and emotional and personality factors are its driving force. Vocal abuse in children takes the forms of loud talking, shouting, screaming, coughing, or throat clearing. The purposes of therapy are to reduce vocal fold trauma through reeducation and to reduce or eliminate emotional and environmental stress.

The therapy of choice in children and adults who have vocal nodules is vocal reeducation rather than surgical removal of the nodules, which may only return if vocal abuse is not reduced. Surgery without treating vocal abuse is now recognized as ineffective, or worse, in the treatment of vocal nodules except in cases of chronic, advanced, mature, fibrous nodules or when a microweb is present. Patients who have not had speech therapy show a higher recurrence rate (Barnes, 1981).

Von Leden (1988) has written that the presence of vocal nodules is not an automatic indication for surgery, particularly in patients who use their voices professionally, and if nodules do not respond to conservative treatment and if surgery is necessary, all efforts must be made to preserve healthy mucous membrane covering the vocal folds. "Stripping" has no place in the removal of vocal nodules because this procedure includes removal of healthy mucous membrane, denuding the vocal folds likely causing scarring, fibrosis, restricted vibratory excursions, and permanent dysphonia. The vocal folds may appear normal on laryngoscopic examination even with magnification; however, stroboscopic examination has shown limitations in the vibratory motions of the vocal folds that are typical in patients who have fibrotic changes. This same precaution to preserve the mucous covering of the vocal folds applies to other benign lesions.

In a survey of 535 otolaryngologists, Moran and Pentz (1987) found that 59% expressed preference for voice therapy as the sole mode of treatment for vocal nodules in children; less than 1% preferred surgery as the sole treatment; 9.4% recommended surgery to be followed by voice therapy; 50% indicated that voice therapy is frequently or always effective in the treatment of vocal nodules in children.

Voice therapy for children who have vocal nodules can be conducted either individually or in small groups. Group therapy has the advantage of heightening competitiveness and, consequently, motivation.

Informational Phase. The child should be given simplified information on the structure and function of the larynx. Drawings, color photographs, slides, models, and motion pictures of the larynx can be used for this purpose. One should explain why the voice is defective by comparing photographs or drawings of the normal vocal folds with those of vocal nodules or general inflammation.

Auditory Discrimination Phase. Using audio or video recordings, one can compare children's normal voices with those who have dysphonia as a result of vocal abuse and can discuss in detail how the voices differ. In group therapy, the children can evaluate one another's voices compared with the normal. Children can use severity rating scales or other means of documenting their reactions.

Voice-Production Phase. By now, the child should know the reason for the voice disorder and its characteristics. Two considerations in the voice-production phase are the following:

1. Situations in which vocal abuse is most likely to occur. The child needs to be made aware of situations in which vocal abuse is likely to occur, for example, yelling during sports activities and other forms of play, airing of conflicts among friends and family, and uncontrolled coughing and throat clearing.

2. Training the child to reduce vocal loudness and glottal attacks is central to direct voice therapy.

   ♦ *Reduce vocal loudness* The child's loudness discrimination abilities can be increased by recording voice at various loudness levels or by using various feedback devices. One should identify a comfortable loudness level and get the child to agree not to exceed this level in outside situations. The child should be told to use alternate signaling devices instead of yelling or be taught to yell by using more abdominal support and less laryngeal constriction.

   ♦ *Reduce sharpness of glottal attack* The child should be taught to produce words beginning with vowels by using a gentle vocal attack. The difference between the sharp or abrupt *coup de glotte* and the easy onset of voicing should be demonstrated. This technique can be illustrated by asking for phonation during sighing, leading into vowels produced with a breathy attack (i.e., beginning with the /h/ phoneme). The child should be made kinesthetically aware of relaxed, easy exhalation along the entire respiratory-laryngeal tract. One should teach the child to be aware of muscle sensation as well as the sound of the voice while developing new habits of phonation.

   ♦ *Discuss personal and family problems* As in all voice disorders, one should try to eliminate underlying causes or aggravating factors. Clinical research has shown that children abuse their voices in the process of acting out their aggressions, thereby discharging emotional tensions. Although many children are insufficiently aware of the emotional aspects of their lives, others have considerable insight and can talk about unpleasant situations, feelings, and attitudes toward friends and family. Time should be given for discussion of anxiety, frustration, anger, and unpleasant experiences. Group therapy is an excellent vehicle for generating discussion among children about their feelings and attitudes. Such discussions can be conducted maturely and without guilt about disclosing personal and family problems. To do so is valuable for the clinician to judge the extent to which the vocal abuse is a component of a larger emotional problem. Discussion with parents, school psychologists, and other professionals in a position to help may be necessary.

Parent Counseling Phase. Parents are an important part of the therapy for vocal abuse. They should be informed as to why voice therapy is being given their child and the alternatives to behavioral management. They should be aware of the potential role of reflux as a causative factor and that it is not uncommon in children. They should know the rationale and the methods being used and, especially, what is expected from the child in the way of self-control. They also should be aware that therapy is generally short-term and if it fails to yield significant changes that surgery may be indicated because of cysts or microwebs. Parental interviews are superior to communicating by letter or telephone. Parents differ in their attitudes toward voice therapy for their children. Many are not aware of the voice disorder—to them the child always sounded that way; that's just "his" voice. Others may not be convinced of the need for a change and resent that their child has been singled out for voice therapy. It is useful, therefore, to clarify objectives and to allow parents to express their attitudes.

Notwithstanding the time-honored concept of vocal nodule as a simple vocal abuse disorder, research studies have now established unequivocally that children who develop vocal nodules often have personality traits that make inhibition difficult and are often in conflict with family members and peers at school. The speech-language pathologist must weigh the factor of vocal acting out because of personality and family conflicts as a cause of the vocal abuse, investigate psychosocial forces at home and at school, and consider appropriate psychologic referral if indicated. One should discuss with parents, as with the child, sources of personal or family conflict that might be producing anger and emotional distress leading to vocal abuse.

Parents want to know whether or not they should remind the child at home about not abusing the voice. There is no firm rule except that the child is responsible for the voice, and the burden of that responsibility needs to be placed primarily on the child. If reminders are necessary, they should be infrequent and should never take the form of nagging. As reminder devices, the child can be given a calendar or other charting device on which to record gradations of voice use and abuse during each day. The child rates the voice according to how much and how loudly it was used. Although such devices are useful as reminders, they should be kept simple. Rewards for progress should be given.

Vocal Nodules in Adults

Vocal nodules in adults produce dysphonia similar to that found in children. It is husky, breathy, hoarse, and of lower than average pitch. Because the cause of vocal nodules in adults is basically the same as in children, so are the principles of therapy. Adults need to be informed of the reasons for the nodules. Graphic illustrations from strobe or other laryngeal exams and technical explanations should be tailored to the patient's background. Advice to reduce abuse of the voice during speaking and singing is usually accepted and implemented by most adults. Singers and professional voice users, as described in a separate chapter, are special cases particularly when the presence of vocal nodules gives the singer the vocal quality with which he or she is identified. Reduction of the nodule changes the vocal characteristics and could ruin his or her career. When singing is suspected as a major or contributory cause, a singing teacher or vocal coach should

be consulted. An assessment needs to be made as to how the voice ought to be used during singing; for example, loudness, background accompaniment (which may be excessive), and appropriate pitch range. The speech-language pathologist, patient, and voice coach all need to work together to determine the best singing practices to avoid vocal problems and aggravation of the nodules.

In all patients, health problems such as LPR and emotional problems paralleling the development of the nodules should be investigated. Many patients develop nodules even though they have not changed their singing or speaking habits. What often emerges during a thorough voice evaluation is that they have experienced an upper respiratory infection or LPR that resulted in irritated tissue and difficulty in producing voice. In many instances, they experienced an emotional upset in their lives that became the tipping point resulting in increased musculoskeletal tension to the point of adding enough frictional trauma to the vocal folds to produce nodules or they experienced the two in concert. The emotional problems may be minor, transient stresses from situational problems at work or at home—or more severe chronic stresses that seriously interfere with the person's sense of well-being. The speech-language pathologist needs to determine how serious these background factors are, and if the patient cannot manage them, she might need to be referred for psychologic or psychiatric consultation.

Adult females with vocal nodules are characteristically extroverts who are active, talkative people. They openly, smilingly, and with a tincture of pride admit they have always liked to talk. Within their ability to do so, they do readily accept advice to limit the amount of their speaking. However, they often have occupations that are not conducive to reduction in vocal output. As in children, adults should be taught to produce voice with less forceful stress or emphasis patterns, which often means lowering vocal intensity, and with easy onset of phonation rather than with a hard glottal attack. Some speech clinicians advocate reducing the pitch level of the voice to an "optimum pitch"; however, the necessity for finding an optimum pitch for reduction of nodules is controversial, as previously discussed in this chapter. Although the pitch is perceived as lower, quantitative measurements of fundamental frequency suggest that the fundamental frequency (Fo) is generally within normal limits. The added mass and abnormal hourglass closure pattern results in a characteristic quality that sounds lower and is only changed by reduction in the size of the nodules. The clinician should help the patient find a comfortable pitch level. The "um-hum" method described previously can be used for this purpose.

If vocal abuse has either caused or maintained the nodule, as is often the case, the voice modifications already mentioned should reduce the size of the nodule and even eliminate it within several weeks, depending upon its size and severity, the patient's ability to comply with therapy, the absence of a laryngeal web, and the size of the larynx. Except for encapsulated nodules, which many laryngologists believe should be removed surgically, voice reeducation is the therapy of choice and should be attempted for 6 weeks before surgery is considered. Patients should be seen periodically on return visits for both laryngoscopic and voice reevaluations to determine whether the effects of therapy are maintained.

One should not hesitate to involve family members in discussions with the patient about habits of voice use and implementation of therapy. Parents, spouses, siblings, and even children can provide objectivity for the adult and can help effect the clinician's recommendations by understanding the objectives of such therapy and feeling like a part of the therapy process.

Electronic devices for measuring vocal load have been used successfully in the treatment of vocal abuse disorders and should be considered as an important adjunct.

Contact Ulcer

Contact ulcers are so called because the granulation tissue occurs on the vocal process of the arytenoids where they make the greatest contact during loud phonation, coughing, and throat clearing. Contact ulcers are thought to result from LPR, abuse, and intubation trauma and result in hoarseness and excessively low pitch. They are rarely seen in females probably because during phonation, females have a posterior glottic gap and do not totally adduct the arytenoids. Therapy aims at reducing LPR and vocal fold trauma through vocal reeducation and eliminating emotional and environmental stress. Prognosis is excellent if the patient is able to reduce reflux and produce voice consistently in the manner prescribed. In cases of large granuloma formation, surgical excision is often necessary. Unless reflux has been managed, however, surgical removal of a contact ulcer is often unsuccessful because the granulation recurs. Clinical evidence shows that healing is best achieved with antireflux regimens and vocal reeducation. Voice therapy begins with an informational phase, during which the patient is given an understanding of the mechanics by which the ulcer has formed, using graphic illustrations. During the auditory discrimination phase, comparisons between the abnormally low-pitched, hoarse dysphonia and normal voice are made. The vocal production phase concerns modification of voice use in daily life. After a thorough analysis of daily dietary habits and voice use and abuse, the patient needs to be informed that until the ulcer heals, the quantity and intensity of voice use has to be modified. Aronson (1990) suggests voice use be reduced ~50% for 1 month, eliminating all but necessary speaking. Silence or whispering is contraindicated because of patient tendency to use stage whispering. Patients are instructed to avoid shouting and communicating over long distances or in high ambient noise levels. Patients can return to normal voice use afterward provided that they follow the additional instructions detailed next:

Anatomical Predisposition   Patients need to recognize that they may have an anatomic predisposition to develop contact ulcers; tissue covering the arytenoids may be thin, tissue may be dry increasing friction during closure, and refractory reflux may irritate the tissue covering the vocal processes. These individuals must be extra cautious how they use the larynx for voice production because without careful use, they are likely to have recurrences.

Produce Words Beginning with Vowels   Because words beginning with vowels may be produced with an explosive

glottal attack, which augments the force of vocal fold adduction and the frictional trauma to the vocal folds, the patient must be trained to produce words beginning with vowels by means of an easy or aspirate vocal attack. The patient should be taught to recognize and to feel the difference between hard and soft glottal attacks. Explosive speech ordinarily used for emphasis needs to be modulated.

Appropriate Pitch Level   Because trauma may result from excessively low pitch, employed because the patient believes it is more authoritative or impressive in the classroom, courtroom, or salesroom, a more appropriate pitch level will need to be taught. The "um-hum" method is advocated for obtaining the most comfortable pitch.

Reduce Coughing   Because frequent coughing or throat clearing not only is damaging to vocal folds but also retards healing of the contact ulcer, the patient needs to reduce these activities. Patients can be taught to swallow hard, sip ice water, or massage the neck when they feel the need to bring up material, or to clear the throat or cough with an easier, more aspirate approach rather than with an explosive glottal attack (i.e., the "silent cough").

Alcohol and Smoking   Because trauma is aggravated by alcohol consumption and smoking, the patient needs to be informed that both substances irritate the vocal folds. For the initial period of 1 month, both drinking and smoking need to be eliminated completely.

Reduce Musculoskeletal Tension   Because patients with vocal abuse disorders have increased musculoskeletal tension, the speech-language pathologist needs to work on reduction of those tensions (see the Musculoskeletal Tension [Vocal Hyperfunction] section of this chapter).

Contact Ulcer Patients   Contact ulcer patients who are hard driving, competitive, angry, and exhibit aggressive traits may be modifiable if the patient is concerned enough about their effects on the voice. If such tendencies are mild, they can be dealt with, but in more severe cases, referral for professional psychotherapy needs to be considered. Vocal abuse often occurs in fundamentally well-balanced people who have allowed themselves to be subjected to tremendous environmental stresses, such as an intensive schedule of speaking under adverse conditions at work, and burdensome extracurricular activities. There needs to be discussion with the patient about refusing to participate in such a vocally demanding schedule. Heavy work schedules that place the patient under extreme pressures resulting in irritability and leading to anger are precursors of the vocal abuse that leads to contact ulcer. The modification of the psychologic environment of some contact ulcer patients may be as important as reflux management and direct voice therapy, and, in fact, one without the other may prove ineffectual.

Conversion Voice Disorders

Conversion reactions produce diverse voice signs: muteness, aphonia, intermittent aphonia, breathiness, hoarseness, excessively high pitch, and falsetto. The abnormal voice, a sign of emotional or interpersonal conflict, has served or continues to serve the purpose of enabling the patient to avoid confrontation with an unpleasant life situation. Also, the voice may be serving the purpose of primary or secondary gain. Conversion aphonia or dysphonia may continue even after conflict resolution.

The voice disorder exists on an unconscious level; the patient is not willfully or volitionally producing the abnormal voice and consciously believes that the disorder is organic, not psychogenic. Even though the neuromuscular system is intact, the patient is unable to phonate voluntarily and is convinced of this inability. The interpersonal problems causing the voice disorder remain unexpressed to the parties concerned, including the clinician from whom the patient has sought help. The likelihood of complete return of the voice via symptomatic voice therapy is excellent if the patient is ready to relinquish the voice sign and to bring the problem causing it into the open. The prognosis is also excellent if the original problem has disappeared. When the conflict has not been resolved, the prognosis is poor for patients who are unwilling to face and deal with the underlying problem causing the voice disorder, in which case either it will be difficult—if not impossible—to improve the voice by means of any therapy or, if improvement does take place, it may be incomplete or short-lived.

Symptomatic voice therapy is subdivided into the following phases: patient education; symptom removal by means of direct voice therapy, manual musculoskeletal tension reduction, catharsis; and psychotherapy when indicated. The efficacy of symptomatic voice therapy is predicated on the following principles:

♦ Reduction of laryngeal musculoskeletal tension will change laryngeal posture and facilitate voice.

♦ Evoking voice by any one of a variety of means will convince the patient of his or her phonatory capability.

Therapy Rationale

Successful therapy for conversion voice disorders begins with the speech-language pathologist taking primary responsibility for patient management. The history of our profession's attitudes toward the treatment of patients with conversion voice disorders has been one of avoidance of this responsibility. It is often reasoned, erroneously, that because the disorder is primarily psychogenic, its treatment should be left in the hands of the psychiatrist or clinical psychologist. Another time-honored belief held by clinicians of all specialties is that symptom removal of a conversion disorder is dangerous if its underlying cause is not treated and that the conversion sign will reappear someplace else. This idea dies hard despite the fact that psychiatrists no longer subscribe to it. Hundreds of cases of conversion symptom removal in many different body parts without adverse effects or subsequent conversions have been documented. The worst result will be failure to relieve the voice sign because of patient unreadiness, undoubtedly a continued defense mechanism. Psychiatrists now believe that reported adverse reactions to attempted symptom removal were caused not by the removal of the conversion itself but by the precipitous and traumatic manner by which it was removed.

Experience with conversion voice disorders shows that premature referral of the patient to the psychiatrist or psychologist is almost a guarantee of failure to improve the voice. The validity of this statement is based on the following reasons:

♦ The voice disorder, a somatic sign, is, in the patient's mind, dissociated from conscious awareness of any emotional problem. This is the reason why most patients whose voices have been treated through traditional "interview" psychotherapy alone have not improved.

♦ Symptom removal in conversion voice disorders requires laryngeal muscular alterations simultaneous with auditory feedback (i.e., treatment directed at the larynx itself).

♦ Despite what might be excellent training in psychodiagnostics and psychotherapy, most psychologists and psychiatrists are not trained to deal with voice disorders.

♦ The unavailability of psychiatric and psychologic personnel and their lack of interest in voice disorders because of the relative mildness of the psychologic problems that underlie most of them make conversion patients less acceptable to such specialists. The psychiatrist and psychologist become most important after the voice disorder has been eliminated or improved. Then, if the emotional factors are sufficiently severe, referral is warranted.

♦ The patient with a conversion voice disorder who is convinced that the disorder is organic more often than not refuses referral to a psychologist or psychiatrist, in the beginning. Only after the voice has returned do such patients become aware of psychologic causes; they are then more receptive to referral.

There is, then, a proper sequence of clinical events that needs to take place in the treatment of conversion voice disorders: laryngologic clearance of organic laryngeal disease and systemic illness; symptomatic voice therapy coupled with ventilation and elaboration of emotional problems, if the patient is capable of doing so; and referral to the psychologist or psychiatrist to achieve a more enduring stabilization of the patient's life adjustment. A mature, cautious, and well-trained speech-language pathologist will not harm the patient. On the contrary, the opportunity given the patient to discuss emotional problems simultaneously while undergoing the more mechanical aspects of voice therapy can only serve to provide that patient with new hope for a better voice. It is for patients such as these that we advocate so strongly the interdisciplinary practice of speech-language pathology in settings that bring psychologist, psychiatrist, laryngologist, and speech-language pathologist together, for such relationships provide a feeling of greater confidence on the part of all clinicians treating such patients.

Patient Education

As in other voice disorders, the first phase of therapy for conversion voice disorders is patient education. After obtaining a complete history and after deciding that a conversion voice disorder exists, if the voice has not improved spontaneously during the history—as it sometimes does as the patient reveals underlying emotional stresses for the first time—the first necessity in therapy is to educate the patient about the cause of the aphonia or dysphonia. Almost universally characteristic is their initial insistence that the disorder is organic. This denial will delay, in many cases, and prevent, in others, successful voice therapy. Time needs to be taken to discuss the beliefs of both laryngologist and speech-language pathologist that the disorder is not due to infection, tumor, or other organic cause and that it is due to excess laryngeal tension. This may be due to emotional stress and/or a habituated pattern of muscle use. How the speech-language pathologist handles this informational phase can determine the difference between continuation on to success or early failure. The difference lies in the manner by which this information is communicated. Many patients previously seen by other clinicians have been told point blank that they needed to see a psychiatrist. Such precipitous revelation of what may be essentially true is almost always indigestible by the patient. On the other hand, a gradual, sympathetic unfolding of this fact through discussion can make the difference between acceptance and rejection of the idea.

The first step is to divest the patient of the notion that the voice disorder is organic by reviewing the laryngologist's findings with the patient. Firmly and authoritatively, the clinician should tell, or preferably read aloud, the laryngologist's report-that the larynx was normal on examination, that no lesions or paralyses were noted, and that the patient has the physical capability to produce normal voice. This information not only serves to start the patient thinking about emotional factors but also relieves anxiety about threatening laryngeal disease, namely, cancer. Patients show visible signs of relief upon hearing this report. Their anxieties about laryngeal disease are real, and with the restatement about the normal laryngologic examination, the patient's mind is cleared of fears of serious illness. The germ of the idea that perhaps the voice is due to emotional causes after all is thus planted. For some patients, this is enough for the moment to begin direct symptom management before dealing more directly with the emotional issues. When the clinician presents the concept, in language appropriate to the patient's educational background, the clinician states that the larynx is a common site for the expression of emotional problems. Most people are already aware of this fact on the basis of lifelong experience. It can be pointed out to them how, in everyday life, we express our emotions—anger, fear, grief—through the larynx, and how it sometimes undergoes violent, uncontrollable muscular reactions that can be felt as well as heard during transient emotional states. The rate of informational exchange, the pacing, and the clinician's finesse develop with practice. It is wise to stop at various points along the way to sample the patient's reactions to this new knowledge. It is always interesting to see how different patients with conversion voice disorders react to the idea of psychogenicity. A few are so threatened and incensed by the idea that they refuse to continue the interview, grabbing for their coats and purses in preparation for terminating the session. Fortunately, although most patients react at first with skepticism, they are willing to listen. Some amiably agree. They "knew it all the time" but needed someone else to confront them with the facts. Once the patient is willing to consider the possibility that the voice disorder is related to emotional conflict or stress, the stage is set for the next phase.

If the patient has not already gained voice, the clinician proceeds to inform the patient that there has been a loss of contact between the desire to produce voice and the voluntary muscular ability to do so. After working with several patients who have conversion voice disorders, the clinician will eventually become convinced that the patient is genuinely under the impression that they are unable to phonate more than they do at the time of examination, even though they have been making audible sounds via throat clearing and coughing, thus failing to appreciate the relationship between those signals and the potential for normal voice (see Chapter 9).

Direct Voice Therapy

During direct voice therapy, all attention is paid to the larynx and voice, and psychologic considerations are set aside. One should test first for the presence and extent of musculoskeletal tension, which almost invariably accompanies conversion voice disorders. The identical procedures for the relief of isolated musculoskeletal tension are employed at this time. Incorporated into the manual relief of such tension are the clinician's instructions to the patient to produce various laryngeal noises—coughing followed by an extension of coughing into continuous voicing, throat clearing, and humming. The purpose of this activity should not be lost on either clinician or patient: it is to convince the patient that there is more voice capability than the patient realized. When increased laryngeal sound occurs, it should be pointed out instantaneously.

Patients vary in their rate of voice improvement and in the acoustic characteristics that accompany such improvement. Those who have had aphonia or dysphonia for long periods of time will go through several stages of dysphonia, which may require as much as an hour of therapy before normal voice is approached. These dysphonic transitional stages can take the form of raucous hoarseness or harshness. They must be recognized as transitional stages and must be worked through to normal voice. Patients react early to voice improvements with much surprise, even astonishment, proving their obliviousness to their actual voice capabilities. Their voice improvements should be met with the clinician's approval and pleasure. Patients who have had conversion voice disorders for shorter periods will often shift from severe dysphonia or aphonia to normal voice within minutes. Others who are not ready for symptom removal either will fail to respond with any voice improvement or will produce varying degrees of voice improvement short of normal and then plateau despite continued efforts at therapy. Such patients are not candidates for further therapy at that point and ought to be asked to return for a second or third try. Some will fail to keep future appointments, for obvious reasons.

Catharsis and Counseling

The next phase of therapy is catharsis and discussion of emotional causes. Upon experiencing a return of their voices, most patients will express emotional relief, usually a mixture of smiling and weeping, which they attribute to their happiness for having been relieved of the burden of the abnormal voice. Such emotional reaction is healthy and is to be encouraged, despite the patient's protestations of embarrassment. One should discuss with them their feelings about the return of the voice while at the same time encouraging them to use the voice to its fullest. This is a good time to get the patient to talk about the frustration, embarrassment, and other effects of the voice disorder. Most will describe considerable inconvenience that they and their families have suffered as a consequence of the disorder. The patient's change of facial expression and general attitude should be noted. The face is less tense, less frowning; there are fewer signs of distress around the mouth and eyes, and a general impression of happiness. The patient's attitude will change to one of increased openness, a willingness to talk more freely, and, most importantly, an apparent improvement of insight and memory for the events, feelings, and attitudes that gave rise to the voice disorder in the first place.

For patients who are receptive to discussion of psychogenic causes, despite earlier denial of them, this is an excellent time to reopen the subject. It is a never-ending source of wonder how often patients become aware of emotional conflicts only after the voice has returned and how they go on to describe acute or chronic stresses and conflicts in their lives, usually of an interpersonal nature and having to do with a breakdown in communication with persons close to them and in whom they have much ego investment. The speech-language pathologist will discover that quite ordinary irritations are, to many patients with psychogenic voice disorders, monumental. One quickly learns that each person responds to life's problems with different degrees of emotional reactivity. Here are some examples: loss of voice after an argument with a relative or friend; loss of voice because of feelings that one's position of authority has been usurped in an office setting; a feeling of having been wronged in the settlement of a family estate; inability to tolerate personal habits in one's spouse and to confront that person with one's feelings; deep frustration, disappointment, or job dislike that one is unable to change for fear of repercussions from employers or family; an engagement or marital relationship that has gone sour in which the patient is unable to express the wish that the relationship be discontinued. A common denominator runs through these themes despite the differences in their specifics: the need to express anger, dissatisfaction, or grief, but an inability to do so. Lifelong, these individuals have never been able to express their feelings openly and directly. Often, the speech-language pathologist is the first person to whom they have had an opportunity to reveal these unspoken and sometimes unspeakable ideas.

Referral

Finally, the speech-language pathologist and patient need to talk about the future. They need to decide whether the orig-

inal emotional problem is still operative, whether it has been resolved or is resolving. With clinical experience, a certain practical sense develops in judging whether or not the patient can benefit from further professional psychotherapy. The decision for referral to a psychologist or a psychiatrist should be bilateral. The patient, however, must make the final decision. Does he or she feel happy or satisfied with life? Is this someone who has long felt the need for professional help but has been too shy, afraid, indecisive, or confused as to how to obtain it? Realistically, not all patients with conversion voice disorders are candidates for psychotherapy. Many are superficial and denying; they either reject such therapy on the grounds of not needing it or, once begun, discontinue. Sometimes, all one can do is carry the person over the crisis by being a listener and a friend. Although speech clinicians do not practice psychotherapy, we have a responsibility for being the "advanced party," for breaking new ground, and for helping the patient to discover, perhaps for the first time, that further help is needed. An impressive number of patients, upon learning that their abnormal voice was a primitive substitute for a more mature solution, will then attack their problems directly. Often, patients will obtain enough insight from voice therapy and discussion alone to make effective changes in their lives, usually those who have sufficient ego reserve and aggressiveness. The passive and dependent types, overwhelmed by life's punishments, cannot seem to get out from under, and for them psychiatric consultation and therapy are indicated and should be advocated as strongly as possible.

The evolution of therapy for conversion voice disorders has arrived at the point where it is now known that mechanical, symptomatic voice therapy must be cradled in kindness, psychotherapeutic counseling, and respect for the unusual nature of conversion itself. The history of treatment of this disorder has been brutal and ineffectual because of the failure to respect and recognize the patient's potential for insight and growth.

The following case studies show the interaction between patient and clinician during interviewing and voice therapy for conversion voice disorders.

Case Study 11.1

A 26-year-old police officer, on the force for 3 years, had never been happy in his work. He had never told anyone about his feelings for fear of disappointing his parents, who were very much in favor of this vocation. He had always been a quiet, unaggressive person who found it difficult to lose his temper, but when he did, he shook and became livid with rage. He found it difficult to reprimand motorists or pedestrians because of a strong need to be liked by everyone. The patient had had several previous episodes of aphonia and dysphonia, which, heretofore, had cleared up spontaneously. At the time of interview, he was aphonic. Laryngologic examination was normal.

Clinician (C): What brings you to this clinic?

Patient (P): (Patient's voice is a complete whisper.) My voice. I haven't been able to talk. It started April 9th; it came back for a few days and then it was gone again. But it was all high-pitched. And then, finally, that went away again. And it has been like this for the last 3 or 4 weeks now. I had a bad cold. It started with laryngitis. And my voice started to come back again. Then, all of a sudden it was gone, just like it is now—completely. Altogether it was about 4 or 5 weeks that I lost it.

C: How did it come back?

P: I coughed and I had a voice back. The next time, it was in either September or October of last year, I had a slight cold—no sore throat or anything—but the next day my voice was gone again. And that lasted only for about 9 days.

C: How did it come back?

P: I can't remember exactly how that one did come back.

C: Are you able to make any sound at all?

P: Once in a while a sound will come out.

C: Before we go any further, I wonder if you would read this aloud for me. (Just before beginning, the patient coughs audibly, but reads the passage in a completely whispered voice.) Now would you cough for me? (Patient coughs repeatedly, each time with an excellent glottal attack and brief audible voicing.)

C: What kind of work do you do?

P: Police officer.

C: How long have you been doing that?

P: Since January of last year.

C: Have you been happy in your work?

P: I wonder . . . if I actually do like the work that I am doing, or if I am just saying I do because I don't want to tell everybody that I would like to quit and that I don't want the police department.

C: Disregarding what other people think, how do you actually feel about the job?

P: Well . . . I have trouble giving somebody a ticket. I have trouble talking to a person.

C: What is there about talking to people that is so difficult?

P: I get nervous. I am always afraid that I am going to say something or do something wrong . . . that's going to get either me or somebody else in trouble. Because if you do one thing wrong in the police department, you might as well forget your job.

C: In other words, when you are talking to a motorist who may have violated a law, you feel under pressure to be correct.

P: I can tell them what they have done wrong, and if they don't start arguing I am all right . . . But once they start arguing, then, well, if I get mad I start to shake when I get nervous like that. Then my words start to get mixed up. I know I shouldn't get nervous. That is our job, and people expect it. It's just something that happens to me. The worst time I got angry, I actually saw red. I got mad once, really mad, while I was in a fight, and a guy bit me; and then I really got mad. I didn't think it was possible to see red, but I saw red.

C: That must have been very frightening.

P: I shook for about an hour and a half after it.

C: Does being a policeman make you uncomfortable because you are in the position of being a disciplinarian?

P: I never thought of that. I don't like people to dislike me.

C: Well, let's say that you have to apprehend a motorist for speeding or some other violation. What are your feelings? What goes through your mind?

P: If we see someone we think is speeding, we get in behind him and clock him with our speedometer . . . If he is speeding, we'll stop the clock which locks the speedometer so that we know what speed he is still going at, and stop the car and go over and tell him, you know, that he has been speeding. Once in a while, you will get a guy who will argue, but usually they will go along with you. Once in a while, you find a guy who is never wrong. His car can't go that fast. And then, we start to argue and then I . . . I don't know, I get flustered . . .

C: You have the evidence there . . .

P: I have the evidence, but yet, I . . . I know I am right and that's what I don't get. I know I am right and yet I am the one that gets nervous. When actually he should be the one. He is getting the ticket . . . I know I am sensitive to other people's feelings about me . . . how people think of me . . . what they think of me. (At this point, discussion was discontinued and voice therapy begun.)

C: I would like to explain something to you. You haven't really lost your voice. You have temporarily lost the knowledge of how to make it function again. But the voice is there, and through certain activities there is a good likelihood that we can get it back. First of all, hum for me. (Clinician demonstrates. Patient does not seem to know how to go about producing a humming noise.) Make a coughing noise. (Patient coughs audibly.) Now do it again, except prolong it this time. (Patient prolongs the cough into a predominately breathy dysphonia.) Now, did you hear that voicing? That's the voice. And I would like you to keep it going. Try it again. (Patient repeats the cough with the breathy prolongation.) Now, try it without the cough. Hum. (Patient begins to produce an intermittent, weak humming noise.) Yes, I hear it now. Again. (Patient repeats. After ~15 seconds of humming at the weak, high pitches, the pitch drops with a marked tremor, at the same time becoming increasingly louder. Suddenly, the patient speaks in a normal voice.)

P: It's back!

C: Well! . . . Very good.

P: Huh! . . . It's back. (Voice quality and loudness are normal.)

C: How does it feel?

P: It feels all right (tentatively). It's not normal. It's higher. A little more gravelly.

C: This is fairly common, and it will come down to where it should be in a reasonably short time.

P: Because, this happened to me before. It was real high, and then it went away again. But it's not as high as it was then.

C: Would you read this out loud for me, to strengthen it a little bit? (Patient reads the passage.)

P: Wonderful! . . . A little funny . . . that it was that easy to get back . . . Would it have come back like this if I had just walked in here, without talking to you fellows? Or is it because I've talked to you and the other doctor?

C: What do you think?

P: I think so . . . I mean I think that I might not have gotten it back.

C: Why do you think that talking to us has played a part in your getting your voice back?

P: Because I know when I was talking to the other doctor (the psychiatrist), there is something that I brought up, that I started feeling funny.

C: What was that?

P: It was about the police department. He asked me about . . . that "you don't really like your job and you are afraid to tell your family this." And I agreed with him, but I felt real funny.

C: Was it true?

P: Yes . . . I have never told anyone.

C: Having talked about it with somebody, how does it make things different?

P: I shouldn't be afraid to tell my family. It's my life. I should enjoy what I am doing. I shouldn't be working for something because they all think I should be working there. I should be doing something that I want to do. And not what they want me to do. That's what I feel, anyway.

C: You feel, then, that having said this to someone else has changed your attitude.

P: Right. Because I had thought of it before, but I had never mentioned it to anybody. You two fellows are the first people I ever told it to.

C: Was it hard for you to think about? To admit it to yourself?

P: Uh huh. I didn't want to admit to myself, you know, that I didn't like the job. Like, me, I am a constant daydreamer, and I dream about it.

C: What would you like to be doing?

P: My old job.

C: Which was . . .

P: Textile chemist.

C: Tell me about that.

P: I'd mix the chemicals, bleach the cloth, dry the cloth . . . I don't know, I just enjoyed working. It was long hours. The pay wasn't that great. But I enjoyed working there.

C: What did you enjoy the most about it?

P: I don't know if it was because I worked alone. I'd maybe say 10 words a day. I didn't mind it. I sing a lot. I'd sing all the time. And I enjoyed it. Or if I wanted to daydream, I could daydream.

C: What do you daydream about?

P: You name it (laughs). Mostly about, oh I don't know, money, being strong, you know, crazy things.

C: How could your loss of voice be related to . . . all this?

P: Well, I don't know . . . Subconsciously, it was the only way I knew of getting away from there . . . maybe rebelling.

C: What do you think would be the solution to the problem of the voice loss?

P: I think it's the job that's causing it. Maybe I'm wrong. Maybe I'd get another job, and it would go away again. I don't think so.

C: Do you really think that you will be able to put into action what you would really like to do?

P: Well, I think that now that I have talked to you fellows, and I know that it's because I don't want to tell my par-

ents, maybe now I can tell my parents. Because I was always shutting it out before. I never wanted to think about it. Maybe it wouldn't bother them half as much as I think it would.

Case Study 11.2

A 46-year-old cosmetologist had been under chronic stress resulting from several sources: her concern about her son, a rebellious, belligerent young man of 25; her unspoken rage at her husband, who had never supported the family completely and usually didn't work at all; and her chronic irritation with her cosmetology-salon employees. She insisted on perfection from them yet was never able to voice her irritations when they fell short. Instead, her voice faltered into an intermittent hoarseness and whisper, and she was overwhelmed with fatigue and usually forced to go home and take to her bed. Her marginal insight into all this was evidenced by her statement that "I am afraid my employees think that I am angry with them when I lose my voice and can't talk." The patient had had many previous brief episodes of dysphonia and aphonia, which had cleared up spontaneously. The most recent one brought her to this clinic because of its unusually long duration (9 weeks). At the time of interview, her voice was an intermittent dysphonia-aphonia. Results of laryngologic examination were negative.

Clinician (C): Is this your first loss of voice?

Patient (P): No, I've had it many times, but I've never had it for more than 14 days.

C: But this last time it's been longer.

P: Started my ninth week yesterday. I know one thing; it seems that I always lose my voice in October. One of my problems is that I have trouble hiring efficient help.

C: Have you felt at all depressed or unhappy whenever you have lost your voice in the past?

P: I've tried to analyze that myself, and I don't come up with the answer. A couple of my better employees say that they think that this directly follows mental strain—if I become upset over something—but I haven't been able to look back and prove to myself that that's true.

C: Does it create any problems, your not being able to use your voice normally?

P: Yes, it makes it so that I'm not really able to cope with my business activities. You can't answer a telephone, people just hang up on you . . . I can't conduct extracurricular activities.

C: What else?

P: (With great emphasis) I can't express myself at all. There is no intonation in your voice at all. You sound like you are angry all the time.

C: Well . . . we would like to help you get your voice back, but we would also like to learn more about you. Would you have any objections to staying on for a few days and being interviewed by some of our psychiatrists?

P: Not at all (surprised). You're not a psychiatrist?

C: No. I am a speech pathologist.

P: You're certainly putting a lot into it, psychology-wise (embarrassed laughter).

C: It's all interrelated, isn't it? Before we arrange these interviews, we would like to help you get your voice back, and I think we can start right away. Would you open your mouth, now, wide as you can? Now say /a:/. (Patient produces a weak, high-pitched, scratchy voice.) Make it louder. Now stick your tongue out, Again, now, /a:/. (Patient produces a harsh voice a shade louder, which has a rapid tremor.) Kind of a tremorous voice, isn't it, but it's there. Try it again. Let's do something else now. Tilt your head back, now open your mouth as wide as you can and stick your tongue way out. Now say /a:/ and keep that up. I want you to listen for that sound and try to keep it going. Try it again, real sharp now. (Patient produces slightly louder tone, momentarily, and is encouraged to listen for it and repeat it.) It sounds worse than it is, doesn't it?

P: It doesn't hurt . . . at all.

C: Can you hum for me? (Patient produces a very clear high-pitched tone on humming.) Oh, very good. Take a deep breath and do that again. Can you do that a little louder? (Tone clearer this time.) Now try /ma:/. (Patient produces a high-pitched, breathy voice, which is an improvement over previous productions. She is asked to repeat this several times.) Let's try /ma:/ again. (Patient produces this equally well.) It's still too high, isn't it? That's not your normal voice.

P: No. But I've never been able to sing for years. (Patient continues to produce a variety of vowels with gradual reduction of breathiness. However, there is a great deal of quavering or tremor to the voice on vowel prolongation.)

C: Let's go down one tone, now. (Patient complies, and the vowel /a:/ is produced at progressively lower pitches. Vocal loudness is also increasing. There is a strained, harsh quality, nevertheless.) Very good. Continue. Now let's make it real smooth . . . Let's try it again. Do you hear the way your voice catches now and then? Do you feel a tightening whenever that happens?

P: I'll . . . take . . . better notice.

C: Now I want you to say this: M-o-n-d-a-y. (Clinician produces it in a monopitch. Patient repeats, "Monday," in a monopitch with fairly good clarity, although with some harshness and voice tremor. She is asked to produce this word at successively lower pitch levels. As she repeats this word, and as the voice quality and loudness improve, she becomes increasingly tearful, and the voice begins to crack.) This improvement in the voice seems to have affected you. True?

P: Yes . . . It relieves me.

C: You notice how your voice has dropped down to a lower pitch? I think that's where it wants to settle. Let's see if it gravitates down in that direction. Try it again. (Patient repeats sentence.) Yes, there it goes down to the lower pitch. That's fine. Continue. (She is then given a passage to read aloud. She does so in a nearly normal voice. As she is reading, the clinician intersperses requests that she speak louder at various points in her reading. With that last reading of the passage, it is apparent to both clinician and patient that the voice is normal or near normal.) How do you feel now?

P: Tired . . . sore . . . but good!

C: Go on.

P: How do I feel? . . . I feel . . . uh . . . sort of exuberant, I am sure . . . it's . . . been a long . . . long time. I feel good. Now my voice sounds more normal. I feel nice. I feel good. (Gives a great sigh.) Now what happens? . . . Is this going to happen every once in a while? When I started talking again, I always just started talking. I never had to struggle like this. I would all of a sudden realize I was talking. I would be whispering and all of a sudden I would be talking. That feels better. It sounds better, too, doesn't it?

C: Is it completely back to normal? Or does it have a way to go yet?

P: Well, I am afraid I have a way to go. My normal voice doesn't take any effort.

C: Does it still take some effort now?

P: Yes, it still takes effort. (Patient resumes practice. Pitch of voice is gradually decreasing, loudness is increasing, and quality is clearing. After this, she is asked to employ spontaneous speech in an effort to enable her to use her voice in more automatic speech situations. She describes the furnishing of her business establishment.)

C: Let's talk about these voice losses. Do you have any warning that you are going to lose it?

P: I do seem to have a warning when I am going to lose my voice . . . I have this tight feeling in my chest. However, I have never associated it with any happening in my life. These are such common, everyday things that it might just take an accumulation to make a person, all of a sudden, fight back some way or another, you see?

C: By "fight back," what do you mean?

P: Well, my husband says, and I think he has got it pretty straight, maybe, that I get so sick and tired of talking to women day in and day out . . . I like my work, but he says I get so sick of women talking and yakking and the daily noise around me, that finally I make up my mind I'm just not going to talk. Well, he might have something there. I don't know. Maybe things pile up on me or something, 'til I'll just fight back by not talking. I'll show them. I don't know. Day in and day out, we have to talk to people and be nice to them, which, of course, we want to be, and, uh, if someone comes in and throws themselves into your chair, starts to be a little bit obnoxious, she's had an argument with her husband, or she didn't like the news on the radio, or one of her children acted up before he got on the school bus . . . You know there is something in the back of her mind, so the first thing you do is try to kind of butter her up a little bit. Now, it's a very very trivial thing, but uh . . . when you've done this about 10 times in 1 day you get sort of sick of it after a while . . . and there is one thing that I cannot do when I don't have a voice, I can't do that!

C: Do you think that your voice loss comes about after a series of stressful events?

P: I have asked myself this same question many times before. As I have said, one of my valuable employees has told me that she has noticed over the years that every time I have a real nervous spell . . . not every time . . . when I have a real nervous time, perhaps not just one day of it, that I oftentimes get laryngitis. So, since she told me that, and I had never heard her voice this until this last siege of laryngitis, I have been trying to think that through and see if she is right. If this is true, I still don't know how to keep from having it happen again. (Patient sent for psychiatric consultation at this point. Resumes next day.)

C: Tell me, what did you do after your appointments yesterday?

P: (Patient's voice virtually normal. She is in good spirits—almost childlike attitude; many pitch and inflectional changes; generally a great deal of melody to the voice.) Well (laughs), we went down to one of the restaurants, had a bit piece of cake, and celebrated, and we made up our minds to hunt for one of my husband's friends living near here. I was tempted to go back to my room and go to bed, but I didn't think that would be smart. I felt that I should keep talking, and driving in my husband's truck I would have to talk loud and keep talking, and so, I just talked over the noise of the motor, and I think my husband helped me along. He asked me everything twice (laughs), on purpose, I think.

C: Is he pleased with your voice?

P: Yes! I should say so.

C: So, you feel that your voice is normal now?

P: Uh huh.

C: You feel well?

P: Uh huh.

C: Is there anything that you would like to ask about?

P: No . . . uh . . . I would like to know about . . . about my psychoanalyst [sic] yesterday . . . I find that very interesting. I'd just like to know a little bit more about myself.

C: I talked with him [psychiatrist], and he confirmed what we had discussed yesterday, that your voice loss is related to your way of reacting to the stresses around you. He thought that you have the habit of bottling up your emotions, instead of allowing yourself to express how you feel, like blowing off steam.

P: That I know about myself.

C: Do you have any idea why you can't?

P: I have always wondered about myself in this respect. I never can express love or emotions of that sort, either, without forcing myself. That's probably why I don't blow up, too . . . Now, I am sure that I feel just as deeply as anyone, but I just don't talk about it.

C: Do you know why this is true?

P: No, unless it's my upbringing. My parents were very close to each other, and they never argued. I never heard them argue in my whole life. I see this as something unusual. However, neither did I ever see my father kiss my mother more than maybe a couple of times in my life. I mean, there was no outward expression of love. I think maybe I was sort of ashamed to express myself. I wasn't brought up to wear my emotions on my sleeve.

C: How do you feel toward people who do express themselves in these ways?

P: Oh! I think it's wonderful! I really do. That is the only way to live.

C: Do you wish, perhaps, that you could live that way?

P: Yes, I think maybe that those around me would like me better.

C: Which of your parents do you think kept their feelings to themselves more?

P: Mother did. Very much.

C: Were you close to your mother?

P: (Emphatically) Yes! My father was 20 years older than my mother. He just worshipped me. I know that. But I was still closer to my mother.

C: Do you feel that you're like your mother?

P: Yes. Uh huh. Everyone does. I mean, in appearance, and they say the older I get the more I look like her and the more I act like her. I always felt that I couldn't be any better than that.

C: Do you think that you are like her also in the respect that you don't show your feelings externally?

P: I suppose you are right! You know, I never thought of that? I never thought of being emotionally like my mother. I presume that I have often expressed the desire to be. Because she was a person who was always so well liked and never seemed to resent anyone. I never heard her say anything unkind about anyone in my whole life. Women would come to our house and gossip, sometimes, and mother would clam right up and not say a word. For a woman not to ever gossip is almost unheard of.

C: Do you think she allowed herself to be taken advantage of?

P: Yes, I think she did.

C: Do you think you are like that?

P: Not as much as she was. I let people run over me at times. That's probably half my trouble in my business. I will let someone keep getting away with something until it builds up too much, I suppose. I should not have let them get away with it to start with. But rather than putting my foot down and saying, "Now look, we don't do things that way," that this is it, I would let them get off easy.

C: Well, why don't you?

P: (Laughs.) I am going to try, I'll tell you.

Mutational Falsetto (Puberphonia)

Despite anatomically and physiologically normal respiratory and phonatory structures, mutational falsetto is produced with the larynx positioned excessively high in the neck and vocal folds lax and stretched thin anteroposteriorly. Phonation is produced with abnormally reduced infraglottal air pressure caused by shallow respiration. The voice is high or intermediate in pitch, weak and thin, breathy, hoarse, and gives the impression of immaturity, passiveness, and effeminacy.

Voice therapy begins with asking the patient to breathe in deeply and to produce a vowel or cough with a sharp glottal attack, as demonstrated by the clinician. The pitch will break abruptly to a lower level. If the sharp glottal attack is unsuccessful, one should manually pull the larynx downward as the vowel is being produced. If these measures fail, while holding the larynx down, one should depress the tongue with a tongue depressor as the patient produces the sharp glottal attack. Alternatively, asking the patient to yell as if he needed someone from the other end of a football field may bring about a lower voice because he can't yell at the high pitch.

The low-pitched voice should be identified immediately for the patient. If the disorder is actually mutational falsetto, it is important to explain early in therapy that the low-pitched voice is the normal one and that the patient must learn to think of it as the target voice in therapy. This information must be conveyed persuasively, because the patient will not be completely convinced until after habituation of the low-pitched voice.

As soon as the low-pitched voice is produced, it should be maintained through repeated vowel production using a sharp glottal attack. The therapy is not a gradual stepwise progression from the high to the low pitch. The break must be sudden and complete. Phonation must be forceful and vigorous. The voice will want to shift up to the falsetto, in which case the patient will need to be reminded to breathe in deeply and then phonate sharply. Increased depth of breathing is fundamental to success in therapy, and the patient needs practice in phonating after deep inhalation. The clinician judges on a moment-to-moment basis how long to remain on vowels before attempting words, sentences, and conversational speech.

In a study of the pitch and quality characteristics of 10 adolescent males aged 13 to 18 years and two adult males, ages 26 and 29 years, who had mutational falsetto, Hammarberg (1987) found that the mean change in fundamental frequency in 10 of the subjects between 13 and 18 years of age before and after therapy was 221 Hz (range, 168 to 288 Hz) and 119 Hz (range, 105 to 135), respectively. In the two males 26 to 29 years of age, the mean fundamental frequency prior to therapy was 198 Hz and after therapy 100 Hz.

A reasonably stabilized voice should be achievable within an hour. Three to five additional therapy sessions are usually necessary to effect habituation. The most difficult phase of the therapy for mutational falsetto is getting the patient accustomed to the low-pitched voice. Gradual guidance into outside activities is necessary. Embarrassment upon returning to school is common among adolescents with mutational falsetto, and for that reason, therapy during vacation is desirable.

Patients who have mutational falsetto, for reasons of immaturity, lack insight into the reason for their voice disorders and even when needed often make poor candidates for counseling and psychotherapy. Fortunately, in most cases the cause is no longer operative by the time the patient comes for voice therapy. A complete and permanent low pitch can be attained without delving into either the psychologic or physiologic reasons for the failure of voice change. Occasionally, despite their ability to produce the low-pitched voice, certain patients will refuse to proceed with the therapy because they are threatened by the prospect of a masculine voice. Discussion with the patient and parents may result in a referral for psychologic or psychiatric therapy. Such patients, however, often return for therapy later after having become accustomed to the idea of the lower pitch.

Case Study 11.3

The typical sequence of events in therapy for mutational falsetto is given in the following study of a 21-year-old male college student.

Patient (P): I guess it was in the ninth grade when my voice first started changing. Seems like it started growing in spurts. The first time I was really aware of it was in stressful situations. We had an English class where you did a lot of book reports, and I'd try to get up and give a report and it would be long periods where it wouldn't break and I couldn't get anything out. I just kept getting worse and worse. At first, it would crack a lot. And a lot of people would say it was so shrill. It would sound just like a girl's, that high. Then through high school, in the tenth grade, it was still the same way, but in the twelfth it got to where it wasn't as shrill and it didn't break quite as much. Like, when a substitute would come and call the roll, and I'd yell "here," it wouldn't even come out; I'd have to try it twice. One guy where I work said, "Whenever you get excited you sound just like a girl." When I was relaxed, it would be hoarse. After swimming, if I was cold, tired, or really nervous, it would get much worse. When I got to college I could try to make it where it wouldn't crack, but it still sounded hoarse.

Clinician (C): Do you have some confusion in your mind as to which is the right voice?

P: Yeah. But the cracking didn't bother me a great deal. We'd moved about six or seven times, and in the seventh grade it was really traumatic. I was extremely shy. I was so shy it was really incredible. I don't think I ever went anywhere in the seventh grade except to school and then straight home. In the eighth grade, I had a pretty low self-image. But I think I've grown out of it a lot. I had a low self-image in the seventh and eighth grades and I was shy, and then it began cracking in the ninth grade and that about shot me down. There wasn't a lot of school-ground taunting, but, like, if you'd answer the telephone, you'd know what people were really thinking.

I put up with it through the whole ninth grade, and then we ended up going to about three or four throat specialists, and they said the voice would change. The last doctor I saw was a year and a half ago; he said it would change, too. Physically I was in real good shape, and I had a real good home life; it was my only refuge. I always wanted to be like my father. Do you think it was a fear of the cracking that made me stay at the high pitch? I think it is possible.

Therapy

C: Have you ever noticed that when you shout, your voice will drop to a lower pitch?

P: Yes, sir, when I shout I've noticed it. I have trouble shouting, though.

C: The first thing I think you ought to know is that the low-pitched voice is the normal voice. For some reason you haven't been using enough muscular effort in exhaling for voice, and if you have a weak flow of air when you speak, it has a tendency to produce this high pitch. But when you get good pressure under it, the voice will go down. There is a second factor—how forcefully you are bringing the vocal folds together. And I'll show you how we can accomplish that. I want you to sit up straight and do this for me. (Clinician demonstrates a sharp glottal attack. Patient repeats, and the voice drops to a low, masculine pitch.) See what I mean? Do it again. Now I want you to hold it out as long as you can. Now produce the old voice. (Patient does at the high pitch level.) Hear the difference? Do you notice how much less effort you have to exert to make the high-pitched voice? Try the low one again, sustaining the vowel. There is an interesting little quiver or warble to the voice which may be a sign that you haven't been using the vocal folds and they are a little bit flabby. Now say "Monday." (Patient says the word, the first syllable at the low pitch, the second at the high. With slightly more effort on the second trial, the entire word is produced at the low pitch.) Say "one Monday," sharply. Now, "one Monday morning"; take a deep breath first. Now we'll do some exercises. (Clinician demonstrates five vowel sounds in short succession, each produced with a sharp glottal attack. Patient repeats all at a low pitch level. This exercise is repeated for several minutes. After that, the patient is asked to count to 10 sharply.) Sound all right? It didn't crack, did it? Now say the days of the week the same way. Notice that when you slack off on the effort, the pitch goes up? Get into the habit of breathing deeply and putting forth effort when you talk. Now, pick up that card and start reading with that voice. (Patient does so with very few falsetto pitch breaks.) Not bad. All right, now let me hear you start counting and see how far you can go. Now I'm going to ask you some questions, and I want you to answer in a low-pitched voice. Remember, sharp and loud. How old are you? (Patient answers 21 in a falsetto voice.) Let's go back to the vowels. Produce them sharply. Now, how old are you? (Patient responds in the low-pitched voice.) Are you getting the feel of it? Now tell me about school, where you go, what subjects you're taking, and so on. (Patient begins to describe his college experience somewhat hesitantly, but in the low-pitched masculine voice.)

C: Well, what do you think of your voice now?

P: Strange. I just can't believe that was it.

C: It sounds completely normal to me, but I know it sounds peculiar to you. It's not cracking, is it? Do you like the new voice?

P: Yeah (somewhat tentatively and quizzically).

C: Well, just keep talking and get some experience with it.

P: I love to play handball. I'm starting to get halfway decent in gymnastics. At first, I was going to be a business major, but it wasn't for me. So I decided on physical therapy. I think I'll be real good at that.

C: A while back you said your mother was an unusual person. Could you tell me more about that?

P: I guess I consider her pretty unusual. I've had a pretty warped view of people in general, twisted, well, not really warped; I saw a lot of cruel things. My mother is real sensitive. She teaches children with learning disabilities. And I think she is probably one of the best in the state. People can be callous and they can be cruel, at school, mostly toward me, but to other people who were shy too. She has a great deal of empathy. She's kind of headstrong though. My father, he didn't have a lot of time, say, when we were growing up. You know, the old deal about making money. And about 2 years ago, he changed more than any person I'd ever seen. He was pretty dogmatic and rigid, and he became more understanding and more open, just less structured, kind of seemed more human. He'd played on a basketball scholarship and I really wanted to be like him,

quite a bit. With my sister, we fought a lot. She is real pretty. The guy she married, we just don't make connections. I'm not kidding, he's really a strange character. (All the above is produced in the low-pitched masculine voice, with few pitch breaks. His rate of speech progressively increases as he becomes more comfortable with the new voice.) We got real close since she has been married. We really have fun with her now. Except, I think she could have reached a higher potential if she had married someone else. She could really write. In English classes, her name would come up a year later when I would take those classes, and her teachers would say, "She could really write. I hope you're as good as she is."

C: You sound as if you are a sensitive person and that you have high standards.

P: I'd like to believe that.

C: Do you think that you're oversensitive?

P: Definitely. As a matter of fact, about 3 months ago, I finally told mother—like that one doctor, he's crazy, thinking that my voice was still going to change, and it got to where I was becoming callous. I'd put up with the voice for 7 years, and I didn't have too much patience with people. It might be that I didn't try to understand them because I was too wrapped up in my own problem. Like the first two doctors, I thought they had to be right, and then the best one in the state said that at 19 I just needed more time! I was pretty well disgusted. Mother asked me once if I ever forgot about my voice, and I said, "No way." (At this point the session was terminated, and the patient was asked to return the following day.)

C: What were your parents' reactions to your voice?

P: Well, I called my mother on the phone and I didn't tell her who I was at first, and when she realized who I was (laughs), she broke down and started crying quite a bit and said that she didn't think she would even recognize me until I told her. I almost didn't sleep last night, and when I woke up this morning I had to concentrate quite a bit to get the voice started. My dad said it was deeper than it was yesterday, and we were outside shopping and it was cold and I said a few words and they came out the old way, but I caught it right away. That was the only time it ever slipped.

C: Does it sound more normal to you now?

P: Yeah. I went over to start talking to Daddy and I almost got lightheaded; I wasn't used to breathing that deeply. I used it in restaurants and shopping. It was fun.

C: Do you have any other impressions of the voice?

P: Not really. I told Daddy the whole story. I just told him I couldn't believe it, and I don't guess he could either. Even he said he couldn't hope for that much. Because they had both been preparing me for partial improvement, maybe having to go home and work at it, and it would take maybe a few months. I thought to myself that I don't know if I'm going to be able to go back and talk to my friends and relatives. I guess it was concern about the hassle of drawing attention to it. Then, I thought that after talking to Mother and Dad, that that's the farthest thing I should be worrying about. In fact, all my aunts and uncles and cousins are coming over Friday, and I can hardly wait. But I had thought about it, that it would be some hassle.

C: Do you feel satisfied?

P: Totally. It's more than you could really hope for in your wildest dreams. When I was in high school, people would treat me like I was a poor little kid. You know, I can't go back to it, but I really could have been a fantastic basketball player. I could have been on a scholarship now, but you know, I just kind of copped out. You know, my mother told me once that she thought I'd gotten used to the voice, and I just couldn't believe it. And I said, "Mother, you've never been to a place where you have to give a speech or talk to a stranger." For a while it dictated my whole life, what I'd do and what I'd try.

The patient's father wrote 2 months later:
Prior to the change in Mike's voice, I felt that he was a shy, sensitive person with a very poor self-image. During Mike's early years, I believe he was what I would call "painfully shy." Mike was not a confiding person, and it was difficult to get him to engage in an open-ended discussion, what I would call a "bull session."

The change in Mike's voice has brought about a profound change in his view of himself and his relationship to other people. Since things are now so much more positive, Mike opens up much more easily and is quite willing to discuss anything and everything.

Prior to Mike's session with you, I was very concerned about his future. I now feel that his confidence and self-image have improved so sharply that he will reach his potential as a person and will have a rewarding life.

Mike now participates in class discussions. He had told us that during 4 years of high school and 3 years of college, he had never before done so.

The patient wrote the following letter 3 months after acquiring his masculine voice:

Most things don't measure up to their expectations. My new voice was one that did. I was in a state of bliss when I returned to _____. When I got home my mother and sister were the first people I talked to. I described every detail and emotion of my trip to the clinic.

When I first came in contact with people outside my family, it was an almost laughable situation. I'd say something and their faces would register shock, but they'd never comment about my changed voice. I assume that in the past, by my action and behavior, it was well understood that my voice embarrassed me and not to mention it. But it was so unusual to me that not a single person outside of my family has ever mentioned or commented on my new voice. And for once in my life I was more than willing to discuss it. As a matter of fact, I wanted to talk about it. I have finally come out and said a few things to my friends, who would immediately be full of questions. We ended up having very enlightening conversations.

The peer pressure was incredible. I've never even so much as flinched before it. Nothing could force me back to the misery that was before my trip. But I can see how powerful role expectations are and to have such a major change in not only voice but identity. Because, too often after hearing my voice people

tacked on behavior traits to me as well. They expected me to act gimpy, since I talked gimpy. I don't know if anyone else can understand how all-encompassing my voice was to me. My father asked me when I had returned if I thought my change of voice would have a very major effect on my life. I could have cried. It was not part of my life, it was my life. Every action I made, every decision, opinion, all of my behavior was what it was because of my voice.

It takes a long time to get everything straightened out. To this day if a phone rings and I'm by myself I'll find myself trying to warm up my vocal cords by talking to myself. The behavior patterns don't fall by the wayside as rapidly or as painlessly as did my voice. There's a whole way of life involved in coping with my voice since it bothered me so much. And it takes effort and desire to overcome that way and replace it with another. In a class once a fellow student made a comment that no one knew what Hell was like. I smiled to myself, because in all honesty and sincerity I felt I was living a Hell and nothing could be worse.

I'll be going to a new school this semester. My whole life is one uphill swing since the clinic. Everything keeps getting better. After visiting four specialists who did nothing, I had a very low opinion of doctors. You raised that opinion, and I thank you for your competence. After saying that it was a living Hell I must also say that my voice gave me a unique perspective on life. I'm glad that I am what I am. I'm thankful that I can relate to unfortunate people—to someone with a handicap. That I'm not someone who has only tunnel vision because they can't see outside of their own experiences.

Spasmodic Dysphonia

One of the most complex voice problems encountered by speech clinicians is spasmodic dysphonia. Because of its complexity, a separate chapter is devoted to description and treatment of its various forms.

Unilateral and Bilateral Vocal Fold Paralysis

Incomplete glottic closure during phonation because of unilateral or bilateral adductor vocal fold paralysis produces variously aphonia, breathiness, hoarseness, excessively low volume, diplophonia, and high-pitched falsetto. Therapy is based on the principle of compensatory glottic closure by capitalizing on the primitive effort closure capabilities of the larynx. In unilateral paralysis, the normal vocal fold is encouraged to cross the midline and contact the paralyzed fold. In bilateral, both folds are forced toward the midline. Voice recovery depends upon the etiology of the paralysis and the position of the paralyzed vocal fold(s). Patients who have degenerative peripheral nervous system diseases are poorer risks than are those with static lesions. Those who have unilateral vocal fold paralyses are better therapy risks than are those who have bilateral paralysis. The closer the paralyzed vocal fold is to the midline, the better the prognosis. Patients who have idiopathic vocal fold paralysis may experience spontaneous return of voice.

Voice Therapy

Behavioral voice therapy for vocal fold paralysis is based primarily on the patient's potential to compensate by means of adduction of the intact vocal fold. The following methods have found widespread support among clinicians:

♦ Effort closure techniques. In Chapter 2 effort closure was described as a primitive reflex mechanism. Stronger glottic closure is facilitated by capitalizing on the effort closure reflex by means of grunting, controlled coughing, laughing, pushing, and lifting. Linking the fingers and pulling in opposite directions while phonating the vowel /i/ and pushing against a table or pulling up on a chair synchronously with phonation are activities that were originally advocated by Froeschels, Kastein, and Weiss (1955). Vowels are introduced with the vowel /u/ having particular value in producing better voice. Progression from vowels to syllables, words, and sentences follows. Singing and humming are additionally helpful. Not all patients who have vocal fold paralysis require strenuous pushing, for many clinicians report that initiating vowels with an abrupt, sharp, or hard glottal attack is often sufficient.

♦ Excessive musculoskeletal tension that may have developed as a secondary reaction should be eliminated (see the Musculoskeletal Tension [Vocal Hyperfunction] section of this chapter).

♦ A trial-and-error search should be conducted for a pitch and loudness level that will yield the best voice quality with the least physical effort. Pinching the wings of the thyroid cartilage together gently during phonation will bring the vocal folds into closer proximity, producing improved voice, which may then be repeated without the therapist's help. Turning the head to the right or left may also improve the voice by increasing the tension on the paralyzed vocal fold.

♦ Sensitizing the patient to improvements in voice during trial-and-error procedures should be emphasized. Moment-to-moment voice changes during therapy need to be pointed out to the patient instantly; otherwise, they will escape notice.

♦ Attention should be paid to secondary personal and emotional problems arising from the voice disorder. One should provide time during each therapy session for discussion of the patient's voice experiences in everyday life, encouraging ventilation of frustrating experiences. It is important to be attentive to more severe emotional reactions, particularly depression, and to be ready to consult with appropriate mental health personnel.

Phonosurgical Treatment

An alternative for patients with unilateral vocal fold paralysis who do not respond to voice therapy is some type of

phonosurgery as described elsewhere in this chapter. Of particular interest to this population are medialization procedures and reinnervation. Although not yet tried in humans, gene therapy has been successfully used to treat laryngeal paralysis in rats (Shiotani, Saito, Araki, et al, 2006).

Following are typical experiences with patients who have had vocal fold paralyses.

Case Study 11.4

A 45-year-old widowed mother of three children, a clerk in a department store, had no previous history of voice disorders, when she awoke one morning with marked hoarseness.

After 2 weeks, she consulted a laryngologist, who found a right unilateral vocal fold paralysis. She had no history of upper respiratory infections or trauma. Neck palpation and chest radiographs failed to reveal any masses. Remaining cranial nerves were normal. The laryngologic diagnosis was idiopathic unilateral vocal fold paralysis.

Her voice was hoarse and diplophonic. Glottal attacks on vowels and coughing were weak. Peripheral speech musculature examination failed to disclose any other abnormalities; neither did the motor speech evaluation. Her voice had not improved during the 2 weeks since onset, and she had taken leave from her job because of difficulty in communicating with customers, especially in noisy settings. She became easily fatigued, both because of the increased vocal effort and because of the need to breathe more frequently owing to air wastage during phonation. She was having trouble talking to her three active children.

A series of voice-therapy sessions was begun, stressing sharp glottal attack activities. She began to show reduced hoarseness and diplophonia while phonating at slightly higher pitch levels. However, when she increased her loudness level beyond a certain point at those pitch levels, diplophonia reappeared, so that therapy necessitated that she learn to modulate the loudness of her voice. A home-therapy program was outlined, and the patient was seen biweekly. During the first month of therapy, her voice underwent stepwise improvements, the first observable change being a disappearance of diplophonia. She returned to work at that point, enduring without undue concern the well-meaning remarks of fellow employees and customers concerning her voice. She managed to communicate with others by standing closer to them while speaking.

Her voice continued to improve during the next 3 months, and 4 months after the beginning of therapy, she was dismissed with mild residual breathiness. Loudness and pitch range had become acceptable, if not normal. The final laryngoscopic examination showed normal bilateral vocal fold movements.

Spontaneous return of voice is common in patients with idiopathic unilateral vocal fold paralysis, although voice therapy may facilitate such recovery. The decision to begin therapy in this case was a precautionary measure predicated on the assumption that the patient might not have had spontaneous improvement.

An experience totally different from the above study is the following.

A 53-year-old housewife and cashier at a coffee shop emerged from anesthesia for thyroidectomy with a severely breathy-hoarse voice that did not improve during the 2-month postoperative period. She returned for laryngologic examination and was found to have a fixed left vocal fold. She returned to work a month after surgery but met with considerable difficulties in her job, being unable to make herself heard in the noisy restaurant and becoming increasingly self-conscious about the steady stream of comments from customers regarding the sound of her voice. She and her husband made no attempt to conceal their hostility and were determined to get help for the voice.

The laryngologist, after explaining to the patient the unavoidability of the paralysis, and after demonstrating much concern over her welfare, referred the patient for voice therapy. On evaluation, she was breathy, bordering on aphonia. She broke down several times during discussion of the effects of her voice on her job and home life, stressing the embarrassment it caused her and how it made her feel self-conscious and "peculiar."

During 4 months of voice therapy, her voice failed to improve. Finally, one day the patient's husband called, saying that his wife had gone on an extended leave of absence from her job and was showing signs of increasing depression and withdrawal.

The patient was referred to a psychiatrist, who believed that the depression was a reaction to her illness, surgery, and voice disorder and placed her on antidepressant medication, agreeing to see her periodically for support. Voice therapy was continued simultaneously, and although she appeared less depressed, her dysphonia failed to improve.

Review of her case with the laryngologist led to the decision to do a Teflon injection of the paralyzed vocal fold. She underwent general anesthesia, during which the left vocal fold was injected. Upon recovery and reexamination 24 hours after surgery, her voice was virtually normal in quality, loudness, and pitch. Her response was ecstatic, her depression had lifted almost instantaneously, and comparison of pre- and postsurgical videotape recordings showed an indescribable difference in facial expression.

The patient returned to work immediately, and her husband reported that her mood had changed back to normal. Six-month and 1-year follow-up examinations showed continuation of normal voice and personal adjustment.

In contrast with the first patient, whose personality strengths and somewhat better voice enabled her to tolerate her dysphonia, the second patient fared less well. In addition to her increasing depression over her voice loss, necessitating psychiatric treatment, her normal vocal fold gave little indication that it intended to compensate. The effects of the Teflon injection, affording a new voice and its concomitant emotional benefits, illustrate the virtue of medialization procedures.

On the pitfalls of injecting Teflon into mobile vocal folds such as for the correction of atrophy and bowing of the folds, Kaufman (1988) wrote:

> Teflon in the mobile vocal cord diffuses and produces a stony-hard cord. The resultant voice may be temporarily improved, but with the passage of time, the voice becomes very poor, indeed worse than prior to injection. Over the past 5 years I have attempted to surgically remove Teflon in six such cases, using the CO_2 laser. The diffusion of the Teflon makes this impossible, and the vocal improvement following removal is modest at best . . . no matter how appealing it may seem to use that technique to correct such cordal defects, no available data supports that practice. Furthermore, irreversibility once Teflon is introduced makes such injections ill advised . . . at present there is no surefire method to correct bowing of the vocal cords, least of all Teflon injection.

Paradoxical Vocal Fold Dysfunction

Paradoxical vocal fold dysfunction (PVFD) occurs when the vocal folds paradoxically close when they should be opening. Paradoxical vocal fold dysfunction (PVFD) occurs when the vocal folds paradoxically close when they shoud be opening. This condition is called by many names including paradoxical vocal cord dysfunction (PVCD), vocal cord dysfunction (VCD), irritable larynx syndrome (ILS), episodic paroxysmal laryngospasm, Munchausen's stridor, factitious asthma, and many other names. The etiology has been attributed to brain-stem problems, performance anxiety, redundant or floppy laryngeal tissue, vagal disturbances, and esophageal reflux (Mathers-Schmidt, 2001; Sandage and Zelazny, 2004). PVFD has occurred in an infant as young as 4 months and in the geriatric population though it is most common in adolescent athletes and women between the ages of 20 and 40. Symptoms may range from mild sporadic breathing problems to complete respiratory obstruction. Approximately 50% of the individuals with PVFD also have asthma. Most paradoxical movements occur during inspiration, but in ~10% of the cases it occurs during expiration. With paradoxical breathing, regardless of etiology or age, patients often experience air hunger and then panic with a fear of impending death. The problem mimics asthma, and commonly patients are referred by allergists reporting that the patient has breathing problems, with or without accompanying hoarseness, that are not responsive to asthma medications. If pulmonary function tests have been ordered, a typical flat inspiratory flow volume loop is observed. When there is not a concomitant medical or psychologic problem, treatment is generally straightforward and successful. Patients are taught to inhale slowly through their nose to maximize glottal opening and exhale through a restricted oral aperture such as created with pursing the lips or producing a soft /s/. Once the patient is aware that he or she can control the airway, the focus of therapy is on teaching abdominal breathing and overall relaxation. In cases where the PVFD is exercise-induced or occurs only during an athletic event, treatment also includes teaching breathing patterns that complement the sport and help reduce anxiety. In those instances when redundant tissue is the cause, surgical expiration of the tissue may be necessary. When anxiety is the primary cause, psychiatric referrals are necessary.

◆ Therapy for Problem Voice Disorders

The therapy principles and methods already described are for those voice disorders about which there is a moderate amount of knowledge and certainty. In this section are discussed voice disorders about which less or little is known.

Neurologic Voice Disorders

Aside from therapy for unilateral and bilateral vocal fold paralysis resulting from lesions of the tenth cranial nerve, which are amenable to surgical and behavioral therapy, most voice disorders due to central nervous system diseases are resistant to modification. In the majority, the dysphonia does not exist alone but is a component of a dysarthria involving resonation and articulation as well. Respiratory weakness and incoordination are inseparable from these defects of phonation and contribute heavily to the voice disorder.

Myasthenia Gravis

Improvement of the breathiness, hoarseness, and insufficient loudness associated with this disease is directly dependent upon alteration of the neurochemistry at the myoneural junction. Patients who respond successfully to the administration of anticholinesterase drugs or to thymectomy will correspondingly experience an improvement in their voices. The velopharyngeal insufficiency of myasthenia gravis can be considerably improved and even eliminated with the use of a palatal-lift prosthesis. Symptomatic voice therapy for patients on maintenance doses of anticholinesterase drugs has not been advocated because of questionable effectiveness; however, more knowledge is needed in this area, and the effects of voice therapy need to be clinically investigated.

Pseudobulbar Palsy

The strained-strangled hoarseness and excessively low pitch of spastic (pseudobulbar) dysphonia, a component of spastic dysarthria, can be a serious obstacle to speech intelligibility. The dysphonia is especially severe when accompanied by a flaccid component in amyotrophic lateral sclerosis. The accumulation of saliva in the pyriform sinuses of the larynx in amyotrophic lateral sclerosis worsens the dysphonia.

Parkinsonism

The breathiness, monopitch, and especially the inadequate voice volume can severely compromise speech intelligibility in this disease. In the not too distant past, the value of voice therapy was considered limited and effective primarily for the mildly impaired. Since the development of the LSVT, this is no longer the case. Many patients undergoing LSVT, drug therapy with L-dopa, and deep brain stimulation experience an improvement in their voices along with improvement of other signs of parkinsonism. A portable, body-worn sound amplifier has been used, as has a vocal intensity controller, with variable success, but as these feedback devices become increasingly sophisticated, this too is likely to change and to complement the other treatments. Some patients can become aphonic. Here, as in other very severe communicative disorders, consideration of a communication aid should be given.

Essential (Voice) Tremor

Although they suffer social embarrassment, patients who have mild to moderate essential (voice) tremor do not usually have an intelligibility problem. Voice therapy is frequently ineffective in reducing the tremor, which is unfortunate, because the tremor is socially restricting for many patients.

Other Less Common Movement Disorders

The waxing and waning laryngeal spasms and uncontrollable pitch changes, which are slower in the dystonias and faster in chorea, generally have not been treated successfully with symptomatic voice therapy.

Gilles de la Tourette's Syndrome

The laryngeal components of this syndrome have been reduced and even eliminated with the administration of the drug haloperidol. The value of voice therapy has not been assessed.

Apraxia of Phonation

Muteness or aphonia as a component of apraxia of speech can be successfully treated by working from primitive, reflexive coughing and throat clearing into humming, vowel production, and, ultimately, word formation, the latter being dependent upon the severity of the apraxic articulatory component.

Voice Disorders Due to Mass Vocal Fold Lesions

Hypothyroidism

The hoarse, low-pitched voice of hypothyroidism improves with the administration of thyroid replacement drugs administered for treatment of the total illness. The pitch of the voice increases and the severity of hoarseness decreases as the patient's thyroxin level approaches normal.

Neoplasms

No rational disorder-specific therapy exists for benign lesions, and therapy depends upon individual circumstances. With this group of patients more than any other, trial-and-error therapy is the order of the day. Different pitch and loudness levels, head positions, and varieties of glottal attack all need to be tried to determine which modes of phonation yield the most audible and aesthetically acceptable voice. Clinician and patient need to be realistic about accepting less-than-desired results.

In patients who possess only one vocal fold because of removal of the other for carcinoma, and in others with severe atrophy, scarring, or other lesions of the vocal folds, ventricular phonation may yield a better voice than voice production with the true vocal fold.

A serious problem is the child who is unable to phonate because of chronic laryngeal obstruction due to congenital or acquired laryngeal stenosis, papilloma, trauma, or subglottal stenosis. A substitute form of communication is mandatory. Children that have had glottic stenoses for long periods, preventing conventional phonation, often spontaneously acquire pharyngeal and buccal speech, gestures, and abnormal breathing patterns. Kaslon, Grabo, and Ruben (1978) advocate alternative approaches to communication, such as sign language, an artificial larynx, communication boards, and esophageal speech. The need for some form of substitute laryngeal sound is especially critical in the very young who are undergoing normal language development, for failure to provide substitute voice will almost assuredly result in delayed speech and language.

Professional Singer and Actor Voice Users

Singers and actors with injured voice present special challenges to voice clinicians. By virtue of their profession, they are required to extend vocal ranges beyond normal use often causing tissue damage in the process. Treatment of singers is discussed in a separate chapter. There is not a separate chapter for the actor because most of the techniques used with the actor who has an injured voice are identical to those used with other patients with a couple of exceptions: they may need to be taught to yell and use unusual voice patterns without causing damage to the tissue; and they may have greater need to work on voice and physical movements together, such as might be necessary in projecting a voice on stage during a sword battle. Actors also may have additional problems related to vocal hygiene that need to be addressed because of working in dusty environments or outdoors with needs to greatly project their voices; eating late at night after performances; or needing to have second itinerate jobs. This suggests that speech-language pathologists working with this special population, and in some cases working with their voice coaches as well, need to know a lot about anatomy and physiology and how various sounds are produced. Clinicians working with actors also need knowledge of the techniques that are used in theater voice training so that they can work better with voice coaches and directors to help modify instruction and performance as needed to produce a healthy voice. Among the numerous theater voice training luminaries, three names that stand out are Alexander, Lessac, and Linklater. The Alexander Technique addresses habits of posture, movement, and relaxation to eliminate inappropriate tension contributing to vocal problems (Conable, 1992). Lessac, as described by Verdolini (1998) ". . . focuses on increasing awareness of potentially numbing habit, then changing them to habitual awareness and active relaxation. Lessac focuses on three actions: structural action, tonal action and consonant action. Structural action relates to lengthening the vocal tract and

releasing tension from the mouth and face to promote easy, free voice. Tonal action focuses on the physical sensations of vibrations in the bones of the palate and skull, creating sound that projects effortlessly and without the likelihood of vocal injury. Consonant action assigns a musical instrument, along with its vibratory characteristics, to each consonant sound. The speaker explores speech sound in such a light, and then brings the fruits of this exploration to the act of communication. Used together in various concentrations, the three actions can lead a speaker to a wide vocal variety, creativity and flexibility." Similarly, Linklater's work on breath and head and neck awareness center around releasing unwanted tension to free the voice (Linklater, 1992). Whereas voice coaches using these techniques often take years of coursework to learn the intricacies of working with actors to bring about the best voice, others with less instruction may also use the technique and benefit from working with speech clinicians who have had more background in behaviors that may result in vocal abuse. Adaptations of these techniques also have been used directly by speech clinicians working with voice disorders.

Transgender Therapy

The majority of individuals who go through gender reassignment procedures are males changing to females (ratio is 4:1). Neither hormones nor genital surgery bring about a feminine voice (Kaira, 1977). Male to female transsexuals believe their voice to be the greatest obstacle to social integration and to succeed changing their identity on completion of their sexual reassignment (Berger, 1988; Neuman, Welzel, Gonnermann, et al, 2002). Therefore, voice treatment is of paramount importance to this population. Voice treatment for transgender individuals may involve surgery, behavioral modification of communication, or a combination of the two.

If the fundamental frequency of an individual falls below 180 Hz, the speaker is likely to be identified as a male. If the speaker appears to be a female but sounds like a male, the voice will call attention to itself. Similarly, if a person's fundamental frequency is above 195 Hz, the individual most often will be identified as a female, particularly if it is accompanied by breathiness. The frequency can be surgically raised by either reducing the size of the vocal folds or increasing the tension. Tension is increased with cricothyroid approximation. Reduction in the size of the vocal fold is accomplished by creating an anterior glottic web to reduce the length of the vocal folds. In isolation, surgery does not necessarily result in a feminine voice because the overall mass of the vocal fold contact area may not be sufficiently changed. Thus, there is more to feminization of voice than changing the fundamental frequency.

Feminization of speaking generally involves a multiprong approach (education, identifying and extending best pitch range, increasing breathiness, inflectional pattern work, articulatory pacing, adjusting language content, and feedback). Education begins with a discussion of vocal fold vibration and demonstrations from movies of individuals who have believably portrayed different gender roles without changing their fundamental frequency. For example, Dustin Hoffman in the role of Tootsie and Robin Williams in the role of Mrs. Doubtfire both accomplish this feat successfully. Improving range is often accomplished by a combination of daily practice of singing and using lip trills up and down the pitch range. Emphasis is placed on achieving a relaxed vocal tract with a wide range of naturally sounding pitches rather than the highest that can be attained, as the higher falsetto levels often sound artificial and with other changes in communication often are not necessary. The goal is to obtain good resonance balance across a range of pitches that do not sound like a male imitating a female. Increasing the breathy quality generally increases the feminization of the voice. This can be done by substituting soft attacks for hard glottal attacks and requesting that the speaker use a softer voice. Also helpful in increasing breathy quality is the use of feedback of either visually monitoring increased opening and change of laryngeal posture or providing visual feedback of airflow. Articulatory pacing focuses on slowing down speech production. Women generally enunciate more clearly and speak more slowly than do men. Memorizing lines from movies and shadow practicing with favorite female stars provides good practice material for this prong of the treatment. Less obvious to many speakers is the need to work on feminization of content (Hooper, 1985). This may include work on modifying body posture and hand gesture, vocabulary and sentence structure, pragmatics, and dress. In her summary of a voice therapy case of a transsexual, Kalra (1997) summarizes the eleven suggestions for feminization of the voice developed by transsexuals and first published by the Looking Glass Society (1997). These self-help suggestions are: (1) sing; (2) raise the position of the laryngeal cartilage; (3) partially open the glottis when speaking; (4) emphasize pitch, not volume; (5) speak slowly; (6) pace speech carefully; (7) use appropriate content; (8) pay attention to tongue position (9); hold mouth in a slight smile with rounder lips and good lip movement; (10) develop head resonance by opening mouth more and pushing voice into the head; and, (11) use feedback from recording samples. Elaboration of these suggestions are found on the Looking Glass Society Web site. Finally, reviewing video-recorded samples of the speaker while reading, conversing with the clinician, and practicing new speech patterns over the telephone provides an opportunity to further shape and feminize communication skills.

♦ Summary

♦ The objective of voice therapy is to return the voice to a level of social and occupational adequacy within the patient's anatomic, physiologic, and psychologic capabilities.

♦ Voice therapy revolves around physiologic principles designed to restore normal biomechanics to the vocal apparatus. In attempting to restore voice, underlying pathology may be revealed as voice problems are often multifactorial. Restoration of the mechanical properties are only part of the treatment. Therapy is also tailored to the voice and personality of the patient and pays attention to emotional as well as the mechanical and acoustic aspects of abnormal voice.

♦ General principles of voice therapy are blended in with the principles and techniques devised for specific voice disorders.

♦ Voice therapy for excess laryngeal musculoskeletal tension is based on the principle of muscle tension reduction and is accomplished by kneading the laryngeal musculature, reducing the elevated position of the larynx, encouraging general relaxation, and alleviating environmental stress.

♦ Voice therapy for vocal abuse is based on the principle of patient reeducation to use the voice more judiciously in everyday life and to reduce those stress factors that drive the patient into patterns of vocal misuse. These principles are implemented by increasing patient awareness of abnormal modes of phonation, teaching modified voice use, and discussing sources of emotional tension.

♦ Conversion aphonia and dysphonia are treated according to the principle of reestablishment of the patient's conscious awareness of greater phonatory capability and discussing the emotional conflicts that have generated the voice disorder, continuously monitoring the possibility of referral for deeper psychotherapy. These principles are implemented by musculoskeletal tension reduction, evocation of increased glottal activity, and encouragement of patient awareness and disclosure of interpersonal conflicts and life stress.

♦ Therapy for mutational falsetto is based on learning to inhale with increased air volume and to exhale with increased force simultaneous with a sharp glottal attack. Laryngeal re-posturing and speaking with increased orality and loudness help facilitate a lower fundamental frequency.

♦ Voice therapy for adductor spasmotic dysphonia has limited value. Phonation with a breathy vocal attack and at elevated pitch can yield reduced laryngospasm under less socially pressured speaking conditions. Botulinum toxin injections reduce symptoms and provide temporary relief but necessitate repeated injections. When combined with voice therapy, the length between treatments is extended. Laryngoplasties have been used with varying degrees of success. Recurrent laryngeal nerve procedures also aid in alleviation of this disorder, but their long-term value is unpredictable.

♦ Therapy for unilateral vocal fold paralysis is based on compensatory glottic closure by the intact vocal fold. Therapy for adductor bilateral paralysis is based on residual adductor vocal fold ability. Both are implemented by effort closure exercises through phonation with a sharp glottal attack during lifting, pushing, and grunting activities. Glottic insufficiency due to vocal fold bowing and disuse are treated similarly. Vocal function exercises and Lee Silverman Voice Therapy also appear to improve closure and function in these populations.

♦ Several voice disorders resulting from central nervous system disease and vocal fold mass lesions are minimally responsive to voice therapy; further research is necessary.

♦ Voice therapy literature that is evidence-based is lacking. Clinicians must be vigilant in their search for verified efficacious treatments. Treatment efficacy is determined by clinical, functional, financial, social, and patient-defined outcomes.

References

Anonymous. feminine voice techniques. Looking Glass Society. October 1997. Available at http://www.looking-glass.greenend.org.uk/voice.htm.

Arnold, G. (1963). Vocal rehabilitation of paralytic dysphonia. IX. Technique of intracordal injection. Arch Otolaryngol 76, 358–364.

Aronson, A. (1990). *Clinical voice disorders: an interdisciplinary approach.* New York: Brian C. Decker.

Araki, K., Shiotani, A., Watabe, K., Saito, K., Moro, K., Ogawa, K. (2006). Adenoviral GDNF gene transfer enhances neurofunctional recovery after recurrent laryngeal nerve surgery. Gene Ther 13(4), 296–303.

Barnes, J.E. (1981). Voice therapy for vocal nodules and vocal polyps. Rev Laryngol Otol Rhinol 102, 99–103.

Bassiouny, S. (1998). Efficacy of the accent method of voice therapy. Folia Phoniatr Logop 50, 146–164.

Behlau, M. (2005). Voice therapy after micro-surgery of the larynx. Proceedings of 10th International Workshop on Laser Voice Surgery and Voice Care. Paris, France.

Behrman, A., Sulica, L. (2003). Voice rest after microlaryngoscopy: current opinion and practice. Laryngoscope 113, 2182–2186.

Berger, R. (1988). Phoniatrische mitbehandlung operierter transsexueller. Praxis 13, 207–210.

Boone, D.R. (1977). *The voice and voice therapy.* Englewood Cliffs, NJ: Prentice-Hall.

Boone, D.R. (1988). Respiratory training in voice therapy. J Voice 2, 20–25.

Boone, D.R., McFarlane, S. (1993). A critical view of the yawn-sigh as a voice therapy technique. J Voice 7, 75–80.

Boone, D.R., McFarlane, S.C., VonBerg, S.L. (2005). *The voice and voice therapy.* 7th ed. Boston: Pearson and AB.

Briess, F.B. (1959). Voice therapy: part II: essential treatment phases of specific laryngeal muscle dysfunction. AMA Arch Otolaryngol 69, 61–69.

Brunning, W. (1911). Ueber eine neue Behandlungsmethode der Rekurrenslaehmung. Verhandl D Ver Deutsch Laryng 18, 93–151.

Chan, R.W. (1994). Does the voice improve with vocal hygiene education? A study of some instrumental voice measures in a group of kindergarten teachers. J Voice 8(3), 279–291.

Cheyne, H.A., Hanson, H.M., Genereux, R.P., Stevens, K.N., Hillman, R.E. (2003). Development and testing of a portable vocal accumulator. J Speech Lang Hear Res 46, 1457–1467.

Cho, S.H., Kim, H.T., Lee, I.J., Kim, M.S., Park, H.J. (2000). Influence of phonation on basement membrane zone recovery after phonomicrosurgery: a canine model. Ann Otol Rhinol Laryngol 109, 658–666.

Colton, R.H., Casper, J.K., Leonard, R. (1990). *Understanding voice problems: a physiological perspective for diagnosis and treatment.* Baltimore: Lippincott Williams and Wilkins.

Colton, R.H., Casper, J.K., Leonard, R. (1995). *Understanding voice problems: a physiological perspective for diagnosis and treatment.* Baltimore: Lippincott Williams and Wilkins.

Colton, R.H., Casper, J.K., Leonard, R. (2006). *Understanding voice problems: a physiological perspective for diagnosis and treatment.* Baltimore: Lippincott Williams and Wilkins.

Conable, B.H., Conable, W. (1995). *How to learn the Alexander technique.* Columbus, OH: Andover Press.

Cooper, M. (1973). *Modern techniques of vocal rehabilitation.* Springfield, IL: Charles C. Thomas.

Cooper, M., Cooper, M.H. (1977). Direct vocal rehabilitation. In M. Cooper, M.H. Cooper, (Eds.), *Approaches to vocal rehabilitation* (pp. 22–41). Springfield, IL: Charles C. Thomas.

Countryman, S., Ramig, L.O., Pawlas, A. A. (1994). Speech and voice deficits in Parkinsonian plus syndromes: can they be treated? NCVS Status and Progress Report, 6, 99–111.

Crumley, R.L. (1982). Experiments in laryngeal reinnervation. Laryngoscope 92(Suppl 30), 1–27.

Crumley, R.L. (1991). Update: ansa cervicalis to recurrent laryngeal nerve anastomosis for unilateral laryngeal paralysis. Laryngoscope 101, 384–388.

Crumley, R.L., Izdebski, K., McMicken, B. (1988). Nerve transfer versus Teflon injection for vocal cord paralysis: a comparison. Laryngoscope 98, 1200–1204.

Dalhoff, K., Kitzing, P. (1989). Voice therapy according to Smith. Comments on the accent method of treating voice and speech disorders [in French]. Rev Laryngol Otol Rhinol (Bord) 110, 407–413.

Davenport, P., Sapienza, C.M. (2004). Pulmonary function and breathing for speech (pp. 331–364). In C.M. Sapienza and J. Casper (Eds.) Chapter 11, 331–364.

Dromey, C., Ramig, L.O., Johnson, A. (1995). Phonatory and articulatory changes associated with increased vocal intensity in Parkinson disease: A case study. Journal of Speech & Hearing Research 38, 751–764.

Durkin, G.E., Duncavage, J.A., Toohill, R.J., Tieu, T.M., Cava, J.G. (1986). Wound healing of true vocal cord squamous epithelium after CO2 laser ablation and cup forceps stripping. Otolaryngol Head Neck Surg 95, 273–277.

Fairbanks, G. (1960). *Voice and articulation drillbook.* New York: Harper & Row.

Ford, C.N. (2004). G. Paul Moore Lecture: lessons in phonosurgery. J Voice 18, 534–544.

Ford, C.N. (2005). Evaluation and management of laryngopharyngeal reflux. JAMA 294, 1534–1540.

Frazier, C.H. (1924). Anastomosis of recurrent laryngeal nerve with descendens noni in cases of recurrent laryngeal paralysis. JAMA 83, 1637.

Froeschels, E. (1952). Chewing method as therapy. Arch Otolaryngol 56, 427–434.

Froeschels, E., Kastein, S., Weiss, D.A. (1955). A method of therapy for paralytic conditions of the mechanisms of phonation, respiration, and glutination. J Speech Hear Disord 20, 365–370.

Goding, G.S. (2005). Laryngeal reinnervation (pp 2207–2221). In: C.W. Cummings, B.H. Haughey, J.R. Thomas, et al (Eds.), *Otolaryngology-head and neck surgery.* St. Louis, MO: Elsevier-Mosby.

Gray, S.D., Pignatari, S.S.N., Harding, P. (1994). Morphologic ultrastructure of anchoring fibers in normal vocal fold basement membrane zone. J Voice 8, 48–52.

Greene, M.C.L. (1972). *The voice and its disorders* (pp. 169–170). Philadelphia: J.B. Lippincott.

Hammarberg, B. (1987). Pitch and quality characteristics of mutational voice disorders before and after therapy. Folia Phoniatr 39, 204–216.

Hoit, J.D. (1995). Influence of body position on breathing and its implication for the evaluation and treatment of speech and voice disorders. J Voice 9, 341–347.

Holbrook, A., Rolnick, M., Bailey, C. (1974). Treatment of vocal abuse disorders using a vocal intensity controller. J Speech Hear Disord 39, 298–303.

Hooper, C. (1985). Changing the speech and language of the male to female transsexual. J Kansas Speech-Language-Hearing Assoc 25, 1–6.

Hoover, C.A., Sataloff, R.T., Lyons, K.M., Hawkshaw, M. (2001). Vocal fold mucosal tears: maintaining a high clinical index of suspicion. J Voice 15, 451–455.

Isshiki, N. (1989). *Phonosurgery-theory and practice.* Berlin: Springer-Verlag, 1989.

Isshiki, N., Taira, T., Kojima, H., Shoji, K. (1989). Recent modifications in thyroplasty type I. Ann Otol Rhinol Laryngol 98: 777–779.

Jacobson, E. (1938). *Progressive relaxation.* 2nd ed. Chicago: University of Chicago Press.

Jacobson, E. (1964). *Anxiety and tension control, a physiologic approach.* Philadelphia: J.B. Lippincott.

Jacobson, E. (1976). *You must relax.* 5th ed. New York: McGraw-Hill.

Jako, G.J. (1972). Laser surgery of the vocal cords. An experimental study with carbon dioxicde lasers on dogs. Laryngoscope 82, 2204–2216.

Jonsdottir, V., Laukkanen, A.M., Ilomaki, I., Roininen, H., Alastalo-Borenius, M., Vilkman, E. (2001). Effects of amplified and damped auditory feedback on vocal characteristics. Logoped Phoniatr Vocol 26, 76–81.

Jonsdottir, V.I., Boyle, B.E., Martin, P.J., Sigurdardottir, G. (2002). A comparison of the occurrence and nature of vocal symptoms in two groups of Icelandic teachers. Logoped Phoniatr Vocol 27, 98–105.

Jonsdottir, V., Laukkanen A.M., Siikki L. (2003). Changes in teachers' voice quality during a working day with and without electric sound amplification. Folia Phoniatr Logop 55, 267–280.

Kalra, M. (1997) Voice therapy in the case of a transsexual. In R. Gemme and C.C. Wheeler (Eds), *Progress in sexology*. New York: Plenum Press. (Presented as a paper at the International Congress on Sexology, University of Quebec, Montreal, Canada, October 27–31, 1976).

Kaslon, K.W., Grabo, D.E., Ruben, K.J. (1978). Voice speech and language habilitation in young children without laryngeal function. Arch Otolaryngol 104, 737–739.

Khidr, A. (2005). A DVD Accent Technique Tutorial. Charlottesville, VA: University of Virginia.

Khidr, A., Lantz, C., Senatore, L. (2005). Evidence-based therapy of dysphonia in singers with functional voice disorders. ASHA Convention Handouts. San Diego, CA, November 18–20.

Korovin. G.S. (2005). Voice res: legend or reality. Proceedings of 10th International Workshop on Laser Voice Surgery and Voice Care. Paris, France.

Kotby, M.N., Shiromoto, O., Hirano, M. (1993). The accent method of voice therapy: effect of accentuations on Fo, SPL and airflow. J Voice 7, 319–25.

Kotby, M.N. (1995). The accent method of voice therapy. San Diego: Singular Publishing Group, Inc.

Kotby, M.N., El-Sady, S.R., Bassiouny, S.E., Abou Rass, Y., Hegazi, M. (1991). Efficacy of the accent method of voice therapy. J Voice 5(4), 316–320.

Koufman, J.A., Amin, M.R., Panetti, M. (2002). Prevalence of reflux in 113 consecutive patients with laryngeal and voice disorders. Otolaryngol Head Neck Surg 123, 385–388.

Koufman, J.A., Aviv, J.E., Casiano, R.R., Shaw, G.Y. (2002). Position statement of the American Academy of Otolaryngology-Head and Neck Surgery on laryngopharyngeal reflux. Otolaryngol Head Neck Surg 127, 32–35.

Koufman, J.A., Belafsky, P.C. (2002). The demise of behavioral voice disorders. Available at http://www.sandiegovoice.org/demise.html.

Koufman, J.A., Blalock, P.D. (1989). Is voice rest never indicated? J Voice 3, 87–91.

Koufman, J.A. (1985). Gastroesophgeal reflux and voice disorders. *The Laryngoscope* 95: 798–801.

Koufman, J. (1991). The otolaryngologic manifestations of gastroesophageal reflux disease (GERD): A clinical investigation of 225 patients using ambulatory 24-hour pH monitoring and an experimental investigation of the role of acid and pepsin in the development of laryngeal injury. The Laryngosocpe 101(53), 1–78.

Linklater, K. (1992). *Freeing the natural voice: imagery and art in the practice of voice and language*. New York: Drama Book Publishers.

Mashima, P.A., Birkmire-Peters, D.P., Holtel, M.R., Syms, M.J. (1999). Telehealth applications in speech-language pathology. J Healthcare Info Managment 13, 71–78.

Mathers-Schmidt, B.A. (2001). Paradoxical vocal fold motion: a tutorial on a comlex disorder and the speech-language pathologist's role. A J Sp-Lang Path 10, 111–125.

McCabe, D.J., Titze, I.R. (2002). Chant therapy for treating vocal fatigue among public school teachers: a preliminary study. Am J Speech Lang Pathol 11, 368–456.

McCloskey, D.G. (1977). General techniques and specific procedures for certain voice problems. In M. Cooper, M.H. Cooper (Eds.), *Approaches to vocal rehabilitation*. Springfield, IL: Charles C. Thomas.

Moran, M.J., Pentz, A.L. (1987). Otolaryngologists' opinions of voice therapy for vocal nodules in children. Lang Speech Hear Services Schools 18, 172–178.

Morrison, M.D., Rammage L. (1993). Muscle misuse voice disorders: description and classification. Acta Otolaryngol 113, 428–434.

Murry, T. (2001). Pre and post-operative phonotherapy. J Sing 57, 39–42.

Murry, T., Rosen, C.A. (2000). Phonotrauma associated with crying. J Voice 14, 575–580.

Neumann, K., Welzel, C., Gonnermann,U., Wolfradt, U. (2002). Satisfaction of MtF transsexuals with operative voice therapy—a questionnaire-based preliminary study. Int J Transgenderism 6, 1–23.

Paniello, R.C. (2000). Laryngeal reinnervation with the hypoglossal nerve: II. Clinical evaluation and early patient experience. Laryngoscope 110, 739–748.

Paniello, R.C. (2001). Laryngeal reinnervation (pp. 189–202). In L. Sulica, A. Blitzer (Eds.), *Vocal fold paralysis*. New York: Springer-Verlag.

Powers, S.K., Howley, E.T. (1990). *Exercise physiology: theory and application to fitness and performance*. Dubuque, IA: Wm. C. Brown Publishers.

Ramig, L.O. (1993). Speech therapy for patients with Parkinson's disease. NCVS Status and Progress Report 5, 83–90.

Ramig, L.O., Countryman, S., Thompson, L., Horii, Y. (1994). A comparison of two forms of intensive speech treatment for Parkinson disease. NCVS Status and Progress Report 7, 41–64.

Ramig, L.O., Countryman, S., Thompson, L., Horii, Y. (1995). Comparison of two forms of intensive speech treatment for Parkinson disease. Journal of Speech and Hearing Research 38, 1232–1251.

Ramig, L.O., Dromey, C. (1996). Aerodynamic mechanisms underlying treatment-related changes in vocal intensity in patients with Parkinson disease. Journal of Speech, Language, and Hearing Research 39, 798–807.

Ramig, L.O., Sapir, S., Fox, C., Countryman, S. (2001). Changes in vocal intensity following intensive voice treatment (LSVT) in individuals with Parkinson disease: a comparison with untreated patients and normal age-matched controls. Movement Disorders 16, 79–83.

Ramig, L.O., Countryman, S., Thompson, L., Horri, Y. (1995). Comparison of two forms of intensive speech treatment for Parkinson disease. J Speech Hear Res 38, 1232–1251.

Ramig, L.O., Pawlas, A.A., Countryman, S. (1995). *The Lee Silverman voice treatment: a practical guide for treating the voice and speech disorders in Parkinson Disease*. Iowa City, IA: National Center for Voice and Speech.

Rattenbury, H.J., Carding P.N., Finn, P. (2004). Evaluating the effectiveness and efficiency of voice therapy using transnasal flexible laryngoscopy: a randomized controlled trial. J Voice 18, 522–533.

Roy, N., Tanner, K., Gray, S., Blomgren, M., Fisher, K. (2003). An evaluation of the effects of three laryngeal lubricants on phonation threshold pressure (PTP). J Voice 17(3), 331–342.

Roy, N., Weinrich, B., Gray, S.D., Tanner, K., Walker-Toledo, S., Dove, H., Corbin-Lewis, K., Stemple, J. (2002). Voice amplification versus vocal hygiene instruction for teachers with voice disorders: A treatment outcomes study. Journal of Speech, Language and Hearing Research 45, 625–638.

Roy, N., Weinrich, B., Gray, S.D., Tanner, K., Stemple, J., Sapienza, C. (2003). Three treatments for teachers with voice disorders: A randomized clinical trial. Journal of Speech, Language, and Hearing Research 46 (3), 670–688.

Roy, N., Gray, S.D., Simon, M., Dove, H., Corbin-Lewis, K., Stemple, J.C. (2001). An evaluation of the effects of two treatment approaches for teachers with voice disorders: a perspective randomized clinical trial J Speech Lang Hear Res 44, 286–296.

Roy, N., Merrill, R.M., Gray, S.D., Smith, E.M. (2005). Voice disorders in the general population: prevalence, risk factors, and occupational impact. Laryngoscope 115, 1988–1995.

Roy, N., Ryker, K.S., Bless, D.M. (2000). Vocal violence in actors: an investigation into its acoustic consequences and the effects of hygienic laryngeal release training. J Voice 14, 215–230.

Roy, N., Weinrich, B., Gray, S.D., Tanner, K, Toledo, S.W., Dove, H., et al. (2002). Voice amplification versus vocal hygiene instruction for teachers with voice disorders: a treatment outcomes study. J Speech Lang Hear Res 45, 625–638.

Sabol, J., Lee, L., Stemple, J. (1995). The value of vocal function exercises in the practice regimen of singers. J Voice, 9:27–36.

Sandage, M.J., Zelazny, S.K. (2004). Paradoxical vocal fold motion in children and adolescents. Lang Speech Hear Services Schools 35, 353–362.

Sapienza, C.M., Crandell, C.C., Curtis, B. (1999). Effects of sound-field frequency modulation amplification on reducing teachers' sound pressure level in the classroom. J Voice 13, 375–381.

Sapir, S., Pawlas, A., Ramig, L., Countryman, S., O'Brien, C., Hoehn, M., Thompson, L. (1999). Speech and voice abnormalities in Parkinson disease: Effect of vocal intensity on articulation. Relation to severity of motor impairment, duration of disease, medication, depression, gender, and age. NCVS Status and Progress Report 14, 149–161.

Sapir, S., Pawlas, A., Ramig, L., Seeley, E., Fox, C., Corboy, J. (1999). Effects of intensive phonatory-respiratory treatment (LSVT) on voice in individuals with multiple sclerosis. NCVS Status and Progress Report 14, 141–147.

Smith, M.E. (2006). Laryngeal reinnervation for unilateral vocal fold paralysis in adolescents and young adults. Paper presented at 9th Biennial Phonosurgery Symposium, July 6–7, 2006, Madison, WI.

Smith, M.E., Ramig, L.O., Dromey, C., Perez, K.S., Samandri, R. (1995). Intensive voice treatment in Parkinson disease: Laryngostroboscopic findings. J Voice 9(4), 453–459.

Smith, M.E., Roy, N., Stoddard, K. (2008). Ansa-RLN reinnervation for unilateral vocal fold paralysis in adolescents and young adults. International Journal of Pediatric Otorhinolaryngology 72(9), 1311–1316.

Smith, S., Thyme, K. (1976). Statistic research on changes in speech due to pedagogic treatment (the accent method). Folia Phoniatrica 28.

Smith, E., Kirchner, H.L., Taylor, M., Hoffman, H., Lemke, J.H. (1998a). Voice problems among teachers: differences by gender and teaching characteristics. J Voice 12, 328–334.

Smith, E., Lemke, J., Taylor, M., Kirchner, H.L., Hoffman, H. (1998b). Frequency of voice problems among teachers and other occupations. J Voice 12, 480–488.

Smith, S., Thyme, K. (1976). Statistic research on changes in speech due to pedagogic treatment: the Accent method. Folia Phoniatr 28, 98–103.

Smith, E., Verdolini, K., Gray, S., Nichols, S., Lemke, H.H., Barkmeire, J., et al. (1996). Effects of voice disorders on quality of life. J Med Speech Lang Pathol 4, 223–244.

Sodersten, M., Granqvist, S., Hammarberg B., Szabo, A. (2002). Vocal behavior and vocal loading factors for preschool teachers at work studied with binaural DAT recordings. J Voice 16, 356–371.

Stemple, J.C., Lee, L., D'Amico, B., Pickup, B. (1994). Efficacy of vocal function exercises as a method of improving voice production. J Voice 8, 271–278.

Thyme-Frøkjær, K. (1998). Results after 1, 2 and 5 years stutter treatment after the accent Method. Proceedings fra den XXIV. Internationale Kongres for Logopædi og Foniatri. Amsterdam: Nijmegen University Press.

Thyme-Frøkjær, K., Frøkjær-Jensen, B. (1987). Analyses of voice changes during a ten month period of voice of training at the education of logopedics in Copenhagen. International Voice Symposium. Edinburgh, Scotland.

Thyme-Frøkjær, K, Frøkjær-Jensen, B. (2001). *The accent method-a rational voice therapy in theory and practice.* Winslow Edition. Oxon, UK: Speechmark Publishing Ltd.

Titze, I.R. (1999). Toward occupational safety criteria for vocalization. Logoped Phoniatr Vocol 24, 49–54.

Verdolini, K. (1998). *Guide to vocology.* Iowa City, IA: National Center for Voice and Speech.

Verdolini, K., Ramig, L., Jacobson, B. (1998). Outcome measurements in voice disorders. In C.M. Frattali (Ed.), Measuring outcomes in speech-language pathology (pp. 1354–1386). New York: Thieme.

Verdolini, K., Ostrem, J., DeVore, K., McCoy, S. (1998). *National center for voice and speech's guide to vocology.* Iowa City, IA: National Center for Voice and Speech.

Verdolini, K., Druker, D.G., Palmer, P.M., Samawi, H. (1998). Laryngeal adduction in resonant voice. J Voice 12, 315–327.

Verdolini, K., Ramig, L., Jacobson, B. (1998). Outcome measurements in voice disorders. In C.M. Frattali (Ed.), *Measuring outcomes in speech-language pathology.* New York: Thieme Medical Publishers.

von Leden, H. (1988). Legal pitfalls in laryngology. J Voice 2, 330–333.

Wang, N.M., Huang, T.S. (1994). A vocal treatment plan for voice disorders after phonosurgery—a preliminary study. Changgeng Yi Xue ZXa Zhi 17, 144–148.

Weiss, D.A. (1971). *Introduction to functional voice therapy.* Basel: S. Karger.

Weitzberg, E., Lundberg, J.O.N. (2002). Humming greatly increases nasal nitric oxide. Am J Respir Crit Care Med 166, 144–145.

Xu, J.H., Ikeda, Y., Komiyama, S. (1991). Biofeedback and the yawning breath pattern in voice therapy: a clinical trial. Auris Nasus Larynx 18, 67–77.

Ye, Q., Yang, Y., Zhao, S., Sun, A., Fan, J. (2002). Voice recovery observation of vocal polyp after operation. Lin Chuang Er Bi Yan Hou Ke Za Zhi 16, 172–173.

Yiu, E.M., Chan, R.M. (2003). Effect of hydration and vocal rest on the vocal fatigue in amateur karaoke singers. J Voice 17, 216–227.

Zealear, D.L., Rodriquez, R.J., Kenny, T., Billante, M.J., Cho, Y., Billante, C.R., Garren, K.C. (2002). Electrical stimulation of a denervated muscle promotes selective reinnervation by native over foreign motoneurons. J Neurophysiol 87, 2195–2199.

Additional Reading

Respiration

Davenport, P., Sapienza, C.M. (2004). Pulmonary function and breathing for speech. In C.M. Sapienza, J. Casper (Eds.), *Vocal rehabilitation for medical speech-language pathology* (pp. 331–364). Austin, TX: Pro-ed. (Read this chapter for a comprehensive review of the respiratory system and how it relates to disordered voice production and how it serves as the basis of many treatment programs.)

Hixon, T.J. (1987). *Respiratory function in speech and song.* San Diego: Singular Publishers. (Hixon provides the underlying physiology of normal respiration for speech and song that serves as the core for assessment and treatment of disordered production.)

Behavioral Voice Therapy

Boone, D.R., McFarlane, S.C., VonBerg, S.L. (2005). *The voice and voice therapy.* 7th ed. Boston: Pearson and AB. (Contains excellent advice on general and specific therapies for virtually all voice disorders.)

Colton, R., Casper, J., Leonard R. (2005). *Understanding voice problems: a physiological perspective for diagnosis and treatment.* 3rd ed. Baltimore: Williams and Wilkins. (Specific treatments are presented from a physiologic perspective.)

Verdolini K., Ramig L., Jacobson B. (1998). Outcome measurements in voice disorders. In C.M. Frattali (Ed.), *Measuring outcomes in speech-language pathology* (pp. 354–386). New York: Thieme Medical Publishers. (Clinicians reading this chapter will have an improved understanding of outcome measures and how they relate to evidence-based practice in voice.)

Verdolini, K., DeVore, K., McCoy, M., Ostrem, J. (1998). *NCVS guide to vocology.* Iowa City: University of Iowa. (This small, beautifully organized book presents a primer on voice disorders and their treatments. It is easy to read, provides an excellent reference list, and serves both as fundamental information for beginners and as a reference or refresher for experienced clinicians. Each of the major laryngeal disorders includes a brief description of the problem and its causes and treatment. For each of the major treatment techniques or programs, the authors have included a paragraph or two describing the treatment and its application, developers, probable underlying mechanism, efficacy studies, and list of usual references.)

Voice Rest

Murry, T. (2001). Pre and post-operative phonotherapy. J Sing 57, 39–42.

Koufman, J.A., Blalock, PD. (1989). Is voice rest never indicated? J Voice 3, 87–91.

Vocal Fatigue

Scherer, R.C., Titze, I.R., Raphael, B.N., Wood, R.P., Ramig, L.A., Blager, R.F. (1987). Vocal fatigue in a trained and an untrained voice user. In T. Baer, C. Sasaki, and C. Harris (Eds.), *Laryngeal function in phonation and respiration* (pp. 533–555). (This study of two speakers provides a good background review of vocal fatigue.)

Reflux

Ford, C.N. (2005). Evaluation and management of laryngopharyngeal reflux. JAMA 294, 1534–1540. (Because laryngopharyngeal reflux (LPR) is a major cause of laryngeal inflammation and presents with a constellation of symptoms that are different from classic gastroesophageal reflux disease, it is essential that practicing speech pathologists understand the problem. This article provides a practical approach to evaluating and managing LPR.)

Koufman, J.A. (1991). The otolaryngologic manifestations of gastroesophageal reflux disease (GERD): a clinical investigation of 225 patients using ambulatory 24-hour pH monitoring and an experimental investigation of the role of acid and pepsin in the development of laryngeal injury. Laryngoscope 101(Suppl), 1–78. (Koufman was one of the first to recognize the causal role reflux plays in voice disorders. This classic articles lays down the foundation for much of the research done on this topic in the subsequent years.)

Vocal Hygiene

Rammage, L. (1997). *Vocalizing with ease: a self improvement guide.* PvCrp Provincial Voice Care Resource Program, British Columbia, Canada. (Self-help book with cartoon illustrations written specifically for patients. Good source of patient homework material and dos and don'ts of vocal hygiene.)

Roy, N., Weinrich, B., Gray, S.D., Tanner, K., Toledo, S.W., Dove, H., et al. (2003). Voice amplification versus vocal hygiene instruction for teachers with voice disorders: a treatment outcomes study. J Speech Lang Hear Res 45, 625–638. (Essential features of vocal hygiene program written in easy language for patients to understand the basic components of vocal hygiene and prevention of voice disorders.)

Hydration

Garcia Real, T., Garcia Real, A., Diaz Roman, T., Canizo Fernandez Roldan, A. (2002). The outcome of hydration in functional dysphonia. An Otorrinolaringol Ibero Am 29, 377–391. (This Spanish article demonstrates on 75 subjects the therapeutic benefit of hydration, with or without voice training, for functional dysphonias.)

Fisher, K.V., Ligon, J., Sobecks, J.L., Roxe, D.M. (2001). Phonatory effects of body fluid removal. J Speech Lang Hear Res 44, 354–367. (This article should help clinicians understand the underlying theories of vocal fold hydration.)

Feedback Devices

Cheyne, H.A., Hanson, H.M., Genereux, R.P., Stevens, K.N., Hillman, R.E. (2003). Development and testing of a portable vocal accumulator. J Speech Lang Hear Res 46, 1457–1467.

Molt, L. (2005). A brief history of assistive devices for treating stuttering. Mankato State University, International Stuttering Awareness Day ONLINE Conference. October 22. Available at www.mnsu.edu/comdis/isad8/papers/molt8/molt8/html. (This paper provides a good review of devices used for auditory, proprioceptive, and kinesthetic feedback.)

Titze, I, Svec, J., Popoto, P. (2003). Vocal dose measures: quantifying accumulated vibration exposure in vocal fold tissues. J Speech Lang Hear Res 46:919–932.

Theater Training

Lessac, A. (1996). *The use and training of the human voice: a practical approach to speech and voice synamics.* 3rd ed. Mountain View, CA: Mayfield Publishing Co.

Linklater, K. (1992). *Freeing Shakespeare's voice: the actor's guide to talking the text.* New York: Theater Communications Groups, Publishers.

Raphael, B.N. (1994). A consumer's guide to voice and speech training. New England Theater Journal 5, 101–114. (This classic article provides an overview of the most common techniques used for voice training and in voice therapy as well as the philosophies of Edith Skinner, Kristin Linklater, and Arthur Lessac.)

Conable, B. (1992). *How to learn the alexander technique.* Columbus, OH: Andover Road Press.

Accent Technique

Khidr, A. (2005). A DVD Accent Technique Tutorial. Charlottesville, VA: University of Virginia. (Didactic presentation of underlying theory and patient demonstration of application of technique.)

Thyme-Frokjaer, K., Frokjaer, B. (2001). *The accent method: a rational voice therapy in theory and practice.* Milton Keynes, UK: Speechmark Publishing Ltd. (This book and accompanying CD provide a thorough description of the evolution of the Accent Method and how it can be used in treating voice disorders.)

Resonant Voice Therapy

Verdolini, K., Druker, D.G., Palmer, P.M., Samawi, H. (1998). Laryngeal adduction in resonant voice. J Voice 12, 315–327.

Lee Silverman Technique

Ramig, L.O. (1995). Voice therapy for neurologic disease. Curr Opin Otolaryngol Head Neck Surg 3, 174–182. (This well-written article addresses the efficacy of voice treatment for neurologic disorders with particular emphasis on evaluation of the treatment efficacy data from the Lee Silverman Voice Treatment.)

Ramig, L.O., Countryman, S., Thompson, L., Horri, Y. (1995). Comparison of two forms of intensive speech treatment for Parkinson disease. J Speech Hear Res 39, 1232–1251.

Ramig, L.O., Pawlas, A.A., Countryman, S. (1995). *The Lee Silverman voice treatment: a practical guide for treating the voice and speech disorders in Parkinson disease.* Iowa City, IA: National Center for Voice and Speech. (These readings are part of a series of papers and studies completed by Ramig and colleagues on the development and efficacy of the Lee Silverman technique.)

Movement Disorders of the Larynx

Blitzer, A., Brin, M., Sasaki, C., Fah, S., Harris, K. (2006). *Neurologic disorders of the larynx.* New York: Thieme Medical Publishers. (This book is revised and updated from the 2nd edition published in 1992. For any speech clinician interested in the diagnosis and treatment of movement disorders, this comprehensive treatise, written by a combination of some of the best clinicians and scientists in the field, seemingly leaves no stone unturned and is a must read. The book will also serve as a valuable reference.)

Paradoxical Vocal Cord Dysfunction

Mathers-Schmidt, B.A. (2001). Paradoxical vocal fold motion: a tutorial on a complex disorder and the speech-language pathologist's role. A J Sp-Lang Path 10, 111–125. (This tutorial provides information of PVFM characteristics, etiologies, differential diagnosis, and medical/psychological intervention.)

Sandage, M.J., Zelazny, S.K. 2004 Paradoxical vocal fold motion in children and adolescents. Lang Speech Hear Services Schools 35, 353–362. (This clinical forum presents a description of the various etiologies, differential diagnosis from asthma, medical and behavioral management, detailed outline of treatment programs, and clinical pathways for working with children with vocal cord dysfunction.)

Vocal Fold Paralysis

The following edited texts provide a comprehensive picture of vocal fold paralysis from a variety of experts.

Sulica, L., Blitzer, A. (Eds). (2006). *Paralysis.* Heidelberg: Springer.

Sulica, L., Myssiorek D. (Eds). (2004). *The otolaryngology clinics of North America. Vocal fold paralysis.* Philadelphia: W.B. Sanders.

Meyer, T., Sulica, L., Blitzer, A. Vocal fold paralysis (pp. 217–234). In A.L. Merati (Ed.), *A voice text.* San Diego: Plural Publishing. (A short but comprehensive discussion of vocal fold paralysis and its evaluation and treatment. Surgical procedures are particularly well illustrated.)

Transsexual

Oates, J.M., Dacakis, G. (1983). Speech pathology considerations in the management of transsexualism: a review. Br J Disord Commun 18, 139–151.

Hooper, C. (1985). Changing the speech and language of the male to female transsexual. J Kansas Speech-Language-Hearing Assoc 25, 1–6.

Adler, R.K., Hirsch, S., Mordaunt, M. (2006). *Voice and communication therapy for the transgender/transsexual client:* a Comprehensive Clinical Guide. San Diego: Plural Publishing. (This textbook provides a comprehensive approach to facilitating communication skills congruent with gender identification in the transgender/transsexual individual.)

Vocal Nodules

Lancer, J.M., Syder, D., Jones, A.S., Le Boutillier, A. (1988). Vocal cord nodules: a review. Clin Otolaryngol 13, 43–51. (This article on vocal nodules is an excellent review of their histology, symptoms, incidence, age and sex distribution, hypothesized causes, occupational background, psychologic factors, and treatment.)

The following two suggested readings are important in understanding how vocal load affects vocal abuse and how monitors might help prevent or reduce vocal nodules.

Titze, I.R., Svec, J.G., Popolo, P.S. (2003). Vocal dose measures: quantifying accumulated vibration exposure in vocal fold tissues. J Speech Lang Hear Res 46, 919–932.

Titze, I.R. (1999). Toward occupational safety criteria for vocalization. Logoped, Phoniatr, Vocol 24, 49–54.

Phonosurgery

Ford, C.N. (2004). G. Paul Moore Lecture: lessons in phonosurgery. J Voice 18, 534–544. (This summary of phonosurgery procedures includes historical milestones in surgery development and pitfalls along the way that have helped improve understanding of what current procedures can and cannot accomplish.)

Friedrich, G., de Jong, F.I., Mahieu, H.F., Benninger, M.S., Isshiki, N. (2001). Laryngeal framework surgery: a proposal for classification and nomenclature by the Phonosurgery Committee of the European Laryngological Society. Eur Arch Otorhinolaryngol 258, 389–396. (This paper provides a precise and descriptive list of definitions and terms of the four types of laryngeal framework surgery developed by Isshiki in the 1970s. The underlying motivation for the paper is to provide a framework to classify current surgical techniques and a framework that can be applied to new procedures.)

Isshiki, N. (2000). Progress in laryngeal framework surgery. Acta Otolaryngol 120, 120–127. (This paper provides a comprehensive review of progress in laryngeal framework surgery over the past 25 years.)

Koufman, J. (1995). *Laryngoplasty phonosurgery. The visible voice.* Winston-Salem, NC: The Center for Voice Disorders of Wake Forest University, 4, 50–58. (Good overview from one surgeon's perspective of laryngoplastic phonosurgery with illustrations that help beginning students see how the various configurations of implants work to medialize the vocal folds. Includes discussion of pitfalls.)

Laryngeal Reinnervation

The following articles provide readers with the historical and current perspectives on reinnervation techniques.

Paniello, R.C. (2004). Laryngeal reinnervation. Otolaryngol Clin North Am 37, 161–181.

Smith, M. Laryngeal reinnervation. Paper presented at the 2006 Bienniel Phonosurgery Symposium, Madison, WI.

Voice Disorders in Children

Gray, S.D., Smith, M.E., Schneider, H. (1998). Voice disorders in children. Pediatr Clin North Am 43, 1357–1384. (This article discusses developmental anatomy and physiology of phonation and resonance and common pediatric disorders of phonation and their evaluation and treatment. It also provides a comprehensive list of suggested readings.)

Sarienza, C. (Ed.). (2008). SIDS III newsletter focus on child voice and its production. Perspectives on voice and voice disorders, American Speech-Language. Hearing Association, Division 3, 12(1). (This special edition is devoted to pediatric voice disorders and presents state-of-the-art information on various upper airway issues in children.)

Chapter 12

Special Considerations for the Professional Singer

Brian E. Petty

The term *professional voice users* is used to denote the segment of the population for whom the voice is used as a primary tool of their occupation. In the United States, this term applies to a staggering 25 to 35% of the national workforce and includes (but is not limited to) such disparate professions as teachers, clergy, radio and television broadcasters, salespeople, politicians, aerobics instructors, auctioneers, cheerleaders, actors, and attorneys (Titze, Lemke, and Montequin, 1997; Wingate, Brown, Shrivastav, Darenport, and Sapienza et al., 2007). Professional singers are a highly visible and specialized subset of individuals within the population of professional voice users and often present an unusual challenge for physicians and speech-language pathologists charged with their care. Although differences exist regarding the specific definition of the term *professional singer* (VanEaton, 1990), for the purposes of this chapter the term will be defined liberally as singers who routinely receive payment for their performances. This chapter will discuss the occupational requirements faced by professional singers, identify specific concerns to be addressed during assessment, and make recommendations regarding treatment and continuing education. Although some of the information at first glance may appear redundant to information provided in other chapters, a closer look reveals the adaptation and elaborations needed to properly assess and treat this special population. Furthermore, whereas professional actors have very specific diagnostic and treatment concerns related to their profession, some portions of this discussion about professional singers may be extrapolated to the acting population as well.

The functional demands that singers place on the laryngeal mechanism in terms of frequency range, amplitude control, acoustic variation, and overall vocal stamina are significant and unique. Because these specific demands vary between singers of various musical traditions and abilities, the risk of vocal impairment or injury is also variable depending on such factors as preferred musical style and performance practices, history of vocal study, general health status, and other influences affecting vocal hygiene (Koufman, Radomski, Joharji, et al, 1996). Singers may be significantly impaired by subtle laryngeal changes that may be considered to be within the normal range of variability within the general population. Conversely, the well-trained singer will also possess a high level of neuromuscular laryngeal control that may lessen (or even eliminate) audible symptoms of some laryngeal pathologies (Elias, Sataloff, Rosen, et al, 1997; Lundy, Casiano, Sullivan, et al, 1999). Therefore, it is imperative that singers receive experienced multidisciplinary medical care from practitioners that are knowledgeable of the functional vocal requirements of singers and sensitive to the particular emotional, physical, financial, and professional concerns that singers may experience as a result of vocal impairment (Sataloff, 2005).

A comprehensive voice evaluation for a professional singer should include a carefully collected and thorough case history (including medical, behavioral, and social information), acoustic and aerodynamic data as appropriate, and visualization of the larynx using rigid and/or flexible fiberoptic endoscopy under halogen and stroboscopic xenon light sources (high-speed laryngoscopy can often be a useful tool if this technology is available). The team should comprise qualified speech-language pathologists, singing teachers, and otolaryngologists who are experienced in treating professional singers. Many professional singers who perform in metropolitan areas prefer to live and raise their families in smaller communities where access to such specialized care is more limited. Because the concerns of the professional singer are unusual and highly specific to their special vocal demands, it is important that they be seen by health care providers who have experience in treating this population. If these specialty services are available within a reasonable travel distance, it is well worth the expense and effort.

◆ Gathering a Comprehensive Case History

When a singer's voice begins to exhibit symptoms of dysphonia, other singers and colleagues are often the first people to notice the problem and offer advice. If the larynx were like a violin, something that the musician could see, touch, and repair, there might not be as much mythology and lore associated with how to take care of it. The traditional methods of singing instruction did not emphasize a comprehensive understanding of laryngeal anatomy and physiology, though in recent years this has become a more widely addressed component of academic music programs. Many remedies that are considered traditional among professional singers have been either proved to be ineffective (Roy, Tanner, Gray, et al, 2003) or have been shown to have adverse effects. It is therefore important to take a thorough case history, including a detailed description of the remedies that

the patient has tried prior to the appointment. Samples of a comprehensive case history form for singers have been published previously (Sataloff, 2000) and may serve as an excellent template for data collection.

One of the first things that a health care provider must do before beginning to treat professional singers is to become familiar with some of the terms that singers use in professional conversation that may not be familiar to nonmusicians. This may seem trivial at first, but displaying poor knowledge of the singer's professional parlance may make it more difficult for the patient to development a feeling of trust and confidence. Michael Trudeau, Ph.D., CCC-SLP, once told a story of a singer who presented to a voice clinic stating that "my voice lacks brilliance," a statement that yielded blank stares from the physician and speech pathologist in attendance. Some simple familiarity with basic terminology will establish rapport and confidence. To that end, **Table 12.1** is a summary of basic musical terms, some of which are contained in this chapter.

Table 12.1   Summary of Basic Musical Terms

Appoggio	The dynamic balance between the inspiratory and expiratory forces in singing.
Aria	An elaborate composition for solo voice with instrumental accompaniment. In opera, the aria represents lyric episodes that temporarily relieve the dramatic tension of the action.
Arpeggio	The notes of a chord played one after another instead of simultaneously.
Chest voice	The vocal register associated with connected speech, or "modal register."
Coloratura	A rapid passage, run, trill, or similar virtuoso-like material, particularly in vocal melodies of 18th and 19th century operatic arias.
Crescendo	Gradual increase in loudness.
Decrescendo	Gradual decrease in loudness.
Dress rehearsal	The rehearsal immediately preceding the first performance of a theatrical production.
Fioritura	Melodic embellishment, either written out or improvised. See *ornamentation*.
Forte	Loud. Notated in musical scores as "f"
Fortissimo	Very loud. Notated in musical scores as "ff."
Green room	A backstage lounge or dressing room used by performers.
Head voice	The upper singing range, which may or may not be used synonymously with *falsetto*.
Legato	Singing (or playing) without any perceptible interruption between the notes.
Melisma	A term originating in medieval Gregorian chant but now used to refer to an expressive vocal passage sung to one syllable, as opposed to the virtuoso-like and frequently stereotyped *coloratura*.
Messa di voce	A special vocal technique of 18th century music, consisting of a gradual crescendo and decrescendo over a sustained tone. Modern singers use it extensively for training but sparingly in performance.
Mezza voce	"Half voice," or singing with restrained volume of tone.
Mezzo forte	Medium-loud. Notated in musical scores as "mf."
Mezzo piano	Medium-soft. Notated in musical scores as "mp."
Opera	A combination of solo vocal, choral, orchestral, and theatrical performance involving music, drama, poetry, acting, dance, stage design, and costuming.
Oratorio	A composition for solo voice, chorus, and orchestra or of religious or contemplative character that is performed in a concert hall or church without scenery, costumes, or action.
Passaggio	Italian word for "passage," used in reference to the transition between vocal registers.
Piano	Soft. Notated in musical scores as "p."
Pianissimo	Very soft. Notated in musical scores as "pp."
Ring	The perceptual term used in reference to the *singer's formant*.
Singer's formant	A strong band of spectral energy found between 2500 and 3300 Hz, associated with a resonant, "well-placed" singing voice.
Staccato	A manner of performance indicated by a dot (or, less frequently, the sign ▶) placed over the note, calling for a 50% reduction of its written duration.
Tech rehearsal	The penultimate rehearsal, not usually costumed, during which the final technical aspects of the performance are finalized.
Vibrato	A scarcely noticeable wavering of the pitch during singing.

Source: Apel, W., Harvard Dictionary of Music. End edition, revised and enlarged. Eighth printing (1974). Cambridge, MA: Belknap Press of Harvard University Press. Permission pending.

Subtlety of Symptoms

Because professional singers may be more attuned to subtle changes in their own vocal quality compared with non-singers, they will often present to the clinic reporting symptoms that are not initially audible in connected speech tasks. Common concerns among professional singers (and amateur singers as well) usually involve issues related to vocal fold closure, pliability, and/or symmetry. The symptoms associated with these areas include difficulty with vocal projection (including vocal fatigue), increased vocal effort during quiet singing, changes to the patient's pitch range, difficulty sustaining longer musical phrases, and/or altered perceptual vocal quality (Dailey, 2005). For the classical or operatic singer, instability in the transition between the modal or "chest" voice and the upper range or "head" voice may be described, resulting in pitch breaks, quality disruption, and/or decreased ability to project the voice in that range. The production and manipulation of the notes within the transition register (also called the *passaggio*, or "passage" in Italian) is one of the more challenging functional goals faced by the singer during formal singing training. When the laryngeal instrument is working optimally and if the singer's technical expertise is well established, the result is perceived as an even, consistent vocal quality throughout the singer's range, without audible transition from chest to head registers. Difficulty negotiating the *passaggio* is often one of the first symptoms reported by singers during the onset of early dysphonia.

Voice Use Patterns Not Related to Performance

The standard case history questions regarding symptoms, time and type of onset, progression of the symptoms since onset, and activities or other factors that influence the symptoms will most certainly apply to the population of professional singers. However, it is important to obtain more specific data to understand fully the nature, etiology, and effect of the dysphonia. One of the first issues to address would be the patient's overall voice use behaviors, during singing engagements as well as nonmusical activities. Many voice problems in singers are the result of nonmusical voice misuse or tissue changes related to other medical issues. Does the patient have another job to supplement his or her music-related income? If so, does that position require a significant amount of voice use (such as sales positions, call center representatives, etc.)? Does this additional job take place in an environment that would be irritating to the larynx (such as smoky bars, restaurants, construction sites, etc.)?

Many professional singers teach singing themselves, placing yet more demands on the laryngeal mechanism. If the patient is a singing teacher as well, how many students will he or she teach in one day? Does the patient often demonstrate for the students by singing him- or herself? How is the studio (teaching space) arranged? Is it ergonomically sound, or is the patient frequently positioned awkwardly in an effort to see the student and play the piano simultaneously? What is the patient's social voice use like? Would the patient describe self- as "extremely talkative"? Does he or she they go to entertainment venues that require speaking in noisy environments (such as bars, clubs, sporting events, etc.)? Does the singer frequently use "character voices" when reading to children, speak for extended periods on the telephone, or frequently raise the voice in anger? Asking multiple open-ended questions regarding voice use patterns outside of the performance venue will provide much more insight into the patient's overall voice use profile and may illuminate significant etiologic factors.

Medications

Part of any comprehensive case history involves obtaining a list of the patient's current medication regimen. Many medications produce a drying effect on the vocal folds, which results in increased phonation threshold pressures and a sensation of increased vocal effort. Medications with drying effects include antihistamines, some acne medications (such as Accutane® [isoretinoin] Roche Pharmaceuticals, Basel, Switzerland), β-blockers, diuretics, diet pills, and high doses of vitamin C. Consultation with the prescribing physician often results in a change to an alternative medication with milder drying effects (Sandage and Emerich, 2002).

Environmental and seasonal allergies are extremely common among the general population and can be diagnosed at any time during the lifespan. Touring singers may be exposed to novel allergens and subsequently experience allergy symptoms that are geographically specific. Although many allergy medications have a drying effect on the vocal folds, it is important to ensure that the airflow through the nose and sinuses is relatively unhindered to help facilitate adequately balanced oral-nasal resonance. Thus it is crucial to adhere to the allergist's recommendations regarding consistent allergy maintenance, even if the patient is initially unenthused about taking medication.

Further environmental factors that may affect the performing artist include substances to which performers are exposed in the workplace. If the patient's onset of voice difficulties coincided with the start of rehearsals or performance for a particular production, he or she should be asked questions regarding the types of sets and props used. For example, Richter and colleagues showed that singers, actors, and other performing artists are occasionally exposed to ambient stage conditions that contain irritating agents such as aromatic diisocyanates used to create a mound as part of the production's set, spore-producing fungi contained in cork granulate, cobalt and aluminum used in paint pigments, and fine quartz sand capable of entering the alveolae (Richter, Löhle, Knapp, et al, 2002). Recent investigations into the harmful consequences of some theatrical special effects have resulted in restrictions being placed by performing artists' unions (such as Actors Equity) on the use of such effects as glycol-based theatrical smoke (Pendergrass, 1999; Rossol and Hinkamp, 2001; Teschke, Chow, van Netten, et al, 2005).

Inhaled medications, often used for treatment of asthma, can cause edema and erythema of the vocal folds, resulting in increased stiffness of the tissues and a subsequent increase in perceived vocal effort (DelGaudio, 2002). The proper diagnosis of asthma in a singer is necessary to avoid unnecessary medications. To optimize pulmonary support for the singing voice in the presence of this condition, collaboration with the pulmonologist is essential in helping the patient to identify the best medication and the minimal effective dose to minimize these effects.

The larynx is a gracefully balanced instrument that is markedly sensitive to endocrine fluctuations in the body. Some female singers report vocal quality changes just prior to starting their menstrual cycle (Davis and Davis, 1993), including thickened laryngeal secretions with subsequent throat clearing, vocal fold edema and stiffness, and increased vocal fatigue. Abitbol and colleagues showed similar thickenings of the endometrial and laryngeal mucosa that are much more pronounced during the premenstrual period, particularly during high-range singing tasks. Accompanying these changes are an increased viscosity and acidity level of the laryngeal secretions, laryngeal edema, and exacerbation of microvarices, resulting in perceptual reports of vocal fatigue, a truncated upper range, decreased ability to produce *pianissimo* notes, effortful vocal projection, and acoustic changes resulting in a "metallic" or "husky" vocal quality (Abitbol, Abitbol, and Abitbol, 1999). Singers may also report voice changes related to menopause (Abitbol and Abitbol, 1998), including a decreased upper range, changes to modal range quality, or decreased control of the *vibrato* (the gentle variation of pitch during sustained sung tones that many classical singers consider to be an inherent by-product of effective singing technique). Under the direction of an experienced endocrinologist, hormone replacement therapy may be indicated for restoring the characteristic *ring* (or *singer's formant*) to the classically trained female singing voice after menopause, depending on the patient's age, family history, and other risk factors (Abitbol, Abitbol, and Abitbol, 1999).

Patients with acute laryngitis occasionally present with a request for a prescription from the otolaryngologist for a corticosteroid such as methylprednisolone (Medrol® [methylprednisolone] Pfizer, Inc., New York, NY). Whereas corticosteroids can be quite useful in obtaining prompt suppression of laryngeal inflammation, they should always be considered carefully. Corticosteroids can interact with some medications such as antibiotics and oral contraceptives (Davis and Davis, 1993), producing an increased risk for side effects, including salt and water retention and decreased glucose tolerance. Increased vascular fragility from corticosteroid use can place some singers at increased risk for vascular injury, including hemorrhage. Discussions regarding the patient's voice type (or *fach* if they are a classical singer) and specific performance demands will help to illuminate the patient's likelihood of developing deleterious consequences from corticosteroid use. In all cases, the duration of the corticosteroid course should be as short as possible. The patient who presents with insistent requests for corticosteroids should be referred to the otolaryngologist to discuss the serious side effects of this powerful class of drugs. The decision to prescribe or not prescribe corticosteroids should be made after an in-depth cost-benefit analysis weighing the risks of the medication against the possible professional or financial impact of cancellation or substandard performance.

The Web site maintained by the National Center for Voice and Speech (www.ncvs.org) offers concise summaries of 200 commonly prescribed medications as well as herbal supplements and their effects on the voice.

Laryngopharyngeal Reflux Symptoms

Gastroesophageal reflux disease (GERD) is one of the most common ailments in the general population (Isolauri and Laippala, 1995) and is a familiar term to many patients. It is important, however, to emphasize the distinction between gastroesophageal and laryngopharyngeal reflux (LPR). Koufman discerned that complaints of throat clearing were significantly more common and complaints of heartburn were significantly less common among patients with LPR compared with patients with GERD (Koufman, 1991). Although laryngeal irritation secondary to LPR is common in at least 50% of patients presenting for evaluation of hoarseness (Koufman, Amin, and Panetta, 2000), the effects of this irritation will be more significant for professional singers due to the nature of the demands they place on the laryngeal mechanism. Although many patients will deny LPR because of the absence of overt heartburn, careful questioning will often reveal several more subtle symptoms consistent with this condition. These symptoms include (but are not limited to) heartburn, hoarseness, dry mouth or throat (despite adequate systemic hydration), chronic dry cough or throat clearing, "morning" voice, nocturnal coughing, persistent and/or thick phlegm in the throat, prolonged warm-up time (especially in the morning), a burning sensation in the throat, a sensation of postnasal drip, occasional regurgitation (sometimes informally described as "hot burps" or "mini throwups"), globus pharyngeus (a "lump" sensation in the throat), and indigestion or "sour stomach."

Gastric reflux is closely associated with athletics and other intense physical activity and is often linked to the length and intensity of the activity (Jozkow, Wasko-Czopnik, Medras, et al, 2006). Placing aside the stereotypical images of the rotund opera singer, it is not surprising to note that professional singers and athletes are similar in this respect. Singers are, by their very nature, more susceptible to LPR because of the prolonged intraabdominal pressures associated with singing (Cammarota, Elia, Cianci, et al, 2003). Furthermore, the lifestyle of the traveling performer puts them at an even higher risk because of the combination of strenuous, prolonged physical exertion during performances followed by relatively late-night meals of often-dubious nutritional value. Therefore, a thorough understanding of the behavioral, dietary, and environmental risk factors associated with LPR is critical to the process of gathering a comprehensive case history. The dietary factors credited with exacerbation of reflux include fried foods, spicy foods, red wine, citrus fruits and juices (including pre-performance lemon juice), tomato-based products (including sauces, soups, and juices), alcohol, caffeine, carbonated beverages, nuts, mint/menthol, and chocolate. Behavioral and environmental exacerbation factors include late eating, obesity, tight clothes or waistbands (including control-top pantyhose), eating shortly before engaging in strenuous exercise (including performances), and smoking. Elimination or moderation of these factors has been shown to be effective in ameliorating symptoms of LPR, independently from medical or surgical intervention (Steward, Wilson, Kelly, et al, 2004).

Emotional Concerns

When discussing the patient's dysphonia, it is important to understand that there is often a significant connection between the singer's voice and his or her self-concept. Singers, especially those who are also singing teachers, will often express feelings of self-blame when they present to the voice clinic, with the assumption that they "should have known better" or have become "lazy with technique." These self-deprecating feelings are often alleviated by the results of the examination, but it is important to acknowledge them and reassure the patient that occasional feelings of guilt are normal sensations among their peers.

Whereas hypochondriasis is rare in professional singers, depression and anxiety are common diagnoses in up to 50% of the general population (Kessler, McGonagle, Zhao, et al, 1994). And although professional singers are indeed a specialized population, they are most certainly affected by psychosocial stressors that have an impact on members of the general population, including anxiety and stress related to social and romantic relationships, financial planning, job security, child welfare, and so forth. It is important to adhere to a holistic patient care paradigm by ensuring adequate consideration of psychosocial factors when indicated. Professional singers and students of singing, it must be realized, are just as susceptible to laryngeal dysfunction associated with psychogenic factors as is the nonsinging population. Therefore, as part of case history taking, the speech-language pathologist absolutely must administer a thorough, probing psychodiagnostic history to determine the presence of interpersonal conflicts involving persons important in their lives, parents, spouses, employers, or anyone else who arouses feelings of anger, anxiety, or depression, producing elevated laryngeal–hyoid musculoskeletal tension (vocal hyperfunction) or even conversion disorder.

The psychosocial history is crucial to a correct diagnosis and appropriate therapy (see Chapters 10 and 11) but is not often addressed because of a lack of training and reluctance to invade that territory of the patient's life. However, when a conflict is addressed by both parties and brought out into the open, the singing difficulty will be much more easily resolved.

I am reminded of a 22-year-old aspirant to an operatic career who found she was unable to practice at home because her father, a frustrated and unsuccessful singer himself, was so jealous of her talent that he sabotaged all her efforts to practice at home. The patient subsequently developed an inability to sing at her full pitch range. When first asked about emotional obstacles in her life, she denied vehemently any such causal factors, but after repeated inquiries into this area she broke down and admitted her father's involvement, having been reluctant to reveal such conflict fearing disloyalty to him. After family therapy, her pitch control problems abated.

Voice Study and Dysphonia History

During the process of gathering a comprehensive case history, it is important to identify what kind of singing training the

patient has had. If the patient has studied singing, then he or she should be prompted to report how long the study lasted, when it occurred, and with whom the patient studied. The patient who underwent formal singing training for 6 years with an experienced teacher at a prominent conservatory with cessation of training a year or two ago will have a much different understanding of his or her instrument than a patient who studied singing for 2 months with a church choir conductor 10 years ago. Additionally, the patient should identify whether or not the voice study was effective in facilitating a solid singing technique, according to the patient's own perception. Making this distinction should certainly not imply that formal training is necessary for one to be a successful and healthy professional singer, but gathering this information will assist the health care provider in planning any future intervention.

If the patient is actively studying voice at the time of the evaluation, and if the patient is comfortable providing the information, it is important to obtain the name of his or her singing teacher and vocal coach. Traditionally, the role of the singing teacher is to facilitate understanding and development of singing technique, with special consideration given to dynamic range, artistic quality, and vocal endurance. The vocal coach is often an experienced pianist serving as a collaborative artist and also instructs the singer in language/ diction, acting/character development, and other forms of performance practice. Collaboration with the singing teacher and vocal coach ensures that the information being presented to the patient is consistent, helps facilitate carryover of therapeutic techniques to functional singing tasks, and establishes a mutually beneficial interdisciplinary relationship between the professions. The American Speech-Language-Hearing Association (ASHA), in conjunction with the National Association of Teachers of Singing and the Voice and Speech Trainers Association, have created a position statement codifying the important roles of these skilled professionals in the process of voice habilitation, which should be read carefully before beginning the collaborative process (Sandage M (ED), Graves-Wright J., Heuer R., Verdolini K., Ferketic M., Westerman-Gregg J., Titze I., DeVore K., Raphael B., and Hooper C., 2005).

Singing Style

Certain vocal styles have been shown to be associated with higher amounts of muscle tension than others, resulting in an increased incidence of dysphonia. Choral music, art song, and opera have been linked to lower amounts of muscle tension than have been jazz/pop, blues, bluegrass/country/ western, and rock/gospel (Koufman, Radomski, Joharji, et al, 1996). It is important to note that many singers perform in more than one style, switching from opera to choral music to jazz depending on the type of venue and the needs of their employer. Even within those styles associated with low amounts of muscle tension, singers may experience challenges when transitioning between styles. For example, opera singers may find it difficult to sing in choirs, reporting that they feel a sensation of "tightness," "constraint," or perceptual respiratory support changes as a result of the singer's attempt to "blend in" with the other voices and not "stick out." Another singer who performs in the bluegrass or gospel traditions may report this this professional culture encourages performers to sing with hyperfunctional technique. He or she may report that "if I'm not hoarse at the end of the performance, then I wasn't really trying." For both groups of these singers, it is important to approach therapeutic intervention with the understanding that treatment will be provided within the context of the musical style in which they are expected to perform. Even within styles that are considered somewhat hazardous from a vocal misuse standpoint (rock, country/western, etc.), there still exists a behavioral margin of improvement that can decrease vocal fatigue and increase perceptual vocal quality. Careful application of techniques learned in behavioral voice therapy, in collaboration with the singing teacher (if applicable), will facilitate improved performance outcomes and patient comfort while still respecting the various stylistic singing traditions.

Smoking

Although not unheard of, smoking has long been taboo among classical singers. In contrast, it is more common among singers of some nonclassical styles, either during the break between sets or during personal time. In addition to gathering information regarding when the patient started smoking and how much he or she smokes, the health care provider should also ask *what* the patient smokes. Marijuana smoking is not usually revealed unless the patient is asked specifically. Because marijuana smoke is significantly hotter than cigarette smoke (depending on the delivery method), it is recommended that the patient (if he or she chooses to continue smoking) use a water-cooling device to cool the smoke and reduce the risk of serious thermal damage to the vocal folds. The patients should be offered information regarding the risks of smoking, as well as referrals to smoking cessation programs if they are interested in quitting. If the patient is touring, he or she may be interested in discussing self-directed smoking cessation methods with the physician, or may wish to receive information about smoking cessation programs located in the city or town in which based. The patient is smoking cessation (whether tobacco or marijuana) is often an ongoing process that requires commitment and perseverance from the patient and support from the health care provider. Although we can never recommend that a patient continue smoking, it is important to avoid making patients feel defensive by encouraging them to pursue cessation at their own pace.

Hydration

Maintaining adequate hydration is important for everyone, but is especially so for the professional singer. An inverse relationship exists between phonatory effort and hydration level, particularly for the high range (Sivasankar and Fisher, 2002). Therefore, if the singer wants to be able to produce high notes with relative ease, he or she must be sure to maintain adequate systemic and superficial hydration. The National Research Council recommends total daily fluid intake of ~12 cups for men and 9 cups for women, in the form of noncaffeinated, nonalcoholic beverages, soups, and foods. Solid foods contribute ~4 cups of water, with an additional cup coming from the water of oxidation (Kleiner,

1999). These daily hydration amounts are recommended for adults with average energy expenditures and environments and must be adjusted depending on individual variability. Because of the particular physical and environmental demands placed on professional singers, it may be extrapolated that they may require more oral hydration than the average sedentary adult (Von Duvillard, Braun, Markofski, et al, 2004). Maintaining an ambient humidity of ~40% may improve superficial hydration of the vocal folds (Lawrence, 1981). Superficial hydration may also be enhanced by emphasizing nasal breathing rather than oral breathing, as nasal breathing warms and humidifies the air before it makes contact with the vocal fold mucosa. This has been shown to result in lower phonation threshold pressures and decreased perceived vocal effort during prolonged reading tasks (Hunter, Svec, Titze, 2006). I also concur with Mary Sandage, M.A., CCC-SLP, who frequently recommends that singers eat less-acidic "wet snacks" backstage in addition to drinking water. Anecdotal evidence suggests that wet-snack consumption results in decreased report of dry mouth and improved patient comfort. Wet snacks can include any nonacidic fruit or vegetable with high water content, such as apple or pear slices, peaches, grapes, melon, or cucumber slices. Acidic foods, such as oranges, grapefruits, lemons (including lemon juice), and limes, should be avoided because of their correlation with reflux exacerbation.

Performance Practices: The Nonclassical Singer

The demands placed on the professional singer depend upon the style of music sung and the type of schedule maintained. Nonclassical singers, such as those who singed gospel, folk, rock, country/western, and so forth, should describe the length of their sets (groups of songs), the number and type of musicians with whom they usually perform, the environments in which they normally perform, and what kind of amplification is used. They should also describe in detail what they usually do between sets; if the singer has a quiet dressing room (or *green room*) in which to relax between sets, it stands to reason that he or she will likely have fewer symptoms related to vocal overuse at the end of the performance than if the singer spends the time between sets chatting with the band, smoking, and drinking caffeine or alcohol. Patients who sing with a band, often will benefit from simple adjustments to the monitors at the foot of the stage that provide feedback to the singer and band members. They may also benefit from in-the-ear monitors, under the supervision of an audiologist experienced in working with musicians. If the performance venue is a smoky bar or club, the singer will often benefit from placing small electric fans on the floor of the stage next to the monitors to create airflow away from the singer.

Performance Practices: The Classical Singer

The performance demands of the classical singer are somewhat different from those of singers of other musical styles. The classical singer is much less frequently amplified, relying more heavily on optimal laryngeal function and the *singer's formant* (Sundberg, 2001). Though the performance venues for classical singers are rarely the smoky clubs endured by rock or jazz musicians, the opera houses and concert halls are usually very large and have acoustic properties that are unique to each location. If the acoustic properties of the venue are suboptimal, it may result in "oversinging," or hyperfunctional vocal projection due to decreased auditory feedback. Performance demands will also change as a function of the size of the orchestra with which the classical singer is performing. If the singer is performing an operatic role, it is important to know whether he or she has performed the role previously or if it is new as well as how much time the singer will be required to spend on stage for the role. Some operatic roles allow for occasional vocal recovery time during costume changes (Angelotti in Puccini's *Tosca* is one example), whereas others require the singer to perform for the majority of a 3-hour production (The Governess in Britten's *The Turn of the Screw*, for example).

Some demands are common among all professional singers of all styles, however. How often does the singer perform? Do he or she employ a consistent warm-up and cool-down exercise regimen? How often, where, and for how long does the singer rehearse? If the singer travels via plane, how soon after the flight will he or she be required to sing? If the singer is a premenopausal woman, is she often required to sing during her premenstrual period? Does the touring performer have "down time," and if so, what does the singer do during that time? All of these factors play an important role in the overall vocal load of professional singers and are critical in understanding the responsibilities and expectations that they face.

Business-Related Concerns

When a singer becomes dysphonic and has to make a decision whether or not to cancel a performance, the decision is usually influenced by business concerns as well as medical factors. Many professional singers are represented by agencies who arrange bookings for performance engagements. Singers who have international careers will sometimes employ agents in several countries who cooperate with the primary agent. Will the cancellation cause financial hardship for the patient as a result of not being paid? Is there a chance of causing difficulty with maintaining agency representations? Will the cancellation produce a perception of unreliability among local booking agents, concert promoters, orchestral conductors, or music festival managers? Will the cancellation result in the forfeiting of monetary deposits for performance venues and merchandising contracts? There are additional concerns regarding long-term effects of proceeding with the performance despite illness. How critical is this performance to the singer's overall career? Will there be press coverage with subsequent performance reviews? Will the concert be recorded for later broadcast or recording sales? Will it be televised? These factors must be seriously considered when formulating a cost-benefit analysis of cancellation versus suboptimal performance or compensatory adjustments to repertoire or range.

◆ Evaluation of the Professional Singer

Auditory-Perceptual Evaluation

The auditory-perceptual evaluation of the professional singer is perhaps the most challenging portion of the examination process for the speech-language pathologist or otolaryngologist who is not a singer him- or herself. The difficulty lies in the extraordinary auditory skills required to detect very subtle changes in timbre, pitch, and stability that in the general population would be considered within the normal range of variability. Usually, one will find that the primary complaints are more subtle among classical singers than among their colleagues who perform in other musical styles.

First, the speech-language pathologist will want to evaluate the patient's voice production during unstructured connected speech and sustained vowel production. This should be accomplished during the initial greeting and casual conversation, as well as during the case history and initial examination phases. Special attention should be paid to perceptions of habitual pitch, speaking rate, overall loudness, roughness (including ventricular phonation or glottal fry), and strain. Be mindful of physical signs of vocal hyperfunction, including furrowed brow, stiff body posture, prominent musculature in the anterior neck, clavicular breathing patterns, clenched jaw, or raised shoulders. Does the patient have adequate prosody? Is the patient's articulatory accuracy within functional limits based on informal perceptual evaluation? When the patient repeatedly produces sustained vowels, do the voice sound stable in terms of pitch, quality, and loudness? If not, then the patient may benefit from a more in-depth clinical oral mechanism and motor speech examination to illuminate or rule out a possible neurologic dysfunction.

Next, attention should be paid to the voice produced during singing tasks. The patient will likely be able to sing a section of a particular piece that demonstrates the problem at hand. He or she may have also brought a recording to demonstrate the singer's typical baseline quality. If the patient cannot adequately demonstrate the voice difficulty, he or she should be asked to produce vocal exercises that will illuminate various aspects of the current vocal quality. Pitch range can be examined using simple scales or slow glides. Control of loudness may be demonstrated using *messa di voce* exercises, using a single breath and a single pitch. This exercise starts with quiet phonation (*piano*) and gradually gets louder (*crescendo*) until reaching a loud phonation (*forte*), then gradually gets softer (*decrescendo*) until the patient is singing quietly again. The crescendo and decrescendo should be well controlled and gradual, and the exercise should be demonstrated on pitches representing the entire pitch range. Voice onset can be evaluated using *arpeggios* on /h/-initial sounds, with short *staccato* production. It is often useful to include all five of the Italian cardinal vowels, /i, e, a, o, u/ when completing multiple repetitions of this exercise, as often singers will report more acute difficulty with certain vowel sounds over others. Throughout the singing examination, listen to ensure that the perceptual vocal quality is consistent throughout the range and that the vibrato (when appropriate) sounds well-controlled. Be sure to examine the patient's physical presentation during this process, ensuring that he or she is performing the exercises without obvious extraneous tension.

Traditional Classification System for Operatic and Classical Singers

For classical singers, it is important to note their *fach*, or "voice type." The *fach* system is the traditional German classification system for classical and operatic singing voices, providing a convenient method for ensuring that singers are not asked to sing operatic roles for which their voice is not suited. The system is used more casually in the United States opera houses than in Europe. There are four primary voice types:

- soprano (the higher female voice)

- mezzo-soprano or alto (the lower female voice)

- tenor (the higher male voice)

- baritone or bass (the lower male voice)

Although the range-specific description of these voice types is somewhat simplistic (the actual pitch ranges of the voice types tend to overlap, requiring classification based on perceived vocal quality in addition to pitch range), it illustrates their most basic differences. Choral singers will often characterize their voices in this way, without additional classification schemes.

Operatic singers, particularly those who maintain international careers, will often use more specific terminology to describe their voice type. It is important to note that modern operatic singers often do not adhere to the confines of the formal *fach* system as strictly as the artists of past generations, but the terminology is nevertheless still in wide use. An abridged summary of the more common terms follows:

Coloratura soprano

- High, light, agile soprano voice

- Must be able to sing very fast and complex progressions of notes

- Examples: Beverly Sills, Edita Gruberova

- *Regnava nel silencio*, from Donizetti's *Lucia di Lammermoor*

- *O luce di quest' anima* from Donizetti's *Linda di Chamounix*

Dramatic coloratura soprano

- "Darker, heavier" sound

- Must still be able to produce very fast, high, complex note progressions

- Examples: Joan Sutherland, Maria Callas

- *Der Hölle rache kocht in meinem Herzen*, from Mozart's *Die Zauberflöte*

- *Casta Diva* from Bellini's *Norma*

Soubrette soprano

- Light, young-sounding voice, with the best quality in the middle range

- No extensive coloratura progressions

- Examples: Kathleen Battle, Dawn Upshaw

- *Batti, batti, o bel Masetto* from Mozart's *Don Giovanni*

- *Mein Herr Marquis* from Strauss' *Die Fledermaus*

Lyric soprano

- Most common female singing voice

- Light, airy voice with equal quality throughout range

- Examples: Renee Fleming, Kiri Te Kanawa

- *Signore, ascolta!* from Puccini's *Turandot*

- *Donde lieta usci al tuo grido d'amore* from Puccini's *La Bohème*

Spinto soprano

- "*Spinto*" means "squeezed" or "throttled" in Italian, and refers to a "richness" or "depth" in perceptual vocal quality

- Same pitch range as the lyric soprano, but "darker" color and more powerful loudness range (especially for high notes); can often sing a mixture of lyric and dramatic roles

- Examples: Leontyne Price, Jessye Norman

- *Es gibt ein Reich*, from Strauss' *Ariadne auf Naxos*

- *Dich, teure Halle! Grüß ich wieder* from Wagner's *Tannhäuser*

Dramatic soprano

- Heavy, brilliant, very loud vocal quality, must carry over large orchestra

- Reports of "thicker, stiffer" vocal folds are not well-documented

- Examples: Birgit Nilsson, Deborah Voigt

- *Starke Scheite schichtet mir dort* from Wagner's *Götterdämmerung*

- *Pace, pace, mio Dio* from Verdi's *La Forza del Destino*

Lyric mezzo-soprano

- Light vocal quality paired with a lower range, roles are often young males

- Must be able to sustain long phrases in upper and lower ranges

- Examples: Denyce Graves, Frederica von Stade

- *Mir ist die Ehre wilderfahren* (duet) in Strauss' *Der Rosenkavalier*

- *Voi che sapete* in Mozart's *Don Giovanni*

Coloratura mezzo-soprano

♦ Similar vocal quality to lyric mezzo-soprano

♦ Must be able to sing very fast progressions of notes, similar to coloratura soprano

♦ Examples: Cecilia Bartoli, Marilyn Horne

♦ *Cruda sorte!* from Rossini's *L'Italiana in Algeri*

♦ *Una voce poco fa* from Rossini's *Il Barbiere di Siviglia*

Dramatic mezzo-soprano

♦ Must be able to project over large orchestra in low range

♦ Most often seen only in operatic performances

♦ Examples: Dolora Zajick, Grace Bumbry

♦ *Entwiehte Götter* from Wagner's *Lohengrin*

♦ *Mon couer s'ouvre à ta voix* from Saint-Saens' *Samson et Dalila*

Tenore leggiero

♦ Light, flexible tenor, especially in comic roles; lightest tenor voice

♦ Must be able to access upper range easily, with great flexibility

♦ Examples: Jerry Hadley, Cesare Valletti

♦ *Il mio tesoro intanto* from Mozart's *Don Giovanni*

♦ *Una furtiva lagrima* from Donizetti's *L'Elisir d'Amore*

Tenore lyrico, or lyric tenor

♦ Male equivalent of "lyric soprano," often romantic lead in Italian opera

♦ Must be able to access full range with similar quality

♦ Examples: Luciano Pavarotti, Enrico Caruso

♦ *Questa o quella* from Verdi's *Rigoletto*

♦ *La fleur que tu m'avais jetée* from Bizet's *Carmen*

Heldentenor, or tenore dramatico

♦ Very strong, "dark," "heavy" sound, mostly heard in Wagnerian opera

♦ Must be able to sustain very loud singing over large orchestra

♦ Examples: Ben Heppner, Jon Vickers

♦ *Los der Anker!* from Wagner's *Tristan und Isolde*

♦ *Ein Schwert verhieß mir der Vater* from Wagner's *Die Walküre*

Lyric baritone

♦ Lighter sound than dramatic baritone, range overlaps somewhat with tenors

♦ Must be able to project modal range while still easily singing high range

♦ Examples: Dietrich Fischer-Dieskau, Thomas Hampson

♦ *Vedro mentre io sospiro* from Mozart's *Le Nozze di Figaro*

♦ *Largo al factotum* from Rossini's *Il Barbiere di Siviglia*

Heldenbariton, or dramatic baritone

♦ Similar to heldentenor, lower range and "darker" vocal quality

♦ Must be able to sustain projection of low to middle voice range very loudly

♦ Examples: Rene Pape, George London

♦ *Wozu die Dienste ohne Zahl* from Wagner's *Tristan und Isolde*

♦ *O du mein holder Abendstern* from Wagner's *Tannäuser*

Bass, or bass-baritone

♦ Low range, "dark" vocal quality; pitch range overlaps with baritone somewhat

♦ Must be able to project lower range over orchestra

♦ Examples: Samuel Ramey, Bryn Terfel

♦ *O Isis und Osiris* from Mozart's *Die Zauberflöte*

♦ *Madamina! Il catalogo il questo* from Mozart's *Don Giovanni*

Acoustic and Aerodynamic Evaluation

Acoustic and aerodynamic data are important tools to document the patient's vocal quality and perceived vocal effort, respectively. Multidimensional voice profiling can document the stability of frequency and amplitude, show the prevalence of voice breaks, and document the noise to harmonic ratio, among many other data points. If the technology is available, it is important to document acoustic data to support the perceptual observations made by the patient and the speech-language pathologist.

One of the more useful applications of acoustic data collection is the voice range profile, or the phonetogram. The phonetogram shows the maximum variation of amplitude (or *dynamic range*) as a function of frequency. In the modal range, the patient should have a quite wide dynamic range. As the patient demonstrates dynamic range near the upper and lower range limits, the range should become smaller. The result will be a data plot that looks roughly like an American football in a normal, healthy singer. There is a difference in phonetogram results as a function of vocal training (Verdolini and Titze, 1994). Disordered singers will show truncated dynamic and/or pitch ranges, depending on their presenting complaints. The phonetogram is a valuable tool to document patient concerns and to show changes made during therapeutic intervention that are easily explained to the layperson. Although the phonetogram can certainly be created using state-of-the-art acoustic analysis equipment, it can also be produced by simply using a simple pitch pipe and a sound-level meter. Therefore, even if the speech-language pathologist does not have access to advanced acoustic equipment, he or she can still produce this very valuable documentation with a minimum of expense.

Phonation threshold pressures are a form of aerodynamic evaluation that document the minimum air pressure required to initiate vocal fold vibration. This measure speaks to the patient's perception of vocal effort, with increased phonation threshold pressure correlating with increased perceived effort. The patient's phonation threshold pressure value will change as a function of hydration (Bless and Hirano, 1993), pitch, and possibly degree of vocal training. Decreased phonation threshold pressure values after behavioral therapy would objectively document progress and would support the patient's perception of improved vocal effort.

Palpation of the Anterior Neck

Palpation of the anterior neck in the area of the laryngeal structures has long been supported as an important part of any voice evaluation (Aronson, 1990; Aronson, Peterson Jr, and Litin, 1964; Roy, Ford, and Bless, 1996), though it may be contraindicated in some specific instances (Angsuwarangsee and Morrison, 2002). For singers, this component may be modified slightly to include palpation during spoken and sung tasks. Whereas moderate pressure may be used when the larynx is at rest (to identify signs of persistent hyperfunction), minimal pressure may be employed during connected speech and simple singing tasks to illuminate any differences in overall laryngeal elevation and extrinsic muscular behavior. The muscles to be palpated include the suprahyoid, thyrohyoid, cricothyroid, and pharyngo-laryngeal (inferior constrictor) muscle groups. Examination should be conducted prior to laryngeal endoscopy to avoid residual muscular tension in these muscle groups as an artifact of the examination process. Patients may report tenderness in these areas, particularly if they are experiencing muscle tension dysphonia. In addition to the tactile, this should also be noted as possible evidence of excess extrinsic muscular tension (Angsuwarangsee and Morrison, 2002). The examiner should remember that hypercontraction of the laryngeal muscles may not be due to a fundamental flaw in the patient's vocal production technique, but may instead be a symptom that appears secondary to internalized anger, anxiety, or depression (Aronson, 2004), which restates the aforementioned recommendation to employ a wholistic approach to patient care.

Indirect Laryngoscopy

Clinical evaluation of the larynx often begins with indirect visualization using a light and a laryngeal mirror. This provides valuable information regarding gross pathology and can also be useful if there are questions regarding color resolution during endoscopy, but this method is not sufficient as the sole source of laryngeal image evaluation. Although visualization of the larynx is greatly improved when using rigid oral endoscopy under a continuous halogen light source, it is critical that the endoscopic examination include images gathered under a stroboscopic xenon light source as well.

Stroboscopic data have been shown to provide important information about subtle laryngeal structure and vibratory dynamics that is easily missed under continuous light source and can be significant enough to alter the medical and surgical treatment plan (Bless, Hirano, and Feder, 1987; Sataloff, Spiegel, and Hawkshaw, 1991; Woo, Colton, and Casper, et al, 1991).

The benefits of indirect laryngeal endoscopy under halogen and stroboscopic xenon light sources have been well documented (Hertegard, 2005) and have since become the standard of care for most comprehensive voice evaluations. It is, however, beneficial to consider the unique needs of this specialized patient population when choosing laryngeal visualization procedures. Rigid oral endoscopy (including endoscopy using visualization angles of 70 or 90 degrees) provides excellent image clarity, allowing for detailed examination of minute laryngeal structure and vocal fold vibratory dynamics. However, this modality only allows for sustained vowel production (usually /i/). To see what the larynx and surrounding structures are doing during functional voice use tasks (speaking and singing), flexible fiberoptic nasal endoscopy must be employed. Standard flexible endoscopes are usually able to provide adequate visualization of the larynx under halogen light, but using a stroboscopic light source to visualize vibratory dynamics is, at the time of this writing, often quite challenging during nasal endoscopy. Furthermore, the image quality during nasal endoscopy is not as precise as that of rigid oral endoscopy, making it rather necessary to employ both modalities to gain a complete impression of functional laryngeal behaviors. It must be noted that distal-chip endoscope technology produces an excellent picture resolution during nasal endoscopy under halogen light source, but connecting this type of nasal endoscope with commonly used stroboscopic equipment and software, at the time of this writing, is often challenging. High-speed oral endoscopy is an extremely valuable tool for identifying subtle anomalies in vocal fold vibratory cycles, particularly in patients who present with irregular or aperiodic vibratory cycles that would confound the standard stroboscopic technology. Continued research and further technologic advances will certainly make high-speed laryngoscopy a more widely available diagnostic tool (Snelgrove, 2006; Yan, Ahmad, Kunduk, et al, 2005).

Whether the voice evaluation consists of standard rigid/flexible endoscopy or includes more technologically advanced imaging techniques, the role of the speech-language pathologist is significant. It is critical to use these images to identify technical or behavioral anomalies that may be influencing the patient's overall voice outcome. The primary goal is to compare the patient's perceptual vocal quality with the images gathered during laryngoscopy. If the images suggest a better laryngeal function than the perceptual quality demonstrates, then a behavioral etiology is indicated. At this point, a treatment plan should be devised that is consistent with the patient's goals and performance schedule. If the patient is able to attend multiple consecutive treatment sessions, the goals for treatment should be written in terms of the desired change in vibratory dynamics, as objectively assessed via laryngoscopy. Examples of such goals are as follows:

The patient will achieve open/closed quotient of 70/30 during phonation using Resonant Voice Therapy as assessed via videostroboscopy.

or

The patient will achieve complete vocal fold closure using Resonant Voice Therapy during sustained /i/ as assessed via videostroboscopy.

This method of writing goals for voice therapy emphasizes the effect of behavioral voice treatment on vocal fold physiology by identifying the targeted physiologic goals needed to improve perceptual vocal quality. The distinction between the role of the speech-language pathologist and the physician in interpreting and implementing the objective videostroboscopic data is also highlighted, providing clear support for the active involvement of the speech-language pathologist in the endoscopic evaluation process. The ASHA and the American Academy of Otolaryngology–Head and Neck Surgery (AAO-HNS) have issued a joint position statement clarifying the roles of the speech-language pathologist and the otolaryngologist in the performance and interpretation of videostroboscopy (American Speech-Language-Hearing Association, 1998). This is available on the ASHA Web site at www.asha.org.

✦ Treatment

Considerations for Treatment

Professional singers who are touring frequently cannot attend multiple treatment sessions. In fact, they often have difficulty returning to the clinic at which they were evaluated, simply because of their traveling schedule. Therefore, it is often necessary to provide the patient with behavioral exercises via a self-directed home practice regimen at the time of the evaluation appointment. For many singers, this involves detailed discussions regarding behavioral and environmental precautions to help control LPR, recommendations for periperformance practices, and establishing consistent warm-up and cool-down exercise regimens that can be reasonably implemented without multiple sessions of therapy.

Given patients' anxiety regarding their dysphonia, it is likely that they will have difficulty recalling some of the information presented to them during the evaluation and therapy processes. Inaccurate recall of medical information may lead to noncompliance with therapy regimens (Behrman and Sulica, 2003). Therefore, it is highly advisable to provide patients with written instructions for all recommendations and behavioral exercises, as well as copies of diagnostic data and reports if available. Because many professional singers use the Internet to maintain communication with family and friends during their concert tours, they will often travel with a laptop or notebook computer. Most patients will appreciate having a copy of their endoscopic video file on CD for their personal medical records, particularly if their follow-up examination will be completed at another clinic.

Indications for Surgery

Most surgeons prefer to exhaust all medical and behavioral options before they will consider performing phonosurgery on a patient who is a professional singer, though this largely depends on the diagnosis. Anxiety among professional singers is a natural reaction, and often the speech-language pathologist is intimately involved in providing information regarding expected outcomes and perioperative behavioral treatment. Because a surgical recommendation usually provides a pause in the patient's touring schedule, preoperative therapy is indicated to train behavioral exercises that will be used postoperatively, as well as to reinforce the surgeon's recommendations regarding postoperative voice rest and realistic expectations.

Because postoperative recommendations for total vocal rest vary somewhat widely between surgeons (Kleiner, 1999), it is important that the communication between surgeon and speech-language pathologist be sufficient to ensure that consistent information is provided to the patient. The preoperative therapy session is also an opportune time to establish plans for postoperative compensatory strategies, including changes to the patient's outgoing message on his or her answering machine or voice mail, procuring materials to support primary written communication, and identifying situations, behaviors, and environments to be avoided during the period of total vocal rest prescribed by the surgeon. It is critical that the recommendations made during this session be provided to the patient in written format for future reference. Postoperative vocal rest may also mean "modified" vocal rest, a period during which the patient is allowed to phonate for conversational speech but is not recommended to resume performance. The period of vocal rest, whether total or modified, should be made on a case-by-case basis, the decision-making process being shaped by the severity of pathology and surgical intervention and by the patient's expected vocal load when resuming performance. Using the analogy of Olympic-caliber athletes being recommended for carefully modified training rather than bed rest after some surgeries, professional singers should not be recommended for a prolonged period of vocal rest simply as a matter of course. They will most often benefit from adjustments to their training to ensure adequate healing of the surgical site while still maintaining the high level of muscle tone and neuromuscular control that the have worked for many years to develop. The surgeon and the speech-language pathologist, through effective communication and collaboration, can create a plan for return to vocal function that strikes a balance between avoiding the deleterious effects of prolonged vocal inaction with the need to maintain a laryngeal environment that will effectively facilitate adequate postoperative wound healing. Research is continuing in the area of vocal fold wound healing at the time of this writing, but it is generally accepted that due to the detrimental effects of scarring on vocal fold viscoelasticity and vibratory dynamics, great care must be taken to minimize the risk of vocal fold scar in the population of professional singers. The current literature does suggest more rapid postoperative reestablishment of the basement membrane zone in an environment of total vocal rest in a canine model (Cho, Kim, Lee, et al, 2000). Branski and colleagues showed in a rabbit model that the wound-healing process was characterized by neo–lamina propria deposition at 3 days postoperatively, with complete epithelial coverage achieved at 5 days, but by the 21-day mark the layered structure of the lamina propria had not yet been regained (Branski, Rosen, Verdolini, et al, 2005). Coupled with the results that Behrman and Sulica found regarding variable postoperative voice rest instructions (Kleiner, 1999), these data show that the optimal recommendation for resuming preoperative vocal load after phonosurgery remains elusive. Until further research provides more definitive guidelines, return to vocal function should be determined after complete evaluation of the extent of the surgical intervention and the patient's expected functional requirements.

Postoperative therapy is also recommended (if possible) to ensure accurate performance of assigned behavioral techniques. Recommended therapy techniques include (but are not limited to) Resonant Voice Therapy (Verdolini-Marston, Burke, Lessac, et al, 1995) and Vocal Function Exercises (Sabol, Lee, and Stemple, 1995; Stemple, 2005; Stemple, Lee, D'Amico, et al, 1994). It is not unusual for professional singers to be unable to participate in behavioral voice treatment for multiple sessions, and the speech-language pathologist is therefore challenged to establish an effective independent practice program in a single session. Although the program should certainly be tailored to the needs of the individual patient, the somewhat structured nature of Resonant Voice Therapy and Vocal Function Exercises can be helpful for instances such as this. And although the literature suggests some degree of individual variability (Blaylock, 1999; Milbrath and Solomon, 2003; Motel, Fisher, and Leydon, 2003; Welham and Maclagan, 2004; Vintturi, Alku, Lauri, et al, 2001), the patient will often benefit from the establishment of warm-up and cool-down exercises to be performed at the beginning and at the end of the day, respectively, particularly for the singer who has not had previous formal singing training. These exercises may often include pitch glide tasks performed using lip/tongue trills (Titze, 1996), *arpeggios*, humming, and *messa di voce* exercises (Titze, Long, Shirley, et al, 1999).

Suggestions for Continuing Education

For the speech-language pathologist who is not a singer him- or herself, it may be challenging to obtain adequate continuing education to develop a sense of confidence with this specialized patient population. For some other subspecialties, there are brief and efficient conferences or certification programs available to provide this education. Working with professional singers is, by contrast, a lifelong educational process. For those who are interested in expanding their competency with professional singers, the following recommendations will likely prove useful:

♦ Take twice-monthly voice lessons for at least a year.

♦ Observe singing lessons in the studio of a master singing teacher. Much can be learned from watching others participate in the training process.

♦ Sit in on rehearsals for choirs (amateur and professional), operas, and musical theater.

♦ Be sure to see the finished product. Musical performances such as operas or musical theater productions are much more engaging in person than on recordings.

♦ Take seminars or classes in bodywork techniques that are commonly used during singing training, such as Lessac, Alexander, or Feldenkreis.

♦ Attend concerts by local bands or singers of various styles or attend regional music festivals.

♦ Read books on vocal pedagogy and singing.

♦ Get a subscription to periodicals that follow the music profession.

♦ Join the Voice Foundation and attend the annual symposium.

♦ Attend meetings of the National Association of Teachers of Singing, the National Opera Association, OperaAmerica, and the Voice and Speech Trainers Association.

♦ Develop collaborative relationships with the singing teachers and arts administrators in your local area.

♦ Apprentice with a mentor.

The professional singer is a challenging, unique, and extremely rewarding patient population. As the collaborative relationships between singers, speech-language pathologists, otolaryngologists, teachers of singing, and voice trainers/coaches continues, the result will be a fruitful merging of art and science that will enhance the professions for the benefit of all.

Acknowledgments   The author wishes to thank Diane M. Bless, Ph.D., CCC-SLP, Mary J. Sandage, M.A., CCC-SLP, Seth H. Dailey, M.D., and Christopher S. Leedy, B.A., for their valuable editorial contributions to this chapter.

References

Abitbol, J., Abitbol, B. (1998). The voice and menopause: the twilight of the divas. Contraception, Fertilité, Sexualité 26, 649–655.

Abitbol, J., Abitbol, P., Abitbol, B. (1999). Sex hormones and the female voice. J Voice 13, 424–446.

American Speech-Language-Hearing Association. (1998). Roles of otolaryngologists and speech-language pathologists in the performance and interpretation of strobovideolaryngoscopy. ASHA 40(Suppl 18), 32.

Angsuwarangsee, T., Morrison, M. (2002). Extrinsic laryngeal muscular tension in patients with voice disorders. J Voice 16, 333–343.

Aronson, A.E. (1990). *Clinical voice disorders*. New York: Thieme Medical Publishers.

Aronson, A.E. (2004). Extrinsic muscular tension in patients with voice disorders. J Voice 18, 275; author reply 275.

Aronson, A.E., Peterson, H.W. Jr., Litin, E.M. (1964). Voice symptomatology in functional dysphonia and aphonia. J Speech Hear Disord 29, 367–380.

Behrman, A., Sulica, L. (2003). Voice rest after microlaryngoscopy: current opinion and practice. Laryngoscope 113, 2182–2186.

Blaylock, T.R. (1999). Effects of systematized vocal warm-up on voices with disorders of various etiologies. J Voice 13, 43–50.

Bless, D.M., Hirano, M. (1993). *Videostroboscopic examination of the larynx.* San Diego: Singular Publishing Group.

Bless, D.M., Hirano, M., Feder, R.J. (1987). Videostroboscopic evaluation of the larynx. Ear Nose Throat J 66, 289–296.

Branski, R.C., Rosen, C.A., Verdolini, K., Hebda, PA. (2005). Acute vocal fold wound healing in a rabbit model. Ann Otol Rhinol Larngol 114, 19–24.

Cammarota, G., Elia, F., Cianci, R., Galli, J., Paolillo, N., Montalto, M., Gasbarrini, G. (2003). Worsening of gastroesophageal reflux symptoms in professional singers during performances. J Clin Gastroenterol 36, 403–404.

Cho, S.H., Kim, H.T., Lee, I.J., Kim, M.S., Park, H.J. (2000). Influence of phonation on basement membrane zone recovery after phonomicrosurgery: a canine model. Ann Otol Rhinol Laryngol 109, 658–666.

Dailey, S.D. (2005). Management of the professional voice user. Presented at University of Wisconsin Department of Surgery, Division of OTO-HNS, UW-Madison; March 23; Madison, WI.

Davis, C.B., Davis, M.L. (1993). The effects of premenstrual syndrome (PMS) on the female singer. J Voice 7, 337–353.

DelGaudio, J.M. (2002). Steroid inhaler laryngitis: dysphonia caused by inhaled fluticasone therapy. Arch Otolaryngol Head Neck Surg 128, 677–681.

Elias, M.E., Sataloff, R.T., Rosen, D.C., Heuer, R.J., Spiegel, J.R. (1997). Normal strobovideolaryngoscopy: variability in healthy singers. J Voice 11, 104–107.

Hertegard, S. (2005). What have we learned about laryngeal physiology from high-speed digital videoendoscopy? Curr Opin Otolaryngol Head Neck Surg 13, 152–156.

Hunter, E.J., Svec, J.G., Titze, I.R. (2006). Comparison of the produced and perceived voice range profiles in untrained and trained classical singers. J Voice 20(4), 513–526.

Isolauri, J., Laippala, P. (1995). Prevalence of symptoms suggestive of gastroesophageal reflux disease in an adult population. Ann Med 27, 67–70.

Jozkow, P., Wasko-Czopnik, D., Medras, M., Paradowski, L. (2006). Gastroesophageal reflux disease and physical activity. Sports Med 36,385–391.

Kessler, R.C., McGonagle, K.A., Zhao, S., Nelson, C.B., Hughes, M., Eshleman, S., et al. (1994). Lifetime and 12-month prevalence of DSM-III-R psychiatric disorders in the United States. Results from the National Comorbidity Survey. Arch Gen Psychiatry 51, 8–19.

Kleiner, S.M. (1999). Water: an essential but overlooked nutrient. J Am Dietetic Assoc 99, 200–206.

Koufman, J.A. (1991). The otolaryngologic manifestations of gastroesophageal reflux disease (GERD): a clinical investigation of 225 patients using ambulatory 24-hour pH monitoring and an experimental investigation of the role of acid and pepsin in the development of laryngeal injury. Laryngoscope 101(4 Pt 2 Suppl 53), 1–78.

Koufman, J.A., Amin, M.R., Panetta, M. (2000). Prevalence of reflux in 113 consecutive patients with laryngeal and voice disorders. Otolaryngol Head Neck Surg 123, 385–388.

Koufman, J.A., Radomski, T.A., Joharji, G.M., Russell, G.B., Pillsbury, D.C. (1996). Laryngeal biomechanics of the singing voice. Otolaryngol Head Neck Surg 115, 527–537.

Lawrence, V.L. (1981). Handy household hints: to sing or not to sing. NATS Bull 37, 23–25.

Lundy, D.S., Casiano, R.R., Sullivan, P.A., Roy, S., Xue, J.W., Evans J. (1999). Incidence of abnormal laryngeal findings in asymptomatic singing students. Otolaryngol Head Neck Surg 121, 69–77.

Milbrath, R.L., Solomon, N.P. (2003). Do vocal warm-up exercises alleviate vocal fatigue? J Speech Lang Hear Res 46, 422–436.

Motel, T., Fisher, K.V., Leydon, C. (2003). Vocal warm-up increases phonation threshold pressure in soprano singers at high pitch. J Voice 17, 160–167.

Pendergrass, S.M. (1999). Determination of glycols in air: development of sampling and analytical methodology and application to theatrical smokes. Am Ind Hyg Assoc J 60, 452–457.

Richter, B., Löhle, E., Knapp, B., Weikert, M., Schlömicher-Their, J., Verdolini, K. (2002). Harmful substances on the opera stage: possible negative effects on singers' respiratory tracts. J Voice 16, 72–80.

Rossol, M., Hinkamp, D. (2001). Hazards in the theater. Occup Med 16,595–608.

Roy, N., Ford, C.N., Bless, D.M. (1996). Muscle tension dysphonia and spasmodic dysphonia: the role of manual laryngeal tension reduction in diagnosis and treatment. Ann Otol Rhinol Laryngol 105, 851–856.

Roy, N., Tanner, K., Gray, S.D., Blomgren, M., Fisher, K.V. (2003). An evaluation of the effects of three laryngeal lubricants on phonation threshold pressure (PTP). J Voice 17, 331–342.

Sabol, J.W., Lee, L., Stemple, J.C. (1995). The value of vocal function exercises in the practice regimen of singers. J Voice 9, 27–36.

Sandage, M. (Ed), Graves-Wright, J., Hever, R., Verdolini, K., Ferketic, M., Westerman-Gregg, J., Titze, I., Devore, K., Raphael, B., Hooper, C. (2005). The role of the speech-language pathologist, teacher of singing, and the speaking voice trainer in voice habilitation. Position statement, American Speech-Language-Hearing Association. Available at www.asha.org./about/publications/leader_online/archives/2002/q3/f020723.htm

Sandage, M.J., Emerich K. (2002). Singing voice: special considerations for evaluation and treatment. ASHA Leader 23 February.

Sataloff, R.T. (2000). Evaluation of professional singers. Otolaryngol Clin North Am 33, 923–956.

Sataloff, R.T. (2005). Arts medicine: an interdisciplinary paradigm. ENT Ear Nose Throat J 84 (8): 462–463.

Sataloff, R.T., Spiegel, J.R., Hawkshaw, M.J. (1991). Strobovideolaryngoscopy: results and clinical value. Ann Otol Rhinol Laryngol 100(9 Pt 1), 725–727.

Sivasankar, M., Fisher, K.V. (2002). Oral breathing increases Pth and vocal effort by superficial drying of vocal fold mucosa. J Voice 16, 172–181.

Snelgrove, S. (2006). A consideration of memory in terms of information giving. Nurs Times 102, 26–28.

Stemple, J.C. (2005). A holistic approach to voice therapy. Semin Speech Lang 26, 131–137.

Stemple, J.C., Lee, L., D'Amico, B., Pickup, B. (1994). Efficacy of vocal function exercises as a method of improving vocal function. J Voice 8, 271–278.

Steward, D.L., Wilson, K.M., Kelly, D.H., Paril, M.S., Sehwartzbaver, H.R., Long, J.D., Welge, J.A. (2004). Proton pump inhibitor therapy for chronic laryngopharyngitis: a randomized, placebo-controlled trial. Otolaryngol Head Neck Surg 131, 342–350.

Sundberg, J. (2001). Level and center frequency of the singer's formant. J Voice 15, 176–186.

Teschke, K., Chow, Y., van Netten, C., Varughese, S., Kennedy, S.M., Brauer, M. (2005). Exposures to atmospheric effects in the entertainment industry. J Occup Environ Hyg 2, 277–284.

Titze, I.R. (1996). Lip and tongue trills: what do they do for us? J Sing 52, 51–52.

Titze, I.R., Lemke, J., Montequin, D. (1997). Populations in the U.S. workforce who rely on voice as a primary tool of trade: a preliminary report. J Voice 11, 254–249.

Titze, I.R., Long, S., Shirley, G.I., Stathopoulos, E., Ramig, L.O., Carroll, L.M., Riley, W.D. (1999). Messa di voce: an investigation of the symmetry of crescendo and decrescendo in a singing exercise. J Acoust Soc Am 105, 2933–2940.

VanEaton, S.F.C. (1990). An investigation of the attitudes of selected professional classical solo singer-actors toward specific concerns of the music profession. Doctoral dissertation, University of North Texas, Denton, TX.

Verdolini, K., Titze, I.R. (1994). Dependence of phonatory effort on hydration level. J Speech Hear Res 37, 1001–1007.

Verdolini-Marston, K., Burke, M.K., Lessac, A., Glaze, L., Caldwell, E. (1995). Preliminary study of two methods of treatment for laryngeal nodules. J Voice 9, 74–85.

Vintturi, J., Alku, P., Lauri, E.R., Sala, E., Sihvo, M., Vilkman, I. (2001). Objective analysis of vocal warm-up with special reference to ergonomic factors. J Voice 15, 36–53.

Von Duvillard, S.P., Braun, W.A., Markofski, M., Beneke, R., Leithauser, R. (2004). Fluids and hydration in prolonged endurance performance. Nutrition 20, 651–656.

Welham, N.V., Maclagan, M.A. (2004). Vocal fatigue in young trained singers across a solo performance: a preliminary study. Logoped Phoniatr Vocol29, 3–12.

Wingate, J.M., Brown, W.S., Shrivastav, R., Davenport, C., Sapienza, C.M. (2007). Treatment outcomes for professional voice users. J Voice 21 (4): 433–449.

Woo, P., Colton, R., Casper, J., Brewer, D. (1991). Diagnostic value of stroboscopic examination in hoarse patients. J Voice 5, 231–238.

Yan, Y., Ahmad, K., Kunduk, M., Bless, D. (2005). Analysis of vocal-fold vibrations from high-speed laryngeal images using a Hilbert transform-based methodology. J Voice 19, 161–175.

Chapter 13

Extended Case Studies in Psychogenic Voice Disorders

History

Ms. R., a 35-year-old single woman, called for an appointment to discuss what she describes as a problem of an excessively loud voice. Ms R., who works for a newspaper, was recently reprimanded for speaking too loudly. This patient describes her inability to keep the intensity of her speech down to appropriate levels as a lifelong problem. She has decided that the time has come when she should do something about this tendency or else review its social and vocational repercussions.

Examination

The patient is a pleasant, obese woman whose voice is somewhat low in pitch and potentially quite loud. However, during the examination, she demonstrated ample ability to maintain a normal loudness level of her voice appropriate to the clinical situation.

Psychosocial examination reveals that the patient is one of six children who had to use her voice and speech as a means of defense while she was growing up. During high school, she was repeatedly reminded she was too loud. She considers that all her life she has been verbally aggressive and defensive. She volunteers that where she is concerned, loudness is equated with anger. Ms. R. has had past psychologic problems of self-acceptance and has had both psychologic and, currently, psychiatric help to learn to accept herself to a greater extent than she has, and not to become angry with herself or to take the blame for all interactions that go bad. During much of this discussion, she cried quietly. Her attitude lifelong has been that "the world is not fair," but she volunteers that she is the one who will have to change. She is aware that she is considerably overweight and has recently become concerned about her personal appearance. She intends to diet and learn to dress in more sophisticated fashion.

Impression

Ms. R. has a problem with poor control over loudness of her voice in the direction of excessive loudness, which appears secondary to personality and adaptation to her environment, traits that she has possessed throughout much of her life. The examining clinician sees her voice disorder as just the surface of a deeper problem of hostile reactions to others, but in a woman who appears to have considerable insight and motivation to change. She believes that the psychotherapy, infrequent as it is, that she has been receiving from her psychiatrist has helped her gain increased self-acceptance and motivation to change.

Therapy

While it appears that Ms. R.'s voice disorder is primarily psychogenic and that a change in the aggressive use of her voice ought to parallel improvement in her self-image and her relationships with others, the need for symptomatic voice therapy to learn control of her loudness level is also evident.

Two years after symptomatic voice therapy, Ms. R., now 37, returns for a brief visit and review of the problem that first brought her to the clinic. Since the initial visit, she has been seeing her psychiatrist, approximately once a month, for depression and to work out some of her interpersonal problems at home. She claims she was able to control her loudness problem until 5 weeks ago when she was reprimanded by her supervisor for speaking "too loudly again" and using the phone too much. The patient says, "That got to me." It is important to note that the patient had been prescribed Valium (diazepam, Hoffmann La Roche, Nutley NJ), which may have resulted in some disinhibition of behavior. Valium was subsequently terminated, and the patient was on Limbitrol (chlordiazepoxide, amitriptyline, ICN Pharmaceuticals, Inc., Costa Mesa, CA) at the time of her subsequent visit.

During this evaluation, the patient's speech is very well modulated, with no signs of loss of loudness control. The clinician and patient discussed the probable atypical situational nature of her loss of loudness control and that no symptomatic voice therapy was indicated. They also discussed the importance of continued psychotherapy with the objective of improving self-understanding. The clinician suggested that she do some reading in the area of interpersonal relations and self-help recommendations that have been reported in the literature. An additional symptom during the current examination was a change in the patient's articulation. The patient's articulation was +1 ataxic dysarthric, very possibly related to her current medication but also could be a sign of neurologic disease. She did not complain of any gait or upper-extremity incoordination. Thus, reassurance appeared to be the method of choice in this situation. The patient was encouraged to remain in touch.

Some months later, Ms. R. called to say that she had completed her psychotherapy, that it had been quite helpful as she had learned to regard herself in a better light, that she does not have to be angry, that she learned where the anger was coming from, and that her generally reduced hostilities reflected itself in much less difficulty with excessive vocal loudness. She felt she was doing quite well both psychologically, with regard to her speech, and in her ability to control her loudness during conversations with others. People have remarked that she is less in evidence: "I don't know where you are anymore," one said. She also reported that she was successful in controlling her loudness during a recent "argument" with a friend. Some days it is an effort to remain aware of the need for control. She continues with her self-improvement plans; has been for "color analysis" wearing different makeup, intends to modify her wardrobe, and to continue working on her obesity. She still sees her psychiatrist, reporting fewer and less intense bouts with depression. She takes lithium. An important clinical insight: her loudness has been the main reason for her previous job/interpersonal failures. It resulted in "punishment" for her, as she puts it, "a self-fulfilling prophecy" that, perhaps, she needed to fail and that her speech was a direct route to alienation of others. She said she no longer needed to do this. At this point, it appeared that she had a good hold on her loudness control and that voice therapy was close to termination. Consequently, she was requested to call again in about 2 weeks for a check on progress and then be terminated from treatment.

Case Study 13.2   Psychogenic Aphonia

History

Miss K. is a 33-year-old, single, remedial reading teacher who had sudden loss of voice associated with laryngitis 1 month prior to examination. Since then, she has been essentially whispering. She has had two to three previous voice losses, which have lasted only a day and which remitted spontaneously. This time, however, it has lasted a month.

Examination

Otolaryngologic examination disclosed normal vocal fold structure and ability to adduct and abduct the vocal folds. During the speech pathologist's voice examination, the patient converses in a strained whisper. She demonstrates +2 musculoskeletal pain in the thyrohyoid space on the left. Her *coup de glotte* was normal again indicating normal vocal fold adduction.

With minimum manual mobilization of the laryngeal-hyoid area, the patient's voice came back within minutes.

The psychosocial history indicates that in all probability, Miss K. was suffering from an accumulation of external pressures or stresses on or about the time she lost her voice a month prior to the evaluation: (1) her mother had entered the hospital, and the patient had become quite worried about her (it turned out that her mother did not have any serious illness); (2) the patient was pressured by an accumulation of paperwork that usually occurs at the end of the school year, but this year it was especially bad because of failure of various test services to return papers to her that she needed for processing; (3) she had been experiencing a flare-up of her multiple schlerosis (MS) consisting of paresthesias of the hands and feet, dizziness, a feeling of thick-headedness, and increased difficulty walking; (4) she has had an ongoing problem with her colleagues who teach regular classes and who resent her small caseload and the interference that they perceive she is creating by taking children out of the classroom for special help.

Impression

Psychogenic (probably conversion) aphonia.

Recommendation

The patient's voice had returned to normal early during this examination. Once voice was achieved, the remainder of the session focused on the relationship between voice losses and external stresses so as to provide somewhat greater insight for the patient, so that if she perceives that pressures are accumulating, she might consider avoiding taking on excessive responsibilities.

Case Study 13.3   Psychogenic Hoarseness

History

A 24-year-old business major was referred by an ear-nose-throat doctor for evaluation of episodic hoarseness and sore throat that was of 6 to 7 years' duration, from which time the patient was a college freshman. She had alternated going to school with working, accounting for the extended duration of her undergraduate years. During the prior few months, voice and throat discomfort worsened.

ENT examination revealed essentially normal-appearing vocal folds except for some erythema in the region of the vocal processes.

Examination

This patient's voice was perceptually normal. However, she felt throat discomfort and described a feeling of a "baseball in my throat sometimes" (globus).

The psychosocial history was highly positive. Over the past 15 years, she had accumulated a tremendous amount of unexpressed anger at her father and especially her stepmother and her stepsisters for the way in which she was treated—made to feel unwanted and creating a "her kids–our kids" conflict. The patient spent a year in another city away from the family, and it seems that since returning more of her angry feelings have come to the surface, and she has been communicating her anger and resentment in a small way toward members of her family. This, however, is very difficult for her because, typically, her entire mode of dealing with others is to suppress anger, which she regards as "scary" and which she equates with "violence and revenge." She freely admitted, "I don't know what to do with anger."

The moment she was asked about her personal life, she began crying and did so on and off for the remainder of the examination. She described her stepmother as "kind of ridiculous as a mother, an alcoholic." The patient was tired of being "treated like dirt." She described years of suppressed pain, "I have a lot of anger but you can't do that." She felt as if she has been "stomped on for years and years." As she cried, she said, "I think I must be upset at myself for taking this for so many years . . . now I feel like I should say stuff, but it's pretty scary." She said she felt better the other day when she was crying and expressing her anger and hurt toward her stepmother but that it happened very infrequently because of her censorship of her feelings. "No one has ever seen me angry or raise my voice."

Possibly contributory has been the fact that she leads a very active life, working hard as a student, holding down a job as a secretary, and admitting that she pushes herself "really hard." In the previous year, she had mononucleosis and did not think she ever recovered completely from that and reported frequently feeling tired and not getting enough sleep.

She saw a psychologic counselor briefly.

Impression

The combination of the erythematous posterior glottis and case history suggest that this patient's episodic dysphonia and throat discomfort may be due to esophageal reflux and musculoskeletal tension. The musculoskeletal tension appears secondary to chronic emotional stress and unexpressed anger, resentment, and hostility toward members of her family, occurring in a young woman whose approach to interpersonal relationships is one of not expressing emotions of anger, particularly because of her perception of its social unacceptability.

Recommendation

The voice clinician devoted a considerable portion of the initial session toward explaining to the patient the relationship between abnormal voice, laryngeal muscle tension, and suppressed emotions, particularly anger. The patient, rather typically, found it difficult, but not impossible, to accept this explanation because of feeling guilty and that to have a physical problem because of emotional difficulties seemed like a sign of "weakness." At the same time, she seemed to recognize the connection, and she was strongly advised to follow an antireflux regimen and to consult with a clinical psychologist or psychiatrist to get out into the open much of the pent-up emotions that she has never fully expressed to anyone.

This case is yet another classic example illustrating that there often is not a single etiologic basis for laryngeal complaints. Determining whether the emotional state was the basis for the reflux, or if the reflux set up the tissue irritation that when combined with musculoskeletal tension caused the globus, or if the conditions were initiated with the mononucleosis and maintained by the musculoskeletal tension secondary to the emotional state, cannot be determined. What can be determined is that there are co-occurring factors that need to be treated concomitantly.

Case Study 13.4   Psychogenic Adductor Spasmodic Dysphonia

This next case history is presented as a transcript of the initial evaluation of a 31-year-old married woman who exhibited the perceptual characteristics of adductor spasmodic dysphonia. She had a strained, strangled voice with frequent voice stoppages. The case is illustrative of how clinicians can ask questions to help patients discover facts about the onset of their voice problems and to uncover the psychodynamics of the individual. It emphasizes the importance of recognizing how difficult it is for patients to accept having a problem related to stress and recommendations to receive psychotherapy. It also suggests clinicians should consider the possibility of muscle tension dysphonia when hearing characteristics of adductor spasmodic dysphonia.

Clinician (C): When did the strained voice first start?

Patient (P): I really became strained I guess 6 to 7 months ago. When I say strained, I mean to the point that words would not come out whenever I tried to express them.

C: But when was the very first change in your voice?

P: Actually a year and a half to 2 years ago. The reason it is so amazing is because it wasn't anything that hit me; it was very subtle.

C: What specifically did you notice a few years ago?

P: Well, that I would wake up and have a gruffness of voice and not have a sore throat or cold.

C: Now, this was 1 to 2 years ago?

P: Yes. About a year and a half, and it would just be maybe a day or two and people would ask me if I had a cold and I wouldn't and then it would and it would just fade away so I never really gave it much consideration.

C: And it was off and on, episodic for the last year, year and a half?

P: Right.

C: And then when did the voice change into a different pattern?

P: I would have to say probably November of last year. That's when I really started noticing that it was sporadic.

C: About 6 months ago?

P: Yes.

C: And what happened then that was different from before?

P: Well it just . . . in conversing, words just would not come out and I think, besides, it was a huge amount of tension or knots in my stomach.

C: Did the voice sound or feel more strained?

P: Yes, strained is a good word. I felt like it was a strain to talk.

C: And did it remain that way throughout the entire 6 months?

P: Well, to me it has gotten worse.

C: But when it started out 6 months ago, how often would you have it?

P: I could get it like 2 or 3 days of talking normal and then maybe a week of not being able to, or just barely being able to talk.

C: And when did it become constant?

P: I would say constant within the past 3 months, constant where it's almost every day. And as I said, there are still points where I have 2 or 3 days where it is perfectly clear.

C: Do you associate those days of clarity with anything else?

P: Not really. It's usually when I'm away from the house.

C: And where would you be?

P: Well, out riding my horse or out visiting with people on the farm or something like that.

C: Your voice would be better in general when you were away from the house.

P: Right. And it is always better in the morning. When I first wake up, I am perfectly clear. And when I have a few drinks of alcohol, it seems to be much clearer.

C: You've been married how long now?

P: Since August; 9 months I guess.

C: Were you having emotional problems 1½ to 2 years ago?

P: No.

C: But you have been over the past 6 months?

P: Yes.

C: Please describe that.

P: I think I've been unhappy in a situation that I haven't done anything about, whereas normally I would. If I'm unhappy in a situation I change it and I just haven't done anything about it. The marriage.

C: When did you become concerned enough about the voice to do something about it, to investigate the voice as a problem?

P: The first time about a month ago.

C: And what did you decide to do then?

P: I went to talk to a specialist; an ear, nose, throat man.

C: And what did that doctor tell you?

P: The only thing that he told me is that he didn't see any damage to the vocal folds. He said that he did see, or

he thought there was a small cyst at the end of my vocal folds and that he recommended I speak to a speech pathologist. He wrote to the speech pathologist that I had spastic dysphonia.

C: What did the speech pathologist do?

P: Well, she told me she didn't think it was spastic dysphonia and she set it up that I would have sessions twice a week, 30 minutes at a time that we never did do, because this doctor had talked to a laryngologist who specializes in spastic dysphonia.

C: So you never had any voice therapy?

P: Right. Never have.

C: Why not?

P: Well, . . . after we talked to this doctor ~30 minutes on the telephone he was ready to do surgery that to me was a turnoff because it just didn't make much sense to have an operation when it hasn't even been investigated. And, a couple of times when I had the appointment set up with the speech pathologist, my husband finally said, "Well, there is no need to even go talk to her." He said "We're going to come up here."

C: You mean on the basis of talking to you on the phone he asked you to come out and have surgery?

P: He was ready to. He said that we would of course do the investigation and think out everything but he said that the only, or in his opinion he was convinced, the only solution was to clip the nerve in the vocal fold and he explained it in detail to my husband and myself. But . . . I haven't had any speech therapy with anyone yet.

C: When you saw the psychiatrist this morning, your voice was worse than it is now?

P: Yes.

C: How much worse?

P: I think it was more difficult to get words out.

C: Much better now or just mildly?

P: Just mildly better.

C: Did it help you to discuss your situation with the psychiatrist?

P: Immensely. And afterwards I discussed it with my husband, which made me feel much better.

C: You felt much better?

P: Yes.

C: What was your husband's reaction?

P: Well, he is very . . . he doesn't want to accept the fact that we don't have a marriage and it's very difficult for him. He doesn't understand a lot of things about it which I understand.

C: What did you tell your husband after you talked with the psychiatrist?

P: Well, I just explained to him what we discussed about marriage and certain reasons why I didn't like marriage. And that I did feel my inward tensions. Because I've never been a nervous person or shaky, you know, about anything, and just since we've been married I've been fighting the divorce or separation. For my husband's sake, I wanted to stay married. And, well I just told him exactly what we discussed and that the psychiatrist had recommended psychotherapy and he also asked that we consider separation. I'm the one that has been worrying about the divorce, you know. Just go ahead and end it and get it over with.

C: The one who has what?

P: Wanted to just end it completely, the relationship and as far as a marriage goes. But, the few options that he mentioned I thought sounded pretty good.

C: And what did you husband think about the possibilities?

P: Well, he would like to discuss it with the psychiatrist and have more insight. I did tell him exactly what was discussed and I think he might want to talk to you, too, which I have no objections to.

C: But is it your interpretation that the psychotherapy is supposed to be some way of forestalling the eventual separation and divorce or is it something you have decided on?

P: Well truthfully, psychotherapy I think is great and I have no objections to it. I don't think that that is needed in my case. I think what I need is probably somebody that knows how to work with someone that has a voice problem. Mentally, I'm very fit. My only discontentment is I'm in a marriage situation that I love the man but I don't want to be married to him.

C: Well, that is a rather interesting split there.

P: Well, yes it is. It's very strange.

C: How do you account for that?

P: I guess I account for it by the fact I don't like the closeness. I've lived 29 years very happily single. I love being single. My favorite things are to ride the horse out in the woods for days or read books. Of course, I love being with people also. I was an executive so I had to be with people but, marriage isn't anything like I thought it would be.

C: What did you think it was going to be like, and how is it?

P: Well, I thought it would be great deal of sharing emotionally and materialistically, all the things that you share, but I didn't think it would be sharing everything, meaning the husband; he doesn't want to do anything unless I am with him. Whether it's golf or whether it's a trip. To me it has been very draining because I've never in my life been, even when I lived with a big family, and we've had all that closeness, I've never had that much closeness in that way; to me it is like 24 hours of . . .

C: Do you feel stifled by it?

P: Yes, and I've told him that and explained it to him and he doesn't do it purposely. I think it's the first time he's ever been in love and he's gotten carried away with it. And the difference being he's a person that needs me and I don't need him. I don't need him in the way, I mean to fulfill my life and that is a big difference in our relationship.

C: Throughout your life, have you been the kind of person who is able to express her emotional feelings freely or have you been the kind who has kept them to herself?

P: I would have to say 50-50. For the past 15 years I would say I've been very outwardly spoken.

C: Did you have trouble confronting your husband with your feelings about the marriage?

P: Not at all. In fact, before we got married, I was really fighting getting married and I expressed that to the psychiatrist and you know he said, "Well, why did you?" And I said I wished I knew because it just happened real sud-denly and my husband is very persuasive person and, I've always really cared for him, too.

C: But you went ahead with it anyway. Did you express your misgivings to your husband before you were married?

P: Very much. I told him I was not a touchy-feely person. I mean I'm loving and I have a lot of love to give, and I can accept love but he is starved for love in the way that he really needs constant patting on the head and a lot of attention and a lot of what I can't, I guess, give, you know, if I were in the right frame of mind. But there are things that I can't give him that he needs. And I don't know if there is any reason for him to lack for that just because of me.

C: May I ask whether you think your voice is better now than when we started?

P: Much better.

C: Do you and your husband have much in common?

P: Oh gosh! We have everything in common. We're both very adventuresome in the way that we love to travel, we love to play golf, we both ski.

C: Do you feel right now as if you have a load off your chest, your mind about this whole thing?

P: Yes.

C: Because there has been some movement here and you've gotten closer . . .

P: Well, I did because I kept rejecting talking to anybody professional about it. I kept thinking, well, whatever it is will go away tomorrow, because tomorrow would be fine. And then, when I finally did get to the point where it was so frustrating not being able to converse and express or even go to a counter and order a bottle of perfume without somebody saying "What are you saying?" When I finally did go to somebody, all it did was confirm my gut feelings, my inner feelings, which were that I felt like it was something to do with keeping things in. In other words, I've always been a happy person, and I'm always jovial and never depressed and just lately I've been in a state of depression.

C: How long?

P: Well, I'd say about 3 or 4 months. And that's when my voice told me that what I'm doing is that I'm fighting myself. I'm not letting myself do what I naturally do, which is always to do whatever makes me happy.

C: Do you think the voice has more or less paralleled the depression?

P: I feel like it has.

C: The more depression the worse the voice?

P: Yes, because I feel like it, in other words, as I said earlier I've never been a nervous person, well lately I'm not nervous but I'm very, very tense. I lay down to go to sleep and try to sleep and then just start thinking. To get to sleep I have to use progressive relaxation techniques. I'll slowly go from toe to head and relax each muscle section of my body.

C: But, how has coming up here and talking to the psychiatrist or to me helped you?

P: Well . . . it isn't a physical thing or I mean I don't have a tumor or I don't have something physical . . . I feel more comfortable about that. I also feel more comfortable because I hadn't talked to anybody at length about this, and after talking to the psychiatrist he suggested psychotherapy and mentioned the fact that we might want to consider a 6-month separation, which I'm open-minded to.

C: Well, what do you want to do?

P: I think it is probably worth a try to first be away from each other for 6 months and for me to seek whatever therapy I need during that 6 months.

C: If you're so convinced that marriage is not for you, what value would separation have?

P: Well, that's a good point, because I'm almost saying a contradiction.

C: . . . prolonging something that you think . . .

P: Well, that was something I talked about when we went back to the room after I talked to the psychiatrist. I told him that as far as I was concerned, a divorce is fine with me, but for my husband's sake if he wanted to make it a 6-month separation possibly I may find out I'm making a bad mistake and want to come back.

C: In other words, there might be some value in separation.

P: Possibly so.

C: You may be 99% sure but you may not be 100% sure.

P: Exactly. That's a very good way of putting it. Like I said to the psychiatrist, I don't want to make it sound like I'm sloughing the voice thing off on the marriage but I know it has gotten increasingly worse and I figured it had something to do with it.

C: The last 6 months that you've had the voice trouble have you been away for any length of time like a couple days or a week?

P: Yes, I went to another city 3 weeks one time.

C: How was your voice then?

P: It was real good.

C: Was it normal or just good?

P: I would say there was only 1 day that it wasn't normal.

C: So the 3 weeks you were away, the voice was essentially normal?

P: Yes.

C: And when you got back home it was bad again.

P: Yes.

C: And how long ago was that?

P: Seems like it was about 3 months ago that I went away.

C: Well, it seems to me that the voice trouble fluctuates so closely with how you are feeling, whether you are relaxed or whether you are anxious, depressed, or anything like that. I don't think voice therapy twice a week is the answer at all. I think the answer is reducing some of that tension in the area of your voice box, and getting some psychological help with the major problem that has caused the voice trouble. In other words, you don't have a habit pattern established here. I believe that voice will return to normal the moment you get out from under stress. And, in the meantime I'll show you today how you might reduce the neck tension. Does that sound right?

P: Most of the time, yes.

C: Right now for example, you are more relaxed and you have put the cards on the table. Your voice is nearly nor-

mal. When you were away for 3 weeks the voice was almost normal because you were away from the situation that was causing you to be tense.

P: The only thing about that is before I was even married I was having problems with the gruffness for no reason, and I don't know if this stems from that or . . .

C: I don't really know. One of our problems is that the farther back you go the harder it is to remember how you were feeling. Now, presumably we're talking about an extension of that earlier problem. It is entirely possible that this is a new disorder and that the other one was related to something else. Did the other one, a couple years ago, sound this way or was it a different sound?

P: No, it was just a bit of a gruffness in the voice.

C: It is conceivable that these are not related and this is a brand new disorder that started during the time of your marriage. But, it is conceivable also that the gruffness that occurred a couple years ago was due to some tension, too. Do you remember having been depressed at that time?

P: Yes, I did go through kind of a move. I had a beautiful condo and I had to sell it and go to work.

Postscript

Manual circumferential therapy was demonstrated to the patient with positive results. She left the session with a normal-sounding voice and claimed the voice was free of tension and that she would follow up with psychotherapy. Three weeks later, the patient's husband called to say that his wife was dissatisfied with our diagnosis, that her spastic dysphonia was worse, and that she thought the cause was organic, not psychologic. She planned to find another ENT specialist for further investigation. Two years later, she returned to the clinic for further consultation. She had found another specialist who injected Botox® (botulinium toxin, Allergan, Irvine, CA) with which she had intermittent success. She terminated that treatment, began psychotherapy, divorced her husband, and developed a near-normal voice. She returned for voice therapy to be reminded how to reduce and/or control laryngeal tension.

Case Study 13.5　Psychogenic Mutational Falsetto (Puberphonia)

History

Dr. L. was a single, 29-year-old resident in dermatology who was referred by an otolaryngologist for the purpose of evaluation of a long-standing voice disorder. Dr. L. believed that he had had a hoarse, high-pitched voice for as long as he could remember. He recently had become concerned over his voice when another resident remarked to him that he was "known by his unusual voice." When he was an intern, he was told by a more senior physician that his voice had a "bad effect" on patients. Were it not for these remarks made within the past few years, and particularly more recently, Dr. L. would not have sought help for his voice. When questioned further about the voice, the patient indicated that he considered it more "hoarse" than high-pitched, and he noted difficulties being understood when having to speak in a noisy environment, such as at parties. His family had never mentioned his voice to him.

Examination

Dr. L. was a very pleasant young man noticeably small and short in stature who spoke in a high-pitched, falsetto voice. Phonation under conditions of maximum inspiration and sharp glottal attack on phonation produced a normally low-pitched voice, indicating normal laryngeal-pharyngeal anatomy for a completely masculine voice and that the falsetto voice was a form of learned behavior.

Psychosocial history was positive and helped to explain the etiology of his falsetto voice. Dr. L. came from a family of modest circumstances, whose parents escaped persecution in Europe. He described his parents as considerably opposite in personality: his mother as highly aggressive and verbal, his father passive, silent, and unassuming. Dr. L., as far back as he could remember, had witnessed considerable family arguments and turmoil. During his early developmental years, he witnessed violent, uncivilized behavior, feeling ashamed over what the neighbors, adjacent to their apartment, would think about his parents' fighting, and often felt like hiding during such conflict to avoid being recognized by his neighbors.

Dr. L. decided to study medicine not only out of his intellectual interest in the field but also because he was determined to bring some happiness and honor to the family, especially in view of his older brother's troubles with drugs and his general failures as a person. Dr. L. completed his premedical studies with high grades and felt "thrilled" to be in medical school.

It is important to note that Dr. L.'s entire approach to communicating verbally with others was one of compliance and compromise. He admitted to difficulty confronting, disagreeing, or arguing with others, preferring to take a conciliatory approach except on matters that clearly indicated the necessity for him to stand his ground. He admitted to a supersensitivity toward others' opinions of him, admitted to a passive approach to people, stated that "confronting creates hostility," and generally feared using speech to express his opinion on issues even of a mundane nature.

Impression

Mutational falsetto (puberphonia), possibly secondary to ambivalence toward confronting others via speech, of long-standing duration.

Recommendation

Direct voice therapy was begun on the morning of the day of his examination, and in a brief period the patient was able to produce a completely normal, low-pitched, reasonably clear voice. He was advised to employ the low-pitched voice over the lunch hour and to return during the early afternoon.

Upon returning for continued therapy, and after having been asked about his experience with the low-pitched voice over the lunch hour, the patient began to express,

using the low-pitched voice, a high degree of anxiety over whether or not he would have the "guts" to return to where he was to continue his residency. He complained that the low-pitched voice took a considerable amount of effort, in spite of the fact that he had been using it for a couple of hours without objective evidence of fatigue. At that point, a considerable amount of time was devoted to discussion of his fears about returning home with his new voice. He frankly admitted that he was "afraid—everybody is used to my old voice," and what would he tell people back home about the ease with which the low-pitched voice was acquired? He even went so far as to suggest he fabricate some diagnosis that he could use in describing the results of the voice examination, one that would indicate an organic cause for his dysphonia, and some medical or surgical therapy resulting in its improvement. He did not like the idea of mutational voice disorder as an explanation because it carried with it too much of the implication of psychogenicity. He was particularly fearful that his new residency chief at the university would think that there was something peculiarly different or wrong with him, even though he admitted that prior to this time he had only met this physician three times and on each occasion the contact was brief. Dr. L.'s concern over his image and future acceptance extended to the point of requesting that the voice clinician not even write a letter back to the referring physician indicating a diagnostic impression, for fear that this information would end up in the patient's medical record and would be prejudicial to him.

In spite of these trepidations, Dr. L. volunteered that, despite his misgivings over returning home with the low-pitched voice, it was imperative for him to do so, because he had become convinced during the treatment sessions that the old, falsetto voice could have long-term negative effects on his professional and social success. The patient was discharged with him using his low-pitched voice and was given a tape to record his voice to return to the voice clinic in 1 month.

Postscript

The 1-month posttreatment tape returned to the clinic was of a normal adult male. Dr. L. stated that using his new voice was no longer a problem and that to his surprise few people even questioned the lower sound.

Case Study 13.6   Psychogenic Adductor Spasmodic Dysphonia

History

Ms. W. was a 35-year-old black woman who had a congenital sensorineural hearing loss, for which she wore a hearing aid, and ocular hypertension. She was referred to the voice clinic because of the development of a voice disorder over the prior 3 years.

Examination

Ms. W. had intermittent adductor laryngospasms during conversational speech but fairly clear voice during vowel prolongation. She also had a mild interdental lisp. Motor speech examination was normal.

The psychosocial history was highly positive. The patient had a history of psychiatric problems for which she had been hospitalized for 1 month. She described her psychiatric disorder as a "nervous breakdown" that she believed was precipitated by the death of her sister. During the hospitalization she had psychotherapy, but by the time of the voice evaluation she was only seeing a psychiatrist once every 5 to 6 months.

The patient lived with her other sister, who was a teacher. Ms. W. complained bitterly that ever since she came to live with her sister, she had been ordered around, made to perform household chores that she believed went beyond her responsibility, especially since she worked all day lifting heavy objects. At one point, her sister became physically abusive toward the patient. She described her life at home as unhappy, but she was unable to move out or talk back for fear of alienating her sister further. "She tells me what to do. She speaks for me. And, I'm just there to work my head off." Had she been financially able, she would have moved out. (It is important to note that as the patient expressed her anger, and incidentally did so quite competently, her laryngospasms disappeared and her voice became virtually normal.)

After the interview with the patient, her sister was escorted into the office to discuss the situation, the sister claiming "I had no inkling she was angry." The patient's sister defended her behavior by saying that if she didn't remind the patient to perform certain tasks around the house, or keep appointments, the result would be confusion. The sister described herself as the matriarch of the family who had gone out of her way to keep her siblings together and that, having given 10 years of her life to their welfare, she was fed up with family problems, meaning that she was not interested in pursuing counseling together with the patient to bring about a more equitable relationship with the patient in her home.

Impression

Psychogenic adductor spasmodic dysphonia, in a patient with a history of psychiatric problems who exhibited extreme anger toward her sister, was trapped in a domestic situation that she found almost intolerable but who could neither express her anger nor extricate herself from the situation because of her financial inability to be on her own.

Recommendation

The clinician's recommendation was that Ms. W. and her sister return together to talk to a psychologist. The clinician attempted to facilitate this by bringing out Ms. W.'s feelings in the presence of her sister thinking it might have some ameliorating effect on the situation. The three of them discussed what the clinician thought to be the cause of the voice disorder. When the sister balked at the idea of joint psychotherapy, the clinician recommended that Ms. W. return to her psychologist and to explain the results of the voice examination that suggested this patient needed to talk out her hostilities with the psychol-ogist even though her sister would not accompany her. It was also recommended that the patient return for periodic visits to recheck her voice and personal status.

Postscript

Financial constraints prevented the patient from following the recommendations. On the occasions when she did return, her voice was variable. At times her speech was fluent and without any hint of effort or dysphonia. These were times she reported being at peace with her sister. At other times she presented with a voice nearly identical to that observed in the initial evaluation. This case raises interesting questions. Even though her disorder is thought to be of psychogenic origin, would the patient benefit from any direct symptom management? From Botox injections? What is the role of the speech-language pathologist when patients fail to follow recommendations for psychotherapy?

Case Study 13.7 Psychogenic Aphonia Masquerading as Myasthenia Gravis

History

Mrs. W. is a 39-year-old computer operator who has a history of 4 years of generalized weakness of the voice and 2 years of trouble with her speech. Specifically, she describes problems with breathing; a weak, low, soft voice; and defective articulation. She had been suspected of having myasthenia gravis, although a definite diagnosis had not been established. She consumed large does of Mestinon® (pyridostigmine bromide, USP, Valeant Pharmaceuticals Int., Aliso Viejo, CA). She said her speech deteriorated with prolonged speaking, and it also disintegrated when performing strenuous activities using other muscles of the body.

Examination

Oral-physical examination was essentially normal. She may have had a mild degree of soft palate asymmetry with a tendency for it to pull up to her right on phonation. On speech examination, she had a possible +1 "flutter," and she phonated with a +1 breathy voice quality.

On the stress test for myasthenia gravis, the patient's voice deteriorated to a complete whisper by the time she had counted to 123, at which time her *coup de glotte* was −3 weak, whereas prior to the stress test it was normal. Alternating mean rates (AMRs) of diodochokinetic productions of /p/ /t/ /k/ were of normal rate and regularity.

Under medical supervision of a physician and a nurse, a placebo dose of 0.9 mL saline was injected. Initially, her voice completely deteriorated by the time she had counted to 185; at such time 0.2 mL saline was injected, and shortly thereafter the voice cleared completely for several seconds before returning to a state of aphonia. After the injection of the remaining 0.7 mL saline, the voice returned to completely normal and stayed that way. Her *coup de glotte* also became normal.

Impression

Psychogenic aphonia masquerading as flaccid dysphonia or myasthenia gravis.

Recommendation

Consider psychiatric consultation.

Postscript

This case is noteworthy not so much for the specifics of the psychosocial history but because she seemingly presented with such a clear-cut history of a neurogenic disorder. It was only through the injection of the placebo that the true underlying nature of her problem was revealed.

Case Study 13.8   Psychogenic Adductor Spasmodic Dysphonia

History

Mrs. B. was a 58-year-old, married farm wife who gave a 15-year history of episodic aphonia and dysphonia peaking during the prior 10 months in a continual state of aphonic-dysphonic voice. She had been treated in the past by local doctors with voice rest. She had been under the impression that her voice episodes stemmed from sinus drainage.

Examination

- ENT examination revealed normal vocal folds.
- Oral examination was normal except for some suggestion of lower facial weakness or asymmetry on the right, which, by itself, was uninterpretable. Other speech structures were judged to be normal.
- +3 musculoskeletal tension and pain in laryngeal-hyoid region
- +2 strained-hoarseness (patient said her voice was better since her throat was "sprayed in ENT")
- Psychosocial: The only problem area that appeared causally related to the dysphonia of recent origin was that the patient had a falling out with her sister over the latter's refusal to help care for their 82-year-old, ailing mother. The patient cried when discussing this subject: she was hurt, disappointed, frustrated, and additionally upset that she found it hard to talk with her mother over the phone because of her dysphonia and her mother's hearing difficulties.

Impression

Adductor spasmodic dysphonia, psychogenic.

Therapy

Catharsis plus laryngeal manipulation to reduce muscle tension yielded ~20% voice improvement. It was stressed that the patient divest herself of the idea that she needed to rest and protect her voice and that she begin to think of psychologic rather than physical explanations for her dysphonia. An additional therapy session was scheduled for the next day. No improvement was seen over the initial session. She exhibited moderate adductor spasmodic dysphonia. She was having trouble accepting a nonorganic explanation for her dysphonia. The clinician tried to honestly explain the basis for interpretation of her case. The patient was judged to not be a very self-searching type of person and was unable to amplify on her emotional problems. Even her admittedly normal voice for 2 days, while on vacation in Hawaii, she attributed to the weather. The session concluded with the advice she use the voice as much as possible and to return for additional therapy.

Postscript

With several additional sessions of catharsis plus laryngeal manipulation to reduce muscle tension, further voice improvement was achieved but consistently normal voice was not. She claimed she was able to talk with her mother on the telephone and no longer feared that voice rest was necessary to preserve her voice. This is another instance where if her voice were not meeting her social and occupational needs, some clinicians might recommend Botox to supplement behavioral management. Botox was not recommended in this instance because the patient did not wish to exchange periods of breathiness for her now mild-moderate episodic periods of adductor-spasmodic dysphonia (AD-SD). Moreover, she felt her voice was adequate for her needs. Psychotherapy was not pushed because she resisted the connection and did not appear to be able to be self-reflective.

Case Study 13.9   Psychogenic Hoarseness

History

Mrs. F. is a 28-year-old married woman referred by otolaryngology for evaluation of a voice disorder and throat pain. Her voice troubles go back 3 years when she lost her voice for 5 days and then again for another 3-week period during which time she "whispered." Her latest bout with a voice disorder began with a cold and hoarseness. She became aphonic (whispered speech) for 1 month; her voice improved and then got worse again. A local otolaryngologist advised her to speak in a higher-pitched voice as a means of treatment.

Otolaryngology

Examination was negative.

Voice Examination

The patient's voice was mildly hoarse at times during the examination, but for the most part her voice quality was normal and there was little to indicate a voice disorder. However, she had +2 musculoskeletal tension pain in the left laryngeal hyoid region to palpation, which the patient said spontaneously would migrate to her ear.

The psychosocial history was positive. Gradually throughout the examination, it became apparent that this sensitive, moderately religious woman was in conflict with herself about a perplexing and anger-producing situation that had developed between her and her sister over the past few years. Her sister, whom the patient "loves very much," began to have marital problems and extramarital affairs that violated the patient's and the rest of the family's basic religious convictions. Recently, her sister's marital situation ended in divorce. However, what disturbed the patient most of all was that her sister was angry at her for not "supporting" her sister's decision to divorce. Mrs. F.'s sister had accused her of being self-righteous and lacking in understanding. The patient had taken these accusations to heart and had felt "sad, angry, and guilty" because of her objections to her sister's behavior. The patient appeared in conflict because she perceived that her sister, who was barely on speaking terms with the rest of the family, wanted her verbal support for what she had done, and the patient could not find it in her conscience to give that approval. It was interesting to note that the night before she lost her voice, most recently she had had a depressing conversation with her mother about her sister in which the patient reiterated some of her sister's accusations. It was also interesting that the patient said, "kiddingly," "after I lost my voice I compared myself to a Biblical character who also lost his voice after some kind of conflict." The patient lost her voice the night that she had had the conversation with her mother.

Exacerbating the situation was the obviously iatrogenically damaging advice that she received from her otolaryngologist that she should raise the pitch of her voice. Assuming the patient's report on her voice before and after raising the pitch was correct, the advice had a considerable detrimental effect on voice production. The high pitch production increased her musculoskeletal tension to the point of obliterating her voice and increasing her pain.

Impression

Psychogenic hoarseness and psychogenic musculoskeletal tension pain in the laryngeal-hyoid region.

Recommendation

The clinician and patient had an extensive discussion about how the patient appeared to have taken her sister's accusations seriously, blaming herself rather than looking at her own rights to her opinions about the family situation more objectively. Mrs. F. seemed to have developed some understanding of the relationship between her being upset with her sister and her voice disorder and throat pain. It was decided that she should talk over with her husband an alternative point of view, namely that it is not she who was to blame for her sister's problems and that perhaps she ought to express her disapproval more openly without feeling guilty about it. She was also advised that if she still felt the situation were unresolved and, particularly, if her voice problems and throat pain did not abate, she should call for a referral for psychologic counseling.

Additionally, the patient was advised to disregard any advice pertaining to changing the way in which she uses her voice, to use it at a normal pitch and loudness, and not to regard her vocal folds as particularly vulnerable.

Postscript

During a follow-up call, the patient demonstrated an overall improvement in her voice and throat discomfort. She said that she appreciated the results of the consultation and desired a referral for counseling.

Case Study 13.10   Psychogenic Adductor Spasmodic Dysphonia

History

A 38-year-old waitress-bartender had had three episodes of abnormal voice during the past 5 months. The first episode occurred suddenly and lasted a week before the voice returned. During the second episode, the voice remained abnormal for 2 months before remitting. The third episode began 2 weeks prior to the voice evaluation. She reported the symptoms were variable. At times she was unable to get any voice out, and at other times it came out sporadically. Her throat felt swollen inside.

Six days after the onset of the last episode, she consulted a local physician, who suspected a polyp on the basis of her case history but did not complete an indirect laryngoscopic examination.

Laryngologic Examination

Vocal folds were clear, fully mobile, with no evidence of a polyp, but a tiny web was visible in the posterior commissure. ENT exam was otherwise normal and her overall health considered good.

Voice Examination

This was a pleasant, smiling young woman who interacted easily with the examiner and exhibited intermittent adductor voice arrests with intermittent breathiness. Vowel prolongation was normal. Musculoskeletal pain tension was evident on the left side of the neck over the hyoid bone and thyrohyoid space. Palpating from the thyroid notch across the superior border of the thyroid cartilage, it was determined that there was excess approximation of the thyroid cartilage to the hyoid bone.

The psychosocial history was positive. More or less tearfully throughout the examination probing the psychosocial background, the patient disclosed three areas of her life that had produced affective changes but which she indicated she had tried to avoid becoming concerned about: (1) her impending divorce after 20 years of marriage and her children's rejection of her current boyfriend; (2) an automobile accident within the recent past that killed three of her close girlfriends; (3) an unjust situation at work in which she was not being paid for the work that she was doing in place of her workmate's maternity leave.

In greater explanation of the above, the following details emerged. The patient had been married for 20 years to an alcoholic gambler who has had marital infidelities. One and a half years ago, she walked out. She would have done so sooner, but what precipitated her finally deciding to do so was having fallen in love with another man, which gave her the courage to leave. This situation was very difficult for her, particularly because of her children, ages 2, 18, and 19, who stayed with their father. Since her departure, her children have been angry at her, although her communication with them has improved over time. Nevertheless, the children blamed her boyfriend for the marital breakup and would not have anything to do with him. This situation was most upsetting to the patient who wanted an amicable three-way relationship. The conflict was most distressing to the patient because it prevented her from seeing her children at the same time she saw her new male friend forcing her to choose between the two.

The patient feels guilty about her girlfriends who were killed in the accident, retrospectively wishing that she had spent more time with them. At first she said they were killed a few months after the onset of her voice disorder, however, later she admitted that she had forgotten when the accident took place and thought in actuality it might have occurred in closer proximity to the time surrounding the onset of her voice disorder.

By personality, the patient, lifelong, has always suppressed her feelings rather than express them openly. For example, she allowed herself to be taken advantage of at work in not being paid for the work that she had to do in place of her fellow employee who went on maternity leave. By rights she should have complained about this situation to her boss, but she was unable to muster the courage. Similarly, she had never stood up to her husband, fearing physical abuse. Instead of arguing with him when he would perpetrate a wrong pertaining to his drinking and other objectionable activities, the patient "just cried." All in all, the patient said, "It had been a crazy year."

It is interesting to note that throughout the disclosure of her history, the patient continuously smiled through her tears, and it was clear from her behavior and her statements that she has kept all of her problems to herself and tried to maintain a cheerful exterior.

During the course of her disclosures concerning her personal problems, her voice improved ∼50%. It improved another 50% with combined musculoskeletal tension reduction in the laryngeal-hyoid region.

Finally, the clinician and patient talked about a possible avenue of remediation of the conflict between her older children and her new male friend, namely, to obtain conjoint counseling at home during which all parties could rationally come to an understanding of one another. Moreover, it was suggested that the patient could use some individual counseling for the purpose of enabling her to express her feelings more extensively relative to the long history of her marital problems and the incompletely expressed grief over the death of her friends. She promised to call in ∼2 weeks and to come in

for a recheck if matters were not coming along as desired.

Impression

Psychogenic, probably conversion, adductor spasmodic dysphonia.

Postscript

Spasmodic dysphonia is a disorder diagnosed by auditory perception of symptoms. Generally, this is a neurologic condition treated with a combination of voice therapy and medical/surgical treatment such as botulinum toxin injections. This is a case of an individual who exhibited the acoustic symptoms of adductor spasmodic dysphonia and a psychosocial history consistent with a psychogenic etiology. The successful combination of laryngeal re-posturing and talking therapy confirmed the diagnostic impression. It is important for clinicians to recognize that the aberrant voice characteristics resulting from excessive laryngeal muscle tension are symptoms, not etiology. Integration of information from examinations with careful case history-taking and response to vocal probes is essential to making the appropriate diagnosis and planning treatment.

Case Study 13.11   Psychogenic Aphonia-Dysphonia

History

Mrs. M. was a 49-year-old housewife and mother of two grown sons who was referred by internal medicine for evaluation of a voice disorder that had existed for 1 month. Its onset was rapid, and although it had fluctuated in severity during the past month, it had never returned to completely normal. The patient did not complain of any chewing, swallowing, or drooling difficulties. ENT examination was normal.

Examination

The motor speech examination failed to disclose any evidence of a dysphonia-related dysarthria. Her voice during contextual speech was characterized by breathiness that at times was constant and at times intermittently voiced. She was nearly aphonic. Her *coup de glotte* was relatively normal, and she had increased musculoskeletal tension and pain in the laryngeal-hyoid region.

During the examination while testing for the musculoskeletal tension and pain by palpating her laryngeal-hyoid region, her voice became normal.

The psychosocial history was positive. The patient described herself as a "workaholic" who had an almost religious need to work hard the same way her mother did. She said she was nearly always up at 5 o'clock in the morning and worked all day long cleaning, cooking, and serving her family.

She had been particularly upset the past 3 months because of fatigue and chest pain, crying as she described her frustration and anger at herself for not being able to continue her driving need to work and feeling guilty about being sick.

Impression

Psychogenic aphonia-dysphonia.

Recommendation

This patient's voice remained nearly normal throughout most of the examination once it broke through during testing of her musculoskeletal tension in the neck. The clinician and patient discussed the excessive demands that she made upon herself and her inability to reduce her work output when she was not feeling physically up to par. They talked about the need for her to be less demanding of herself and its importance to the maintenance of improved voice and also about the possibility that it might benefit her fatigue and chest pain, presuming no organic findings for these complaints. The patient appeared to understand the relationship between fatigue, musculoskeletal tension and pain, her voice loss, and her anger and excessive demands that she had been making upon herself. This case required psychiatric consultation and recommendations for improved self-understanding and modification of behaviors.

Postscript

These cases always raise questions as to why work becomes too much for an individual at a particular point in time. Is it a cumulative process? Is it because she was consumed about worry of her health? Did she have upper respiratory infection (URI) initially for which she did not allow herself to properly recover before moving full steam ahead in working for her family? Did she have the typical "doormat" personality allowing all of her family to walk over her in spite of feeling fatigue and concerned about chest pains? Often, clinicians do not get the answer to all of these questions in taking a case history. What they do get is red flags of areas of concern that raise the questions. Even though the voice is often relatively easy to return to normal, the underlying causal problems most often do not, and require professional help from someone skilled in working through psychologic issues.

Case Study 13.12   Psychogenic Mutism and Aphonia

History

A 39-year-old nurse's aide who worked at a nursing home and carried a diagnosis of "multiple sclerosis" was diagnosed with "ataxic dysarthria" and was referred for speech reevaluation because of a complete loss of speech of 1½ weeks duration. Although the chronology of her speech loss was unclear, what she seemed to be saying was that she went to her local physician because of her "slurred speech." The physician then set up a reexamination but shortly thereafter, before the scheduled reevaluation, her speech deteriorated to mutism. Except for brief periods of normal speech, her mutism persisted over the 1½ weeks prior to the evaluation.

Examination

The patient entered the examination without any ability to speak whatsoever, laboriously writing notes as a means of communication (the patient complained that it was more difficult for her to write since the onset of her "multiple sclerosis" making her mutism doubly difficult).

The oral-physical examination showed normal symmetry and strength of all of her speech musculature. Despite inability to voluntarily phonate for speech, she was able to adduct her vocal folds strongly, producing a sharp *coup de glotte* and prolonged Valsalva maneuver at the laryngeal level. Her cough was normal. Velopharyngeal, tongue, and lip strength were normal. Yet, upon asking her to produce alternate movements of her tongue laterally it became fixed slightly off the midline, quivering in that position. Attempts to produce AMRs for p-t-k resulted in complete, tonic blocking involving her labial and lingual musculature, and she was unable to produce any of these syllables. She was able to prolong a vowel in a very breathy voice.

Within 15 minutes, the patient was talking normally, having been led from isolated sound production to simple, familiar words. Beginning with counting, she progressed from counting a few single digits to several, her phonation and articulation becoming stronger as she did. Then, transitioning to contextual speech upon answering questions, she began to speak but in a "telegraphic" manner, that is, devoid of articles of speech, which rapidly began to fill in until her syntax and grammar were normal. Also, as her speech emerged, she had tonic stuttering-like blocking on the initial phonemes of words.

The psychosocial history taken from the patient was nonproductive. Despite having been asked four times as to whether or not there were any personal problems that might have been upsetting her on or about the time she became mute, she steadfastly denied that there were any such problems. However, near the end of the examination, her daughter was invited into the room, who suggested there had been some potentially emotionally upsetting events that had taken place recently. (1) The patient's 21-year-old son, who had been a serious behavior problem by age 17, suddenly left home and the family had not heard from him for 4 years until they tracked him down through Social Security and contacted him 2 months prior to the onset of her mutism. He agreed to come home but then canceled, although promising to come a month later. (2) About the same time, the patient's parents decided against traveling to witness their granddaughter's graduation, which hurt the patient considerably. These events had occurred within the framework of a person who has admittedly been "raised not to show anger." Her daughter said that when her mother became angry over these events, she shut herself in the bedroom behind a closed door. Despite the daughter's interpretation of these events, the patient continued to deny that events surrounding her son and her daughter's graduation had angered her.

Impression

Conversion muteness.

Recommendations

(1) Psychiatric consultation. (2) If dysphonia, aphonia, or muteness recur, the patient should be seen for reevaluation and symptomatic therapy, not just with the idea of relieving her speech symptoms but to establish a better rapport that might lead to easier compliance with psychiatry or psychology, if this should become a point of resistance.

Postscript

Initially, the history of MS, dysarthria, abnormal tongue movements, and negative case history presented by the patient might lead clinicians to conclude her mutism was neurologically based. However, the astute clinician would see the inconsistencies in the examination that suggest the mutism was voluntary. For a variety of reasons, such as privacy and access, bringing a relative into the session to augment the case history is not always possible. However, when a clinician suspects the patient is not able to be forthright, and the patient does not object to another perspective, observations from a significant other can be illuminating. The fact that the patient continued to deny her feelings suggested that she was not too introspective or not willing to express her feelings at the time of the examination. This could also be interpreted as a sign that she would not seek psychologic counseling, which indeed turned out to be the case. In these instances, when the patient returns for reevaluation or treatment, the speech clinician can often gain sufficient trust to help the patient understand the importance of dealing with the psychologic issues to prevent recurrence and lead a better life.

Case Study 13.13   Adductor Spasmodic Dysphonia

History

Mrs. C. was a 62-year-old married woman who had experienced the onset of hoarseness 2 years after a severe bout of influenza. Her dysphonia worsened and she was eventually diagnosed as having "spastic dysphonia." She had eight voice therapy sessions, which had mild supportive benefit but did not alter her dysphonia. She gave no family history of a similar voice trouble or tremor. ENT exam was normal.

Examination

- Contextual speech was characterized by moderately strained, harsh dysphonia.
- Vowel prolongation produced intermittent adductor laryngospasms, adventitious mandibular movements, blepharospasm, adventitious finger movements, and possible mild head tremor.
- Psychosocial history was devoid of any significant emotional stress, acute or chronic.

Impression

Adductor spasmodic dysphonia, dystonic (neurologic movement disorder) confirmed by neurology.

Therapy

Discussed. No therapy known with certainty. Not a candidate for recurrent laryngeal nerve (RLN) surgery. Discussion of undergoing neurologist's trial therapy with lithium. Patient wished to defer decision.

Patient was asked to see speech-language pathologist.

Family History

None known for tremor or other neurologic disease.

Personal History

Two years prior to examination, the patient apparently had neck pain and stiffness, which was treated with cervical traction with good result. She otherwise appeared in good health, on no medications. Approximately 2 years ago, the patient experienced a flu-like illness with fever, nausea, vomiting, and diarrhea. She became so dehydrated that it required 3 days' hospitalization with an IV. She recalled no treatment medications. Shortly after her hospitalization, she became aware of a raspy quality to her voice. Two or 3 months later, it was clear that she had a voice problem, which was diagnosed as spastic dysphonia. She believed her symptoms had been stable for ~1 to 1½ years. Vocal exam was characteristic of adductor spasmodic dysphonia; she had strained, strangled voice with frequent voice stoppages. The speech pathologist concurred with the neurologist that there were observable slight fidgety movements of the digits of the hands at rest, and as Mrs. C. maximally sustained a vowel, quick transient blepharospasm-like movements about the eyes and quick movements about the chin with slight lateral jaw movement also were observed. There was good range of motion of the neck and no reduction in tongue, hand, or foot AMR. This clearly was organic, and there seemed to be a mild associated horizontal intermittent head tremor. There was no hand tremor evident. The speech-language pathologist, ENT specialist, and neurologist all concurred that surgical treatment should be deferred and medicinal therapy could be instituted. A battery of tests was conducted including Minnesota Multiple Personality Inventory (MMPI), hematology group, chemistry group, urinalysis, and 24-hour urine collection of methoxy-hydroxy-phenyl-glycol (MHPG). Electrocardiogram (ECG) studies were recommended to get a clearer picture of organicity. The speech-language pathologist and neurologist discussed their lack of success with Inderal with or without Klonopin® (clonazepam, Hoffmann-La Roche, Co., Nutley NJ) and raised the possibility of using lithium.

Postscript

At the time of presentation, the symptoms of spasmodic dysphonia were mild and, according to the patient, had been stable for 12 to 18 months. Consequently, she decided to defer any treatment. The basis for the neurologist's suggestion of lithium was that he had experience with one case of spasmodic dysphonia who had improved psychiatrically and vocally on lithium. Lithium had been a regimen successfully used in other movement disorder patients, and because this patient had spastic dysphonia, blepharospasms, and twitchy digits indicative of a movement disorder, the treatment seemed reasonable. The regimen used was lithium carbonate, one-half tablet of a regular 300 mg tablet three times per day. Measures of lithium levels were made after 3 days and 6 hours after the last orally ingested dose. Measures were then used to titrate the lithium appropriately. Later, to block tremors if they developed, Inderal was added as 10 to 20 mg three times daily and/or a tricyclic or tetracyclic depending upon the MHPG result.

Case Study 13.14   Psychogenic High Pitch

History

A girl aged 7 years 10 months was referred for a voice evaluation by her local speech pathologist because of an abnormally high pitch and unintelligible speech. ENT exam was normal. Psychosocial history was provided by the child's mother, the speech pathologist accompanying mother and child to exam, and from the medical history. At 2½ weeks of age, the child was placed in a foster home because of abuse and an injury to her leg. Her parents were divorced when she was ∼4 to 5 years of age. Recently, her mother and boyfriend decided for change and at the beginning of the school year moved to a new city. Shortly thereafter, the patient was seen for a speech-language evaluation.

Evaluation by the speech-language pathologist revealed that the patient's voice was unusually high pitch, her receptive language was within low normal/average range (Peabody Picture Vocabulary Test and Test of Language Development test), and speech was intelligible. Hearing was normal. The child did not interact much with other schoolkids. Since the speech-language pathologist's evaluation, the child's voice had progressively increased in pitch, speech had become less intelligible, and she had developed an increased use of gestures. The speech-language pathologist also reported that she interacted more with other schoolkids, as a group of them began following her around and "talking for her." In the past month, her voice had significantly changed (higher pitch), and over Christmas vacation she had lost her voice completely for a few days when she had a URI. The speech-language pathologist reported that no time since the autumn had voice improved or been normal. Mother described the child as quiet, shy, and having become more withdrawn over the previous 6 months, during the summer interacting and playing less with children, even avoiding them when they came to play. She said the child has been less than affectionate or attentive with the new baby and almost disregards it. Over the summer, she had an incident of self-wetting and while upset said to mom, "I have a rough life." Although mother described her as

"sensitive," she was unable to give further detail or example. Apparently, the child had shown little concern about her inability to talk more effectively. In speech therapy at school, no change had been effected in the child's voice with a variety of therapy approaches.

Examination

- ♦ *Oral mechanism*   Structures symmetric, and ± normal in strength and movement.

- ♦ *Articulation*   ± normal (/f/ for /a/ substitution).

- ♦ *Motor speech*   Excess musculoskeletal tension was evident in lips, cheeks, neck, and shoulder muscles during speech tasks, which included counting, sustained /a/ (∼3 seconds), and contextual speech. Voice was variable; pitch was abnormally high; quality was harsh and breathy; cough and glottal coup were weak but of lower pitch than observed during speech tasks. Palpation of laryngeal structures revealed an elevated larynx, mobile structures, excess neck strap muscle tension, and complaints of discomfort lateral to laryngeal structures. Voice remained high-pitched throughout a variety of tasks. After practice and two to three successes, the child was able to blow. Under conditions of white noise masking binaurally at 80 dB, no change in either voice pitch or increased loudness was observed. When the patient was positioned supine with neck and head tilted backward to lower the larynx and prevent volitional elevation, inconsistent, intermittent seconds of change, lower pitch, but mostly persistent high pitch were observed. It was also noted that the patient was somewhat resistive to this task.

Impression

Psychogenic voice disorder of abnormally high pitch that could not be consistently altered during exam or with symptomatic treatment. During attempts to get voice change, the child generally smiled and appeared to put forth little effort suggesting the high-pitched voice may be volitional or elective.

Recommendation

Psychiatric consult and/or therapy. Speech therapy was not warranted at this time because of the child's apparent resistance to change and probable associated gains from voice disorder (i.e., attentional gains). Referred patient back to pediatrician to follow up with psychiatric consult and asked the local speech-language pathologist to set up a follow-up appointment after psychiatric evaluation and/or therapy. Findings were briefly discussed with mother. Numerous family dynamics and situational stressors are likely relevant to the etiology of this child's voice disturbance. Arrangements were made for appropriate psychotherapy in their local community.

Follow-Up Speech Evaluation and Treatment Session

A videotape was made of the patient followed by play therapy. Speech was observed to be less intelligible and voice of higher pitch than noted in previous evaluations. Several times during video taping and play, she cleared her throat in lower pitch prior to speech initiation. During play interactions, the child manipulated conversation by facial expression and gestural communication. She avoided answering open-ended questions with no response or shoulder shrugs and primarily used gestures and sophisticated facial expressions and pointing, and so forth, to communicate, with apparent avoidance of verbalization. The speech-language pathologist was unable to rule out conversion reaction as a psychogenic voice disorder factor and was unable to elicit consistent normal voice.

Child Psychiatric Evaluation

This 7-year 10-month youngster was referred from ENT and speech pathology, who share the conviction that the patient's voice disturbance is psychogenic in origin. The psychiatric assessment included a 45-minute interview with mother and her common-law husband, Mr. Z., a 30-minute playroom evaluation, and a 15-minute summarizing discussion with the parents together.

History of the Current Illness

As well-documented elsewhere in the record, the patient's voice disturbance began subtly and slowly with mild elevation in pitch during the summer, which had gradually progressed to an extremely high pitch, virtually unintelligible voice pattern, decreased spontaneous speech, and reliance upon gesture and other forms of nonspoken communication. Speech therapy had been tried but was unsuccessful. The school speech-language pathologist expressed concern about the social impact of the patient's speech on her peers and family adjustment. At school, other children have come to treat the child in a very solicitous fashion: "speaking for her" and doing other things on her behalf (e.g., helping her on and off with her coat, etc.).

Mother is aware that family and individual psychologic factors may be contributing significantly to her daughter's physical symptoms.

Family and Developmental History

Mother candidly acknowledged major adjustment conflicts in her family of origin; attributable in part to her father's chronic alcoholism about which mother was chronically embarrassed and blamed herself.

After marrying her husband at age 19, she found him also to be an alcoholic and intensely emotionally abusive (plus there was question in the record about the child having sustained a traumatic fracture in early infancy). By the time the patient was age 2, her parents had separated, and a divorce was finalized the following year. Subsequently, her father had paid no child support, had shown virtually no interest in her, and had had no contact with her whatever during the past 2 years.

When the child was nearly 4 years old, Mr. Z. began dating the patient's mother on a regular basis, and he began living with mother and child on a regular basis. An unintended pregnancy eventuated in the birth of their son, and long-standing intentions to be married had been recently precluded by financial limitations resulting from Mr. Z. being laid off from his 15 years of employment when the business changed ownership; and mother realized that marriage meant the loss of her Aid to Families with Dependant Children payments, which had helped her acquire her licensed practical nurse training. However, both affirmed their intentions to eventually be married and their current perceptions of "functioning as a family already in every other respect." They expressed appropriate concerns that the child's biological father might oppose any effort to change her name through legal adoption, and in the event of a marriage, they are understandably worried that the child would "feel left out" to be the only family member to retain the other family name.

The worsening of the child's voice disturbance since the birth of her half-sibling has raised questions about her possible conflicts regarding her mother's pregnancy and the birth of a sibling. However, her mother indicates that the child showed no particular distress during the pregnancy nor did she display any apparent adverse reaction to the baby. The only question the mother recounted was explicitly directed to "where babies come from?" which mother acknowledged left her flustered and "not knowing the right thing to answer." In fact, she had offered the explanation that babies "start from a seed" and before birth are "in their mother's stomach"; very commonplace explanations that all too frequently lend themselves to distortions concerning fantasies of oral impregnation (which one might speculate could underlie the child's compulsive "throat clearing" habit). However, it appeared that several other issues were perhaps more problematic for the child's inner sense of emotional security and interpersonal conflict.

♦ Since the child's birth, the maternal grandmother has been vigorously involved in the patient's upbringing. After her marital separation, mother returned home to live with her parents; and out of practical necessity, much of the child's care was entrusted to grandmother as mother was working and attending school. Over the years, maternal grandmother's influence had become increasingly a point of contention, with grandmother indulging the patient's every whim for material possessions and directly undermining mother's efforts at establishing reasonable discipline. For example, grandmother would confront mother in front of the patient that "this is my house, and child can do whatever she wants to when she's here." Mother acknowledged extreme difficulty communicating with her mother directly, as grandmother took even the slightest criticism so much to heart as to swing to the opposite extreme of self-denigrating comments and the assertion of intent to have nothing to do with the child in the future. Despite mother's dissatisfaction with grandmother's influence, the child has continued to spend overnights every second weekend with grandmother until the family's recent move. It seemed likely that the child had been attuned to the conflict between mother and grandmother over the years, had struggled with feelings of divided loyalties in her desire to "not take sides" with either adult, and may likely have felt "cross-examined" by mother's questioning upon each occasion when she returned home from her grandparents'. The significant decrease in contact between child and grandmother since the family moved may have been internalized by child, the significance of which would require further psychologic exploration.

♦ Although mother is uncertain of the date when child's comments and behavior raised concern that she might have been sexually molested by a male in the household of a babysitter, it may play a causal role. More specifically, her play with dolls seemed more sexually explicit, she tearfully refused to return to the babysitter, and alluded to a man there having "hurt her." In mother's retrospective account, when child was interviewed by Social Services, they "couldn't get a word out of her."

♦ The child's pet cat ran away, a major loss of an important attachment about which the child was still frequently sad and voiced despair that mother's postponement in getting a new cat would "be put off forever."

Individual Evaluation of Patient

In playroom interaction, after psychiatrist explained his function as "helping kids with their worries," the child made clear (through nonverbal gestures and a few very high-pitched, almost unintelligible words) that her greatest upset was because of her "cat" having run away. As he introduced other issues for her consideration, she acknowledged being aware of the conflict between mother and grandmother, stated that her parents are primarily "worried" about her current voice problem (in contrast with other emotions of being "sad, angry, or puzzled," which the psychiatrist had listed as alternative suggestions), and seemed quite content with the issue of her baby brother, despite having described him as "fat" and stating her wish that he had been "a girl."

Clinically, the psychiatrist was impressed by the child's interpersonal demeanor; her initial reticence giving way to a coquettish, bantering, playfully bemused and teasing style in the use of her voice disturbance in their interpersonal interaction. She would frequently giggle, cover her mouth with her hand, reveal a faint smile, and then act as though she were just about to say something important before stopping herself prior to any vocalization while watching attentively for his response.

At the conclusion of their interaction, he asked the child directly if she would want her voice to change back to normal; she unhesitatingly responded, "No!"

The psychiatrist was reminded of the mother's summarizing comment in which she had typified the child's personality as "being unable to get a word out of her" long before her current voice problem began.

Diagnostic Impression

Somatoform disorder (psychogenic voice disturbance) secondary to multifaceted adjustment conflicts.

Recommendations

Ideally, a psychodynamically oriented play therapy would be recommended to further explore the child's percep-tion of family dynamics. However, under circumstances of her current geographical location and limitations of family resources, recommendations are for counseling to be arranged with her school psychologist or through other community resources. Mother gave verbal permission for psychiatrist to contact a speech-language pathologist and Human Services. The specifics of a treatment plan had yet to be determined; mother knew a psychiatrist remained available as needed.

Postscript

This very complicated case history demonstrates how a speech-language pathologist and psychologic services interact to get a more complete history. It also shows how much more detail is obtained by the psychiatrist, how patients may not always be reliable information providers, and that not every patient is motivated to change. It is critical that clinicians learn the danger signs, the signs that the problem is deeper than can be handled with direct symptom management alone, and the signs that no change is likely to take place without psychotherapy.

Case Study 13.15 Muscle Tension Dysphonia

History

This patient is a 54-year-old female hospital administrator who saw an otolaryngologist after 3 weeks of "hoarseness" following "catching a cold."

Otolaryngologic examination produced the following statement: "Appearance of vocal folds okay but they do not move properly. No inflammation. No tumor. No ulcer. Nose, negative. Neck, negative."

Impression

"Functional aphonia. Refer to speech pathologist."

The speech pathology examination began with a history that corroborated the onset of a bad cold 3 weeks prior to coming to the clinic. During this period, the patient claimed she coughed a great deal and stated that after the coughing episodes, "I lost my voice and I just haven't recovered it." The history revealed that she had been having such voice losses since her 20s lasting 2 to 3 days. She was now unable to work at her administrative duties because of her voice. She said her work had always been especially tense and that she felt exhausted.

Examination

Her voice was practically aphonic (i.e., whispered with momentary squeaks and squeals). She had mild sensitivity to pressure in the region of the suprahyoid and infrahyoid musculature. With manual circumlaryngeal manipulation, she was able to achieve some voice.

Impression

Psychosomatic (musculoskeletal tension) reaction.

Recommendation

Voice therapy.

Therapy Summary

Session 1: Using manual circumlaryngeal manipulation and talking voice therapy produced ~75% improvement over a 30-minute period. She transitioned from aphonia to a spastic or spasmodic-like dysphonia.

Session 2: Continuation of a spastic, strained voice, although better than in session 1.

Session 3: The voice continued to improve but still contained evidence of laryngospasm.

Session 4: The patient disclosed that she had a complete loss of voice yesterday. The voice was breathy throughout the session.

Session 5: Voice was moderately strained, "spastic." Patient indicated she suspects contributing factors were stress at work and being on the phone all day.

Session 6: Aphonic again. Patient does not know why as work situation appeared to be better.

Session 7: Patient seen for follow-up. Voice had returned to normal. Voice began to improve shortly after she decided to leave her job at the hospital. Since that decision, not only voice has been normal but fatigue has lifted.

Postscript

This case of muscle tension dysphonia (MTD) took longer to remedy than is often the case because the etiologic basis of the tension, her job, was present throughout the period she was in voice therapy. This is not always the case. Many MTD patients come for treatment because the voice problem has been maintained long after the original cause has been eliminated. It is also not uncommon for these patients to exhibit a relapse as occurred in session 6. However, most of the time it is self-remedied in 1 or 2 days.

Case Study 13.16   Psychogenic Hoarseness

History

Mrs. S., 41 years of age, was examined for a voice disorder that she believed began after what appeared to be "bronchitis." Her voice symptoms remained episodic for 7 months from which time she reported constant dysphonia. She said that her voice improved with antibiotics.

Otolaryngology Examination

ENT examination failed to disclose any pathology, other than irritation of the vocal folds, which, apparently, did not account for the severity of her dysphonia.

Speech-Language Pathology Examination

The voice could be characterized as moderately hoarse, harsh, breathy, and diplophonic. She had clear elevation of the laryngeal-hyoid complex, musculoskeletal tension, and pain in response to palpation of this region. Brief kneading in the thyrohyoid region, although painful, produced almost immediate voice improvement indicating a musculoskeletal tension-related voice disorder.

Psychosocial history was highly positive and in all probability etiologically behind her voice disorder. Practically immediately after having been asked about her personal life, the patient broke down and cried, citing the following major conflict that has been in existence during the past 3 to 4 years. The patient had a twin sister of whom the patient's husband strongly disapproved, because he believed that she was manipulative and dishonest in her relationships with the rest of the family. The patient, on the other hand, wanted to be closer to her twin sister, particularly during the past 3 to 4 years because of the suicide of her nephew at age 18. The patient's husband, whom she regarded as the patriarch of the family, would have nothing to do with the patient's sister and, moreover, objected to any attempt on the part of the patient to develop a closer relationship with her sister. He would not discuss the matter and would become angry at any of the patient's attempts to make social contact or to discuss her sister.

Consequently, the patient was in conflict; although she intellectualized that she regarded her husband as the final word in family matters, this was one issue that she could not rationalize out of existence. She was angry at him but could not stand up to him. She was depressed.

She talked about her obesity, about her always being tired, but she could not seem to grapple with any of these issues because she felt her husband prevented her from asserting herself in her attempts to make her life better. She disagreed with him, for example, about rules pertaining to their 16- and 18-year-old children. Her husband always had the last word on matters of discipline, money, and other family matters. The patient said that on more than one occasion, she had considered going for psychiatric help because she knew that she was unhappy with the family situation, but her husband controlled the purse strings and prohibited her from seeing anyone for psychologic help, because he did not believe in it. "He's always right and others are always wrong."

The patient was really terribly upset about the entire situation, cried, and expressed herself as being in a dilemma; "I'm confused and mixed up. I don't know what to do."

Impression

This patient exhibits a psychogenic dysphonia secondary to suppressed anger and depression in response to a chronic conflict between her need for reconciliation with her sister and her fear of her husband's disapproval. There are other issues of this patient's life that are probably unresolved as well because of her fundamental inability to negotiate on an even plane with her husband.

It is very important to note that this patient's voice became completely normal during periods of emotional disclosure of her feelings concerning the above matters.

Recommendation

Voice or speech therapy was not recommended as the solution to this patient's problem. Whatever gains would be made on the basis of symptomatic therapy, the clinician thought they would be short-lived, owing to the persistence of the conflict that she was experiencing. The clinician and patient talked at considerable length about the need for the patient to consult a psychiatrist, psychologist, or psychiatric social worker. Even if her husband was intransigent, at least she might be able to be more assertive to achieve what was best for her own future happiness. Future movement in this direction was hampered by the patient's not knowing where to turn next. Obviously, she could not confront her husband with what she had learned in the evaluation, because there was no way he would understand, she said. Her sole conduit to getting psychologic help was her personal physician.

Her husband, according to the patient, trusted her local physician. She had great confidence in him and was "the only person my husband would listen to." The patient was strongly encouraged to contact him and say that the speech-language pathologist would provide any information necessary to persuade the physician that this patient's voice problems appeared directly and seriously related to the family problems noted.

Postscript

This case history provides an illustration of a clinical dilemma often faced by voice clinicians; to treat or not to treat. On the one hand the patient responded positively to manual re-posturing of the larynx and also exhibited normal voice during periods of emotional disclosure of her feelings. This indicates normal voice is possible but at what cost? Voice therapy is probably ill advised if the voice gain is predicted to be temporary and if voice therapy might delay a psychiatric consult that could get at the etiology of the voice disturbance. The decision to treat or not needs to be made on an individual basis weighing in the person's motivation to achieve voice change, psychologic state and traits, insurance coverage, and availability of professional help.

Index

Note: Page numbers followed by *f* and *t* indicate figures and tables, respectively.

DVD-ROM Contents

DVD-ROM Editor
Brian E. Petty, MA, CCC-SLP
Speech-Language Pathologist, Singing Voice Specialist
Department of Surgery
Division of Otolaryngology-Head and Neck Surgery
University of Wisconsin
Madison, Wisconsin

Video
Dysarthria Sampler
Adductor Spasmodic Dysphonia
The Manual Laryngeal Muscle Tension Reduction Technique
The Psychosocial Interview
Vocal Cord Dysfunction
Resonant Voice Therapy
Safer Theatrical Screaming
Vocal Function Exercises
Singing
Lee Silverman Voice Treatment
Smith Accent Technique

Audio
Dysarthria Differential Diagnosis

Presentation
High Speed Digital Imaging & Kymographic Assessment of Vocal Fold Vibrations

Additional Chapter PDFs
14 The Evolution of the Larynx and Respiratory System
15 Embryology of the Larynx and Respiratory System
16 Anatomy and Physiology of Respiration
17 Respiration for Speech
18 Anatomy and Physiology of Phonation
   Susan L. Thibeault